Medical Management of Diabetes Mellitus

Clinical Guides to Medical Management

Consulting Editor

BURTON E. SOBEL, M.D.
Medical Center Hospital of Vermont
University of Vermont
Burlington, Vermont

Medical Management of Heart Disease, edited by Burton E. Sobel

Medical Management of Rheumatic Musculoskeletal and Connective Tissue Diseases, edited by Jan Dequeker, Gabriel Panayi, Theodore Pincus, and Rodney Grahame

Medical Management of Atherosclerosis, edited by John LaRosa

Medical Management of Liver Disease, edited by Edward L. Krawitt

Medical Management of Pulmonary Diseases, edited by Gerald S. Davis; Associate Editors: Theodore W. Marcy and Elizabeth A. Seward

Medical Management of Diabetes Mellitus, edited by Jack L. Leahy, Nathaniel G. Clark, and William T. Cefalu

ADDITIONAL TITLES IN PREPARATION

Medical Management of Kidney and Electrolyte Disorders, edited by F. John Gennari

Medical
Management
of
Diabetes
Mellitus

edited by

Jack L. Leahy
Nathaniel G. Clark
William T. Cefalu

University of Vermont College of Medicine
Burlington, Vermont

MARCEL DEKKER, INC.   NEW YORK · BASEL

ISBN: 0-8247-8857-5

This book is printed on acid-free paper.

Headquarters
Marcel Dekker, Inc.
270 Madison Avenue, New York, NY 10016
tel: 212-696-9000; fax: 212-685-4540

Eastern Hemisphere Distribution
Marcel Dekker AG
Hutgasse 4, Postfach 812, CH-4001 Basel, Switzerland
tel: 41-61-261-8482; fax: 41-61-261-8896

World Wide Web
http://www.dekker.com

The publisher offers discounts on this book when ordered in bulk quantities. For more information, write to Special Sales/Professional Marketing at the headquarters address above.

Current printing (last digit):
10 9 8 7 6 5 4 3 2 1

PRINTED IN THE UNITED STATES OF AMERICA

Program Introduction

A salutary revolution is taking place in the management of diabetes mellitus. Diverse pharmacological agents in novel classes are now available for favorable modification of both altered mediatary metabolism and insulin resistance, recognized to be pivotal in the pathophysiology of type 2 diabetes, the dominant form in the population. Accordingly, the publication of *Medical Management of Diabetes Mellitus,* the most recent entry in the Clinical Guides to Medical Management program, could not be more timely.

In this monograph edited by Drs. Leahy, Clark, and Cefalu, the field is reviewed in depth. It begins with the perspective of Doro Sims, a unique individual who has experienced the disorder and lived in the forefront of its elucidation as Dr. Ethan Sims' partner in life. The first part of the book, Overview, describes the impact of diabetes on our population, mechanisms contributing to its occurrence, standards of care and self-management, the nature of insulin resistance, and challenges confronting patients with diabetes in the managed care environment. In the second part, Signs, Symptoms, Diagnosis, and Diabetes Types, type 1 and type 2 diabetes mellitus are differentiated and described in detail as well as diabetes in pregnant women, in those afflicted with secondary forms or, with specific genetic syndromes giving rise to diabetes, and in children and adolescents. Part 3, Therapies, covers not only the key role of nutrition and exercise but also the use of oral pharmacological agents, conventional and novel insulin regimens, and the use of insulin pumps and pancreatic transplantation. Part 4, Complications, deals with complications encountered, often the features that bring the presence of diabetes to the attention of the patient and the physicial. Complications are described not only phenomenologically but also in terms of mechanisms responsible and responsivity to therapeutic interventions. The last part of the book, Special Settings, addresses diabetes in the elderly, obese subjects, hospitalized patients, diabetic patients undergoing surgical procedures, and women with a polycystic ovary syndrome who require special consideration.

Clinical Guides to Medical Management volumes are designed to bring a "consultant" to the elbow of the physician treating patients in the office, the clinic, the hospital, and emergency facilities. The concept underlying the series is that cardinal features of disease including prominent signs and symptoms must be recognized and appreciated appropriately to initiate definitive diagnosis. Only then can optical treatment be initiated and optimal surveillance pursued. This new volume should serve physicians and their patients well because of its comprehensive nature, the recent advances that are addressed so elegantly by the editors and contributors, and the remarkably increased opportunity to provide effective treatment to afflicted patients.

Burton E. Sobel, M.D.

Preface

A worldwide health care crisis looms in the form of diabetes mellitus and the associated illnesses of insulin resistance. Diabetes is the leading cause of blindness, kidney failure, and nontraumatic limb amputation in U.S. adults, as well as a leading cause of death overall. Similar statistics are found for most developed nations, and many third world nations, that are rapidly catching up because of the skyrocketing incidence of obesity and physical inactivity that accompany Westernization. Nearly 20 million persons in the United States are affected with diabetes, and many remain undiagnosed. Complicating the latter issue, the incidence of diabetes is highest in the disadvantaged and minority populations who have the least access to the medical system. Moreover, the rising frequency of obesity in children of all ethnic groups, combined with our lengthening lifespan and the startling extent of glucose intolerance (nearly 50% of the U.S. population above the age of 65 have diabetes or impaired glucose tolerance), portend a worsening situation for the future.

Countering this discouraging picture, the last decade has seen an explosion of new therapies for many of the troublesome aspects of clinical diabetes care. ACE inhibitors and the quantification of microalbuminuria have revolutionized diabetic nephropathy, as have laser therapy for retinopathy and microsurgical bypass operations for nonhealing foot ulcers. The critical importance of near-normal blood sugar control, in terms of preventing the microvascular complications of diabetes and maximizing successful pregnancies, has been clearly demonstrated. Clinical guidelines for virtually all aspects of diabetes care have followed, as well as major developments in our ability to attain tight glycemic control. The last few years have seen the release of thiazolidinediones and the first insulin analog. In addition, α-glucosidase inhibitors and metformin have made it to the U.S. market, and insulin pen systems are now widely available. As such, the outlook for patients, and for their ability to live a healthy life unencumbered by end-organ complications from diabetes, is better today than ever before. Moreover, the promise for even more effective therapies in the future is strong as noninvasive glucose monitors, insulin delivered by means other than injection, islet transplantation, and prevention strategies for types 1 and 2 diabetes, move toward becoming clinical realities.

Primary care providers face a difficult challenge. They are the liaisons between patients and the diabetes research community. They are expected to be familiar with, and expert in the use of, new clinical information as it appears. No physician is exempt. Diabetes mellitus affects all ages, races, ethnic backgrounds, and socioeconomic groups. Moreover, the multiorgan nature of the micro- and macrovascular complications means that practicing physicians in all areas of medicine, from the most general to the most specialized, are likely to see patients with diabetes.

The current volume is intended to bridge that gap by providing a comprehensive, up-to-date overview of diabetes mellitus for practicing providers and physicians in training. The format differs from most diabetes textbooks, which are often encyclopedic, trying to comprehensively cover physiology, biochemistry, anatomy, and molecular biology, and how they relate to diabetes. This book is more of a ''how to'' manual which has been written by experts in their fields with strong clinical and teaching backgrounds. Their charge was to outline the most effective diagnostic and therapeutic approaches to clinical problems within their respective realms.

The book is divided into five parts. Part I, Overview (Chapters 1–7), provides a background into the general subject. What is diabetes mellitus? How is it diagnosed? What are the standards of care? The term diabetes mellitus represents a constellation of disorders with different signs, symptoms, clinical characteristics, and therapies depending on the pathogenesis, clinical setting, and age of the patient. Part II, Signs, Symptoms, Diagnosis, and Diabetes Types (Chapters 8–14), focuses on the unique characteristics of the different entities and clinical settings in which they occur. Part III, Therapies (Chapters 15–20), provides an overview of the therapeutic modalities. What are their mechanisms and rationale for use? How are they used? When, and in whom? What are the expected outcomes and how are they tracked? Part IV, Complications (Chapters 21–34), focuses on the end-organ complications. It is these complications that patients fear most, and some of the most spectacular successes in the last decade have been with their early detection and therapy. Individual chapters cover the pathogenesis, clinical presentation, diagnosis including specialized laboratory tests, and therapy of the various diabetic complications. Finally, Part V, Special Settings (Chapters 35–42), addresses management of diabetes mellitus and associated illnesses in specialized clinical settings.

We thank the many contributors to this volume, without whose diligence, effort, and commitment it would not exist. We dedicate it to the patients we have known over the years who daily face the struggle of living with an illness that robs them of many of the freedoms most of us take for granted. Further, we particularly acknowledge Doro and Ethan Sims, each of whom has contributed to the effort against diabetes in a profound way. Doro has lived with type 1 diabetes for more than 40 years with grace and humor, and has been a role model for countless persons with diabetes, as well as a national leader in the development and implementation of programs to help patients live successful, independent lives. Ethan has been a leading researcher and clinician in the disciplines of obesity and insulin resistance. We are indebted to Doro for her reflections that begin this book.

Jack L. Leahy
Nathaniel G. Clark
William T. Cefalu

Contents

Contributors

Andrew J. Ahmann, M.D. Division of Endocrinology, Diabetes, and Clinical Nutrition, Oregon Health Sciences University, Portland, Oregon

Ronald E. Aubert, M.S.P.H., Ph.D. The Prudential Center for Healthcare Research, Prudential Healthcare, Atlanta, Georgia

Paul J. Beisswenger, M.D. Dartmouth Medical School, Hanover, and Dartmouth–Hitchcock Medical Center, Lebanon, New Hampshire

Caroline S. Blaum, M.D. Department of Internal Medicine, and Geriatrics Center, University of Michigan, Ann Arbor, Michigan

Patrick J. Boyle, M.D. Department of Internal Medicine, University of New Mexico Health Sciences Center, Albuquerque, New Mexico

Michael Camilleri, M.D. Gastroenterology Research Unit, Mayo Clinic and Mayo Foundation, Rochester, Minnesota

William T. Cefalu, M.D. Division of Endocrinology, Diabetes, and Metabolism, Department of Medicine, University of Vermont College of Medicine, Burlington, Vermont

Debasish Chaudhuri, M.D. Cardiology Unit, University of Vermont College of Medicine, Burlington, Vermont

Nathaniel G. Clark, M.D. Division of Endocrinology, Diabetes, and Metabolism, Department of Medicine and Pediatrics, University of Vermont College of Medicine, Burlington, Vermont

Bernard Coulie, Ph.D., M.D. Gastroenterology Research Unit, Mayo Clinic and Mayo Foundation, Rochester, Minnesota

John T. Devlin, M.D., F.A.C.P. Maine Center for Diabetes, Maine Medical Center, Portland, Maine

Peter D. Donofrio, M.D. Department of Neurology, Wake Forest University School of Medicine, Winston-Salem, North Carolina

Andrea Dunaif, M.D. Department of Medicine and Department of Obstetrics and Gynecology, Brigham and Women's Hospital, Boston, Massachusetts

Richard Eastman, M.D. National Institute of Diabetes and Digestive and Kidney Diseases, National Institutes of Health, Bethesda, Maryland

Steven V. Edelman, M.D. Division of Endocrinology and Metabolism, Department of Medicine, University of California, San Diego, and VA Medical Center, San Diego, California

George S. Eisenbarth, Ph.D., M.D. Barbara Davis Center for Childhood Diabetes, University of Colorado Health Sciences Center, Denver, Colorado

Michael M. Engelgau, M.D. Division of Diabetes Translation, Centers for Disease Control and Prevention, Atlanta, Georgia

Jorge Calles Escandón, M.D. Division of Endocrinology, Diabetes, and Metabolism, Department of Medicine, University of Vermont College of Medicine, Burlington, Vermont

Suzanne S. P. Gebhart, M.D., F.A.C.P. Division of Endocrinology and Metabolism, Department of Medicine, Emory University School of Medicine, Atlanta, Georgia

Linda S. Geiss, M.A. Division of Diabetes Translation, Centers for Disease Control and Prevention, Atlanta, Georgia

Gary W. Gibbons, M.D. Boston University Medical School, Boston Medical Center, Boston, Massachusetts

Craig M. Greven, M.D. Department of Ophthalmology, Wake Forest University School of Medicine, Winston-Salem, North Carolina

André Guay, M.D., F.A.C.P., F.A.C.E. Endocrinology Section, Lahey Clinic Northshore, Peabody, Massachusetts

Burritt L. Haag, M.D., F.A.C.E.   Division of Endocrinology, Diabetes, and Metabolism, Baystate Medical Center, Springfield, Massachusetts

Geoffrey M. Habershaw, D.P.M.   Department of Podiatry, Beth Israel Deaconess Medical Center, Boston, Massachusetts

Jeffrey B. Halter, M.D.   Department of Internal Medicine, and Geriatrics Center, University of Michigan, Ann Arbor, Michigan

William H. Herman, M.D., M.P.H.   Departments of Internal Medicine and Epidemiology, University of Michigan, Ann Arbor, Michigan

Virginia L. Hood, M.B.B.S., M.P.H.   Nephrology Unit, University of Vermont College of Medicine, Burlington, Vermont

William E. Hopkins, M.D.   Department of Medicine, University of Vermont College of Medicine, Burlington, Vermont

Karen Hugo, M.D.   Sansum Medical Research Institute, Santa Barbara, California

Alan M. Jacobson, M.D.   Joslin Diabetes Center, and Department of Psychiatry, Harvard Medical School, Boston, Massachusetts

Lois Jovanović, M.D.   Sansum Medical Research Institute, Santa Barbara, California

Frank P. Kennedy   Division of Endocrinology, Metabolism, and Nutrition, Mayo Clinic, Rochester, Minnesota

Carolyn H. Kreinsen, M.D.   Division of Women's Health, Department of Medicine, Brigham and Women's Hospital, Boston, Massachusetts

Jack L. Leahy, M.D.   Division of Endocrinology, Diabetes, and Metabolism, Department of Medicine, University of Vermont College of Medicine, Burlington, Vermont

Paul B. Madden, M.Ed.   Joslin Diabetes Center, Boston, Massachusetts

Melinda Downie Maryniuk, M.Ed., R.D., C.D.E., F.A.D.A.   Affiliated Programs, Joslin Diabetes Center, Boston, Massachusetts

M. Molly McMahon, M.D.   Division of Endocrinology, Metabolism, and Nutrition, Mayo Clinic and Mayo Foundation, Rochester, Minnesota

Shirwan A. Mirza, M.D.   Division of Endocrinology, Diabetes, and Metabolism, Department of Medicine, University of Vermont School of Medicine, Burlington, Vermont

Sri Prakash L. Mokshagundam, M.D.   Division of Endocrinology, Department of Medicine, University of Louisville, Louisville, Kentucky

Muriel Helene Nathan, Ph.D., M.D.   Division of Endocrinology, Diabetes, and Metabolism, Department of Medicine, University of Vermont College of Medicine, Burlington, Vermont

Daniel J. Nigrin, M.D.   Department of Medicine, Children's Hospital, and Department of Pediatrics, Harvard Medical School, Boston, Massachusetts

K. Patrick Ober, M.D.   Section on Endocrinology and Metabolism, Department of Internal Medicine, Wake Forest University School of Medicine, Winston-Salem, North Carolina

Alan N. Peiris, Ph.D., M.D., M.R.C.P.   Department of Internal Medicine, James H. Quillen College of Medicine, East Tennessee State University, Johnson City, Tennessee

Bharat Raman, M.D.   Division of Endocrinology, Metabolism, and Hypertension, Wayne State University School of Medicine, Detroit, Michigan

John R. T. Reeves, M.D.   Division of Dermatology, Department of Medicine, University of Vermont College of Medicine, Burlington, Vermont

Matthew C. Riddle, M.D.   Division of Endocrinology, Diabetes, and Clinical Nutrition, Department of Medicine, Oregon Health Sciences University, Portland, Oregon

Ernst J. Schaefer, M.D.   Division of Endocrinology, Diabetes, Metabolism, and Molecular Medicine, Department of Medicine, New England Medical Center and Tufts University, Boston, Massachusetts

Elizabeth R. Seaquist, M.D.   Division of Endocrinology and Diabetes, Department of Medicine, University of Minnesota, Minneapolis, Minnesota

Leo J. Seman, Ph.D., M.D. Division of Endocrinology, Diabetes, Metabolism, and Molecular Medicine, New England Medical Center and Tufts University, Boston, Massachusetts

Rishi Sikka, M.D. The Prudential Center for Healthcare Research, Prudential Healthcare, Atlanta, Georgia

Kenneth J. Snow, M.D. Joslin Clinic, Boston, Massachusetts

James R. Sowers, M.D. Department of Internal Medicine, Wayne State University School of Medicine, Detroit, Michigan

Elizabeth Stephens, M.D. Division of Endocrinology, Department of Medicine, University of Colorado Health Sciences Center, Denver, Colorado

David E. R. Sutherland, Ph.D., M.D. Department of Surgery, University of Minnesota, Minneapolis, Minnesota

Christine T. Tobin, R.N., M.B.A., C.D.E. Health Care Consultant, Atlanta, Georgia

Katie Weinger, Ed.D., R.N. Joslin Diabetes Center and Department of Psychiatry, Harvard Medical School, Boston, Massachusetts

Joseph I. Wolfsdorf, M.B. Division of Endocrinology, Children's Hospital, Boston, Massachusetts

Bernard Zinman, M.D.C.M., F.R.C.P.(C), F.A.C.P. Banting and Best Diabetes Center, University of Toronto; Division of Endocrinology and Metabolism, Department of Medicine, Mount Sinai Hospital; and The University Health Network, Toronto, Ontario, Canada

Introduction: Medical Management of Diabetes 1916–1999: A Personal Perspective

I. INTRODUCTION

I am privileged to offer a perspective on the diagnosis and treatment of diabetes based on more than 80 years' personal experience of living with the disease. My years as a paraprofessional health educator provide another view of the skills that are essential for persons with diabetes in order to reach beyond illness.

In 1916, when I was born, my sister developed diabetes at age 2 before the availability of insulin. Our mother struggled with her child's hunger on Dr. Allen's starvation diet, which was the only treatment available at the time. My sister died at age 4.

By 1955, when I developed autoimmune type 1 diabetes at the age of 38, what was the approach of professionals to the person with diabetes? My physician, in all good faith, told me to follow a rigid daily routine that included frequent urine testing, which was the best indicator we had at that time. Attempts to control blood glucose with one shot of NPH insulin were common practice. Dietitians were scarce, and American Diabetes Association (ADA) dietary guidelines began with the word *no*: no sugar, no variation in time or content of meals. Exercise was considered dangerous. If there was difficulty as suggested by ongoing diabetes symptoms or persistence of glycosuria, it was often assumed that we had been "cheating" or were noncompliant by temperament.

We have now learned that diabetes is not a single disease with a common etiology. Treatments, which differ markedly for each type of diabetes, enable full and productive lives. There is a wide choice of human insulins and oral agents that can be variously combined to suit individual needs as required by the type and stage of the diabetes. Insulin pumps and even pancreatic transplants are increasingly in use for type 1 diabetes. Regular exercise is an important element for both types of diabetes, especially in type 2 to assist in modifying insulin resistance. Physical activity, such as climbing stairs and walking to the store, may be the most appropriate way to make changes in some persons' lifestyles. This approach may be as effective as, and less expensive or intimidating than, formal programs several times a week. In the case of type 1 diabetes, it is inspiring to see so many members of the International Diabetic Athletes Association running in marathons (and other kinds of extreme activities) and enjoying their experiences. In addition, the team approach to care is common practice and includes certified diabetes educators and dietitians as well as nurse practitioners.

Also, we have learned that diabetes is not merely abnormal blood glucose values, but a whole-body disease. Furthermore, we have learned that persons' needs in terms of diabetes management change as their bodies change over the normal course of life in all its stages.

II. NEW CHALLENGES FOR US ALL

These remarkable advances pose new challenges for those who care for people with diabetes as well as those who live with it. For one thing, there is much more information to absorb, to learn, and to teach, let alone keeping up with ongoing developments.

Most importantly, there has been a change in the relationships between care-givers and patients, moving gradually toward collaboration as equals in a shared adventure. The technological advance in the early 1970s that enabled this new relationship was patients' ability to test their own blood glucose levels and provide a record of the results. It has taken about 20 years to adapt to this change so that glucose monitoring is finally almost universal. In addition, the Diabetes Control and Complications Trial (DCCT) sharpened everyone's perspective on the efficacy of keeping the blood glucose level as close to normal as possible. The goal is to postpone and minimize the complications from inexorable damage to small blood vessels in the kidney and eyes. Now there is comparable information for type 2 diabetes from the United Kingdom Prospective Diabetes Study (UKPDS).

III. PERSONAL EXPERIENCE OF TYPE 1 DIABETES

I am unusually fortunate in being married to a forward-looking endocrinologist (Ethan Sims) who cares about me as a person. That is why I have tripled the number of survival years, beyond the 15 I was offered in 1955, to 44 years. We soon recognized that because I am a "brittle type 1," one shot of NPH a day would not work for me. We moved promptly to two injections. Then we had several strenuous years of pinpointing my allergy to the impurities in the insulins of the time. This produced bodywide hiving, which disappeared in 24 hours when we switched to the purer NOVO insulins from Denmark. From 1965, we imported Novo-Nordisk insulins until human insulins became available here. Currently, my daily plan includes three injections of Humalog before meals and the addition of Humulin Lente at supper. Dosage varies according to needs, totaling 20–30 units a day.

The keys to our success are teamwork and staying up-to-date. We've had some fun along the way. We have collaborated on writing for medical journals and books, making use of our different perceptions of the issues. Ethan is there for me when the chips are down, but we are not codependent. For many years he has been my guide, philosopher, and friend.

The philosopher aspect of Ethan is as important to me as his medical expertise. He has allowed me to take risks, to lead my own life outside the family. Together we chose safeguard procedures that let us hike in the Yosemites, cruise in our sailboat, and cross-country ski. In the 1970s, when the children were grown, I began to volunteer at several levels in the ADA. I served on the National Diabetes Advisory Board at the National Institutes of Health in 1981–1985. My efforts there centered on establishing National Standards for Patient Education Programs for self-care. I am lucky to have had the opportunity to travel to 22 states as a nonprofessional advocate for education for self-care, for both types of diabetes, which is now accepted as vital to survival as insulin and oral agents. Insurance reimbursement for education is mandated in many states because it helps avoid costly hospitalization. Along the way, I have met dedicated caregivers and ingenious patients to inspire me.

IV. NEW RESPONSIBILITIES SHARED IN COMMON

What interests me is the degree to which patients and professionals now share many responsibilities. One of the most rewarding aspects is recognizing that we all need to redefine our expectations of ourselves and one another. If we respect that task in a mutual manner, we are on our way to fruitful dialog. If we identify and are open about what we do not know or cannot control, we bypass the traditional guilt and confrontation sequence. Frustration will always be there, but we are freer to work together on what really matters.

V. FAMILY MATTERS AND THE STAGES OF ADAPTATION TO DIABETES

What really matters most over the long term are the daily decisions about basic everyday life activities that are often in conflict with managing blood glucose concentrations: food, physical activity in any form, and unavoidable changes in schedule. The atmosphere around the daily choices affects the whole family. What time is supper? Can we go out to eat? What kind of vacation will work for the person who has diabetes? It is here that the physician has a golden opportunity to bring family members into discussions with members of the health care team who can offer them support and invite them to define their own roles in living with a chronic disease.

It is here also that the normal stages of adaptation to chronic disease show up. They include astonishment, anger, fear, denial, rebellion, and jealousy. They vary from individual to individual, and the cycles recur. Loss of spontaneity is one of the hardest to bear. For me, the goal has been to accept diabetes as a companion, not an enemy. Acceptance differs from resignation, which is often passive and unhappy. Acceptance opens the door to persistent, responsible negotiation.

In the 1950s, we used glass syringes and boiled them every time. This was not handy on a hike. We sharpened steel needles on my husband's oilstone. Things are much better now, but as Ethan watched me doing yet another of the 4000-plus per annum skin punctures, he said, "It never lets up, does it!" Even HbA_{1c} results may be all very well for the medical record, but they do not tell what it is like to jump from a blood glucose value of 50 to one of 300 in a day for no discernible reason. They do not describe the fatigue from gradually advancing neuropathies that blunts awareness of hypoglycemia and disrupts sleep.

People ask "Why do you keep trying to control your blood glucose" when it is so difficult with current methods of treatment? There are two motivations, and they do not come from "compliance." First, we are more alive, full of energy, fun to be with, visually viable, sexually healthy, and able to enjoy living fully each moment of the day. For me, the practice of Yoga and Zen meditation helps me live each moment and converse with my body in a practical, but appreciative manner. Second, we hope to keep damage to our blood vessels and nerves at bay as long as possible. Persons who have type 1 diabetes are more at risk because of hypoglycemia. But when we succeed, we obtain positive feedback soon. We simply feel better, even if only for that day. People with type 2 diabetes also have demanding self-care tasks. But they may not feel rewarded for their disciplines with regard to food and exercise-promoting weight loss for as long as weeks or months. These ups and downs recur in both types of diabetes. We will always need support and encouragement.

VI. CONTINUITY OF CARE

Given the relentlessness of diabetes, ongoing access to different levels of care throughout the lifespan is necessary. How can it best be provided now? Continuity of care was easier to achieve in times past when neither professionals nor patients moved as often as they do today. Costs have risen as interventions have multiplied. So have our expectations of what is ours by right. The referral process has become uncomfortable and complex. However, in the human physician–patient encounter, opportunity abounds to develop trusted habits of communication. Experienced, perceptive physicians often say that they can tell a lot about a patient's needs just by the manner in which they enter the office. The experienced patient acquires the same capacity to notice the attitudes of physicians at their desks. They recognize which physicians are able to refer to clinics that specialize in diabetes and related disorders to expand their own observations of changes in their patients. Making a conscious effort to maintain open communication channels will always be essential, and one hopes this will be aided as computer technologies for the transfer of information further develop.

VII. GIFTS THAT COME FROM LIVING WITH DIABETES

We choose to go on learning and changing, to roll with the punches. It keeps the brain active into the ninth decade. "Use it or lose it" is a valuable slogan. It sustains our endurance. We must acquire decision-making skills and assume responsibility for seeing them through. That is an excellent attribute to highlight when seeking employment.

We become aware of the intricate marvels of body systems, complete with interactions and alternative fail-safe mechanisms. We are equipped to appreciate deeply all advances in research, and we learn to be thankful for much that we always took for granted. We are grateful for health professionals who are teachers and friends as well as medical experts. We know that we can never pay our debt for the Gift of Life.

Doro F. Sims

1

The Burden of Diabetes Mellitus

Michael M. Engelgau and Linda S. Geiss
Centers for Disease Control and Prevention, Atlanta, Georgia

I. INTRODUCTION

In 1997, an estimated 15.7 million Americans, or 5.9% of the population, had diabetes mellitus. Among this group, 10.3 million persons had diagnosed diabetes and 5.4 million had undiagnosed diabetes. Diabetes is a complex and costly disease that can affect nearly every organ in the body and result in devastating consequences. The leading cause of nontraumatic lower extremity amputations, renal failure, and blindness in working-age adults, diabetes is also a major cause of premature mortality, stroke, cardiovascular disease, peripheral vascular disease, congenital malformations, perinatal mortality, and disability. The economic impact of diabetes is tremendous and parallels the morbidity and mortality pattern of the disease.

II. CLASSIFICATION, DIAGNOSIS, AND TESTING

Before 1979, neither a standard classification scheme nor uniform diagnostic criteria existed for diabetes. In 1979–1980 the National Diabetes Data Group (NDDG) in the United States and the World Health Organization (WHO), in parallel efforts, reviewed the available scientific knowledge and developed and disseminated recommendations for the classification and diagnosis of diabetes. These recommendations were accepted worldwide and contributed significantly to a tremendous expansion in knowledge about diabetes that began in the 1980s and continues today.

During 1995–1997, the International Expert Committee on the Diagnosis and Classification of Diabetes Mellitus convened and revised the NDDG–WHO

1

Table 1   Classification of Diabetes Mellitus

Type 1: Characterized by β cell destruction leading to absolute insulin deficiency. Can
  be immune-mediated or idiopathic.
Type 2: Characterized by metabolic states that range from predominantly insulin resistance
  with relative insulin deficiency to a predominantly secretory defect with insulin resistance.
Other specific types: Include genetic defects of beta-cell function, genetic defects in insulin
  action, infections, chemical- or drug-induced, diseases of the exocrine pancreas, endocrinopathies, uncommon forms of immune-mediated diabetes, and other genetic syndromes
  that can be associated with diabetes.
Gestational

---

recommendations for the classification and diagnosis of diabetes and also made
recommendations for testing for diabetes. The committee recommended that diabetes be classified as type 1, type 2, other types, or gestational (Table 1). The
type 1 designation was chosen to replace the designation of insulin-dependent
diabetes mellitus (also called juvenile-onset diabetes); the type 2 designation
replaced the designation of non–insulin-dependent diabetes mellitus (also called
adult-onset diabetes). Type 1 diabetes is characterized by an absolute deficiency
of insulin. Type 2 diabetes is characterized by insulin resistance (i.e., ineffective
use of insulin in target tissue), inadequate compensatory insulin secretory response, or both. Other types of diabetes include disorders or factors such as
endocrinopathies, genetic syndromes, pancreatic disease, and exposure to diabetogenic drugs, toxins, and chemical agents. Gestational diabetes develops during
pregnancy, after which it normally resolves.

Following careful review of data from three population-based studies, the
committee also recommended new diagnostic criteria (Table 2). When typical
diabetes symptoms are present (i.e., polyuria, polydipsia, or unexplained weight

Table 2   Criteria for the Diagnosis[a] of Diabetes

---

1. Symptoms of diabetes[b] and a casual[c] plasma glucose ≥ 200 mg/dL (11.1 mmol/L)
2. Fasting plasma glucose ≥ 126 mg/dL (7.0 mmol/L)
3. 2-hr plasma glucose in an oral glucose tolerance test ≥ 200 mg/dL (11.1 mmol/L)

---

[a] Needs to meet only one criterion. Test must be repeated and remain positive on a separate day
  except when symptoms of unequivocal hyperglycemia with acute metabolic decompensation are
  present.
[b] Polyuria, polydipsia, and unexplained weight loss.
[c] Anytime during day without consideration of the time since the last meal.

loss), a casual (i.e., anytime during the day without regard to the last meal) plasma glucose level of 200 mg/dL (11.1 mmol/L) or higher, confirms the diagnosis. In addition, the diagnosis can be made with fasting or glucose tolerance test measures. The fasting diagnostic criterion, plasma glucose level of 140 mg/dL (7.7 mmol/L) or higher, was lowered to 126 mg/dL (7.0 mmol/L), or higher. The oral glucose tolerance test (OGTT) 2-h value of 200 mg/dL (11.0 mmol/L) or higher was retained, but because the OGTT (requiring a plasma glucose measurement 2 h after consumption of a 75-g glucose meal) was deemed more difficult and more expensive to perform than the fasting glucose test, its routine use was eliminated. The committee advised that subjects with only one positive diagnostic test should have a repeat test on a different day to confirm the diagnosis.

The committee also recommended consideration of diabetes testing for all persons aged 45 years or older and repeat testing at 3-year intervals. For persons who are considered to be at high risk for diabetes, testing should be considered at a younger age and or be performed more frequently. Those at high risk include persons who are obese, are hypertensive, or have a blood lipid abnormality; who have a family member with diabetes; who belong to a high-risk racial or ethnic group (African Americans, Hispanics, American Indians); or who either have delivered an infant weighing 9 lb or more or had gestational diabetes diagnosed.

III. PREVALENCE AND INCIDENCE

In 1988–1994, the prevalence of diabetes among persons 20 years of age or older in the United States was 7.8% (5.1% diagnosed, 2.7% undiagnosed). An estimated 798,000 new cases occur each year.

A. Type 1 Diabetes

Type 1 diabetes accounts for 5–10% of all diagnosed diabetes. It is one of the most frequent chronic diseases in children. About 40% of persons with type 1 diabetes are younger than 20 years of age. About 30,000 new cases of type 1 occur each year.

Most of the information about the incidence and prevalence of type 1 diabetes in the United States comes from population-based type 1 diabetes registries. Registries and special studies have found considerable racial and ethnic variation in the incidence of type 1 diabetes. The highest incidence tends to occur in white populations. For example, the incidence per 100,000 population for children younger than 14 years of age is 18.1 for whites and 10.2 for blacks in Allegheny County, Pennsylvania. In Colorado, the incidence per 100,000 population among Hispanic children in this age group is 9.7. There are also gender differences. In Allegheny County among whites, boys have a slightly higher incidence of type

1 diabetes than girls. Among nonwhites, in contrast, girls have a slightly higher incidence than boys. The age at onset among children peaks during puberty (10–14 years of age) and tends to be slightly younger among girls. There is a seasonality of onset: the peak incidence of type 1 diabetes occurs in late winter and early spring. Some European countries recently reported an increasing incidence of type 1 diabetes. The incidence of type 1 diabetes in the United States has been relatively stable over the past several decades, except for sporadic peaks. For example, a marked rise in 1983 in Birmingham, Alabama, was coincident with an epidemic coxsackievirus infection.

B. Type 2 Diabetes

Type 2 diabetes accounts for 90–95% of the diabetes in the United States. Much of the information about type 2 diabetes comes from national surveys, such as the National Health and Nutritional Examination Surveys (NHANES) and the National Health Interview Surveys (NHIS). These surveys collect self-reported information from a representative sample of the U.S. population. The NHANES also performs biochemical and clinical measurements. Both type 1 and type 2 diabetes cases are included in these surveys. However, because 90% or more of

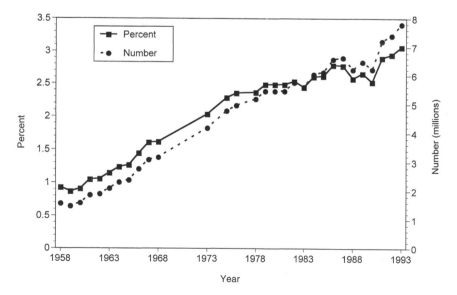

Fig. 1   Number and percentage of the population with diagnosed diabetes, United States, 1958–1993.

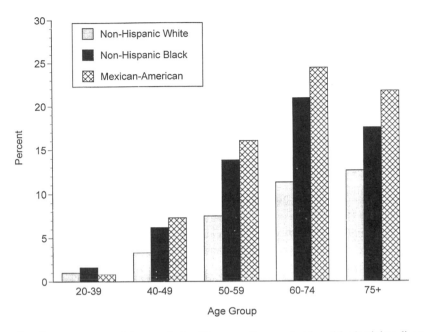

Fig. 2   Percentage of the population 20 years of age and older with physician-diagnosed diabetes by age and by race/ethnicity, United States, 1988–1994.

diabetes is type 2, the NHANES and NHIS largely track the course of type 2 diabetes.

Data from the NHANES and NHIS show that diabetes has become more and more common over the past four decades (Fig. 1). From 1980 to 1994 the number of persons with diagnosed diabetes grew by 2.2 million. The largest increase in prevalence occurred among persons 45 years of age or younger (34%). The prevalence of type 2 diabetes increases with age (Fig. 2). There tends to be only minor differences in prevalence by gender; particularly when differences in age between genders are taken into account. Between 1980 and 1994 the incidence of diabetes increased substantially. Adjusted for age changes in the population, the rate of new cases increased 49% from 2.36:1000 to 3.51:1000 population.

C.   Ethnic Differences

There is tremendous variation in the diabetes burden among the different racial and ethnic groups. Among all adults with type 2 diabetes in the United States, 70% are non-Hispanic white, 20% are non-Hispanic black, 4.8% are Mexican

American, and 5.4% are of other racial and ethnic groups. Most adults with type 1 diabetes are non-Hispanic whites (92%). Even though most of the total diabetes burden is present in the white population, minority populations are disproportionately affected. Compared with their non-Hispanic white counterparts of similar age, blacks and Hispanics are more likely to have diabetes than their non-Hispanic white counterparts (see Fig. 2). The prevalence of diagnosed diabetes in persons 45–74 years of age was 10.1% and 14.3% in Mexican Americans and Puerto Ricans, respectively, compared with 5.9% in non-Hispanic whites.

The prevalence of diabetes among Asian and Pacific Island populations residing in the United States also tends to be higher than the prevalence among whites. For example, second-generation Japanese Americans, 45–74 years of age, had a prevalence of 13.2% in men and 8.3% in women, both figures higher than among whites in the United States. Moreover, this age group of Japanese Americans was more likely to have diabetes than their counterparts in Tokyo. Few studies are available on Pacific Islander populations, but among Hawaiian and American Samoan populations, risk factors for diabetes, such as obesity, have increased and diabetes tends to be more prevalent than among their white counterparts.

The prevalence of diabetes is high among most American Indian and Alaskan Native populations. A special medical expenditure survey of persons 19 years of age or older, who were eligible for Indian Health Services benefits, found a prevalence of 12.2% among American Indians, compared with the rate of 5.2% among the general U.S. population. There is also dramatic variation in the prevalence of diabetes from tribe to tribe; whereas some tribes are no more likely to have diabetes than their white counterparts, others have some of the highest rates of diabetes in the world (50% prevalence among Pimas aged 30–64 years).

D. Geographic Variation

The prevalence of diagnosed diabetes in the United States also varies markedly by geographic region (Fig. 3). Taking age differences into account, western states tend to have a lower prevalence of diabetes and the southern and eastern states tend to have a higher prevalence.

IV. DEMOGRAPHICS AND SOCIOECONOMICS

Persons with diabetes, on average, are older than the general population. Almost 60% of adults with diabetes are 60 years of age or older, compared with 22% of the U.S. population. As would be expected, major differences in the age exist

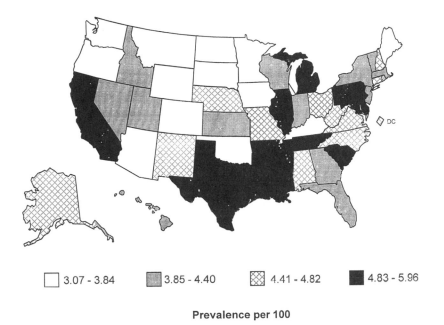

| | 3.07 - 3.84 | | 3.85 - 4.40 | | 4.41 - 4.82 | | 4.83 - 5.96 |

Prevalence per 100

Fig. 3 Age-standardized prevalence of diagnosed diabetes per 100 adult population, by state, United States, 1994.

between persons with type 1 and type 2 diabetes; the median age for persons with type 1 diabetes is 32 years and for type 2 diabetes is 64 years.

The mean age at diagnosis for persons with type 1 diabetes is about 16 years and for type 2 diabetes about 51 years. There are considerable racial and ethnic variations in age at diagnosis among persons with type 2 diabetes. The average age at diagnosis is 52 years among non-Hispanic whites, 49 years among non-Hispanic blacks, and 45 years among Mexican Americans. The mean age at diagnosis does not differ between genders. The white population with type 2 diabetes tends to be older than either the black or the Hispanic population with this disorder.

Persons with type 2 diabetes tend to be from low socioeconomic groups. Accounting for age differences within the general population, persons with type 2 diabetes have less education and lower income levels and are less likely to be employed than persons without diabetes. Among adults with type 2 diabetes, only 21% have some college education and only 16% have family incomes of $40,000 or more, compared with 40% and 33%, respectively, of persons without diabetes.

V. COMPLICATIONS

The devastation of diabetic complications has several dimensions, including premature mortality; acute metabolic complications, such as diabetic ketoacidosis;
and long-term complications affecting the microvascular (eye, kidneys, and
nerves) and macrovascular (cardiovascular, cerebrovascular, and peripheral vascular) systems. These complications can create significant disability and lower
the quality of life, consume excessive medical care resources, and place a heavy
economic burden on society.

A. Mortality

Diabetes is one of the leading causes of mortality in the United States, and deaths
attributed to diabetes are on the increase. In 1994, diabetes was the seventh
leading cause of death (Table 3). There are significant racial, ethnic, and gender
differences in the ranking of diabetes as a cause of death. The disease is the
seventh leading cause among whites, blacks, Chinese Americans, and Filipino
Americans; the sixth-leading cause among Japanese Americans; the fifth among
Hawaiians; and the fourth among American Indians. Regardless of race, diabetes
ranks higher as a leading cause of death among females than among males.

Between 1980 and 1994, the annual number of deaths for which diabetes
was the underlying cause increased from 35,000 to 57,000. Accounting for age
changes in the population during this period, the diabetes death rate increased
27% (from 15.3:100,000 to 19.5:100,000 population).

Among persons with type 1 diabetes, mortality in males is 5 times higher
and in females, 11 times higher than the mortality expected in the U.S. population.
In addition, the life expectancy of persons with type 1 diabetes is reduced by at

Table 3 Ten Leading Causes of Death in the United States, 1994

  1. Diseases of the heart
  2. Malignant neoplasms, including neoplasms of lymphatic and hematopoietic tissues
  3. Cerebrovascular disease
  4. Chronic obstructive pulmonary diseases and allied conditions
  5. Accidents and adverse effects
  6. Pneumonia and influenza
  7. Diabetes
  8. Human immunodeficiency virus infection
  9. Suicide
 10. Chronic liver cirrhosis

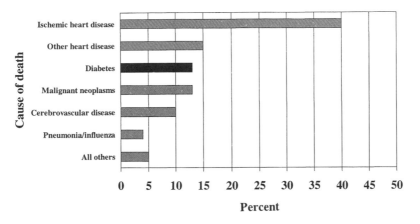

Fig. 4   Approximate distribution of causes of death in persons with diabetes in the United States.

least 15 years. Persons with shorter duration of disease (< 30 years) tend to die of renal or noncardiovascular disease causes of death; those with longer duration tend to die of cardiovascular disease.

  Type 2 diabetes is estimated to account for 17% of all deaths among persons aged 25 years or older. The overall mortality, adjusted for age, is approximately twice that of persons without diabetes. Among middle-aged populations, life expectancy is reduced by 5–10 years. This reduction in life expectancy decreases with increasing age at onset. In addition, females tend to have a greater reduction in life expectancy than males. The leading causes of death among persons with type 2 diabetes are cardiovascular disease, diabetes, malignant neoplasms, and cerebrovascular disease. Ischemic heart disease alone accounts for roughly 40% of all deaths and together with other heart disease and cerebrovascular disease accounts for 65% of all deaths (Fig. 4). Persons with diabetes have a risk of developing or dying of cardiovascular disease that is two to four times higher than that of persons without diabetes.

B.   Morbidity

1.   Cardiovascular Disease

Cardiovascular disease is also a major cause of morbidity and tends to occur at a younger age among persons with diabetes than among their counterparts without diabetes. Although the overall prevalence of cardiovascular disease increases with age for both persons with and without diabetes, the differential in cardiovascular

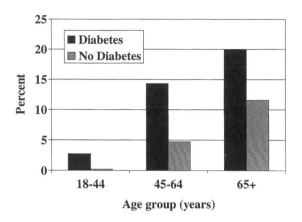

Fig. 5 Prevalence of self-reported ischemic heart disease in adults by diabetes status, United States, 1989.

disease prevalence is greatest among persons younger than 65 years of age. The 1989 NHIS found that, compared with persons without diabetes, the prevalence of self-reported ischemic heart disease among persons was about 14 times higher among those aged 18–44 years (2.7 vs. 0.2%); about 3 times higher among those aged 45–64 years (14.3 vs. 4.7%); and almost twice as high among those aged 65 years or older (20 vs. 12%; Fig. 5). Women with diabetes tend to be affected by cardiovascular disease almost as often as men.

In 1994, 33% of all the diabetes-related hospitalizations, a total of 1.1 million, had cardiovascular disease as the primary diagnosis. Older persons were more likely to be hospitalized with cardiovascular disease; among persons with diabetes, those aged 75 years and older were almost ten times more likely to be hospitalized for cardiovascular disease than those younger than 45 years of age.

Stroke is also a major cause of morbidity among persons with diabetes and is more common in persons with diabetes compared with their nondiabetic counterparts. For example, the proportion reporting a history of stroke was higher among persons with diabetes 45–64 years of age than in the general population of similar age (8.4 vs. 1.7%). The 1989 NHIS found that 9% of all adults with diabetes had a medical history of stroke. For both persons with and without diabetes, stroke was more common in older persons than in younger persons.

2. Retinopathy

Visual impairment and blindness are major disabling diabetic complications. Retinopathy, cataracts, and glaucoma can lead to blindness in persons with diabetes.

Diabetic retinopathy, the leading cause of blindness (visual acuity $\leq$ 20/200) in persons aged 20–74 years, causes from 12,000 to 24,000 new cases of blindness each year in the United States. An estimated 12% of all new cases of blindness are due to diabetic retinopathy. The proportion of new cases of blindness caused by diabetic retinopathy is about 12% among persons aged 20–44 years, about 19% among persons aged 45–64 years, and about 8% among persons aged 65 years or older.

3. Renal

The leading cause of end-stage renal disease (ESRD) in the United States, diabetes accounts for about 40% of all new cases of ESRD. Persons with diabetes are the fastest-growing group of recipients for kidney dialysis and transplantation. New cases attributed to diabetes increased from an estimated 7,000 in 1984 to almost 31,000 in 1996 (Fig. 6). The rate of increase in the incidence of ESRD attributable to diabetes increased with age among persons with diabetes. Between 1984 and 1993, the incidence increased 5% among persons younger that 45 years of age, more than 100% among persons aged 45–64 years, and more than 200% among persons aged 65 years or older. Several factors may account for the increase in incidence, including a true increase in the incidence, an increase in the recognition of the etiological role of diabetes, an increase in the use of treatment, or a combination of these factors.

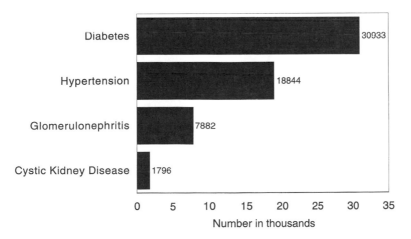

Fig. 6 Number of new cases of treated end-stage renal disease for the top four primary diagnoses, United States, 1996.

Among persons with diabetes, the incidence of ESRD differs considerably among racial and ethnic groups. In 1993, compared to their white counterparts, both black males (511:100,000 vs 220:100,000) and black females (439:100,000 vs. 184:100,000) were more than twice as likely to have a diagnosis of ESRD.

4. Foot Ulcers and Amputations

Lower extremity ulcers and amputation are an increasing problem among persons with diabetes. Diabetic foot ulcers are common and estimated to occur in 15% of all persons with diabetes during their lifetime. Studies have found that, depending on the severity of the ulcer, from 6 to 43% of persons with diabetes with ulcers will ultimately have an amputation. Among persons with diabetes who have had an amputation, as many as 85% may have had a preceding foot ulcer.

More than half of all nontraumatic lower extremity amputations occur in persons with diagnosed diabetes. Among persons with diabetes, the number of amputations increased from 36,000 in 1980 to 67,000 in 1994. In 1994, hospitalizations for amputations among persons with diabetes accounted for 984,000 hospital days. Rates of amputation increase with increasing age. Fifty-five percent of all diabetes-related amputations occur in persons aged 65 years or older. Adjusting for age differences, from 1980 to 1994 the rates of amputation have been higher among men than women and higher among blacks than whites (Fig. 7).

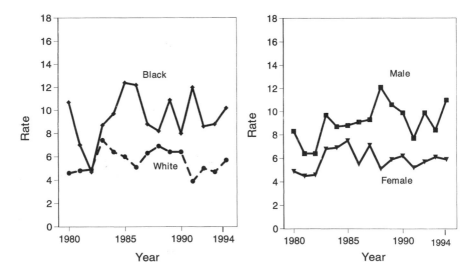

*Age-adjusted to 1980 diabetic population

Fig. 7   Age-adjusted hospital discharge rate for nontraumatic lower extremity amputation per 1000 diabetic population by race and by sex, United States, 1980–1994.

Studies have shown that among persons with diabetes-related amputations, 9–20% may experience a second amputation within 12 months, and 28–51% within 5 years of the first one.

5. Diabetic Ketoacidosis

Diabetic ketoacidosis (DKA) is an acute metabolic complication of diabetes that may require hospitalization and can result in death. In population-based studies, the incidence of DKA ranged from 5:1000 to 8:1000 person-years, although the rate was much higher (13:1000 person-years) in persons whose age at diagnosis was younger than 30 years (mostly type 1 diabetes). In these studies, DKA was the initial manifestation of diabetes in 20–25% of the cases. Among patients who did not initially present with DKA, the median duration from their diagnosis of diabetes to DKA was 4.6 years.

The number of hospitalizations in the United States owing to DKA rose from 59,000 in 1980 to 89,000 in 1994. Hospitalization rates for DKA are similar for males and females. Compared with whites, blacks have more than twice the age-adjusted rate of DKA hospitalizations (15.7:1000 vs. 6.8:1000 diabetic population).

Deaths due to DKA are relatively rare and have been declining. From 1980 to 1994, the age-adjusted DKA death rate declined 34% (30.8:100,000 to 20.2:100,000 diabetic population). The rates are highest among younger persons ($\leq$ 44 years of age) and older persons ($\geq$ 75 years of age). There is also racial variation in DKA death rates: rates are highest among black males, followed by black females, and then by white males and white females. For example, the age-adjusted DKA death rate for black males was almost twice that of white males (38:100,000 vs. 20:100,000 diabetic population) in 1994.

6. Disability and Quality of Life

Persons with diabetes experience much greater levels of disability and a lower quality of life than the general population. Rates of activity limitation (e.g., unable to or limited in ability to perform a major activity, such as attending school, working, doing housekeeping, or performing other activities of daily living) and restricted activity days (e.g., bed days, work loss days, school loss days) are two to three times higher among persons with diabetes than among counterparts without diabetes. The age-adjusted proportion of persons with type 2 diabetes reporting activity limitation was 50% and with type 1 diabetes was 42% compared with 16% among persons without diabetes. The proportion reporting restricted activity days with type 2 diabetes was 22%, and with type 1 diabetes, was 21% compared with 10% among persons without diabetes. Rates of activity limitation and restricted activity days are generally higher among females than among males and higher among blacks than among whites.

Unemployment may be a manifestation of disability. It is difficult to determine the effect of disability among persons with type 2 diabetes because a large proportion are not in the labor force. Among persons enumerated in registries of type 1 diabetes, about half of those who are disabled are not working, manifesting a proportion of unemployment almost two to three times that of persons without disability.

7. Pregnancy and Diabetes

Both gestational diabetes and pregnancy with preexisting diabetes (either type 1 or type 2) can influence pregnancy outcomes. Estimates of the prevalence of gestational diabetes, which are highly dependent on screening methods, diagnostic criteria, and detection practices, range between 2 and 5%. The rate of perinatal mortality does not appear to increase with this condition. The major morbidity of gestational diabetes is macrosomia and associated obstetrical morbidity. By contrast, pregnancies with preexisting diabetes can have a 1.5- to 2-fold higher perinatal mortality and 3- to 5-fold higher rate of preterm delivery and cesarean delivery. Spontaneous abortions and major malformations also occur at higher rates than in pregnancies without diabetes.

VI. UTILIZATION OF HEALTH CARE

Persons with diabetes use more health care resources than persons without diabetes. Resources include medications and health care services through telephone calls to care providers, doctor's office visits, hospital outpatient clinic and emergency room visits, and hospitalizations. In 1993, persons with diagnosed diabetes made an estimated 121 million contacts with physicians, or an average of about 16 contacts per person. About half of the contacts were for office visits for an average of 8 visits per person. After adjusting for age, females had more contacts and office visits (17.1 and 9.9) than males (14.3 and 6.8). From 1983 to 1993, the age-adjusted number of contacts and office visits rose about 40% for females and 10% for males. Among visits to physicians for diabetes, 72% were to primary care physicians (family practice, general practice, internal medicine, and pediatrics), 8% were to diabetologists or endocrinologist, and 20% were to other specialists or subspecialists (e.g., surgeons, ophthalmologists, cardiologists, nephrologists).

A significant portion of the health care utilization by persons with diabetes is for inpatient and emergency room care. Data from the 1989 NHIS showed that during one year, 24% of persons with diabetes are hospitalized at least once, compared with 8% of persons without diabetes. In 1994, 3.5 million diabetes-related hospitalizations accounted for 24.7 million hospital days. The age-adjusted diabetes-related hospitalization rate increased 10% from 1980 to 1994 (from 387:1000 to 427:1000 diabetic population). In 1992, 12% of persons with diabetes had an emergency room visit ($n = 877,000$) which was related to their diabetic condition.

VII. HEALTH COVERAGE AND ECONOMICS

Among adults with diabetes, 92% have some form of health insurance and 41% have coverage from more that one source. Almost 600,000 adults with diabetes have no medical care coverage. Government-funded programs (Medicare, Medicaid, military benefits, other public sources) provide coverage for 58% of adults with diabetes, including 96% of those aged 65 years and older. Among this group, about 95% are covered by Medicare, 70% by private insurance, 5% by military benefits, and 15% by Medicaid or another public source.

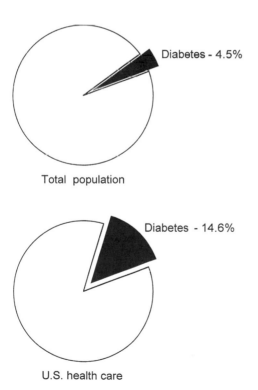

Fig. 8 Health care expenditures for persons with diabetes, United States, 1992.

Several studies have estimated health care costs related to diabetes, and each has reported a substantial economic burden. One effort estimated the total cost of health care (both diabetes-related and non–diabetes-related) in 1992 for persons with diabetes at $105 billion, or 14.6% of the U.S. health care expenditures that year (Fig. 8). Persons with diabetes incurred health care costs that were 3.6 times higher than costs incurred by persons without the disease ($9493 vs. $2604/person). A more recent study estimated the direct cost (cost of medical care and services) and indirect cost (cost of short-term disability, permanent disability, and premature death) attributable to diabetes. This study determined the fraction of all health care costs that are due specifically (attributable) to diabetes and estimated a direct cost of $44.1 billion and an indirect cost of $54.1 billion in 1997.

VIII. SUMMARY

Diabetes imposes a tremendous burden on the population. In recent decades, both the number of cases and the prevalence of diabetes have increased substantially. Diabetic complications are common and can have devastating consequences in terms of disability and quality of life. Several minority groups are disproportionately affected by the disease. Finally, persons with diabetes consume a vast amount of health care resources, and the economic consequences of diabetes are substantial.

BIBLIOGRAPHY

American Diabetes Association. Economic consequences of diabetes mellitus in the U.S. in 1997. Diabetes Care 1997; 21:296–309.
Centers for Disease Control and Prevention. Diabetes Surveillance, 1997. Atlanta, GA: U.S. Department of Health and Human Services, 1997.
Centers for Disease Control and Prevention. National Diabetes Fact Sheet, 1997. Atlanta, GA: U.S. Department of Health and Human Services, 1997.
Engelgau MM, Smith PJ, German RR, Aubert RE, Herman WH. The epidemiology of diabetes mellitus and pregnancy, United States, 1988. Diabetes Care 1995; 18: 1029–1033.
Flegal KM, Ezzati TM, Harris MI, Haynes SG, Juarez RZ, Knowler WC, Perez-Stable EJ, Stern MP. Prevalence of diabetes in Mexican Americans, Cubans, and Puerto Ricans from the Hispanic Health and Nutrition Examination Survey, 1982–84. Diabetes Care 1991; 12(suppl. 3):628–638.
Fujimoto WY, Leonetti DL, Kinyoun JL, Newell-Morris L, Shuman WP, Stolov WC, Wahl PW. Prevalence of diabetes mellitus and impaired glucose tolerance among second-generation Japanese-American men. Diabetes 1987; 36:721–729.

Fujimoto WY, Leonetti DL, Bergstrom RW, Kinyoun JL, Stolov WC, Wahl PW. Glucose intolerance and diabetic complications among Japanese-Americans women. Diabetes Res Clin Pract 1991; 13:119–130.

Harris MI, ed. Diabetes in America. 2nd ed. Washington DC: National Institutes of Health. NIH publication 95-1468, 1995.

Harris MI, Cowie CC, Eastman R. Health insurance coverage for adults with diabetes in the U.S. population. Diabetes Care 1994; 17:585–591.

Harris MI, Flegal KM, Cowie KK, Eberhart MS, Goldstein DE, Little RR, Weidmeyer HM, Byrd-Holt DD. Prevalence of diabetes, impaired fasting glucose, and impaired glucose tolerance in U.S. adults. The third National Health and Nutritional Examination Survey, 1988–1994. Diabetes Care 1998; 21:518–524.

Johnson AE, Taylor AK. Prevalence of chronic diseases: a summary of data from the survey of American Indians and Alaska Natives. National Medical Expenditure Survey Data Summary 3, Agency for Health Care Policy and Research publ. 91-0031. Rockville, MD: Agency for Health Care Policy and Research, 1991.

Karvonen M, Tuomilehto J, Linman I, LaPorte R. A review of the recent epidemiological data on the worldwide incidence of type 1 (insulin-dependent) diabetes mellitus: World Health Organization DIAMOND Project Group. Diabetologia 1993; 36: 883–892.

Knowler WC, Saad MF, Pettitt DJ, Nelson RG, Bennett PH. Determinates of diabetes mellitus in the Pima Indians. Diabetes Care 1993; 16(supp 1):216–227.

Rubin RJ, Altman WM, Mendelson DN. Health care expenditures for people with diabetes mellitus, 1992. J Clin Endocrinol Metab 1994; 78:809A–809F.

Songer TJ, LaPorte RE, Dorman JS, Otchard TJ, Becker DJ, Drash AL. Employment spectrum of IDDM. Diabetes Care 1989; 12:615–622.

The Expert Committee on the Diagnosis and Classification of Diabetes Mellitus. Report of the Expert Committee on the Diagnosis and Classification of Diabetes Mellitus. Diabetes Care 1997; 20:1183–1197.

2

Type 1A Diabetes as an Immunological Disorder

Elizabeth Stephens and George S. Eisenbarth
University of Colorado Health Sciences Center, Denver, Colorado

I. INTRODUCTION

Insulin-dependent diabetes, or more specifically, type 1A, results from immune-mediated destruction of insulin-producing beta cells of the pancreas. In this chapter we will review the autoimmune process and genetics of type 1A diabetes, followed by a discussion of the prediction and diagnosis of type 1A diabetes in both children and adults. We will also review associated autoimmune processes that should be considered when caring for a patient with this type of diabetes and ongoing trials for diabetes prevention.

II. PATHOGENESIS

Although type 1A (immune) diabetes was previously thought to develop suddenly, it is now understood to be a chronic process that evolves over months to many years (1). Histologically, there is destruction of beta cells, whereas other islet cells, such as alpha cells (which secrete glucagon) and delta cells (which produce somatostatin), are left intact. On examination, the involved islets contain cells with enlarged nuclei, variable numbers of degranulated beta cells, and a chronic inflammatory infiltrate that is known as insulitis. This infiltrate is composed of T lymphocytes, most of which are CD8 and CD4, as well as natural killer cells and macrophages (2). The involvement of islets is variable. Within the same pancreas there are areas of complete destruction of beta cells, other islets with inflammation surrounding beta cells, and areas where islets appear normal. This variability may explain the slow progression to overt hyperglycemia commonly seen with type 1A diabetes, especially in adults. Overall symptomatic diabetes occurs when there has been destruction of over 80% of beta-cell volume, at which point exogenous insulin is required (2).

III. GENETICS

Type 1A diabetes is a genetically determined disorder, as evidenced by the increased frequency of disease in monozygotic twins and first-degree relatives. For identical twins, the risk of developing diabetes approaches 70% with long-term follow-up, and approximately 1 : 20 first-degree relatives develop diabetes in contrast to a U.S. population risk of 1 : 300 (3). The genes primarily responsible for the familial aggregation of diabetes are within the major histocompatibility complex located on chromosome 6, also called the HLA locus. At least 40% of the familial aggregation of type 1A diabetes is accounted for by major histocompatibility complex (MHC) genes, in particular the HLA class II molecules, DQ and DR (3). Class II molecules function by binding short peptides and presenting them to CD4-positive T cells. Each class II allele is composed of two chains, α and β, and is classified with a unique number. In DQ molecules, both the α- and β-chains are polymorphic, so that the description of a DQ molecule requires two numbers (e.g., DQA1*0501, DQB1*0201). For DR molecules the α-chain is constant, so designation includes only a number for the β-chain (e.g., DRB1*0301). Certain combinations of these DQ and DR alleles are associated with both a higher risk of the development of type 1A diabetes as well as protection from disease. For example, 2% of children born in the United States are DR3/4 heterozygotes with DQA1*0501, DQB1*0201, and DQA1*0301, DQB1*0302 (e.g., DRB1*0301/DRB1*0401), whereas these individuals constitute approximately 40% of all children developing diabetes (4).

The HLA alleles are also associated with protection from diabetes. The most common and most protective HLA DQ allele is DQA1*0102, DQB1*0602. This allele occurs in more than 20% of individuals from the general population, but in less than 1% of children who develop type 1A diabetes (3). Table 1 gives a listing of the HLA alleles associated with both risk of and protection from diabetes.

The familial aggregation of type 1A diabetes is partly explained by MHC alleles, but clearly other genetic loci are involved. A second susceptibility gene that has been identified is the INS (insulin) region on the short arm of chromosome 11. However the association between INS and the development of diabetes is much weaker than that with HLA (5), and the mechanism by which it is involved

Table 1 HLA Haplotypes (DR and DQ) and Diabetes Risk

DRB1	DQA1	DQB1
High risk		
0301 ("DR3")	0501	0201
0401, 0402 ("DR4")	0301	0302
04	0301	0401
0801	0401	0402
1601	0102	0502
Moderate risk		
0401, 0402 ("DR4")	0301	0301
0901	0301	0303
1302	0102	0604
Low risk		
0403 ("DR4")	0301	0302
0701	0201	0201
1101	0501	0301
Strongly protective		
1501 ("DR2")	0102	0602
1401	0101	0503
0701	0201	0303

remains to be determined. In addition, nongenetic factors are thought to be important in the initiation of the autoimmune process and insulitis development. Environmental factors have been implicated, particularly infectious processes. For example, children with congenital rubella have a high risk of developing diabetes and thyroiditis (5). Another possible initiating factor suggested is dietary protein, which has been associated with the development of diabetes in mouse models. Bovine milk is an example of a possible protein trigger of autoimmunity; however, a prospective study did not find an association between milk ingestion and the development of autoimmune diabetes.

IV. ASSOCIATED DISEASES

It is now well recognized that individuals with type 1A diabetes are at increased risk for the development of other immune diseases including Addison's disease, celiac disease, autoimmune thyroiditis, and pernicious anemia. When caring for a patient with immune diabetes, screening for these associated conditions is recommended. In the presence of an associated autoimmune disorder, patients with type 1A diabetes are frequently asymptomatic, and may unknowingly suffer consequences that will be discussed in the following.

Addison's disease or primary adrenocortical insufficiency is a progressive disorder that is now recognized to most commonly result from autoimmune adrenalitis. Antiadrenal antibodies (21-hydroxylase, or 21-AA) are found in more than 90% of those with the disease, and they tend to be more common in patients with a shorter duration of disease. Addison's disease is much more common in patients with type 1A diabetes, being found in 1:200 patients with diabetes compared with 1:20,000 in the general population. Screening patients with diabetes has revealed that 2% have 21-AA, which correlates with their increased frequency of Addison's disease (6). In addition to screening for antibodies, genotype is important in establishing risk for development of Addison's disease in those with diabetes. A recent study of patients with type 1A diabetes indicated that among those with 21-AA, DRB1 subtyping helped in predicting those at risk for Addison's disease. In this population of diabetics with adrenal antibodies, Addison's disease was diagnosed in 90% of those having DRB1*0404, DQB1*0302 haplotype. This was in contrast to patients with diabetes and 21-AA, but without Addison's disease, in which 90% expressed either DRB1*0401 or DRB1*0402 (7). This data suggests that risk for Addison's disease may depend on DRB1 subtype, with an allele associated with disease (*0404) and others potentially protective (*0401 or *0402). Also, patients with type 1 diabetes who develop Addison's disease can present with severe hypoglycemia before the development of hyperpigmentation. In these patients, determination of 21-AA and adrenal function testing should permit earlier diagnosis of adrenal insufficiency.

Celiac disease (CD) or gluten-sensitive enteropathy is a disorder involving the small intestinal mucosa. Celiac disease is increased in patients with type 1A diabetes. In celiac disease, antiendomysial (EMA) and transglutaminase autoantibodies (TGAA) are produced that react with the enzyme transglutaminase (TG). Transglutaminase functions by catalyzing the cross-linking of proteins with glutamine. Ingested gliadin, which triggers the formation of these antibodies, is an abundant source of glutamine and is an excellent substrate for transglutaminase. Sensitive assays for TGAA (both IgA and IgG) are now available and are used to identify those at risk, but confirmation of disease requires an intestinal biopsy (6). Among those with type 1A diabetes, the prevalence of CD ranges from 2.3 to 7% in children and approximately 4.5% in adults (8). Interestingly, the individuals found to have positive antibodies and celiac disease on biopsy are often completely asymptomatic. This is important to recognize because CD is associated with an increased risk of growth impairment and defects in bone mineralization in children. In adults with asymptomatic CD, osteopenia can develop from chronic malabsorption (5). In patients with symptomatic celiac disease, there is an increased incidence of gastrointestinal malignancies, including mouth, pharynx, esophageal cancers, and lymphoma. To identify patients with type 1A diabetes who are at risk for CD, antibody evaluation for EMA and TGAA are useful. In a study of 93 patients with diabetes, EMA had an 86% positive predictive value for celiac disease (8), and in a separate study, those with high TGAA values (greater than 0.75) all had a positive intestinal biopsy results (6). Susceptibility to celiac disease is associated with certain HLA alleles, including DQA1*0501, DQB1*0201, and DQA1*0301, DQB1*0302 (8).

Thyroid autoimmune disease (TAI) is found more frequently in patients with type 1A diabetes. The prevalence of thyroid autoantibodies in those with immune diabetes from differing populations has ranged from 5 to 40%, a prevalence two- to fivefold greater than the general population (9). Despite increased frequency of thyroid antibody formation in these patients with type 1A diabetes, multiple studies have failed to document a clear association with HLA alleles. With the increased risk of thyroid disease in those with immune diabetes, it is currently recommended that yearly screening of TSH be performed to determine the presence of hypo- or hyperthyroidism. In women of childbearing age with type 1A diabetes it may be useful to determine thyroid autoantibodies. It has been described that women with TAI and immune diabetes often have poorer glucose control during pregnancy (9), and a higher incidence of spontaneous abortion. In this particular population, evaluation of thyroid autoantibodies in addition to TSH may be useful.

V. ANTIBODIES

Over the past 20 years, autoantibodies have been identified that are both diagnostic and predictive for type 1A diabetes. Initially, autoantibodies to islets were identified by indirect immunofluorescence using human pancreas (3). This test has been difficult to standardize. Subsequently, several specific antigens were identified, including the enzyme GAD65 and ICA512 (also called IA-2). These antigens are not specific for the islet cell, as both are also found in other neuroendocrine cells and tissues, and additional islet autoantigens remain to be identified. The only beta–cell-specific antigen is insulin. Currently, there are the three autoantigens (GAD65, ICA512, and insulin) for which reproducible and convenient autoantibody assays are available. Autoantibody testing is typically performed by using cloned DNA to produce labeled GAD65, ICA512, and insulin. Fluid-phase radioimmunoassays to identify the presence of autoantibodies have high specificity and sensitivity. These autoantibody assays can be set with quantitative "cutoffs," such that less than 1:100 normal individuals express a single autoantibody and less than 1:300 more than a single autoantibody (6).

The evaluation of first-degree relatives of patients with type 1A indicates that the presence of two or more defined autoantibodies confers a greater than 80% 10-year risk of diabetes versus less than 20% risk with only one defined antibody (10). Most individuals expressing multiple autoantibodies do not have protective HLA alleles. For the rare relative with multiple autoantibodies and the protective allele DQB1*0602, it is not yet possible to assess diabetes risk.

Expression of antibodies and HLA typing provides important prognostic information, but does not define the time course to onset of hyperglycemia. In these circumstances, the first-phase insulin release (FPIR) rate after intravenous glucose can be a useful adjunct. The FPIR is generally calculated as the sum of the plasma insulin levels on samples drawn at 1 and 3 min after a standard intravenous glucose injection during an intravenous glucose tolerance test (IVGTT). In the presence of autoantibodies, this evaluation of FPIR during an IVGTT is the best predictor of time to onset of diabetes, and it should be repeated yearly to achieve the greatest sensitivity. There has been controversy over the chronology of FPIR loss in the years before the diagnosis of overt diabetes, as there can be considerable variations among individuals. However, severe abnormalities have a high positive-predictive values, whereas normal FPIR has a high negative-predictive value (5). Overall, those with an FPIR higher than the tenth percentile rarely progress to having diabetes within 1 year of follow-up (5). Of note, high levels of insulin antibodies often predict a more rapid decline in beta-cell function and onset of diabetes.

How antibodies can be used in the diagnosis of type 1A diabetes will be discussed further in the next section.

VI. ISSUES IN DIABETES DIAGNOSIS

A. Type 2 Diabetes

Recently, new issues in the diagnosis of diabetes have become apparent. One such issue has been the rising prevalence of type 2 diabetes in the young. In the past, when children or younger adults presented with the signs or symptoms of diabetes, it was assumed that, because of their age, the etiology was type 1 diabetes requiring insulin. However, with the rising incidence of obesity in the young has also come an increase in insulin resistance and type 2 diabetes. In a recent study of a pediatric population with diabetes in Cincinnati, the number of individuals with a new diagnosis of type 2 diabetes rose from 4% before 1992, to 16% in 1994 (ages 0–19); among those aged 10–19, type 2 diabetes accounted for 33% of those with a diagnosis of diabetes in 1994 (11). As expected, these patients also had an elevated body mass index (BMI), with a mean of 37.7 ± 9.6 kg/m^2 (for reference, the 90th percentile of BMI for the pediatric population as a whole is 27 kg/m^2), and also suffered from conditions associated with obesity and insulin resistance, including hypertension (17%), sleep apnea (6%), and hypertriglyceridemia (4%) (11).

In a child or young adult with an elevated BMI and hyperglycemia, the possibility of type 2 diabetes needs to be considered. To help diagnose these individuals, determination of anti-islet autoantibodies is useful. Autoantibodies to GAD65, ICA512, and insulin are commonly found at the time of diagnosis of type 1A diabetes (10). Therefore, if antibodies are not identified in the young patient with hyperglycemia, it makes the diagnosis of type 1A diabetes much less likely.

Family history can also be a factor to assess in the obese child with hyperglycemia. In the Cincinnati group, 85% of the children with a type 2 diabetes diagnosis had either a first- or second-degree relative with type 2 diabetes (11), whereas most cases of type 1A diabetes occur in the absence of any family history. In addition, ethnicity needs to be considered, as the incidence of type 2 diabetes is higher among African American and Mexican American children. This was found in the Cincinnati study, in which African American children accounted for 70–75% of type 2 diabetes patients, and in a separate study of Mexican American children from Ventura, California (31% of those younger than 17 had a diagnosis of type 2 diabetes; 12).

Given the comorbidities associated with insulin resistance, it is important to accurately diagnose a pediatric patient with type 2 diabetes; it is also useful for treatment and management. In a patient with insulin resistance, oral medications, such as metformin or sulfonylureas, may be more appropriate therapy than insulin.

A second group of patients has also been identified with an early-onset form of diabetes. Maturity-onset diabetes of the young (MODY) is a monogenic form of diabetes that has been intensively studied. It is characterized by familial diabetes, with an early age of onset (childhood, adolescence, or young adulthood), autosomal dominant inheritance, and a primary defect in insulin secretion (13). There is variability in the phenotype of subjects with MODY, and further studies have isolated some of the specific gene defects involved. These include mutations in genes on chromosome 20q (designated MODY1/hepatic nuclear factor-4_α; HNF-4_α), 7p (MODY2/glucokinase), and 12 q (MODY3/HNF-1_α; 13). MODY 2, which results from a defect in the glucokinase gene, results in mild postprandial hyperglycemia caused by reduced pancreatic beta-cell responsiveness to glucose and decreased accumulation of hepatic glycogen and increased hepatic gluconeogenesis after eating. MODY 1 and 3 are characterized by severe insulin secretory defects, with associated fasting hyperglycemia and microvascular complications (13). Other MODY genes are likely to be identified in the future, as there are families who appear to have MODY, but do not have recognized mutations. The prevalence of MODY has been suggested to be 2–5% of those with type 2 diabetes (13). Patients with MODY can often be identified by the strong family history of diabetes and negative anti-islet autoantibodies.

Other rare forms of diabetes need to be considered when evaluating a patient with diabetes, especially patients who are anti-islet autoantibody-negative. These include Wolfram syndrome, which is a gradually progressive neurodegenerative disorder, with a nonautoimmune loss of beta cells, and diabetes caused by mitochondrial DNA mutations that are frequently associated with deafness.

B. Type 1 Diabetes in Adults

Classification of children with diabetes has become increasingly difficult as the prevalence of type 2 diabetes in that population increases. Adults can be equally if not more, difficult to categorize as either type 1 or 2. It is now recognized that adults with an initial diagnosis of type 2 diabetes, but requiring insulin therapy, are often reclassified as type 1A diabetes, and they usually require insulin therapy within 3 years of the diagnosis. Unlike children with immune diabetes who usually have more rapid onset of disease, adults frequently have significant variability in diabetes progression. This is supported by finding that beta cells disappear during the first 12 months of diabetes in patients younger than 7 years of age, whereas in adults, beta cell function can be detected for much longer periods. The presence of anti-islet antibodies is useful in the classification of diabetes type. In a Swedish study, the presence of islet cell antibodies (ICA) and GAD65 antibodies in patients previously thought to have type 2 diabetes was strongly correlated with future insulin treatment and likely identified patients with type 1A diabetes. Data from this study found 74% with positive ICA or GAD65 becoming insulin-dependent, compared with 12% in those not requiring insulin (14). Another study evaluating type 2 diabetes and antibody production found that approximately 85% of patients with type 2 diabetes who were ICA-positive eventually required insulin treatment (15). Other features that have been suggested to distinguish between type 2 and type 1A diabetes include low or normal body weight, reduced C-peptide levels, HLA-DR3 or DR4, and other autoimmune diseases or antibodies (15).

The identification of a patient as having either type 1A or type 2 diabetes also has important therapeutic implications. In the early stages of the immune destruction of the beta cells, an adult with type 1A diabetes can often be adequately controlled with oral diabetes medications. However, there is a suggestion that initiating insulin therapy sooner in these patients may preserve beta-cell function. The benefit of prolonged beta-cell function and endogenous insulin production has been suggested in studies that document lower hemoglobin A_{1c} values and fewer microvascular complications in those who secrete C peptide compared with those who do not (15).

VII. PREVENTION STUDIES

Currently, human trials are evaluating agents that have been demonstrated to prevent disease in animal models of type 1A diabetes. The two largest trials will be briefly discussed here.

Nicotinamide is a derivative of vitamin B_3, nicotinic acid, which in NOD mice limits the development of diabetes. The mechanism of action is unclear, but may involve protection of cells from lysis after exposure to oxygen radicals or on blockage of lymphokine-mediated islet destruction. Studies from New Zealand that used nicotinamide have reported a 50% delay in progression to diabetes in those who were ICA-positive compared with a nonscreened and non-treated group (3). These trials have led to randomized studies being conducted in Europe, including the Deutsche Nicotinamide Trial (DENIS) and the European Nicotinamide Diabetes Intervention Trial (ENDIT). This latter study has screened a large population to identify 500 with positive ICA who are randomized to treatment with nicotinamide or placebo for 5 years. This study is currently in progress. The smaller DENIS trial was stopped, with no beneficial effect of nico-tinamide observed.

The association between high titers of insulin antibodies and the develop-ment of diabetes suggests that insulin is an important element in the immune response that leads to beta-cell destruction. From this recognition came specific interest in insulin as an antigen to be used to prevent the development of diabetes. In the BB rat model, high doses of subcutaneous insulin prevented the develop-ment of diabetes. From this finding, developed the theory that the administration of insulin may induce beta-cell "rest" and, subsequently, slow or prevent the immune-mediated destruction that results in diabetes. A pilot trial was designed to examine this hypothesis in 12 high-risk persons with positive antibodies (IAA and ICA) as well as diminished first-phase insulin response. Of the 12, 7 chose not to be treated with exogenous insulin, and all developed diabetes within 3 years. Of the 5 who selected insulin treatment (intravenous infusion daily for 5 days every 9 months and daily subcutaneous insulin), only 1 developed diabetes within 3 years (1). The results of this preliminary study have led to a multicenter, National Institutes of Health-sponsored clinical trial called the Diabetes Preven-tion Trial (DPT-1), which will screen ICA antibody-positive individuals for entry into either the subcutaneous or oral insulin arms. This study is currently under way.

VIII. FUTURE DIRECTIONS

The development of type 1A diabetes involves a combination of genetics, autoim-munity, and environmental factors. Together, these three influences result in a disease process with extremely high health and economic costs. The prevention studies that are currently underway will probably not provide the final answer to the question of immune diabetes prevention, but will, we hope, better define individuals who are at risk and identify potential therapies. The success of diabetes prevention in animal models makes us optimistic that the same will be possible in humans. However, it is recognized that there is still a great deal to be unraveled before the definitive treatments are discovered.

REFERENCES

1. Sperling MA. Aspects of the etiology, prediction, and prevention of insulin-dependent diabetes mellitus in childhood. Pediatr Clin North Am 1997; 44:269–284.
2. Atkinson MA, Maclaren NK. The pathogenesis of insulin-dependent diabetes mellitus. N Engl J Med 1994; 331:1428–1436.
3. Gottlieb PA, Eisenbarth GS. Diagnosis and treatment of pre-insulin dependent diabetes (IDDM). Annu Rev Med 1998; 49:391–405.
4. Rewers M, Bugawan TL, Norris JM, et al. Newborn screening for HLA markers associated with IDDM: diabetes autoimmunity study in the young (DAISY). Diabetologia 1996; 39:807–812.
5. Verge CF, Eisenbarth GS. Natural history of autoimmunity in type I diabetes mellitus. In: LeRoith D, Taylor SI, Olefsky JM, eds. Diabetes Mellitus: A Fundamental and Clinical Text. Philadelphia: Lippincott–Raven, 1996:287–297.
6. Yu L, Eisenbarth GS. Immunology of type 1 diabetes and related endocrine disorders. Clin Endocrinol Update 1998; 257–266.
7. Yu L, Brewer KW, Gates S, et al. DRB1*04 and DQ alleles: expression of 21-hydroxylase autoantibodies and risk of progression to Addison's disease. J Clin Endocrinol Metab 1999; 84:328–335.
8. Vitoria JC, Castano L, Rica I, Bilbao JR, Arrieta A, Garcia-Masdevall MD. Association of insulin-dependent diabetes mellitus and celiac disease: a study based on serologic markers. J Pediatr Gastroenterol Nutr 1998; 27:47–52.
9. Fernández-Castañer M, Molina A, López-Jiménez L, Gómez JM, Soler J. Clinical presentation and early course of type 1 diabetes in patients with and without thyroid autoimmunity. Diabetes Care 1999; 22:377–381.
10. Gottlieb PA, Eisenbarth GS. Mouse and man: multiple genes and multiple autoantigens in the aetiology of type I DM and related autoimmune disorders. J Autoimmun 1996; 9:277–281.
11. Pinhas-Hamiel O, Dolan LM, Daniels SR, Standiford D, Khoury PR, Zeitler P. Increased incidence of non-insulin dependent diabetes mellitus among adolescents. J Pediatr 1996; 128:608–615.
12. Rosenbloom AL, Joe JR, Young RS, Winter WE. Emerging epidemic of type 2 diabetes in youth. Diabetes Care 1999; 22:345–354.

13. Velho G, Froguel P. Genetic, metabolic and clinical characteristics of maturity onset diabetes of the young. Eur J Endocrinol 1998; 138:233–239.
14. Littorin B, Sundkvist G, Hagopian W, et al. Islet cell and glutamic acid decarboxylase antibodies present at diagnosis of diabetes predict the need for insulin treatment. Diabetes Care 1999; 22:409–412.
15. Leslie RD, Pozzilli P. Type I diabetes masquerading as type II diabetes. Possible implications for prevention and treatment. Diabetes Care 1994; 17:1214–1219.

3

Type 2 Diabetes: Where Have We Been, Where Are We, and Where Are We Going?*

Richard Eastman
National Institute of Diabetes and Digestive and Kidney Diseases, National Institutes of Health, Bethesda, Maryland

I. EPIDEMIOLOGY AND DEMOGRAPHICS

Diabetes is one of the most common chronic diseases. In the United States today, 5.9% of the population has diabetes, or about 15.7 million people, and about 800,000 new cases are diagnosed annually. Although most have type 2 diabetes, and are the focus of this chapter, type 1 diabetes is a very significant disease and is a major health issue for the population. Of those with diabetes, it is estimated that it has been diagnosed in 10.3 million persons, whereas it has yet be diagnosed in the remaining 5.4 million persons. Most patients in whom it is undiagnosed have type 2 diabetes. The diagnostic criteria have changed recently with diagnosis based on a fasting plasma glucose level. This should increase the proportion of those in whom diabetes is diagnosed.

Studies of the demographics of diabetes show that the disease increases with age; 18.4% (6.3 million) of those 65 years old or older, 8.2% (15.6 million) of those age 20 or older, and 0.16% (123,000) younger than 20 have diabetes. The number of males and females with diabetes is approximately equal. Minority populations carry an extra burden of diabetes, which begins earlier in life and is

---

* This contribution is an official contribution of the National Institutes of Health, and cannot be copywrited. This material does not represent an official policy of the National Institutes of Health or other agency of the U.S. Federal government.

associated with higher rates of complications; 7.8% of non-Hispanic whites (11.3 million), 10.8% of non-Hispanic blacks (2.3 million), and 10.6% (1.2 million) of Mexican Americans have diabetes. Other Hispanic–Latino groups are also about twice as likely to have diabetes as non-Hispanic whites. Diabetes is also much more common among American Indians, Alaskan Natives, Asian Americans, and Pacific Islanders.

Trends in diabetes in the population are ominous. Diabetes prevalence has increased steadily since monitoring began in 1953. This trend is likely to continue, as older Americans and minorities constitute a greater proportion of the population. Recent data suggest an increase in type 2 diabetes in youth.

Diabetes is a major risk factor for vascular disease. Heart disease and stroke are two to four times more common than in nondiabetics, and 60% of patients with diabetes have hypertension. Diabetes is the leading cause of blindness in adults age 20–74, with up to 24,000 new cases annually. It is also the leading cause of end-stage renal disease (40% of cases); 27,851 persons with diabetes developed kidney failure in 1995. In the same year, 98,872 persons with diabetes were receiving dialysis or received a kidney transplant. Neuropathy is another common complication of diabetes, and is a major risk factor for lower-extremity amputation; about 67,000 nontraumatic amputations are performed each year in the United States. Diabetes is also a major cause of periodontal disease, and of major congenital malformations. Hypoglycemia, ketoacidosis, and hyperosmolar coma are life-threatening, acute complications of diabetes, with significant morbidity and mortality.

The cost of diabetes is estimated to be $98.2 billion annually in the United States. This includes $54.1 billion annually in disability, work loss, and premature mortality, and the cost of treating diabetes and its complications. In addition, other studies suggest that the cost of caring for non–diabetes-related illnesses in persons with diabetes is twice as great as in nondiabetic patients. Thus, the health and economic burden of diabetes is staggering.

II. PATHOGENESIS AND NATURAL HISTORY

Many different causes of diabetes have been identified. Specific mutations in the insulin and insulin receptor gene, the glucokinase gene, in genes for hepatic nuclear factors (HNF-1_α and 4_α), and in mitochondrial DNA have been identified in patients with type 2 diabetes. Most recently, a mutation has been discovered in a transmembrane protein leading to diabetes and optic atrophy (Wolfram syndrome). These defects account for only a small proportion of the cases of diabetes, and the genes for the common form remain to be discovered. Insulin resistance is found in most, but not all, individuals with type 2 diabetes. It predates the development of diabetes, and is similar in magnitude to the insulin resistance seen in obese individuals without diabetes. Although insulin resistance is important in the pathogenesis of type 2 diabetes, it is not invariably present, and it is not the cause of diabetes per se. The defect is in insulin-mediated glucose disposal through nonoxidative pathways. Recent data show that activation of a nuclear transcription factor PPAR-γ in adipose tissue leads to reduced insulin resistance in muscle, probably through changes in lipid metabolism.

Decreased insulin secretion, usually coupled with preexisting insulin resistance, is a critical feature in the development of diabetes. Insulin secretion is initially able to compensate for insulin resistance, resulting in normal glucose tolerance. With development of impaired glucose tolerance (IGT), insulin levels after a glucose load may be higher than in a normal individual, but are clearly inadequate to overcome the degree of insulin resistance. Thus, relative deficiency in insulin secretion is an early feature in the natural history of the disease. Indeed, first-phase insulin secretion is abnormal in people with IGT. Abnormalities in the pulsatile secretion of insulin are also present early in the natural history.

The progression from IGT to diabetes is usually due to a further decline in insulin secretion, although absolute insulin levels may remain elevated relative to those without diabetes. The pathogenetic mechanisms underlying this loss of insulin secretion are largely unknown. Glucose toxicity may be an important factor, because beta cells are rapidly and reversibly desensitized to glucose-stimulated insulin secretion in the presence of high glucose concentrations. Degenerative changes, perhaps on a genetic basis, may play a role. Lipotoxicity is increasingly implicated in the loss of insulin secretion. In addition, in some populations, 10–15% of persons who have the phenotype of type 2 diabetes have evidence of islet-cell autoimmunity in the form of antibodies to islet cell autoantigens. Early requirement for insulin is a feature of this variant of type 2 diabetes.

Further deterioration in beta-cell function is characteristic of the natural history of diabetes. In addition, insulin resistance increases after development of diabetes, with glucose toxicity playing a major role. The deterioration in beta-cell function is reflected by the need to change treatment as the duration of diabetes increases. Early in the natural history, lifestyle change may be effective. As time goes on, more and more patients require oral antidiabetic agents, and many patients subsequently require insulin to maintain glycemic control. Increasingly complex and expensive regimens are needed to maintain glycemic control as the disease progresses, and treatment is often accompanied by weight gain.

Several factors can exacerbate diabetes, or even transiently cause diabetes. These include lack of exercise and weight gain, pregnancy, stress (particularly infections and operative stress), endocrinopathies, and many commonly used pharmaceutical agents (steroids, thiazide diuretics, calcium channel blockers, diphenylhydantoin, and others). Avoidance or correction of these risk factors can significantly improve the diabetic state, reducing the requirement for pharmacological treatment in many patients, and even eliminating the need for drug therapy in some.

III. PREVIOUS MAJOR CLINICAL TRIALS

Several landmark trials sponsored by the National Eye Institute were conducted in the 1970s and 1980s to determine the optimal treatment of diabetic retinopathy (Table 1). The Diabetic Retinopathy Study, Early Treatment of Diabetic Retinopathy Study, and the Diabetic Retinopathy Vitrectomy Study demonstrated tremendous benefits of early detection and appropriate treatment of sight-threatening retinopathy. Implementation of these treatments in the health care system can eliminate 95% of blindness caused by proliferative retinopathy and about half of the cases of blindness caused by macular edema. Macular edema is the predominant cause of vision loss in type 2 diabetes.

Success has also been shown in delaying renal failure in patients with established clinical nephropathy. Use of angiotensin-converting enzyme inhibitors (ACRI) in patients with proteinuria significantly reduces the risk of developing renal failure and death in patients with type 1 diabetes. In the United Kingdom Prospective Diabetes Study no difference was seen in the effects of beta-adrenergic blockers and ACEI in patients with type 2 diabetes, but the study may not have been powerful enough to see a difference in rates of renal disease.

Table 1 Major Diabetes Trials: Past, Present, and Future

Past trials
  Diabetic Retinopathy Study
  Early Treatment of Diabetic Retinopathy Study
  Diabetic Retinopathy Vitrectomy Study
  ACE Inhibitors in Diabetic Nephropathy Trial (Lewis Trial)
  Diabetes Control and Complications Trial
  United Kingdom Prospective Diabetes Study
Ongoing trials and future trials
  Diabetes Prevention Program—Primary Prevention of Type 2 Diabetes
  Canadian and European Trials of Diabetes Prevention
  Appropriate Blood Pressure Control in Diabetes Trial
  Veterans Affairs Cooperative Study on Glycemic Control and Complications in Type
    II Diabetes (VA CSDM)
  Prevention of Cardiovascular Disease in Diabetes Mellitus
  Study of Health Outcomes of Weight Loss (SHOW) Trial

Before 1993, there was a lack of consensus that hyperglycemia was the major cause of microvascular complications of diabetes, and that intentionally lowering glucose concentrations would reduce the risk of these complications. The Diabetes Control and Complications Trial (DCCT) clearly demonstrated that controlling blood glucose markedly reduces the risk of developing these complications, and the rate of progression of existing complications. Evidence from basic and clinical studies, observational studies, and a clinical trial in Japanese, led authorities to conclude that the benefits of glucose control are the same for all persons with diabetes, regardless of the underlying etiology of the disease.

A consensus developed over the ensuing 5 years after the DCCT, that maintaining good glucose control should be the goal of treatment for all persons with diabetes. In 1998 the National Institute of Health (NIH) and the Centers for Disease Control and Prevention (CDC) announced a National Diabetes Education Program (NDEP). The program is a collaborative effort between government agencies and the private sector, with over 100 organizations involved in its planning and implementation. The program will carry the message to patients, providers, and policy makers that glucose control can lead to very significant reductions in the risk of diabetes complications.

The evidence supporting the benefits of glycemic control greatly increased in 1998 with the announcement of the results of the United Kingdom Prospective Diabetes Study (UKPDS). The UKPDS began in 1974, and was designed to see if glycemic control reduces the risk of diabetes complications in persons with newly diagnosed type 2 diabetes. The median follow-up of patients was 10 years (range 6–20). Patients were randomly assigned to intensive or standard treatment. The trial showed that lowering glycemia from a glycosylated hemoglobin (HbA_{1c}) of 7.9% in the standard treatment group to 7.0% in the intensive group significantly reduces the risk of diabetes-specific complications, with the greatest reduction in microvascular complications. The reduction in risk was similar to that observed in the DCCT, with a reduction of about 35% in relative risk for a 10% lowering of HbA_{1c}.

Whether glycemic control reduces macrovascular disease is more controversial. The DCCT and the Japanese trial in type 2 diabetes showed a nonsignificant reduction in cardiovascular disease (CVD) in intensively treated patients. Observational studies, including the Framingham Study, Wisconsin Epidemiologic Study of Diabetic Retinopathy (WESDR), and the San Antonio Heart Study, showed significant associations between glycohemoglobin and CVD risk. Studies in other countries have shown similar findings. However, these studies show association only, not causation. The DIGAMI study showed a 34% reduction in 1-year mortality in patients treated intensively with insulin and glucose at the time of myocardial infarction (MI).

The UKPDS did not prove conclusively that controlling glucose reduces cardiovascular risk, but it was not designed to ascertain effects on single endpoints, such as myocardial infarction. In the main randomization of the trial, there was a trend in the risk of myocardial infarction (16% risk reduction in those under better glucose control), but diabetes-related death and all-cause mortality were not significantly affected. A substudy with metformin in obese subjects show a significant reduction in cardiovascular disease morbidity and mortality, and patients did not gain as much weight as those receiving insulin or sulfonylureas. These results are offset to some extent by an increase in diabetes-related death and all-cause mortality among patients receiving combination sulfonylurea and metformin treatment. Further study is needed on the benefits and risks of metformin therapy, particularly in combination with sulfonylureas.

The absence of an increased risk of vascular disease in patients receiving insulin and sulfonylurea in the UKPDS should help dispel concerns about cardiovascular toxicity of insulin and sulfonylureas. Long-term follow-up of the UKPDS cohort is planned, and future intention-to-treat analysis of the data has the potential to establish significant benefits of glycemic control on CVD morbidity and mortality. Given what we know today, it seems imperative that health care systems implement intensive treatment of type 2 diabetes.

IV. THE FUTURE

Research efforts in diabetes are evolving in many directions. On the basic science side, major initiatives are underway to find the molecular mechanisms underlying insulin resistance and beta-cell failure. Expressed sequence-tagged libraries of beta cells and other tissues of relevance to diabetes are an important first step, and full-length sequence libraries from these tissues are likely to emerge in the near future. These efforts include efforts to find the underlying genes for diabetes, and the genes that predispose individuals to diabetes complications. Consortia of investigators will probably be needed to answer these difficult questions by using standard methods and pooling results from different data sets. Identifying these genes is expected to lead to new diagnostic tools to identify individuals at risk for diabetes for early intervention. In addition, understanding the molecular pathogenesis of diabetes could lead to the development of novel therapeutic approaches, including different pharmacological agents and gene therapy approaches.

In the clinical arena, a large multicenter clinical trial is underway to see if diabetes can be delayed or prevented. The Diabetes Prevention Program (DPP) is recruiting high-risk individuals with impaired glucose tolerance, who are randomized to an intensive lifestyle program, or to a standard lifestyle intervention plus metformin or metformin placebo. Preventing diabetes has the potential to reduce diabetes-related morbidity and mortality by shortening or eliminating the lifetime exposure to hyperglycemia, hypertension, and dyslipidemia that characterize the disease. The DPP is specifically targeting recruitment of minorities into the program, so that the results will apply to the populations in the United States that are disproportionately affected by diabetes. To date, the DPP has recruited about 45% of the trial participants drawn from Hispanic–Latino, black, Asian, and Pacific Islander populations. The trial is scheduled to conclude and report results in 2002. Trials to prevent diabetes with disaccharidase inhibitors and sulfonylureas are underway in Canada and Europe.

Many clinical trials are addressing the efficacy of various approaches to treating dyslipidemia and hypertension. For example, the ABCD trial, for appropriate blood pressure control in diabetes, is examing intensive blood pressure control in patients with type 2 diabetes. Numerous studies are underway to examine treatment of dyslipidemia in diabetes.

What future trials are needed? Analyses of the data on ethnicity and diabetes indicate that poor glycemic control, blood pressure control, and smoking underlie the higher rates of complications in minority populations, although the increased risk is not explained in all populations by these factors. In general, health care access by minorities is not the problem, because it is similar in minority and nonminority populations. This suggests that the effectiveness of care is less in some populations. Studies are clearly needed to understand why care is less effective, and to develop more effective interventions. A Federal Government Initiative to Eliminate the Health Disparities in Minorities was announced by President Clinton, and had been incorporated into the long-range plans of the Department of Health and Human Services Agencies. This initiative has set the goal of eliminating the racial disparity in diabetes by the year 2010.

Future trials will also examine the efficacy of other therapeutic agents and approaches to preventing type 2 diabetes.

There is a great need for health care delivery and outcomes research. Trials need to be done to determine the optimum way of treating patients at various stages of the disease, and of the best way to deliver care so that all patients can benefit from scientific advances in the treatment of diabetes. Many questions are unanswered. Reducing the cost of diabetes is a priority, both for diabetes-related costs and non–diabetes-related health care costs, which are double those in the nondiabetic population.

The effect of glycemic control on macrovascular disease remains an important issue. The enthusiasm for eliminating hyperglycemia would likely be much greater if this treatment were proved to significantly reduce macrovascular disease risk. Physicians may be reluctant to implement complicated and costly treatment regimens in patients with vascular disease when the benefit is proved only for microvascular complications. One hopes that continued follow-up of the UKPDS cohort will answer the question definitively. In the interim, other clinical trials may be started to study the benefits and risks of glycemic control for macrovascular disease prevention.

Such trials will likely focus on very tight glycemic control, because data from observational studies suggest that even modest elevations in glucose, for example, as seen with IGT, increase CVD risk. Because the UKPDS was not highly powered to detect differences between therapeutic agents, there is continued interest in the question whether hyperinsulinemia or insulin resistance is important in the pathogenesis of vascular disease in diabetes. Thus, future trials may compare regimens that raise insulin levels (insulin, sulfonylureas) or maintain or reduce insulin levels (biguanides, disaccharidase inhibitors, thiazolidinediones).

As of this writing, several trials are under serious consideration or are planned. The Veteran's Administration is planning a full-scale trial of the effects of glycemic control on macrovascular outcomes in patients with type 2 diabetes. The National Heart, Lung, and Blood Institute is considering a trial of glycemic control on macrovascular outcomes in patients with type 2 diabetes who have evidence of existing cardiovascular disease. Comparison of agents that raise and lower insulin is planned. The National Institute of Diabetes, Digestive, and Kidney Diseases is also planning a trial of the effects of intentional weight loss on cardiovascular disease in patients with type 2 diabetes who have evidence of preexisting vascular disease. Thus, considerable information on the role of weight loss and glucose control in preventing cardiovascular disease will come to light in the next decade.

BIBLIOGRAPHY

Abraira C, Colwell JA, Nuttall FQ, et al. Veterans Affairs Cooperative Study on glycemic control and complications in type II diabetes (VA CSDM): results of the feasibility trial. Diabetes Care 1995; 18:1113–1123.

American Diabetes Association. Metabolic control matters—nationwide translation of the diabetes control and complications trial: analysis and recommendations. Clin Diabetes 1993; 11:91–96.

American Diabetes Association. Economic consequences of diabetes mellitus in the U.S. in 1997. Diabetes Care 1998; 21:296–309.

Andersson DKG, Svardsudd K. Long-term glycemic control relates to mortality in type II diabetes. Diabetes Care 1996; 18:1534–1543.

Early Treatment Diabetic Retinopathy Study Research Group. Phococoagulation for diabetic macular edema. Early Treatment Diabetic Retinopathy Study report number 1. Arch Ophthalmol 1985; 103:796–806.

Early Treatment Diabetic Retinopathy Study Research Group. Early photocoagulation for diabetic retinopathy: ETDRS report no. 9. Ophthalmology 1991; 98:765–785.

Klein R. Hyperglycemia and microvascular and macrovascular disease in diabetes. Diabetes Care 1995; 2:258–268.

Malmberg K on behalf of the DIGAMI Study Group. Randomized trial of insulin-glucose infusion followed by subcutaneous insulin treatment in diabetic patients with acute myocardial infarction (DIGAMI study): effects on mortality at 1 year. J Am Coll Cardiol 1995; 26:57–65.

National Diabetes Data Group, eds. Diabetes in America. 2nd ed. Bethesda, MD: National Institutes of Health, National Institute of Diabetes and Digestive and Kidney Diseases, 1995; 782 pp (NIH publ. 95-1468).

National Diabetes Education Program Home Page. HTTP://www.NIDDK.NIH.GOV/health/ndep

National Diabetes Information Clearinghouse. Diabetes Statistics. U.S. Department of Health and Human Services, Public Health Service, National Institutes of Health. NIH publication 96-3926, 1998. Updated statistics available at http://www.niddk.nih.gov American Diabetes Association.

Ohkubo Y, Kishikawa H, Araki E, et al. Intensive insulin therapy prevents the progression of diabetic microvascular complications in Japanese patients with non–insulin-dependent diabetes mellitus: a randomized prospective 6-year study. Diabetes Res Clin Prac 1995; 28:103–117.

The Diabetes Control and Complications Trial Research Group. The effect of intensive treatment of diabetes on the development and progression of long-term complications in insulin-dependent diabetes mellitus. N Engl J Med 1993; 329:977–986.

The Diabetic Retinopathy Study Research Group. Photocoagulation treatment of proliferative diabetic retinopathy. Clinical application of Diabetic Retinopathy Study (DRS) findings, DRS report no. 8. Ophthalmology 1981; 88:583–600.

The Diabetic Retinopathy Vitrectomy Study Research Group. Early vitrectomy for severe vitreous hemorrhage in diabetic retinopathy. Arch Ophthalmol 1985; 103:1644–1652.

United Kingdom Prospective Diabetes Study (UKPDS) Group. Glyccmic control final results. Lancet 1998; 352 (Sept 12); Blood pressure control final results. Br Med J 1998; 317 (Sept 12). For further information contact http://www.drl.ox.ac.uk

Villarosa IP, Bakris GL. The appropriate blood pressure control in diabetes (ABCD) trial. J Hum Hypertens 1998; 12:653–655.

Wei M, Gaskill SP, Haffner SM, Stern MP. Effects of diabetes and level of glycemia on all-cause and cardiovascular mortality. The San Antonio Heart Study. Diabetes Care 1998; 21:1167–1172.

4

Standards of Care in Diabetes

Nathaniel G. Clark
University of Vermont College of Medicine, Burlington, Vermont

I. INTRODUCTION

Because of the huge financial and health care burden of diabetes in the United States and worldwide, standards of care for persons with diabetes has become an extremely important topic. For several years the American Diabetes Association (ADA) has published *Clinical Practice Recommendations.* The issue of standards of care has grown increasingly important over the last number of years as a large body of government regulatory agencies and groups to promote quality health have adopted in large part the ADA's recommendations. Included at this time are the ADA, National Committee for Quality Assurance (NCQA), Health Care Financial Administration (HCFA), and Foundation for Accountability (FACCT). All these associations have come together in a collaborative mode and agreed on a single set of *measures* (not guidelines). The Diabetes Quality Improvement Project (DQIP) has delineated six measures (Table 1) that reflect key components of diabetes care. As stated by the DQIP committee "the DQIP measures are NOT guidelines for care and do not reflect either the minimal or maximal level of care that should be provided to the individual patient with diabetes. The measures are indicators or tools to assess the level of care provided within systems of care to populations of patients with diabetes." In several instances the DQIP "measures" differs from the "standards" described in this chapter. These measures will be used to evaluate health plans as part of the HEDIS (Health and Employer Data and Information Set) system. The measures are indicators or tools that assess the level of care provided within a system of care. In the future, individual physicians may be judged based on the extent to which their care conforms to established guidelines. The Provider Recognition Program which is cosponsored by the ADA and NCQA is a program whereby individual physicians or groups of physicians

Table 1   Synopsis of the DQIP Initial Measure Set[a]

Accountability set	Quality improvement set
1. Percentage of patients receiving ≥ 1 glycohemoglobin (HbA$_{1c}$) test per year	1. HbA$_{1c}$ levels of all patients reported in six categories (i.e.,
2. Percentage of patients with the highest risk HbA$_{1c}$ level (i.e., HbA$_{1c}$ > 9.5%)	< 7.0%, 7.0–7.9%, 8.0–8.89%, 9.0–9.9%, ≥ 10.0%, no value documented)
3. Percentage of patients assessed for nephropathy	
4. Percentage of patients receiving a lipid profile once in 2 years	
5. Percentage of patients with a low-density lipoprotein (LDL)[b] < 130 mg/dL	2. Distribution of LDL values[b] (i.e., < 100, 100–129, 130–159, > 159 mg/dL, no value documented)
6. Percentage of patients with blood pressure[b] < 140/90 mmHg	3. Distribution of blood pressure values[b] (i.e., < 140, 140–159, 160–179, 180–209, > 209 mmHg systolic; < 90, 90–99, 100–109, 110–119, > 119 mmHg, no value documented)
7. Percentage of patients receiving a dilated eye examination (see description for frequency)	
8. Foot examination	4. Proportion of patients receiving a well-documented foot examination to include a risk assessment

[a] Some of the measures have exclusions based on comorbidity or based on the results from a previous examination. All measures apply to persons between 18–75 years of age with diabetes, regardless of type of diabetes, and measures 1, 2, and 7 can be applied to children 10–17 years old as well. See following pages for details.

[b] For all measures requiring a value (e.g., LDL-C, blood pressure), the most recent test result will be used.

prospectively evaluate the care of their patients and submit this data to achieve this measure of national recognition.

A second significant issue relative to standards of care is that, despite the existence of the ADA standards and studies indicating that most providers are familiar with them, studies conducted in a variety of practice types (HMO, fee-for-service) have demonstrated that adherence is extremely poor. In the HMO setting Peters has documented that during a 1-year period only 44% of patients received at least one hemoglobin A$_{1c}$, 56% had a total cholesterol determination (only 31% with an low-density lipoprotein [LDL] level documented), 48% a urine protein measurement, and 6% a documented foot examination. In the fee-for-service setting patients were not receiving quality diabetes care either. The Provider Recognition Program gathered data from providers (primary care and endocrinologists) in all practice settings to set their standards for recognition. They chose for each measure the level at which 50% of the pilot sites had achieved their standard. For selected measures (for which the recommendation is one test per year), the results were:

Eye examination	40%
Urinary microalbumin determination	31%
Lipid profile	52%

Of note, there was no difference in the results when analyzed for practice type or training of the provider (endocrinologist vs. primary care). Clearly, we are not being successful in implementing the existing standards. There is a growing body of literature examining what the barriers are to successful implementation of standards of care in diabetes that include provider, health care system, and patient barriers. Defining the standards, however, is an important first step toward implementation.

This chapter will contain a summary of the current standards of care in diabetes as published by the ADA for 1999. A rationale is provided for each standard plus how it was developed and details on its implementation will be provided.

II. DIAGNOSIS OF DIABETES MELLITUS

In June of 1997 revised criteria for the diagnosis of diabetes were released. Diabetes mellitus is now diagnosed by one of three criteria:

1. Typical symptoms of diabetes with a casual (random) plasma glucose level higher than 200 mg/dL. *Casual* (or random) was defined as any time of day without consideration of the time of the last meal. Classic symptoms of diabetes include polyuria, polydipsia, and unexplained weight loss.
2. A fasting plasma glucose level of 126 mg/dL or higher. This criterion is the most significant change from prior criteria and was intended to be the major diagnostic criterion to eliminate confusion over the role of fasting plasma glucose versus an oral glucose tolerance test (OGTT). The level of 126 was chosen over the previous 140 to be consistent with the standard OGTT criteria. The decision was made to reduce the

level for fasting plasma glucose from 140 to 126 mg/dL, because, as a rule, patients without diabetes had fasting levels lower than 110 mg/dL.

3. A 2-h plasma glucose level higher than 200 during a 75-g oral glucose tolerance test. It was felt that the performance of a glucose tolerance test should rarely be necessary, as the diagnosis could most typically be made on the basis of either of the first two criteria.

One important aspect of the new diagnostic criteria was the inclusion of revised criteria for the diagnosis of "impaired glucose tolerance." It is believed that most patients who go on to develop type 2 diabetes mellitus, go through the stage of impaired glucose tolerance during which plasma glucose levels are significantly higher than they are in any person with fully normal glucose tolerance, but yet they are not high enough to make the diagnosis of diabetes. Criteria for impaired glucose tolerance were specified using either the fasting plasma glucose or the 2-h value from a 75-g oral glucose tolerance test. Using the fasting plasma glucose level, if the value was less than 110 mg/dL this was considered to be a *normal* fasting glucose level. If the level was 110–125 this would constitute *impaired fasting glucose.* If the fasting plasma glucose was 126 mg/dL or higher, this would support the diagnosis of diabetes. When using the 2-h postload glucose level from an OGTT, if the value was less than 140 mg/dL this was considered to be normal glucose tolerance. If the value was 140 mg/dL or higher, but less than 200, this constituted impaired glucose tolerance. If the value was 200 or higher, this supported the diagnosis of diabetes. Specific recommendations for screening for diabetes using these new criteria were also included.

It is hoped that the use of these new criteria will significantly lower the high percentage of patients who have diabetes, but are undiagnosed at this time (30–50% of affected persons). Also, there is clear evidence that patients with impaired glucose tolerance have increased risk for the complications of diabetes, and it behooves physicians to identify patients with abnormal glucose tolerance of any degree and aggressively treat using standard guidelines for atheriosclerotic cardiovascular disease (ASCVD) prevention. The current National Institutes of Health (NIH)-sponsored multicentered research trial, The Diabetes Prevention Program (DPP) is examining the effect of various interventions in patients with impaired glucose tolerance on decreasing the rate of their developing diabetes.

III. A GLYCEMIC CONTROL

To assist practitioners and patients in understanding what constitutes good blood glucose control, the following standards have been suggested (Table 2). The goal for the preprandial glucose is 80–120 mg/dL. Action is suggested if the level is

Table 2 Guidelines for Diabetes Care

Assessment	Frequency	Goal	Action required
Glycated hb			
HbA$_{1c}$	Every 6 mo if at or less than action-required level; every 3 mo if greater	≤ 7%	> 8%
Other	Yearly or more often as necessary	≤ 1% above upper limit of normal	> 2% above upper limit of normal
LDL-C			
CAD absent		< 100 mg/dL	> 130 mg/dL
CAD present		< 100 mg/dL	> 100 mg/dL
HDL-C	Yearly	> 35 mg/dL (males)	—
		> 45 mg/dL (females)	—
TG	Yearly or more often, as necessary	< 200 mg/dL	> 400 mg/dL
Urinary microalbuminuria	Yearly in all patients with diabetes except: those with type 1 within 5 yr of diagnosis, age < 10 y or overt proteinuria	< 30 mg/g creatinine	1. Consider ACE inhibitor 2. Maximize BP control 3. Maximize glycemic control
Dilated eye examination	Yearly dilated funduscopic examination in all patients with diabetes except those with type 1 within 5 yr of diagnosis or age < 10 yr		
Blood pressure	Minimum every 6 mo (or more often as necessary)	< 130/85[a]	1. Consider ACE inhibitor
Foot examinations	Minimum every 6 mo by provider or more often as necessary	1. Teach patient to do self-examination	
Smoking assessment	Yearly; if current smoker, counseling or referral for cessation	Strongly encourage patient to quit	1. Medications 2. Counseling

[a] Or age-appropriate standard in children (see text).

less than 80 or higher than 140 mg/dL. The goal for the bedtime glucose level is 100–140 mg/dL, with action suggested if it is less than 100 or higher than 160 mg/dL. The goal for HgA$_{1c}$ (see Table 2) is less than 7%, with action suggested if the value is higher than 8%. This standard is based on the assumption that the range for nondiabetic persons (in your assay) is up to 6%.

When translating these goals to individual patients, it is extremely important to remember that diabetes care must be individualized to the patient. The foregoing goals represent the ideal, which may not be optimal for every patient. When one looks, for example, at the stated goal for HgA$_{1c}$ being less than 7%, one must realize that in some patients, to achieve a HgA$_{1c}$ lower than 7% one may increase the risk of hypoglycemia to a nonacceptable level. The HgA$_{1C}$ (or glycosylated hemoglobin) level should be obtained on a regular basis. In most patients it should be obtained every 3 months unless there have been no changes in the treatment regimen, and the patient has an established record on the current treatment regimen of achieving and maintaining excellent blood glucose control. If the treatment regimen is stable and goals are being achieved, every 6 months is reasonable.

IV. LIPID LEVELS

Adult patients with diabetes should be tested annually for lipid disorders with a full lipid profile (see Table 2). Optimally, these should be determined on a fasting specimen, although some have argued that using a nonfasting specimen will increase compliance to the standard, and if a nonfasting specimen puts the patient within the target range then the patient could be spared having to make an extra visit in the fasting state for blood work.

The goals for lipid levels have traditionally divided patients into those with no known cardiovascular disease by history, and those who have a significant history in this area. In defining the goal for low-density lipoprotein (LDL) cholesterol, NCEP guidelines state that the goal should be less than 130 mg/dL in those without a history of cardiovascular disease and less than 100 mg/dL in those with such a history. Many leaders in this field, however, have argued that the patient with diabetes should be considered in the same category as a person without diabetes with a positive history of cardiovascular disease. Studies looking at the risk of cardiovascular events have found that the risk in a patient without diabetes and a positive history of prior cardiovascular disease is the same as a person with diabetes, but no known history. In the 1999 Clinical Practice Recommendations, 100 mg/dL became the LDL goal in all patients with diabetes. The goal for triglycerides (TG) is a level of less than 200 mg/dL. High-density lipoprotein (HDL) cholesterol should be higher than 35 mg/dL in men and 45 in women. A lipid profile should be performed on children older than 2 years of age after diagnosis and once glucose control is established. The goal in those with risk factors in addition to diabetes is an LDL lower than 110 mg/dL. Lipid profiles should be repeated every 5 years if goals are met, or yearly if not.

V. URINARY MICROALBUMINURIA

Patients should have their urine screened for albuminuria on a yearly basis starting at diagnosis, in those with type 2 diabetes, and after 5 years of diabetes in those with type 1 (see Table 2). A yearly urinalysis should be performed and if proteinuria is documented its extent should be quantitated. If the urinalysis is negative for protein an assessment for microalbuminuria should be performed. Multiple studies have documented that diabetic kidney disease is a progressive disorder that begins with microalbuminuria. The amount of protein in a given urine specimen can be highly variable based on time of day, recent strenuous activity, and presence of a urinary tract infection. Ideally, one might collect a 24-h urine specimen and analyze it for protein and creatinine. However, this technique has proved to be very cumbersome for patients and can decrease compliance significantly. Most laboratories can now analyze a spot (random) urine sample for microalbumin and creatinine and calculate the albumin/creatinine ratio as a measure of urinary protein excretion rate as if a 24-h urine sample had been collected. Laboratories differ slightly in terms of what they define as a normal level of albuminuria, but most standards have chosen either 20 or 30 mg of albumin per gram creatinine as the upper limit of normal. Instead of sending urine samples to the laboratory to be analyzed there are now some highly sensitive dipsticks that can detect microalbuminuria. These are generally used for screening, rather than as accurate measures of albumin excretion rate. However, it must be remembered that *traditional* dipsticks are of little value in screening for microalbuminuria, as a positive result indicates macroalbuminuria.

The importance of screening for microalbuminuria is not merely to document patients who may be developing future renal disease, but to identify who might benefit from intervention. When a patient is identified as having persistent microalbuminuria, it is strongly suggested that (a) the patient be considered for use of an angiotension-converting enzyme (ACE) inhibitor, (b) that blood pressure be carefully controlled, and (c) that glycemic control be maximized. Obviously, blood pressure and glycemic control are important even in the absence of microalbuminuria.

VI. RETINOPATHY SCREENING

Patients with type 1 diabetes should have an initial dilated eye examination beginning at age 10 and approximately 5 years after the onset of their diabetes and yearly thereafter (see Table 2). Patients with type 2 diabetes should be examined at the time of their diagnosis and then yearly thereafter. It is recommended that the eye examination be performed by an ophthalmologist or optometrist who is knowledgeable and experienced in diagnosing diabetic retinopathy and its treatment. Although it may be true that if the primary care provider is interested and skilled in performing dilated retinal examination the goal of the standard could be met, most standards require an examination by an eye professional. There is a growing body of literature that dilated 7-standard field fundoscopic photography maybe more sensitive at detecting retinopathy than the clinical examination alone. Future standards may evolve in this direction.

VII. BLOOD PRESSURE

The primary goal of therapy for blood pressure for adults should be to maintain a blood pressure lower than 130 systolic and 85 mmHg diastolic (see Table 2). In children, for those with isolated systolic hypertension higher than 180, a goal for blood pressure would be less than 160. Use of the age- and sex-specific 90th percentile is felt to be a reasonable upper limit. The recent UKPDS trial has supported the importance of blood pressure control in reducing complications.

VIII. FOOT EXAMINATIONS

Feet should be examined every 6 months by the health care provider and more often as necessary (see Table 2). Documentation of the foot examination is essential noting high-risk areas. Patients should be instructed to examine their feet daily. If foot lesions are detected as early as possible, the rates of serious sequelae, including amputation, will be decreased significantly.

IX. SMOKING

Smoking status should be documented at every visit and all means to allow the patient to quit smoking (counseling, hypnotism, medications) should be employed (see Table 2). Smoking is a major risk factor for many of the complications of diabetes.

X. FUTURE

Standards of care for patients with diabetes have been proposed by the ADA and have now been codified by multiple governmental groups. The challenge we face is how to implement these standards in caring for our patients. The use of flow sheets and a computerized database in clinical settings have proved to be very useful. A wider implementation may be useful, although flowsheets are limited as they are used only when the patient presents for care. A computerized database allows patient population data to be continually queried to identify patients who are not achieving treatment goals or not meeting established standards of care. Whatever patient care techniques are employed, standards must be met if our patients are to receive optimal care.

BIBLIOGRAPHY

American Diabetes Association (ADA). Standards of medical care for patients with diabetes mellitus. Diabetes Care 1999; 22:S32–S41.

ADA. Diabetic retinopathy. Diabetes Care 1999; 22:S70–S73.

ADA. Diabetic nephropathy. Diabetes Care 1999; 22:S66–S69.

ADA. Management of dyslipidemia in adults with diabetes. Diabetes Care 1999; S56–S59.

Bennett PH, Haffner S, Kasiske BL, et al. Screening and management of microalbuminuria in patients with diabetes mellitus: recommendations to the Scientific Advisory Board of the National Kidney Foundation From and Ad Hoc Committee of the Council on Diabetes Mellitus of the National Kidney Foundation. Am J Kidney Dis 1995; 25:107, 112.

Peters AL, et al. Diabetes Care 1996; 19:601–606.

The Expert Committee on the Diagnosis and Classification of Diabetes Mellitus. Report of the Expert Committee on the Diagnosis and Classification of Diabetes Mellitus. Diabetes Care 1998; 21:S5–S19.

5
Diabetes Self-Management Education and the Diabetes Team

Christine T. Tobin
Health Care Consultant, Atlanta, Georgia

Diabetes patient education has evolved to "diabetes self-management education and training" an integral component of diabetes care and treatment. The goal of diabetes self-management education is to enable the person with diabetes, through motivation to use knowledge and skills to become an active participant in their diabetes care and treatment. In fact, the clinical management of diabetes relies on the ability of a person with diabetes to make lifestyle changes to control his or her diabetes. Living well with diabetes requires a positive psychosocial adaptation to, and effective self-management skills of, the disease. Diabetes self-management education is associated with improved patient outcomes and reduces costs. The fundamental importance of diabetes skills and knowledge to care and treatment makes self-management education and training a cornerstone of diabetes management.

Diabetes self-management education is a series of planned-learning experiences, including a combination of teaching, counseling, and behavior modification, that influence the patient's knowledge, skills, health behaviors, and health outcomes. Diabetes self-management education is a complex process that consists of:

- Assessment of educational needs
- Planning the teaching–learning process
- Implementation of the educational plan
- Documentation of the process
- Evaluation based on outcome criteria

Diabetes self-management education is individualized for the patient, and occurs in a variety of settings, depending on the needs of the patient, the practice of the educator, and the local external environment. Inpatient, outpatient, home care, and telephonic settings are used effectively for both individual and group education. Education should always complement and enhance the treatment plan determined by the diabetes health care team.

Diabetes self-management education is most effectively and efficiently provided by a qualified diabetes educator as part of a diabetes team. Diabetes educators collaborate with the multidisciplinary team of health care professionals and integrate their knowledge and skills to provide a comprehensive educational experience. The makeup of the diabetes team will vary considerably, depending on the health care setting. The minimal number of health care providers on the team would typically be a physician, a registered nurse, and a registered dietitian. The team ideally includes the patient in decision making and goal setting. The patient who is an active participant on the team manages daily diabetes care and treatment most effectively. Adherence or compliance with prescribed diabetes care and treatment improves when the patient is included in the goal setting. A more comprehensive diabetes team could include a social worker, psychologist, exercise physiologist, pharmacist, physicians' assistant, podiatrist, or certified nurse practitioner. Qualified health care providers for the diabetes team are essential to the success of the diabetes self-management education and training. All diabetes educators should have sufficient educational background and expertise. American Diabetes Association (ADA) identifies *qualified personnel* as skilled and experienced health care professionals with recent education in diabetes, education principles, and behavior change strategies. Diabetes educators must have a thorough and current knowledge of basic principles of diabetes treatment and care. Education principles include a basic understanding of learning and teaching, communication, and counseling skills. Diabetes educators must have an understanding of various behavior modification techniques because of the patient's age, type of diabetes, psychosocial circumstances, and economic status.

A clearly defined team for diabetes self-management is the gold standard for all patients with diabetes. Clarification of the role of diabetes team and role of the members is necessary for effective utilization. The scope of practice for educators has changing dimensions because of the multidisciplinary nature of the health care professionals who provide education. To aid in understanding who is the diabetes educator, the following is a list of titles that may be present on a diabetes team:

> *Diabetes educator:* Any one involved with the education of patients including, but not limited to, the registered nurse, registered dietitian, physician, pharmacist, social worker, psychologist, exercise physiologist, and podiatrist.
>
> *Diabetes teaching nurse:* A nurse who spends most his or her time in diabetes education.

Diabetes nurse clinician: Provides care, management, and instructional services. The title implies specialized training, although it may be on-the-job-training. Most clinicians have at least an undergraduate degree.

Diabetes nurse specialist or diabetes clinical specialist: Advanced level of practitioner. These individuals have at least Master of Science degree in a specialized area of study. They have the training, expertise, and autonomy to provide most clinical management responsibilities, including patient and professional education.

Certified Diabetes Educator: Diabetes educators who pass a certification examination become a certified diabetes educator (CDE). CDE is then added after their name and degree. Certified diabetes educators must pass a certification examination every 5 years to maintain certification. CDE implies a minimal standard of knowledge, expertise, and skills in all aspects of diabetes education.

The primary responsibilities of the diabetes educator are the education of patients, their families, and appropriate support systems about diabetes self-management and related issues. The contents of this educational experience should include, but are not limited to, the following:

Diabetes mellitus overview
Stress and psychosocial adjustment
Family involvement and social support
Exercise and activity
Nutrition
Medications
Relation among nutrition, exercise, and activity, medication, and blood glucose levels
Self-monitoring for glycemic control and use of results
Prevention and management of acute complications
Prevention and management of chronic complications
Foot, skin, and dental care
Behavior change strategies, goal-setting, risk factor reduction, and problem-solving skills
Benefits, risks, and management options for improving glucose control
Preconception care, pregnancy, and gestational diabetes
Use of health care delivery systems and community support services

The goal of diabetes team management is to individualize care and treatment to maximize patient adherence to the recommended treatment, thereby, decreasing morbidity and mortality of diabetes to the patient. A coordinated team approach is necessary due to the multidisciplinary nature of the treatment. Team management is crucial to share information gained from individual patient assessments (e.g., medical, nursing, and nutrition). To obtain this goal the team uses diabetes self-management education coupled with these evidence based strategies:

Expert adjustment of medication
Reinforcement of learned behaviors
Effective behavior change strategies
Instruction in the use of self-monitoring of blood glucose (SMBG) data

The literature demonstrates that incorporation of these elements by the diabetes team are associated with reduced hospitalizations for diabetes-related problems, which reduce diabetes-related health care costs.

Under most circumstances the diabetes team works under the auspices and direction of the physician. This is necessary to meet standards of care and for reimbursement of services. Educators are "physician extenders" offering initial education and training, then follow-up teaching to support the patient in the home setting. The need for diabetes self-management is lifelong owing to the chronicity of the disease. Making an educator part of the team, or by referring patients to a diabetes educator can produce many results:

Individualized and comprehensive patient education and follow-up
Retention of knowledge and skills
Motivation, and support using problem solving
Continuity of care
Facilitation of communication within a multidisciplinary team by acting as
    coordinator of care
Information on sources of insurance and reimbursement, diabetes supplies,
    and community agencies for the patients.

Ultimately a diabetes educator can decrease the number of phone calls to the physician, office visits, emergency room visits, and hospital admissions. These results make the diabetes educator an integral part of the diabetes health care team. The benefits of a coordinated team approach to diabetes care and treatment has been well documented in the literature.

Many physicians do not have access to a diabetes team in their health care setting. Physicians can develop a team approach by collaborating with diabetes educators. Calling the American Association of Diabetes Educators (AADE) Hotline Number 1-800-TEAMUP4 will provide you with names and phone numbers of up to three diabetes educators in your local area for referrals. American Diabetes Association (ADA) number 1-800-676-4065 will provide the name and number of local diabetes education programs that meet The National Standards for Diabetes Self-Management Education and have received ADA recognition.

Regardless of practice setting or environment, providers should understand and incorporate basic diabetes self-management skills when instructing patients with diabetes in the office. Although a referral to a team or a diabetes educator is desirable, the basic education or ''survival skills'' may be taught by office staff in some health care environments. Survival skills are those minimum skills necessary for the person with diabetes to manage at home. The survival skills for the person with type 2 diabetes includes eating healthy, general diabetes information, medications, monitoring, hypo- or hyperglycemia, and use of the health care system. The specific instructions include:

1. Healthy eating: Explain the relation of food, insulin, activity, and blood glucose. Explain the type of food, the amount, and timing of the meal or snack.
2. General information: Explain the relation between food, exercise, activity, medication if any, and blood glucose levels.
3. Medications: Explain the action, dose, timing, and how to store prescribed medications. Describe likely side effects. Tell patient where to obtain medication.
4. Monitoring: Demonstrate how to perform accurate SMBG. Explain how to use the information. Tell patient who to call and when with the data.
5. Hyperglycemia and hypoglycemia: Differentiate the signs and symptoms of high or low blood glucose levels. Explain the action to take for each situation. Explain when to seek immediate medical help for an illness, hyperglycemia, or hypoglycemia.
6. Use of the health care system: Identify how to obtain supplies, who to call for professional advice, and who to call in an emergency.

For the person with type 1 diabetes, survival skills instruction in addition to the type 2 should include:

1. Medications: Explain insulin is necessary for life. Demonstrate the proper insulin dosage, correct injection technique, and how to handle and store the insulin and supplies. Explain the action of insulin and timing of the dose.
2. General facts: Explain the need for daily insulin injections and that treatment of diabetes will include insulin, meal planning, exercise and activity, and SMBG.
3. Nutrition: Explain the relation of food, insulin, activity, and blood glucose. Explain type of food, the amount, and the timing of a meal or snack to maximize blood glucose control.
4. Exercise: Explain the relation of activity, food, and insulin and how to prevent hypoglycemia from exercise.
5. Monitoring: Demonstrate accurate SMBG and urine ketone testing.

These constitute the bare minimum of skills and knowledge that must be taught to the person with diabetes. The complexity of the diabetes treatment regimen and the support they receive will influence the patients' ability to self-manage, making diabetes education and training an ongoing process.

There are a variety of printed materials that can be used to reinforce instruction or serve as reminders. Bear in mind that the average reading level for the American public is fifth grade, which makes much of the print material ineffective. When reviewing materials, there are a few tips to keep in mind. Printed material should be black print on white. A print size of 14 pt in lower-case letters, avoiding fancy typeface, is preferable. Graphics should be simple, line drawings that show shape and texture. Use a lot of white space to reduce eye distraction for poor readers and those with visual acuity problems. Also, you may not be aware that a patient is a nonreader, for this is usually a well-kept secret. Materials such as food models and labels, samples of diabetes products, audio and visual tapes can enhance learning.

The more senses you can relate to and incorporate, the more effective the learning of a skill. Health professionals have no difficulty using verbal or written messages. But, sometimes we forget to have the patient repeat a skill demonstration as we rush to the next patient. Allow adequate time for discussion, looking for understanding and how the patient is feeling. Increased anxiety is associated with a decrease retention of learning. When planning teaching, use the smallest amount of content possible for a given session. Limit content concepts to three to four items at one session. Make points vivid. Specific instructions, rather than general rules, are better retained by patients. Ask patients to demonstrate skills and provide feedback. Review repeatedly while instructing, then reward and encourage. There are several sources that can provide office staff with useful and current diabetes self-management education information these include the following:

The American Diabetes Association (ADA). National Standards for Diabetes Self-Management Programs and American Diabetes Association Review Criteria. Diabetes Care 1998; 2(suppl 1) which can be valuable in determining the level of patient training to be provided.

ADA. Medical Management of Type 1 Diabetes. 3rd ed. 1998.

ADA. Medical Management of type 2 Diabetes. 4th ed, 1998.

The American Association of Diabetes Educators (AADE). A Core Curriculum for Health Education. 3rd ed. 1998. This is an up-to-date-reference tool for diabetes education. This resource includes self-management guidelines, reflecting the latest diagnostics, meal planning, monitoring, education, and psychosocial issues. Call AADE at 1-800-338-3633, press 1, and enter document no. 9001 to request a product order form.

Clement S. Diabetes self-management education [technical review]. Diabetes Care 1995; 18(2).

Funnell, MM, Haas LB. National standards for diabetes self-management education programs [technical review]. Diabetes Care 1995; 18(1).

6
Insulin Resistance

William T. Cefalu
University of Vermont College of Medicine, Burlington, Vermont

I. INTRODUCTION

The very concept of "insulin resistance" originated with the availability of insulin therapy for treatment of diabetes well over 50 years ago. At that time, clinical observations suggested that there were two groups of diabetic patients who were roughly divided by their response to the glucose-lowering effects of exogenously administered insulin. These two groups generally corresponded to the present-day classifications of type 1 and type 2 diabetes. The term *insulin resistance* was then coined to describe diabetic patients who had a markedly elevated exogenous insulin demand (e.g., requiring more than 200 U of insulin a day), often in association with antibodies induced by the insulin preparations available at the time (e.g., bovine and porcine insulin). The term continued to evolve with the use of the radioimmunoassay for insulin in the 1960s, which distinguished type 1 diabetic patients, with an absolute insulin deficiency, from type 2 patients, who have relatively normal or elevated levels. It soon became apparent that there were many individuals with normal glucose levels, but relatively high insulin levels. Further research conducted in the 1970s and 1980s (with in vivo metabolic techniques that assessed glucose uptake during insulin infusions and with tissues from insulin-resistant patients studied ex vivo) demonstrated conclusively that insulin resistance was due to an impaired insulin action in peripheral tissues such as fat, muscle, and liver. These studies have led to the current-day definition of insulin resistance as a *clinical state in which a normal or elevated insulin level produces an impaired biological response.*

Insulin is a growth factor and elicits a myriad of biological responses. In theory, the biological response measured could be a metabolic process (changes in carbohydrate, lipid, or protein metabolism) or a mitogenic process (alterations

57

in growth, differentiation, DNA synthesis, or regulation of gene transcription). Although insulin resistance could apply to any of these pleiotrophic effects of insulin, the term is classically applied to insulin's ability to stimulate glucose uptake because this is the biological response most directly relevant to the clinical manifestations (e.g., hyperinsulinemia and impaired glucose tolerance). However, insulin resistance, although generally referring to the glucose–insulin relation, should not be confused with the concept of the "insulin resistance syndrome," which applies to additional biological actions of insulin, including its effects on lipid and protein metabolism, endothelial function, and gene expression. Indeed, the insulin resistance syndrome consists of a cluster of disorders and biochemical abnormalities, and this particular syndrome has been given the name "syndrome X," or "the deadly quartet." The associated clinical and laboratory abnormalities that represent this syndrome consist of type 2 diabetes mellitus, central obesity, dyslipidemia (increased triglycerides, decreased HDL, and increased small dense LDL), hypertension, increased prothrombotic and antifibrinolytic factors (i.e., hypercoagulability), and a predisposition for heart disease (Fig. 1). Furthermore, there are several other conditions associated with insulin resistance that refer to specific clinical presentations, such as the polycystic ovarian syndrome, pregnancy, or glucocorticoid therapy, that may include some or none of the features of the insulin resistance syndrome or so-called syndrome X.

II. INSULIN RESISTANCE IN THE NATURAL HISTORY OF TYPE 2 DIABETES

Insulin resistance is an integral part of the natural history of type 2 diabetes and has been observed to be present many years before development of the disease. Studies in families and populations that have a high incidence of type 2 diabetes have shown that reduced insulin-dependent glucose transport is frequently found in nondiabetic relatives and offspring of patients with type 2 diabetes mellitus. The presence of this abnormality in these subjects suggests that insulin resistance may be a primary factor in the development of type 2 diabetes and the early development of accelerated atherosclerosis. As recently reviewed from the Consensus Development Conference on Insulin Resistance (1998), it is well established that plasma insulin levels, whether measured fasting or postprandially, are a predictor for the risk of developing type 2 diabetes, and this risk appears independent of obesity or waist circumference. In addition, this risk is particularly strong for individuals with a known family history of type 2 diabetes.

Current concepts in the development of type 2 diabetes indicate that glucose and fasting insulin levels may be normal for many years before the development of the disease. In the presence of obesity and a family history of diabetes, insulin resistance typically is present. The individual will increase insulin secretion, par-

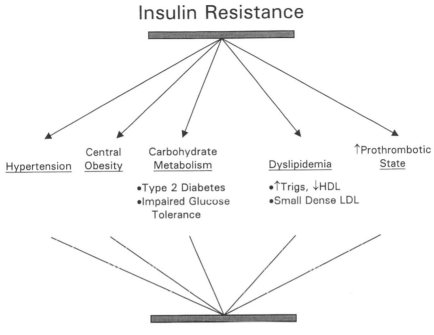

Fig. 1 Schematic demonstrating conditions associated with the insulin resistance syndrome.

ticularly after meals, to compensate for the insulin resistance. In this way, glucose levels remain normal. As long as the individual continues with this compensatory hyperinsulinemia as necessary to overcome the resistance, normal glucose levels are maintained. However, as beta cell dysfunction becomes manifest, leading to a "relative" decrease in insulin, the individual is unable to compensate for the insulin resistance, and fasting blood sugars begin to rise, such that the clinician now makes the diagnosis of type 2 diabetes mellitus. This period in the patient's life associated with insulin resistance and impaired glucose tolerance is felt to represent the prediabetic phase. Indeed, it is at this stage in the natural history of type 2 diabetes that prevention trials are currently addressing the need to reduce the insulin resistance, by both pharmacological and nonpharmacological means, in the hope that type 2 diabetes can be prevented or delayed. It is also at this stage in the natural history of type 2 diabetes when the clustering of risk factors or the so-called cardiovascular dysmetabolic syndrome, (e.g., deadly quartet) is

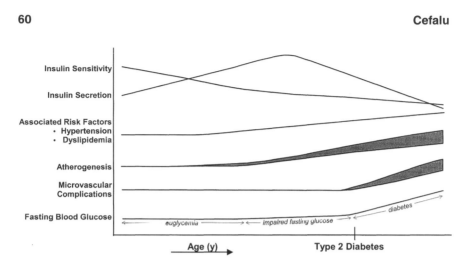

Fig. 2   Proposed metabolic observations in the natural history of type 2 diabetes.

observed. Therefore, we now recognize that insulin resistance occurs many years before the diagnosis of type 2 diabetes is made and is associated with a clustering of risk factors that predisposes a patient to accelerated atherosclerosis. A schematic representing insulin resistance and compensatory hyperinsulinemia, associated risk factors, and when a diagnosis of type 2 diabetes is likely to be made is outlined in Fig. 2 (as adapted from the results of the Paris Prospective Study).

III.   CELLULAR EVENTS OF INSULIN ACTION

Understanding the cellular mechanism of insulin resistance would be important in identifying its genetic basis and would allow both the development of effective therapies and optimal use of current therapies. As stated, the aspect of insulin resistance that has been the most well described is the inefficient glucose uptake and utilization in insulin-stimulated conditions. In in vivo conditions, this is represented by a reduction in the insulin-stimulated storage of glucose as glycogen in both muscle and liver. It has been described that the primary mechanism in muscle appears to be a block in the glucose transport and phosphorylation step, and both genetic and environmental factors appear to induce this defect. To have an understanding of the potential cellular abnormalities that predispose an individual to insulin resistance, a brief overview of the cellular factors regulating insulin action will be presented.

Insulin action in peripheral tissues begins with specific binding of insulin to high-affinity receptors on the plasma membrane of the target tissues (Fig. 3). The insulin receptor is a large transmembrane protein consisting of two α- and β-subunits. Insulin initiates its cellular effects by binding to the α-subunit of its receptor (the structure of which establishes the specificity for insulin binding), and this binding leads to the autophosphorylation of specific tyrosine residues of the β-subunit. The β-subunit possesses tyrosine kinase activity, and this process enhances the tyrosine kinase activity of the receptor toward other protein substrates. Considerable evidence demonstrates that activation of insulin receptor kinase, one of the earliest postbinding events in insulin action yet recognized, plays an essential role for many, if not all, of the biological effects of insulin. Furthermore, insulin receptor tyrosine kinase plays a major role in signal transduction distal to the receptor, as the primary event leads to subsequent phosphorylation of cytoplasmic proteins, called insulin receptor substrate proteins (IRS-1 and IRS-2). The IRS proteins are cytoplasmic proteins, with multiple tyrosine

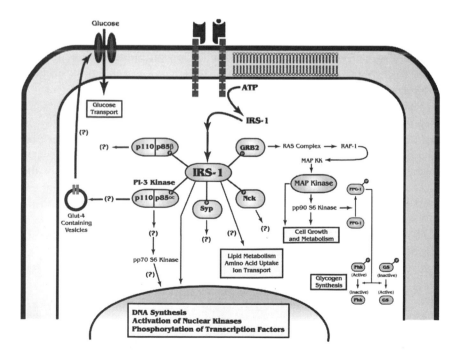

Fig. 3 Schematic demonstrating proposed intracellular events for insulin action.

phosphorylation sites, and phosphorylation of the IRS proteins has been implicated as the first postreceptor step in insulin signal transmission. Following insulin stimulation, these sites serve as "docking sites" for cytosolic substrates that contain specific recognition domains, termed SH2 domains. These structural domains on the IRS proteins provide an extensive potential for interaction with downstream-signaling molecules by the multiple phosphorylation motifs, including $p85\alpha/\beta$, $p55^{PIK}$, GRB-2, SHP-2, and nck. As described, the divergence of insulin-signaling pathways within the cell may reside at the level of the IRS-docking proteins and, therefore, the IRS proteins have been referred to as the *metabolic switch* of the cell.

The explanation provided for insulin's effect on glucose uptake is less well defined, but involves the enzyme phosphatidylinositide-3 kinase (Pl-3 kinase). Insulin stimulation increases the amount of Pl-3 kinase associated with IRS, and its activity is directly activated by docking. Activation of the Pl-3 kinase appears to be critical for transducing the metabolic effects of insulin, as inhibition of Pl-3 kinase activation blocks insulin's ability to stimulate glucose transport. However, other growth factor receptors activate Pl-3 kinase to the same extent as the insulin receptor, but they do not stimulate glucose transport. Therefore, it appears that although Pl-3 kinase is necessary for the action of insulin, it is not sufficient, in and of itself, to account for the glucose uptake process. The additional factors that are responsible for the stimulation of glucose transport are still unknown. In summary, current evidence suggests that IRS proteins, in their phosphorylated form, may regulate insulin signaling by acting as a docking site by binding to and regulating intracellular enzymes containing SH2 domains that allow the insulin signal to "diverge" throughout the target cell.

After the generation of the second messengers for insulin action, glucose transport into the cell is activated. This effect of insulin is brought about by the translocation of a large pool of glucose transporters from an intracellular pool to the plasma membrane. Glucose transporters reside almost exclusively in the intracellular membrane pool and, in response to insulin, translocate from this pool to the plasma membrane where they become the predominant glucose transporters. There are several isoforms of glucose transporters, depending on the tissue studied; the major insulin responsive glucose transporter isoform is termed GLUT-4 and is predominantly expressed in insulin target tissues, such as skeletal and cardiac muscle and adipose tissue.

A. Mechanisms for Impaired Insulin Action

With the foregoing overview of normal insulin action, one can now appreciate that defects in any one of the multiple steps of the insulin-signaling cascade can induce an insulin-resistant state. Alterations in insulin production, insulin binding, or intracellular signaling, all have the potential to induce an insulin-resistant state.

For example, a mutation in the gene coding for the insulin molecule can give rise to an abnormal beta-cell product, which is associated with a decreased biological effect. These clinical conditions have been referred to as *mutant insulin syndromes,* whereby single amino acid substitutions in regions of the molecule that interact with the insulin receptor with reduced affinity ultimately result in an impaired biological action. An example of an acquired defect associated with insulin resistance is anti-insulin antibodies. In this state, antibodies directed against the insulin molecule can complex with insulin and reduce the amount available to target insulin receptors. Fortunately, high titers of insulin antibodies are now rare owing to the common use of recombinant human insulin. Such examples as just cited are referred to as *prereceptor* causes of insulin resistance, for these defects occur before or at the binding of insulin to the receptor. The insulin resistance most commonly observed clinically is referred to as a *postreceptor* defect because insulin signaling or effective glucose transport after insulin binding (e.g., intracellular events) is attenuated.

Insulin resistance may be secondary to overproduction of counterregulatory hormones, such as cortisol, epinephrine, and growth hormone. As such, clinical conditions of acromegaly, Cushing's syndrome, and pheochromocytoma are associated with attenuated insulin action and may present with hyperglycemia. There have been described various other human diseases and conditions characterized by insulin resistance and, as recently reviewed by Hunter and Garvey (1998), these are listed in Table 1.

As understood from a clinical perspective, the aspect of insulin resistance most studied is the defective insulin-mediated glucose uptake and utilization. In patients, this defect is manifest by a reduction in glycogen synthesis in muscle and liver. With the observation that the rate-limiting role in cellular glucose metabolism is the plasma membrane transport, GLUT-4 defects have the potential to readily result in insulin resistance at the level of the glucose transport effector system. A decrease in gene expression (i.e., protein content), diminished functional capacity, or impaired translocation of GLUT-4 to the plasma membrane are defects that may explain the diminished transport. However, this defect in glucose transport cannot be explained by a reduction in the total number of glucose transporter units, and studies have not defined whether the intrinsic activity of the glucose transporter is impaired, or whether there is a defect in translocation.

Whether defects in intracellular signaling are the cause for the resistance has been argued to be very likely, but a specific defect in any one signaling pathway to explain insulin resistance has not been observed. It has been described that a critical threshold level of IRS activity is necessary to maximally stimulate Pl-3 kinase, and that IRS proteins play a major role in insulin-stimulated glucose uptake. But precise and specific intracellular defects to account for most cases of insulin resistance are not yet described. It is highly likely, however, that the molecular basis of insulin resistance is polygenic, and the relative contribution

Table 1 Human Diseases and Conditions Characterized by Insulin Resistance

Insulin resistance may be primary	Insulin resistance may be secondary	Insulin resistance associated with genetic syndromes
Type 2 diabetes mellitus	Obesity	Progeroid syndromes (e.g.
Insulin resistance syndrome	Type 1 diabetes	Werner's syndrome)
(syndrome X)	mellitus	Cytogenetic disorders (Down,
Gestational diabetes	Type B severe insulin	Turner, and Klinefelter)
mellitus	resistance	Ataxia telangiectasia
Type A severe insulin	Hyperlipidemias	Muscular dystrophies
resistance	Pregnancy	Friedreich's ataxia
Lipoatrophic diabetes	Acute illness and	Alstrom syndrome
Leprechaunism	stress	Laurence-Moon-Biedl
Rabson-Mendenhall	Cushing's disease and	syndrome
syndrome	syndrome	Pseudo-Refsum syndrome
Hypertension	Pheochromocytoma	Other rare hereditary
Atherosclerotic	Acromegaly	neuromuscular disorders
cardiovascular disease	Hyperthyroidism	
	Liver cirrhosis	
	Renal failure	

Source: Hunter and Garvey, 1998.

of any one signaling defect varies greatly among individuals. It is further suggested that the additive effects of several mild alterations of signal transduction is needed to induce insulin resistance.

The studies, as outlined in the foregoing, have provided valuable information on the proposed mechanism by which insulin exerts its effect. Yet the understanding of specific defects of in vivo signaling processes that contribute to insulin resistance in humans is currently unknown, and this remains an area of very active human investigation.

IV. CLINICAL CONDITIONS ASSOCIATED WITH INSULIN RESISTANCE

The "cardiovascular dysmetabolic syndrome," or "syndrome X," encompasses various clinical and biochemical abnormalities that are associated with insulin resistance. Frequently, cause and effect is difficult to establish. The relation of insulin resistance to each condition is described.

A. Obesity

Most clinicians will recognize that obesity is associated with chronic diseases such as type 2 diabetes, coronary heart disease, and dyslipidemia. Yet the mechanisms underlying these clinical observations are poorly understood. Recent studies have suggested that insulin resistance may play a major role in the pathophysiology of these observed metabolic abnormalities and their associated morbidity. These observations are supported by the fact that insulin resistance is frequently observed in obese subjects and is known as an independent risk factor for the development of both type 2 diabetes and coronary artery disease. Although it is established that insulin resistance and other obesity-related metabolic abnormalities are associated with overall accumulation of fat in the body, there is now substantial evidence that the distribution of fat may have an additional role. This is supported by evidence that excessive accumulation of fat in the upper body's so-called truncal region, or central obesity, is a better predictor of morbidity than excess of fat in the lower body, the so-called lower body segment obesity. These types of body composition have been clinically separated based on a waist-to-hip circumference ratio, and individuals are referred to as having "apple"- or "pear"-shaped bodies. The study of this type of body composition is not new, as over 40 years ago Vague (1947) noted that the incidence of metabolic complications among equally obese subjects varied depending on their physique. Morbidity was shown to be higher in "android-type" obesity than in "gynoid-type" obesity. This heterogeneity is supported by several recent findings on the metabolic characteristics of adipose tissue, for fat tissue isolated from subcutaneous abdominal regions has a higher metabolic activity than that isolated from lower body subcutaneous regions. This heterogeneity of fat distribution has led investigators to accept the concept of morbid regional adiposity (i.e., that accumulation of fat in certain adipose tissue regions appears to be more deleterious than accumulation of fat in other adipose tissue regions). The hypothesis that has been put forward is that mesenteric adipose tissues constitute the morbid areas of the body and accumulation of fat in these regions has major implications for metabolism and, particularly, for insulin sensitivity.

If fat distribution, particularly in the central area, is vitally important, a precise measure of these fat depots would be necessary. Sonography has been used for the evaluation of intra-abdominal tissue; however, comparisons of ultrasounds with computed tomography (CT) scans have shown poor correlation between the two methods. In addition, the accuracy and precision of ultrasound for this use has not been determined. However, both CT and magnetic resonance imaging (MRI) allow direct visualization of internal adipose tissue compartments, and both MRI and CT scans have been tested and validated in human subjects for assessment of intra-abdominal fat stores. Studies that have used MRI have demonstrated a very significant relation of intra-abdominal fat to the development of insulin resistance. In particular, when evaluating the insulin resistance of aging, which appears to be associated with changes in body composition, insulin resistance related more to the visceral fat depot than to the subcutaneous fat depot. However, studies that have used the hyperinsulinemic euglycemic clamp technique to measure insulin sensitivity in men reported that the visceral fat depot did not play a major role, and that subcutaneous abdominal fat had the strongest relation with peripheral insulin sensitivity, independently of the effects of generalized adiposity. Thus, although it is well established that obesity, in particular central obesity, appears to be the more morbid condition, and this condition is associated with insulin resistance, it is not conclusively established whether it is the visceral (i.e., intra-abdominal) or subcutaneous abdominal adipose tissue that accounts for most of the variability in insulin resistance.

B. Lipid Abnormalities

The increased risk for cardiovascular disease, as observed with insulin-resistant states, may be explained partly by unfavorable changes in lipoproteins. Specifically, the major quantitative change associated with the insulin resistance syndrome is an elevation in triglyceride-rich lipoproteins, often accompanied by a decreased HDL cholesterol level. This observed abnormality in the natural history of type 2 diabetes may be present many years before glucose abnormalities are detected. Although the levels of LDL cholesterol are similar to those seen in the general population, LDL compositional differences may make these particles more atherogenic. Specifically, hyperinsulinemia predicts the development of both quantitative changes (e.g., increase triglycerides, high apo-B, low apo-A_1 levels) in the lipoproteins and also qualitative changes (e.g., low LDL cholesterol–apo B and low HDL cholesterol–low apo A_1). It is further established that insulin levels appear not to be associated with the absolute concentration of the LDL cholesterol, but are associated with the relative decrease in the small, dense LDL particles termed LDL subclass pattern B. Insulin resistance has also been associated with this preponderance of small dense LDL particles. It is the presence of small, dense LDL particle that has been suggested to be the more atherogenic LDL. These abnormalities in the LDL may indeed be reversed by specific insulin sensitizers, such as troglitazone. Although the ratio of LDL to HDL cholesterol may not change with treatment with insulin sensitizers, the qualitative properties of LDL may change with their use: large, (buoyant) LDL is increased and small, dense LDL is decreased. Whether the compositional change in LDL is indeed secondary to improvement in insulin resistance or secondary to other characteristics of insulin sensitizers (e.g., antioxidant effect) is an area of great debate because there appeared to be no relation between the effect of troglitazone on lipoproteins and the effect on insulin sensitivity.

C. Endothelial Function

The vascular endothelium modulates the underlying blood vessel tone by producing various vasoconstrictors and vasodilators. Agents that preferentially dilate the vascular wall include nitric oxide (NO), prostacyclin, bradykinin, and endothelium-derived hyperpolarization factor. Agents that constrict blood vessel tone include endothelin, superoxide anion, endothelium-derived constricting factor, locally produced angiotensin II, and thromboxane. These agents have been described to not only control and regulate arterial tone, but also to affect other parameters that may contribute to atherosclerosis, such as platelet adhesion, aggregation, and thrombogenicity of the blood. Therefore, if damage to the endothelium results in more production of vasoconstrictors and less of the latter, particularly NO, circulating platelets may aggregate in these particular areas, releasing cytokines and growth factors and may initiate the inflammatory reaction. After the initial inflammatory reaction, LDL cholesterol is taken up into the vessel wall by a direct mechanism, or possibly in the form of foam cells (lipid-laden macrophages), resulting in the formation of a fatty streak. Ultimately, vascular smooth-muscle cells migrate into the intima, proliferate, and increase their production of extracellular matrix proteins, resulting in the formation of organized atherosclerotic plaque. Therefore, from the foregoing discussion, one can appreciate that the endothelium has great potential to participate in cell proliferation contributing to the development and progression of atherosclerosis.

Insulin resistance and hyperinsulinemia, in addition to other components of the cardiovascular dysmetabolic syndrome, enhance many of the alterations in the vessel wall that contribute to atherosclerosis. As such, hyperlipidemia, hyperglycemia, hypertension, smoking, and homocysteine have been reported to damage the endothelium, which now leads to an imbalance in the endothelial production of the vasoconstrictors versus the vasodilators. With such an association, studies have evaluated pharmacological and nonpharmacological regimens in treatment of the endothelial dysfunction. In particular, a study evaluated the role of an insulin sensitizer in patients who were felt to be impaired glucose tolerant and insulin resistant, and who had attenuated brachial artery vasoactivity. After 2 months of therapy with an insulin sensitizer, vasoactivity improved and appeared to normalize after 4 months. Although this demonstrates that pharmacological treatment of insulin resistance may have favorable effects on endothelial dysfunction, this should not imply that insulin resistance is the sole factor in the development of such dysfunction. Lipids, glucose, hypertension, and smoking, all damage the endothelium, and in studies that have treated these particular components, there have been favorable effects on endothelial dysfunction.

D. Atherosclerosis

Although it is still unclear whether insulin itself is a pathogenic factor in the development of atherosclerosis, it is clear from epidemiological studies that insulin levels are associated with coronary artery disease. There have been several large-scale prospective trials that have shown that insulin levels correlate with coronary artery disease in multivariate analyses (see Welborn and Wearne, 1979; Pyörälä, 1979; Ducimetiere et al., 1980.) A prospective study of men in Quebec found that fasting insulin levels were indeed associated with ischemic heart disease, after adjustment for coexisting factors, such as hypertension, medications, family history, and lipid levels. In the Multiple Risk Factor Intervention Trial (MR-FIT), fasting insulin levels were a risk factor for coronary artery disease only in men with a certain lipid phenotype (apolipoprotein E3/2 phenotype). However, in the Caerphilly Prospective Study, the effect of insulin levels on heart disease event rates appeared to be present only in the setting of hypertriglyceridemia. Therefore, the possibility exists that hyperinsulinemia is a risk factor only in certain ethnic groups or in patients with certain risk factor abnormalities. Another explanation is that it may simply be a marker for insulin resistance.

Despite the conflicting data with insulin levels, insulin resistance appears to be a better correlate with coronary artery disease. Although it is argued that the number of patients studied to date with direct measurement of insulin action is small, many of these studies have shown a relation of insulin resistance to specific measures of atherosclerosis, such as arterial lesion size. In particular, the Insulin Resistance and Atherosclerosis Study (IRAS) measured insulin resistance in three groups of patients: Hispanics, non-Hispanic whites, and African Americans. Insulin resistance correlated with carotid intimal medial wall thickness in non-Hispanic whites after adjustment for factors such as smoking, lipids, hypertension, medications, and gender. This suggested that insulin resistance had an independent effect on the development of atherosclerosis. In African Americans, however, there appeared to be no detectable relation between insulin resistance and the carotid intimal wall thickness. Another report from the same group of investigators demonstrated an association between insulin resistance and definite coronary artery disease, even after adjusting for demographics, hypertension, smoking, and dyslipidemia.

Importantly, from the effects of the IRAS, over 50% of the subjects in the study were women, therefore, providing substantial evidence that insulin resistance and coronary artery disease are indeed related in women. Most of these women reported were postmenopausal. Taken together, the observations, as outlined in the foregoing, indicate that a more precise measure of insulin action is critical for investigating and defining the relation between insulin resistance and coronary artery disease.

E.   Hypertension

The relation between hypertension and insulin resistance has been well observed, but correlation between blood pressure and plasma insulin levels is inconsistent and relatively weak. Some of the evidence that would argue against the direct relation of insulin to hypertension is the observation that administered exogenous insulin has a direct vasodilatory and not a vasoconstricting effect. In addition, blood pressure has not been elevated in patients with insulinoma, a tumor of the pancreas producing elevated levels of insulin. Moreover, in type 1 patients who are receiving insulin therapy and have yet to develop nephropathy, blood pressure is not consistently elevated. Finally, studies suggest that the relation appears weak in those individuals who are insulin resistant without a family history of hypertension.

In summary, although insulin resistance and hypertension appear to be very much associated, a direct effect of insulin on mediating defects of hypertension has not been consistently observed.

F. Prothrombotic Activity

The accelerated atherosclerosis observed with type 2 diabetes cannot be fully explained; conventional risk factors, such as smoking, obesity, blood pressure, and serum lipids, fail to fully explain this risk. Additional mechanisms, such as a hypercoagulable state, are postulated to contribute, as disturbance of the fibrinolytic system favors the development of vascular damage and the final occlusion event in the progress of coronary heart disease.

The fibrinolytic system limits thrombosis and is responsible for dissolution of thrombi after vascular repair has occurred, and a balance exists between plasminogen activators and inhibitors. As such, diminished fibrinolysis secondary to elevated concentrations of plasminogen activator inhibitors may help explain the exaggeration and persistence of thrombosis observed in acute events. Impaired fibrinolysis can be caused by either a diminished release of tissue plasminogen activator (t-PA) or increased levels of plasminogen activator inhibitor (PAI)-1 (Fig. 4). PAI-1, a major regulator of the fibrinolytic system, is a serine protease inhibitor and binds to and inhibits t-PA and urokinase plasminogen activator (u-PA). Sources of PAI-1 include hepatocytes, endothelial cells, adipocytes, and smooth-muscle cells. PAI-1 is present in the alpha-granules of platelets.

Defective fibrinolysis, caused by elevated PAI-1 activity or reduced t-PA, not only predisposes individuals to thrombotic events, but it also plays a role in the development and progression of atherosclerosis. Increased production of PAI-1 has been demonstrated in components of the atherosclerotic plaque. This vessel wall PAI-1 appears to modulate vessel wall proteolysis. Decreased vessel wall proteolysis may predispose to accumulation of extracellular matrix. Moreover, cell migration is dependent on cell surface expression of u-PA. Thus, overexpression of PAI-1 in the vessel wall may limit migration of smooth-muscle cells and limit their migration into the neointima. This limitation of migration may

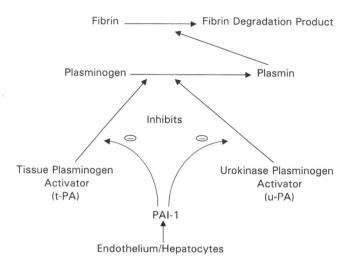

Fig. 4   The fibrinolytic system and the proposed role of PAI-1 in this process.

predispose to the development of a thin cap overlying the lipid core, a feature associated with increased risk of plaque rupture.

It seems well established that PAI-1 levels are elevated in patients with insulin resistance. It has been observed clinically in cross-sectional studies that the fibrinolytic parameters (PAI-1 and t-PA antigen) are strongly associated with insulin, insulin resistance, triglycerides, HDL, body mass index, waist/hip ratio, and blood pressure. The link between insulin resistance and PAI-1 or t-PA antigen levels that has been observed cross sectionally has also been confirmed in intervention studies aimed at reducing insulin resistance. The improvement in insulin resistance occurs in parallel with improvement of the metabolic abnormalities in the concentration of the parameters. Among those patients who manifest insulin resistance and parameters related to the syndrome (i.e., excess body weight, increased waist/hip ratio, hypertension, and elevated lipids), treatment of these conditions is associated with a decrease in PAI-1 and improvement of the fibrinolytic activity in most of these studies.

V. HOW DOES ONE MEASURE INSULIN RESISTANCE?

A variety of procedures have been developed to detect the presence of clinical insulin resistance. The most-studied and specific measure is a technique called the *euglycemic hyperinsulinemic clamp*. A second, less invasive, method is the *frequently sampled intravenous tolerance test,* or the so-called minimal model. The third, and simplest from a clinical perspective, is the fasting insulin level. Studies that have used any or all of these techniques have demonstrated that there is a wide range of insulin sensitivity in normal individuals, and these values overlap with similar values in type 2 diabetics. Therefore, it is very difficult to distinguish between nondiabetic and diabetic individuals on the basis of insulin resistance.

The most widely accepted research gold standard is the euglycemic hyperinsulinemic clamp technique. In this procedure, exogenous insulin is infused to maintain a constant plasma insulin level above fasting, while glucose is infused at varying rates necessary to keep glucose within a fixed range. The amount of glucose that is infused over time (M value) is an index of insulin action on glucose metabolism. Therefore, the more glucose that has to be infused per unit time, the more sensitive the patient is to insulin. With this procedure, the insulin-resistant patient requires much less glucose to maintain its basal level. This technique, however, has several limitations. Most importantly, the procedure's complexity and cost make it unrealistic for clinical practice or large population-based studies; therefore, its use is limited to research laboratories.

A second, and more practical, method that can be applied to larger populations is a procedure known as the minimal model, or the frequently sampled intravenous glucose tolerance test. With this procedure, glucose is injected as a bolus and both glucose and insulin levels are frequently assessed from an indwelling catheter over the next several hours. The results are entered in a computer model that generates a value that is an index of insulin sensitivity, termed S_1 units. This measure of insulin resistance correlates well with the euglycemic hyperinsulinemic clamp in nondiabetic subjects, but its accuracy deteriorates in diabetics because the immediate plasma insulin response to the glucose challenge, a major determinant for this analysis, is diminished. This problem has been addressed in diabetic patients by giving exogenous insulin or a secretagogue (i.e., tolbutamide) during the early parts of testing. However, from a clinical perspective, the most practical way of assessing insulin resistance is the measurement of plasma insulin levels. This is suggested to be done in the overnight-fasting condition, because in the postprandial state glucose levels are changing rapidly and the variable levels of glucose confound the simultaneous measure of insulin. There is a significant correlation between fasting insulin levels and insulin action as measured by the clamp technique. In addition, it is generally true that very high plasma insulin values in the setting of normal glucose tolerance are very likely to reflect insulin resistance, and high insulin levels are a predictor of the development of diabetes. The value of a fasting insulin is limited because, again, there is considerable overlap between insulin resistant and normal subjects, and another major limitation is the lack of standardization of the insulin assay procedure. However, if the assay for insulin is reliable, it may be useful to detect the insulin resistance early and before clinical disease appears.

VI. SHOULD INSULIN RESISTANCE BE TREATED FOR PRIMARY PREVENTION OF DIABETES?

It is well observed that insulin resistance is associated with much morbidity and mortality, but it has not been proved that improvement of insulin resistance will prevent mortality and morbidity resulting from the insulin-resistant state. This is further complicated because a clinically practical test for insulin resistance or a way to follow clinical resistance in a prospective study is not well established. However, it is well established that there are various interventions that do reduce insulin resistance. These interventions include a calorie-restricted diet, weight reduction, exercise, and pharmacological intervention with metformin and troglitazone. There are probably few clinicians now who have not observed the beneficial effect of a calorie-restricted diet on clinical insulin resistance. For those patients who do comply, insulin resistance is significantly reduced within a few days of instituting the diet, and this reduction is observed even before significant weight loss has occurred. Clinically, this is reflected either by an improvement in glycemic control, a markedly decreased exogenous insulin requirement, or the need to rely on higher doses of oral antidiabetic medications to maintain glycemic control. It has also been firmly established that weight reduction over a longer time frame continues to improve insulin sensitivity. Should the patient not be able to lose weight, avoiding the excess weight gain may provide the most efficient means to prevent insulin resistance and worsening morbidity. Although considerable research has evaluated distribution of calories on these effects, it appears that the total caloric intake, rather than distribution among carbohydrates and various fats, is the critical parameter.

Insulin sensitivity is significantly improved with exercise, for vigorous exercise reduces resistance, even in elderly patients. Unfortunately, the effect on insulin resistance diminishes quickly (within 3–5 days) after stopping the exercise. However, long-term exercise would result in little weight reduction unless caloric intake is also part of the regimen.

Pharmacological treatment of insulin resistance is an area of great debate. Over the last several years there have been two specific pharmacological approaches available to reduce insulin resistance. A class of compounds, called biguanides, as represented by the agent metformin, has a predominant effect to diminish hepatic glucose production and has modest effects on insulin resistance. On the other hand, a class of drugs referred to as thiazolidinediones, represented by the agent troglitazone, is considered a true "insulin sensitizer" by enhancing insulin-stimulated glucose disposal in muscle. Although both drugs are currently available in the United States for treatment of the type 2 diabetic condition, neither agent is approved to treat insulin resistance in the absence of the type 2 diabetic state. For the immediate future, several other agents in the thiazolidinedione class that are classified as insulin sensitizers will be released for general use.

Both classes of drugs have been postulated to be beneficial in either delaying or preventing the progression to type 2 diabetes, and they will be evaluated in national trials. In particular, the National Institute of Health's study termed the Diabetes Prevention Program (DPP) is designed to determine if any treatment (nutrition, exercise, pharmacological treatment) is effective in the primary prevention of type 2 diabetes in persons who have a diagnosis of impaired glucose tolerance. As originally designed, there was to be a control group that employed intensive lifestyle changes and was designed to effect an approximately 7% reduction in body weight through caloric restriction and exercise. The second and third groups were to consist of pharmacological treatments to reduce insulin resistance, mainly metformin and troglitazone. At the writing of this chapter, the troglitazone arm of study will not be evaluated, yet it is expected that by late spring of 1999 an additional primary prevention study with thiazolidinediones will be initiated through support of a pharmaceutical company.

It is not currently recommended that a patient receive pharmacological treatment for insulin resistance outside of the diabetic state. Depending on the outcome of the current prevention trials, this may be a recommendation in the near future. However, until the results of the prevention trials are known, it is extremely reasonable and recommended that the clinician offer nonpharmacological treatments to the patient in hopes of reducing insulin resistance and preventing the disease. Candidates for such therapy include those who are overweight (particularly with central obesity) and those who have a strong family history of diabetes or gestational diabetes, a condition termed impaired fasting glucose, or other clinical reasons that are associated with insulin resistance (hypertension, dyslipidemia).

VII. SUMMARY

It is now well recognized that insulin resistance precedes the diagnosis of type 2 diabetes and contributes greatly to metabolic abnormalities that cluster with this particular diagnosis. With such an understanding, prevention trials designed to improve insulin resistance and determine if type 2 diabetes can be prevented or delayed are currently ongoing. Whether treatment of insulin resistance with pharmacological agents outside the diabetic state is to be recommended will depend on the outcome of the current trials.

BIBLIOGRAPHY

Abate N. Insulin resistance and obesity. The role of fat distribution pattern. Diabetes Care 1996; 19:292–294.

Avena R, Mitchell ME, Nylen ES, Curry KM, Sidawy AN. Insulin action enhancement normalizes brachial artery vasoactivity in patients with peripheral vascular disease and occult diabetes. J Vasc Surg 1998; 28:1024–1031.

Cheatham B, Kahn CR. Insulin action and the insulin signaling network. Endocrol Rev 1995; 16:117–142.

Consensus Development Conference on Insulin Resistance. 5–6 November 1997. American Diabetes Association. Diabetes Care 1998; 21:310–314.

Després JP, Lamarche B, Mauriège P, Cantin B, Dagenais GR, Moorjani S, Lupien PJ. Hyperinsulinemia as an independent risk factor for ischemic heart disease. N Engl J Med 1996; 334:952–957.

Ducimetiere P, Eschwege E, Papoz L, Richard JL, Claude JR, Rosselin G. Relationship of plasma insulin levels to the incidence of myocardial infarction and coronary heart disease mortality in a middle-aged population. Diabetologia 1980; 19:205–210.

Eschwege E, Richard JL, Thibult N, Ducimetiere P, Warnet JM, Claude JR, Rosselin GE. Coronary heart disease mortality in relation with diabetes, blood glucose and plasma insulin levels. The Paris Prospective Study, ten years later. Horm Metals Res Suppl 1985; 15:41–46.

Fontbonne AM, Eschwege EM. Insulin and cardiovascular disease. Paris Prospective Study. Diabetes Care 1991; 14:461–469.

Grundy SM. Small LDL, atherogenic dyslipidemia, and the metabolic syndrome. Circulation 1997; 95:1–4.

Haffner SM, Valdez RA, Hazuda HP, Mitchell BD, Morales PA, Stern MP. Prospective analysis of the insulin-resistance syndrome (syndrome X). Diabetes 1992; 41:715–722.

Haffner SM. The insulin resistance syndrome revisited. Diabetes Care 1996; 19:275–277.

Hansen BC, Bodkin NL. Primary prevention of diabetes mellitus by prevention of obesity in monkeys. Diabetes 1993; 42:1809–1814.

Howard G, O'Leary DH, Zaccaro D, Haffner S, Rewers M, Hamman R, Selby JV, Saad MF, Savage P, Bergman R. Insulin sensitivity and atherosclerosis. The Insulin Resistance Atherosclerosis Study (IRAS) investigators. Circulation 1996; 93:1809–1817.

Hsueh WA, Quinones MJ, Creager MA. Endothelium in insulin resistance and diabetes. Diabetes Rev 1997; 5:343–352.

Hsueh WA, Law RE. Cardiovascular risk continuum: implications of insulin resistance and diabetes. Am J Med 1998; 105:4S–14S.

Hunter SJ, Garvey WT. Insulin action and insulin resistance: diseases involving defects in insulin receptors, signal transduction, and the glucose transport effector system. Am J Med 1998; 105:331–345.

Juhan-Vague I, Alessi MC, Vague P. Thrombogenic and fibrinolytic factors and cardiovascular risk in non–insulin-dependent diabetes mellitus. Ann Med 1996; 28:371–380.

Kaplan NM. The deadly quartet. Upper-body obesity, glucose intolerance, hypertriglyceridemia, and hypertension. Arch Intern Med 1989; 149:1514–1520.

Opara JU, Levine JH. The deadly quartet—the insulin resistance syndrome. South Med J 1997; 90:1162–1168.

Panahloo A, Yudkin JS. Diminished fibrinolysis in diabetes mellitus and its implication for diabetic vascular disease. Coronary Artery Dis 1996; 7:723–731.

Pyörälä K. Relationship of glucose tolerance and plasma insulin to the incidence of coronary heart disease: results from two population studies in Finland. Diabetes Care 1979; 2:131–141.

Quyyumi AA. Endothelial function in health and disease: new insights into the genesis of cardiovascular disease. Am J Med 1998; 105:32S–39S.

Reaven GM. Banting lecture 1988. Role of insulin resistance in human disease. Diabetes 1988; 37:1595–1607.

Schneider DJ, Nordt TK, Sobel BE. Attenuated fibrinolysis and accelerated atherogenesis in type II diabetic patients. Diabetes 1993; 42:1–7.

Tack CJ, Smits P, Demacker PN, Stalenhoef AF. Troglitazone decreases the proportion of small, dense LDL and increases the resistance of LDL to oxidation in obese subjects. Diabetes Care 1998; 21:796–799.

Vague J. La différenciation sexuelle facteur déterminant des formes de l'obésité. Presse Med 1947; 55:339–340.

Welborn TA, Wearne K. Coronary heart disease incidence and cardiovascular mortality in Busselton with reference to glucose and insulin concentrations. Diabetes Care 1979; 2:154–160.

Yamashita S, Nakamura T, Shimomura I, Nishida M, Yoshida S, Kotani K, Kameda-Takemuara K, Tokunaga K, Matsuzawa Y. Insulin resistance and body fat distribution. Diabetes Care 1996; 19:287–291.

7
Diabetes in Managed Care

Ronald E. Aubert and Rishi Sikka
The Prudential Center for Healthcare Research, Prudential Healthcare, Atlanta, Georgia

William H. Herman
University of Michigan, Ann Arbor, Michigan

I. INTRODUCTION

A health care system consists of the arrangements and processes by which a society organizes health care services. The major parties in any health care system include the purchasers (governments, employers, individuals), the payers or financial intermediaries (government agencies, insurance companies), providers (hospitals, physicians, nurses, dietitians, and others), and patients. Traditional indemnity health insurance plans have offered patients unrestricted choice of health care providers and reimbursed on a free-for-service basis. In general, such plans have done little to ensure appropriate utilization of preventive services and little to restrict inappropriate utilization of health services or to manage patients with chronic diseases.

Under indemnity insurance, the U.S. health care system has been oriented toward reactive treatment of disease. As a result, the costs of health care have been largely driven by illness-related care. It has been estimated that 70% of the burden of illness and its associated costs are due to preventable disease (1). Even in the absence of a diagnosed medical condition, individuals with behavioral risk factors, such as obesity, physical inactivity, smoking, alcohol use, and seatbelt nonuse, utilize more health services than those without behavioral risk factors (2). Such findings have contributed to the belief that health promotion and disease prevention interventions can improve health and reduce cost.

Under indemnity insurance, wide variations in rates of medical procedures have also been observed in the U.S. health care system (3,4). This variation has been attributed to both uninformed consumers and provider uncertainty about the best clinical practices. Lacking good and complete information, consumers demand services that may be ill-suited to their needs or in quantities that are inappropriate to their needs. In addition, lacking good evidence for which of the possible approaches in a given clinical situation will be most effective, physicians may recommend unnecessary procedures. Indeed, a substantial portion of all medical care has been inappropriate or unnecessary (5–10). Such findings have contributed to the belief that demand management strategies can improve health and further reduce cost (11).

Finally, under indemnity insurance, proved-effective interventions are sporadically and inconsistently applied. Indeed, despite the proved effectiveness of interventions to delay or prevent the complications of diabetes mellitus, their application is more the exception than the rule (12,13). Although slow diffusion of new medical knowledge contributes to the slow adoption of new and effective interventions (14), lack of proactive management systems also contribute. Such findings have further strengthened the belief that comprehensive disease management strategies might improve health and reduce cost.

The past decade has witnessed a surge in the growth and prevalence of managed care. By 1993, 75% of practicing physicians had at least one managed care contract (15). Indemnity insurance decreased from 73% of the private health insurance market in 1988 to 33% of the market by 1993. In contrast, health maintenance organization (HMO) enrollment grew from 29 million in 1987 to more than 45 million in 1993. Preferred provider organization (PPO) membership increased from 12 million in 1987 to 77 million in 1993 (16).

In contrast with indemnity insurance, managed care plans furnish a comprehensive set of health services, including health promotion, demand management, and disease management services; use explicit criteria to select health care providers; and provide significant financial incentives for members to use providers and services associated with the plan. Managed care organizations (MCOs) generally possess sophisticated information systems that integrate patient, provider, and utilization data and have formal programs for ongoing quality assurance and utilization review. Utilization review is a process of examining the care provided to individual consumers with the goal of improving the quality and decreasing the costs of health care (17). Utilization review has been adopted throughout the health care industry. In 1990, 85% of indemnity insurers had some form of utilization review (15). If one considers any type of managed intervention within the delivery of health care, then to some degree, almost all third-party payers could be considered managed care organizations (18).

II. TYPOLOGY OF MANAGED CARE

Traditionally, managed care refers to three distinct delivery systems of care: preferred provider organizations (PPOs), health maintenance organizations

(HMOs), and point-of-service plans (POS). Preferred provider organizations contract with a limited number of providers for health care services. The preferred providers are reimbursed on a discounted fee-for-service basis. Consumer members of PPOs pay less for health care received from a preferred provider than for care received from other providers. In this type of delivery environment, implementing system-wide quality improvement efforts is often difficult.

Health maintenance organizations encompass the role of insurer and provider under the umbrella of prepaid health care. HMOs vary according to the nature of the relations between insurance entity and the provider:

1. In a staff model HMO, the HMO employs providers and usually owns the facilities. Physicians typically are reimbursed by salary. In this type of health care delivery environment, physicians follow the policies established by the HMO, and systems-based quality improvement interventions tend to be easier to implement. There are usually common and shared automated data systems that allow identification of high-risk patients and targeting of interventions. One disadvantage perceived by purchasers is that this model of health care delivery offers a limited choice of physicians and facilities.

2. In a group model HMO, the HMO contracts with a multispecialty provider group. It is an exclusive contract in which the physician group agrees to provide services to only HMO members. The provider group establishes the practice policies and procedures. Because of the exclusive nature of the contract between the HMO and the provider group, systems-based intervention efforts tend to be relatively straightforward, similar to those for the staff model HMO. The perceived disadvantage of this model is that it is very limiting in choice of physicians and facilities.

3. The network-model HMO expands on the concept of the group model HMO. Network model HMOs contract with one or more multispecialty provider groups on a nonexclusive basis. This allows the provider groups to contract with additional HMOs and to care for other patients. In this health care delivery environment, quality improvement efforts originating from the health plan or HMO tend to be more difficult to implement to the extent that they are unique and might apply to only a part of the provider's patient population. The perceived advantage of this model is that it offers greater choice and flexibility for the consumer.

4. In an independent practice association (IPA) model HMO, the HMO contracts with multiple individual providers or provider groups. These providers typically practice in their own offices and are permitted to establish contracts with multiple HMOs. The challenges for implement-

ing interventions in this environment are similar to, or even more complex than in the network-model HMO. The perceived advantage of this model is that it offers the greatest flexibility and choice of physicians and facilities to the consumer.

IPA model HMOs are currently the dominant HMO model. In 1988, 42% of HMO members were enrolled in staff and group model HMOs. In 1994, staff and group model HMOs constituted only 31% of HMO membership. In contrast, during the same time period, IPA model HMOs have increased their market share from 43 to 50% (19). This growth is driven by the growing demand of purchasers and consumers to have a greater choice in selecting their physicians, and the growing cost of maintaining group and staff-model HMOs. The decreasing market share of group and staff model HMOs has alarmed some advocates of quality. However, there is no conclusive evidence that staff or group model HMOs are more effective than network or IPA model HMOs (20).

Point-of-service (POS) plans like HMOs may adopt staff, group, network, and IPA models. In HMOs, members must bear the full cost for any medical services delivered by non-HMO physicians. Point-of-service plans mitigate this financial burden by allowing members to receive care from physicians outside the HMO network. Point-of-service members pay higher premiums and have to pay a greater portion of the costs for self-referred and out-of-network coverage. Nevertheless, they are provided greater autonomy and flexibility.

Reimbursement methods vary among the different model HMOs and POS plans. However, most nonstaff model HMOs reimburse physicians on a capitated basis. In a capitation contract, the individual physician or medical group receives a fixed reimbursement on a per member per month basis, regardless of the amount of services provided. This type of financial arrangement allows the medical group or individual physician to share financial risk with the HMO. In 1989, 35% of HMOs paid primary care physicians with capitation. By 1994, half of all HMOs were using capitation to reimburse primary care providers (19). In other instances, providers are reimbursed on a discounted fee-for-service basis.

These trends in increased risk parallel other changes within HMOs. For-profit HMOs have had significant growth in the marketplace. Currently, most HMO members are enrolled in for-profit organizations. From 1988 to 1994, membership in for-profit HMOs increased by over 91%, compared with a 25% non-profit HMO membership increase (19).

III. THE EVOLUTION OF HEALTH MANAGEMENT

Critics argue that managed care reimbursement mechanisms and controls, such as utilization review, promote undertreatment and discrimination against consumers with costly medical conditions. Some argue that cost-containment strategies, such as utilization review, undermine the clinical autonomy of physicians, deter them from recommending services, and compromise quality of care (21,22).

In contrast, proponents believe that given appropriate resources, managed care may both improve the quality and control the costs of health care in the United States. The reasons for this are first, that managed care organizations (MCOs) must weigh and balance the interests of all of the major parties in the health care system, particularly those of purchasers and patient and, second, MCOs compete among themselves on the basis of both quality and cost; thus, they have developed systems to measure performance and improve quality of services. One of these systems, the Health Plan Employer Data and Information Set (HEDIS) was developed jointly by purchasers, patients, and MCOs under the guidance of the National Committee for Quality Assurance (NCQA), an accrediting organization for HMOs. Third, federal and state regulatory agencies impose external systems of measurement on MCOs.

In the sections that follow, we review how MCOs have brought together three concepts—health promotion, demand management, and disease management—into proactive programs to improve quality and control costs. These have been termed health management programs. These programs are applied to individuals across the wellness–illness spectrum to improve the health of the population. They require collaboration and cooperation among payers, the health plan, physicians, and patients.

Health promotion involves the use of health promotion and disease prevention strategies to keep healthy people healthy. The effectiveness and cost-effectiveness of some health promotion interventions, such as influenza immunization, have been well documented. Unfortunately, however, until recently, there was little evidence for the benefits of behavioral health promotion and disease prevention interventions. More recently, studies in California (23,24), Minnesota (25,26), and Finland (27) have demonstrated that community-based interventions to improve health can be effective. In a 1993 report summarizing the influence of worksite wellness programs on health and costs, 23 studies were identified from the previous 2 years, and all but 1 were found to be effective and cost-effective (28). Most such programs have attempted to identify the risk status of individuals in the population and then provide them with, and encourage them to take advantage of services most relevant to them.

Managed care organizations have employed a variety of strategies for health promotion. Often times, pediatric and adult preventive care guidelines have served as the basis for these activities. Claims-based prediction models incorporating age, gender, and historical service utilization have been used to assess risk. Self-administered health risk appraisals have been used to assess behavioral risk factors. Clinical screenings conducted through primary care providers or worksite wellness programs have also been used to directly assess risk factors, including overweight, inactivity, hypertension, dyslipidemia, and substance abuse.

Population-based interventions have included direct mailings to members to promote health promotion and disease management strategies, such as healthy eating and physical activity. In addition, targeted mailings have been sent to members reminding them of the availability of specific services particularly appropriate to them. For example, such mailings have reminded smokers of the availability of smoking cessation interventions. Several plans have employed lifestyle change ''coaching.'' Such programs are initiated through outbound telephone calls inviting members to take advantage of telephone-based services of a nurse counselor who works with the member and his or her primary care physician to develop and implement a risk reduction plan. Preventive service reminder systems, such as postcard immunization reminders, have also been used to help members remember to seek the right preventive care at the right time. Clinical preventive service profiling has been used to monitor and provide feedback to physicians concerning their preventive care practices relative to preventive care guidelines. Plans have also successfully developed and implemented worksite wellness initiatives in partnership with employers. Finally, plans have partnered with local weight management programs and health clubs to offer discounted programs for dietary modification, weight loss, and exercise.

Demand management involves use of self-management education and decision support services to encourage appropriate utilization of services. Better-informed patients tend to choose interventions that are more in keeping with their own preferences (29–33). Such interventions have also reduced unnecessary visits to physicians and admissions to hospitals and improved functional status (34–36).

Health plans have used a variety of strategies to influence demand. Plans have used direct mailing to members to encourage appropriate use of services according to clinical practice guidelines. Plans have distributed books to members in which they can look up a symptom, find a complete explanation of probable causes, how serious they are, and how they might be relieved at home. Such books also provide easy-to-follow decision charts that instruct the patient when to see a doctor (37). Other plans have used nurse-counseling telephone services to educate and support persons in making appropriate choices about health and medical care. In some instances, such service provides preprovider (triage) decisions concerning acute minor illnesses and injuries. Other plans have used nurse triage lines to further assist patients with decisions about when and where to seek care (at home, in the physicians office, or in the emergency room). Demand management strategies have been integrated with traditional utilization management strategies, clinical practice guidelines, and critical pathways to guide major therapies and hospital care.

Disease management brings together a variety of strategies to help physicians and patients better manage chronic diseases. Disease management programs have generally focused on common chronic conditions in which there is substantial practice variation and for which interventions have improved outcomes. Such conditions include, for example, diabetes mellitus, asthma, and congestive heart failure. A variety of approaches have been employed ranging from individual, reactive strategies, to population-based, proactive strategies. Individual, reactive strategies have built on traditional utilization management. For example, patients hospitalized for diabetic complications might be identified by utilization management nurses and provided a visiting nurse after discharge. Population-based, proactive strategies have used systematic evaluations of available administrative data to identify members for active disease management.

Most population-based disease management programs have begun with the establishment of a population-based registry. Registries have generally been developed on the basis of available administrative data, including demographic data collected at enrollment, reports of outpatient encounters and inpatient hospitalization, laboratory data, pharmacy claims, and claims for supplies and durable medical equipment. In some instances, data from health risk appraisals, member surveys, providers, and utilization management nurses have been used. In general, combinations of claims data are used to define members with diabetes and the sensitivity and specificity of different definitions are assessed against a gold standard, such as self-report or medical record review. Many plans have simply used the HEDIS definition, which defines diabetes on the basis of a prescription for a diabetes drug, a primary diagnosis of diabetes during an inpatient admission or emergency room visit, or two separate outpatient visits with a primary diagnosis of diabetes. Once a registry is developed, it is possible to assess the current processes of care to identify opportunities for improvement.

Clinical practice guidelines are then developed to identify "best practices." Clinical practice guidelines have been based on recommendations of the American Diabetes Association (ADA; 38). Others have adopted an evidence-based approach (39) and focused on cardiovascular risk factor detection and control, prophylactic use of aspirin, diabetic retinopathy, diabetic nephropathy, diabetic neuropathy, and glycemic control (40). In general, clinical practice guidelines are developed with coordinated input from physician leaders from throughout the managed care network (41).

A variety of implementation strategies have been used to encourage and support the incorporation of these recommended best practices into day-to-day medical practice. Plans have mailed self-care guides and educational materials to members on the registry (42,43). In addition, plans have sent service reminders, for instance, for retinal examinations or influenza immunizations, to members on the registry. Some plans have refined their reminder systems by sending reminders only to members overdue for the services. Plans have also disseminated clinical practice guidelines to providers and then used provider profiling systems to inform contracted physicians of their members with diabetes and their adherence to the processes of care outlined in the clinical practice guidelines. Plans have also coordinated guidelines with benefit coverage to ensure that administrative and financial barriers to recommended services are minimized or eliminated. Lack of knowledge or misunderstanding of covered benefits on the part of both patients and providers may be a barrier to appropriate care. In other instances, plans have followed up with primary care providers to ensure provision of supplies and tools, such as glucose reflectance meters and self-monitoring supplies to selected members. Plans have also encouraged referral of selected members to outpatient education programs, dietitians, and specialists.

Comprehensive, population-based strategies have attempted to provide tiered services to members identified on the disease registry. One proposed model for diabetes disease management provides three levels of care. Level 1 care is proactively offered to everyone on the registry. The focus of level 1 care is assessment of educational needs to promote positive self-care behaviors, monitoring of glycemic control, and systematic screening for diabetic complications and cardiovascular risk factors. Results of the educational assessment and tests are provided to members and a report is generated for the primary care physician with interpretation and guideline-based recommendation for follow-up. Level 2 care involves nurse case management to assist patients and primary care physicians to achieve the goals established in the level 1 care plan. Level 2 care is subdivided to address short-term and long-term patient needs. Implementation of minor adjustments in medical therapy and acute health care problems are indications for short-term care management. Complex intervention plans or medical treatment regimens, or multiple intercurrent conditions represent indications for long-term care management. Specific examples of appropriate candidates for short-term care management are patients with a new diagnosis of diabetes, patients newly identified with diabetic complications requiring intervention, and patients starting new treatments. Examples of patients appropriate for long-term care management include those unable to meet glycemic goals, despite intensified treatment, those with complications or comorbidity requiring ongoing therapy, and patients with frequent utilization of emergency or inpatient services. Level 3 care represents diabetes subspecialty care. Its focus is on optimizing glycemic control using complex treatment regimens, interventions for advanced diabetic complications and comorbidity, and coordination of multispecialty care. Level 3 care is generally applied to a small minority of diabetic subjects who, because of complex psychosocial issues or medical conditions, exceed the scope of services provided in primary care practice.

IV. PHYSICIAN-DIRECTED NURSE CARE MANAGEMENT INTERVENTIONS

A growing number of observational and randomized studies have demonstrated that physician-directed nurse case management programs are associated with improved glycemic control and improved processes of diabetes care. Peters et al. (44) examined the use of specially trained nurses to assist people with diabetes to achieve better glycemic control. They found that nurse implementation of algorithms with computerized tracking methods and follow-up among high-risk patients achieved an average decline of HbA_{1c} of 3.0% over a 1-year period. In a subsequent analysis, Peters and Davidson (45) compared the physician-supervised nurse managed group with a group of similar patients in a local group model HMO. They found that the patients in the nurse-managed group showed significant improvement in glycemic control when compared with the group model HMO patients, and this improvement was sustained over 3 years of follow-up. In addition, patients in the nurse management program with hypercholesterolemia were more likely to have their cholesterol lowered than patients in the comparison population. Improvements were seen in process measures, such as annual measurement of HbA_{1c} levels, lipid levels, and foot and retinal examinations, and occurred more frequently in the physician-directed nurse management group.

In a group model HMO, a randomized, controlled trial demonstrated nurse case management that included close follow-up, continuous reinforcement of meal planning and exercise, and systematic treatment adjustments was effective in improving patient outcomes (46). In this latter study by Aubert et al., potential study participants were identified through a database registry used to support quality improvement activities. Members in the plan who had diabetes were included in the database if they had a visit to the doctor for diabetes (ICD-9 code of 250.0 to 250.9), had a hospital claim processed for diabetes, were seen by the utilization management nurse, or had a referral to the ophthalmologist for a diabetic retinal examination. The registry was updated annually.

The nurse case manager was a registered nurse and certified diabetes educator. She was trained to follow a set of detailed management algorithms under the direction of a board-certified family medicine physician and an endocrinologist who were responsible for all diabetes management decisions for patients in the intervention group, but were not the primary providers for these patients. The algorithms were specific for type of diabetes and were developed by a multidisciplinary team that represented endocrinology, family medicine, nursing, pharmacy, health services research, and epidemiology. The algorithms progressively moved a patient toward improving glycemic control through adjustment in medication, meal planning, and exercise reinforcement (Fig. 1).

Members randomized to nurse case management met with the nurse for an initial assessment, were instructed on a blood glucose-monitoring schedule, and returned for a follow-up visit in 2 weeks. This initial visit with the nurse case manager was on average 45 min in length. During the 2-week follow-up visit the nurse reviewed the blood glucose log, explained the algorithm step to which the patient had been assigned, and used this information as the baseline for subsequent medication adjustments, meal planning, and exercise reinforcement. Mem-

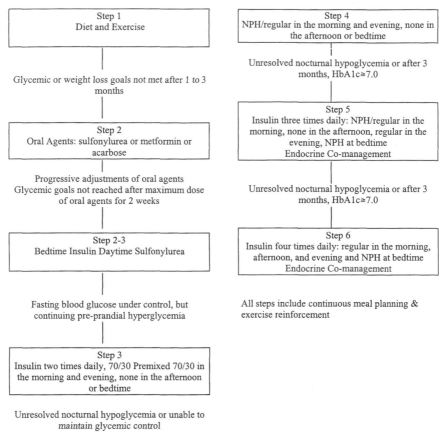

| Step 1
Diet and Exercise | Step 4
NPH/regular in the morning and evening, none in
the afternoon or bedtime |

Glycemic or weight loss goals not met after 1 to 3 months

Unresolved nocturnal hypoglycemia or after 3 months, HbA1c≈7.0

Step 2
Oral Agents: sulfonylurea or metformin or acarbose

Step 5
Insulin three times daily: NPH/regular in the morning, none in the afternoon, regular in the evening, NPH at bedtime
Endocrine Co-management

Progressive adjustments of oral agents
Glycemic goals not reached after maximum dose of oral agents for 2 weeks

Unresolved nocturnal hypoglycemia or after 3 months, HbA1c≈7.0

Step 2-3
Bedtime Insulin Daytime Sulfonylurea

Step 6
Insulin four times daily: regular in the morning, afternoon, and evening and NPH at bedtime
Endocrine Co-management

Fasting blood glucose under control, but continuing pre-prandial hyperglycemia

All steps include continuous meal planning & exercise reinforcement

Step 3
Insulin two times daily, 70/30 Premixed 70/30 in the morning and evening, none in the afternoon or bedtime

Unresolved nocturnal hypoglycemia or unable to maintain glycemic control

Move to Step 4

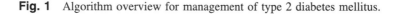

Fig. 1 Algorithm overview for management of type 2 diabetes mellitus.

bers were also referred to a 5-week, 12-h diabetes education program, which included individual counseling by a dietitian, an exercise therapist, and group diabetes education classes. Subsequent in-person follow-up occurred quarterly.

Members who were taking insulin received a follow-up telephone call weekly. After a review of the blood glucose log and discussion of values with the patient, medication adjustments were made if necessary and meal planning and exercise were reinforced. Members on oral agents or diet and exercise regimens received only a follow-up telephone call every 2 weeks. The nurse case manager met at least biweekly with the family medicine physician and endocrinologist to review patient progress, medication adjustments, and any other pertinent issues related to the diabetes care of the patients. All medication adjustments or changes were communicated back to the patients' regular primary care physician.

Change in HbA_{1c} after a 12-month follow-up period was the primary outcome measure. In addition, health-related quality of life was assessed using four generic questions developed by the Centers for Disease Control and Prevention (CDC) for the Behavioral Risk Factor Surveillance System.

Of the 545 members in the diabetes registry, eligibility and recruitment information was confirmed for 480. Eligibility status was established for 92% of these. Of the 208 members who met eligibility criteria for randomization, 34% did not appear for their scheduled appointments; therefore, they were not randomized, and 66% were randomized to nurse case management or usual care. Of the 138 members randomized into the study, 100 (72%) provided 12-month follow-up data.

Most baseline characteristics were similar in the two treatment arms, but the nurse case management arm had slightly fewer ethnic minorities, more smokers, and more patients treated with insulin. Of the patients in nurse case management, 17% had type 1 diabetes, as compared with 8% in the usual care arm. The median baseline HbA_{1c} in the nurse case management arm was similar to the usual care arm (8.8 vs. 8.4%). The median baseline fasting blood glucose level for both arms was also quite similar (194 mg/dL vs. 191 mg/dL).

The nurse case management group showed a greater drop in HbA_{1c} than the usual care group. The average change in HbA_{1c} in the nurse case management group was − 1.7% (9.0–7.3%) compared with − 0.6% in usual care (8.9–8.3%) (p < 0.001). On average, patients in nurse case management had a decrease of 48.3 mg/dL in fasting blood glucose compared with a decrease of 14.5 mg/dL in usual care (p = 0.003). There were no statistically significant differences between nurse case management and usual care relative to changes in systolic or diastolic blood pressure, serum cholesterol and triglycerides, or weight. Although both groups reported an improved perception of health status after 12-months, patients in nurse case management were more than two times as likely to report improved health status than patients in usual care (p = 0.02).

Observational studies, clinical trial, and this randomized, controlled clinical trial demonstrated the effectiveness of a nurse case management diabetes program that included close follow-up, continuous reinforcement of meal planning and exercise, and systematic treatment adjustments. Hemoglobin A_{1c} levels declined significantly in patients randomly assigned to the nurse case management intervention. This decline was consistent across the spectrum of baseline HbA_{1c} levels greater than 7.0 and was consistent in both type 1 and type 2 diabetic subpopulations. We observed maximum effect size after 6 months of follow-up, and the effect of the intervention was sustained after 12 months. Patients in the nurse case management arm perceived greater improvement of general health status than those receiving usual care.

In a subsequent analysis of the benefits of nurse case management, Sikka et al. (47), found a higher adherence to ADA recommendations for renal function assessment. Patients randomized to nurse case management were 65% ($p < 0.05$) more likely to have quantitative protein testing and 60% ($p < 0.05$) more likely to have microalbumin testing done compared with patients in usual care. This is additional evidence that with appropriate clinical support and information systems, physician-directed nurse management interventions can produce better outcomes for people with diabetes.

V. COST-EFFECTIVENESS OF DIABETES DISEASE MANAGEMENT INTERVENTIONS

Despite the increasing evidence demonstrating the effectiveness of diabetes disease management programs, little is known about their cost-effectiveness to a health care system or purchasers of health care services. In an era of heightened cost consciousness, beneficial outcomes alone are insufficient criteria for the adoption of such programs. The success and broad implementation of comprehensive diabetes disease management programs rest in their potential to deliver positive results in an environment of limited resources. Understanding the resources and costs associated with a diabetes disease management intervention is the first step in assessing the cost-effectiveness and feasibility of such programs.

We have assessed the resources used for a nurse case management (NCM) intervention to improve diabetes care. Specifically, we enumerated the direct medical costs of the NCM intervention for diabetic patients in a group model HMO. Data were collected during the randomized, controlled trial of NCM intervention. The costs of both medical care and the intervention were considered. Medical care costs were divided into categories of pharmacy, blood glucose monitoring, and outpatient visits. Programmatic costs associated with the intervention included salary, fringe benefits, equipment, telephone, and diabetes education. The probability of patients attending the diabetes education program was based on chart review, for the education program was offered at a hospital outside of the primary care environment. The cost of education was based on unit cost and actual utilization.

Others have shown that resource utilization varies by duration of diabetes. In the evaluation of nurse case management resource utilization was determined by duration of diabetes and patient enrollment in either NCM or usual care. Unit costs were derived from the prevailing costs during the study period and were chosen to reflect what an item would cost a single-payer health system. Costs were calculated as the product of resources used, and unit costs and are reported in 1994 dollars.

The annual treatment cost of comprehensive diabetes care with NCM was approximately $300 greater than the costs of comprehensive care without NCM. The largest differences in costs were observed in pharmacy and self-blood glucose monitoring subcategories. Patients in NCM also had a greater probability of participating in the formal diabetes education program than patients in usual care. Nurse case management was about 22% more expensive than usual care, but the benefits may make this marginal difference a good value.

To compare the lifetime benefits and costs of usual care and nurse case management, we used a Monte Carlo simulation of diabetes complications that is described elsewhere (48,49). In brief, the model projects the incidence of microvascular, neuropathic, and cardiovascular complications in a hypothetical sample of 10,000 persons with type 2 diabetes. Diabetes-related morbidity is categorized, using 12 states of health, grouped according to the major complications of retinopathy, nephropathy, and neuropathy.

At each point in time, a patient is in one of five retinopathy health states, one of four nephropathy health states, and one of three neuropathy health states. The probability of advancing to a given health state is a function of (a) the epidemiology of diabetes in populations assumed to receive the standard of care prevailing in the United States over the preceding two decades; (b) the patient's gender, race, and duration of diabetes; (c) the level of glycemic control.

The model begins by randomly selecting an individual from a sample representing the demographic characteristics of patients with diabetes in the Jacksonville study population. The patient's demographic profile and level of glycemic control determine the baseline health state in each of the three diabetic complications. The model then simulates the course of diabetes-related complications over their lifetime. The ocular, renal, and neurological health states are advanced in parallel and on an annual basis.

The costs associated with diabetic complications, hypoglycemic events, laboratory, and nondiabetes medical care, were based on published data or prevailing Medicare reimbursement rates. The model was augmented to accrue the unique direct medical costs associated with the management of diabetes in the study cohort. The nurse case management (NCM) simulation included a per member per year cost and enrollment probability associated with NCM. The fixed costs of the NCM intervention include salary, fringe benefits, and equipment. We assumed that the nurse case manager oversaw a population of 300 persons with diabetes, consistent with previous studies.

In our preliminary analysis, we ran one usual care and one nurse case management simulation of 10,000 people each. The inputs for the two simulations differed in three respects: (a) the levels of glycemic control in each simulation reflected the level of control as observed in each cohort in the randomized trial;

(b) the short-term cost drivers in each simulation reflected the actual resource utilization observed in the trial; (c) the NCM simulation reflected the additional programmatic costs and probabilities associated with the intervention.

In the reference case analysis, comprehensive care with nurse case management reduced proliferative retinopathy 57%, end-stage renal disease 67%, and lower extremity amputation 15%. Using a 3% discount rate the expected lifetime cost of comprehensive diabetes care with NCM was approximately $7000 greater than comprehensive care without NCM. When the incremental benefits of comprehensive diabetes care with NCM are compared with the incremental costs of a NCM comprehensive care program, NCM intervention costs less than $20,000 per quality-adjusted life year. The results of the simulation indicate that the cost-effectiveness ratio for comprehensive diabetes care with nurse case management is well within the range to represent a good value.

VI. CONCLUSION

In this chapter we have described diabetes care in the changing environment of managed care, discussed the evolution of health management strategies, and provided an example of one rigorously evaluated program that appears to be cost-effective.

The existence of an organized system of health care delivery and a centralized database that includes enrollment, inpatient and outpatient encounters, pharmacy and laboratory data, facilitate the implementation of health management strategies. Whether these and other interventions are cost-effective, affordable, and can be easily adapted to the different managed health care delivery environments are questions to be answered by future investigation.

In addition it remains to be seen whether the promise of managed care to provide more comprehensive coverage, innovative services, or other desirable products at a competitive price, will actually be realized. The quality measurement efforts such as HEDIS and others, such as the Diabetes Quality Improvement Program initiated by ADA in collaboration with NCQA, will perhaps provide the surveillance capacity to monitor the improvement in diabetes care during this period of rapid change in the U.S. health care system.

REFERENCES

1.   Fries JF, Koop CE, Beadle CE, Cooper PP, England MJ, Greaves RF, Sokolov JJ, Wright D. Reducing health care costs by reducing the need and demand for medical services. The Health Project Consortium. N Engl J Med 1993; 329:321–325.

2. Yen LT, Edington DW, Witting P. Corporate medical claim cost distributions and factors associated with high-cost status. J Occup Med 1994; 36:505–515.

3. Wennberg JE, Freeman JL, Shelton RM, Bubolz TA. Hospital use and mortality among Medicare beneficiaries in Boston and New Haven. N Engl J Med 1989; 321: 1168–1173.

4. Welch WP, Miller ME, Welch HG, Fisher ES, Wennberg JE. Geographic variation in expenditures for physicians' services in the United States. N Engl J Med 1993; 328:621–627.

5. Chassin MR, Kosecoff J, Solomon DH, Brook RH. How coronary angiography is used. Clinical determinants of appropriateness. JAMA 1987; 258:2543–2547.

6. Kahn KL, Kosecoff J, Chassin MR, Solomon DH, Brook RH. The use and misuse of upper gastrointestinal endoscopy. Ann Intern Med 1988; 109:664–670.

7. Leape LL, Hilborne LH, Park RE, Bernstein SJ, Kamberg CJ, Sherwood M, Brook RH. The appropriateness of use of coronary artery bypass graft surgery in New York State. JAMA 1993; 269:753–760.

8. Hilborne LH Leape LL, Bernstein SJ, Park RE, Fiske ME, Kamberg CJ, Roth CP, Brook RH. The appropriateness of use of percutaneous transluminal coronary angioplasty in New York State. JAMA 1993; 269:761–765.

9. Bernstein SJ, Hilborne LH, Leape LL, Fiske ME, Park RE, Kamberg CJ, Brook RH. The appropriateness of use of coronary angiography in New York State. JAMA 1993; 269:766–769.

10. Kleinman LC, Kosecoff J, Dubois RW, Brook RH. The medical appropriateness of tympanostomy tubes proposed for children younger than 16 years in the United States. JAMA 1994; 271:1250–1255.

11. Chassin MR, Glavin RW. The urgent need to improve health care quality. Institute of Medicine National Roundtable on Health Care Quality. JAMA 1998; 280: 1000–1005.

12. Kenny SJ, Smith PJ, Goldschmid MG, Newman JM, Herman WH. Survey of physician practice behaviors related to diabetes mellitus in the U.S. Physician adherence to consensus recommendations. Diabetes Care 1993; 16:1507–1510.

13. Beckles GLA, Engelgau MM, Venkat Narayan KM, Herman WH, Aubert RE, Williamson DF. Population-based assessment of the level of care among adults with diabetes in the U.S. Diabetes Care 1998; 21:1432–1438.

14. Stross JK, Harlan WR. The dissemination of new medical information. JAMA 1979; 241:2622–2624.

15. Eisenberg JM. Economics. JAMA 1995; 273:670–671.

16. Weiss B. Managed care: there's no stopping it now. Med Econ 1995; (Managed Care suppl), March 13:4–12.

17. Harris J, et al. Prevention and managed care: opportunities for managed care organizations, purchasers of health care and public health agencies. MMWR Morbid Mortal Wkly Rep 1995; 44:1–12.

18. Bischof RO, Nash DB. Managed care: past, present and future. Med Clin North Am 1996; 80:225–244.

19. Gabel J. Ten ways HMOs have changed during the 1990s. Health Affairs 1997; 16: 134–145.

20. Miller RH, Luft HS. Managed care plan performance since 1980: a literature analysis. JAMA 1994; 271:1512–1519.
21. Institute of Medicine. Controlling costs and changing patient care? The role of utilization management. Washington, DC: National Academy Press, 1989.
22. Halm EA, Causino N, Blumenthal D. Is gatekeeping better than traditional care? JAMA 1997; 278:1677–1681.
23. Farquhar JW, Fortmann SP, Flora JA, Taylor CB, Haskell WL, Williams PT, Maccoby N, Wood PD. Effects of community-wide education on cardiovascular disease risk factors. The Standford Five-City Project. JAMA 1990; 264:359–365.
24. Taylor CB, Fortmann SP, Flora J, Kayman S, Barrett DC, Jatulis D, Farquhar JW. Effect of long-term community health education on body mass index. The Standford Five-City Project. Am J Epidemiol 1991; 134:235–249.
25. Murray DM, Kurth C, Mullis R, Jeffery RW. Cholesterol reduction through low-intensity interventions: results from the Minnesota Heart Health Program. Prev Med 1990; 19:181–189.
26. Jeffery RW, Hellerstedt WL, Schmid TL. Correspondence programs for smoking cessation and weight control: a comparison of two strategies in the Minnesota Heart Health Program. Health Psychol 1990; 9:585–598.
27. Vartiainen E, Paavola M, McAlister A, Puska P. Fifteen-year follow-up of smoking prevention effects in the North Karelia youth project. Am J Public Health 1998; 88: 81–85.
28. Pelletier KR. Clinical and cost outcomes of multifactorial, cardiovascular risk management interventions in worksites: a comprehensive review and analysis. J Occup Environ Med 1997; 39:1154–1169.
29. Randall T. Producers of videodisc programs strive to expand patient's role in medical decision making process. JAMA 1993; 270:160–162.
30. Grimshaw JM, Russell IT. Effect of clinical guidelines on medical practice: a systematic review of rigorous evaluations. Lancet 1993; 342:1317–1322.
31. Grimshaw JM, Hutchinson A. Clinical practice guidelines—do they enhance value for money in health care? Br Med Bull 1995; 51:927–940.
32. Grimshaw JM. Towards effective professional practice. Therapie 1996; 51:233–236.
33. Bero LA, Grilli R, Grimshaw JM, Harvey E, Oxman AD, Thomson MA. Closing the gap between research and practice: an overview of systematic reviews of interventions to promote the implementation of research findings. The Cochrane Effective Practice and Organization of Care Review Group. Br Med J 1998; 317:465–468.
34. Vickery DM, Kalmer H, Lowry D, Constantine M, Wright E, Loren W. Effect of a self-care education program on medical visits. JAMA 1983; 250:2952–2956.
35. Lynch WD, Golaszewski TJ, Clearie AF, Snow D, Vickery DM. Impact of a facility-based corporate fitness program on the number of absences from work due to illness. J Occup Med 1990; 32:9–12.
36. Vickery DM, Lynch WD. Demand management: enabling patients to use medical care appropriately. J Occup Environ Med 1995; 37:551–557.
37. Vickery DM, Fries JF. Take Care of Yourself. The Complete Guide to Medical Self-care. Redding, MA: Addison-Wesley, 1994.
38. American Diabetes Association: Clinical Practice Recommendations 1998. Diabetes Care 1998; 21(suppl 1).

39. U.S. Preventive Services Task Force. Guide to Clinical Preventive services 2nd ed. Baltimore: Williams & Wilkins, 1996.

40. Vijan S, Stevens DL, Herman WH, Funnell MM, Standiford CJ. Screening, prevention, counseling, and treatment for the complications of type 2 diabetes mellitus. Putting evidence into practice. J Gen Intern Med 1997; 12:567–580.

41. Wise CG, Billi JE. A model for practice guideline adaptation and implementation: empowerment of the physician. Joint Commission J Quality Improv 1995; 21: 465–476.

42. Brisco P. Diabetes. Questions You Have—Answers You Need. Allentown, PA: People's Medical Society, 1997.

43. Centers for Disease Control and Prevention. Take Charge of Your Diabetes, 2nd ed. U.S. Department of Health and Human Services, Centers for Disease Control and Prevention, National Center for Chronic Disease Prevention and Health Promotion, Division of Diabetes Translation, Health Communications Section, 1997.

44. Peters AL, Davidson MB, Ossorio RL. Management patients with diabetes by nurses with support of subspecialists. HMO Pract 1995; 9:8–13.

45. Peters AL, Davidson MB. Application of a diabetes managed care program. The feasibility of using nurses and a computer system to provide effective care. Diabetes Care 1998; 21:1037–1043.

46. Aubert RE, Herman WH, Waters J, et al. Nurse case management to improve glycemic control in diabetic patients in a health maintenance organization. Ann Intern Med 1998; 129:605–612.

47. Sikka R, Waters J, Moore W, Sutton DR, Herman WH, Aubert RE. Renal assessment practices and the effect of nurse case management of health maintenance organization patients with diabetes. Diabetes Care 1999; 22:1–6.

48. Eastman RC, Javitt JC, Herman WH, et al. Model of complications of NIDDM. Diabetes Care 1997; 20:725–734.

49. DCCT Study Group. Lifetime benefits and costs of intensive therapy as practiced in the Diabetes Control and Complications Trial: an economic evaluation. JAMA 1996; 276:1409–1415.

8
Type 1 Diabetes

Paul J. Beisswenger
*Dartmouth Medical School, Hanover, and Dartmouth–Hitchcock
Medical Center, Lebanon, New Hampshire*

I. INTRODUCTION

Persons with type 1 diabetes are dependent on injected insulin to prevent hyperglycemia and ketosis and to preserve life. This diabetes type is characterized in
its complete state by insulinopenia and virtually complete destruction of the beta
cells, although there may be preketotic, non–insulin-dependent phases earlier in
the natural history of the disease.

Over the past four decades, we have been experiencing a virtual epidemic
of type 1 diabetes in the Western world with increases of three-4 to fivefold
occurring in many European countries. In the United States, a total of 30,000
new cases of type 1 diabetes occur each year. There are 120,000 individuals with
diabetes in the younger than 20-year-old group, and the most common age of
onset is between 12 and 16, which coincides with peak pubertal ages for both
boys and girls. In the United States there are between 300,000 and 500,000
individuals with type 1 diabetes, but based on the finding that 10% of those who
develop diabetes beyond age 30 have detectable anti-islet cell antibodies (a marker
for type 1 diabetes), it is possible that another 500,000 adults may also have this
type.

There are considerable racial and ethnic differences in the propensity to
type 1 diabetes in children, with the highest incidence of 17.3 cases per 100,000
occurring in the white populations and in Hispanic populations of Puerto Rican
origin. Somewhat lower figures are seen for African American (12.1 : 100,000)
and Mexican American populations (8.8 : 100,000), and it is rarely seen in Native
Americans and Asian American populations. International studies have also
shown dramatic geographic variation in risk for type 1 diabetes, with very low

rates observed in China and Japan (0.7–2.0 cases per 100,000 per year) and 50-fold higher rates in Finland (35.3 : 100,000).

II. TIME COURSE OF ONSET OF TYPE 1 DIABETES

The primary lesion responsible for type 1 diabetes is a destructive process involving the insulin-secreting beta cells, manifested by a mononuclear infiltrate and beta cell lysis in the islets of newly discovered type I diabetics (insulitis). This infiltrate comprises cytotoxic T cells (CD4 and CD8), suggesting that an infectious or autoimmune process has initiated the damage, with the eventual outcome of complete beta-cell destruction and insulin deficiency (1). Significant beta-cell damage is already present at the onset of type 1 diabetes, and up to 75% of islet function is lost before significant fasting hyperglycemia occurs. Some patients

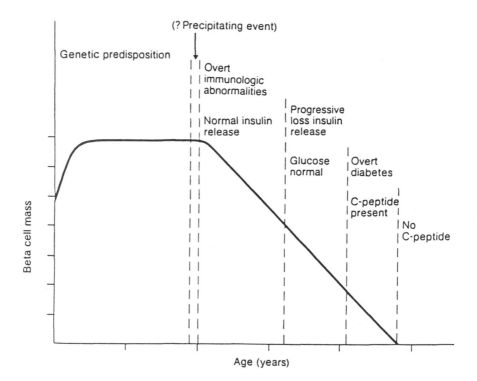

Fig. 1 Proposed stages in the development of type I diabetes (from left to right). Also plotted is "hypothetical" beta cell mass versus age (from Ref. 1).

with type 1 diabetes may demonstrate residual beta-cell function for substantial time periods, whereas others may show more acute destruction. Although many cases of type 1 diabetes seem to be of sudden onset, it is apparent that a long period of gradual beta-cell destruction precedes the onset of overt diabetes with signs of beta-cell autoimmune damage occurring up to 8 years before its onset.

III. PATHOGENESIS OF TYPE 1 DIABETES

A. Genetic Factors

At the time of presentation of type 1 diabetes more than 80% of those so afflicted have no known first-degree relative with diabetes. In spite of this fact, there are important genetic factors that appear to play a role in the pathogenesis of this syndrome (2).

When one uses the family history to predict type 1 diabetes, an individual with an affected parent, sibling, or child has a roughly 5% lifetime chance of becoming diabetic. On the other hand, if one identical twin has type 1 diabetes, the other twin has only a 30–50% of developing this form of diabetes. This suggests that the development of type 1 diabetes is not solely due to genetic factors, for which one would predict a 100% concordance. For two parents with type 1 diabetes the association is (30–50%) similar to that seen with an identical twin sibling. A mother with diabetes has a 2% chance of transmitting it to her offspring, whereas a father with diabetes has a 6% risk.

Association with certain HLA antigens is also a powerful predictor for the development of type 1 diabetes. An initial association was found with the class I HLA alleles B-8 and B-15, whereas a negative association has been demonstrated with HLAB-7. With the definition of the class II HLA (immune responsiveness complex), stronger positive associations have been demonstrated between HLA DR3 and DR4 and type 1 diabetes. Ninety-five percent of type 1 diabetes patients carry DR3, DR4, or both, compared with 45% in the general population. More recent data have suggested that another class II allele in the DQ group may be the primary class II antigen associated with type 1 diabetes. Each DQ gene expresses an α- and β-protein chain on cell surfaces that together are responsible for presentation of antigens to immunologically active T cells. The structure of these antigen-presenting sites, and more specifically the amino acid composition of the β-chain, seems to be important in determining the risk of developing type 1 diabetes. The presence of an aspartic acid residue at position 57 of the DQ β-chain (non–Asp-57) is protective for the development of type 1 diabetes, and most individuals who develop type 1 diabetes have another amino acid, such as alanine at this position. Also the presence of an arginine residue at position 52 of the α-chain of the DQ (DQ* Arg-52) increases diabetes risk, whereas a nonarginine at this position decreases risk. Inheritance of a combination of DQ* non–Asp-57 and DQ* Arg-52 seems to be particularly diabetogenic, with two-thirds of the risk of type 1 diabetes being explained by the presence of these two antigens in most populations. Because the presentation of antigens to T cells is dependent on the structure of α- and β-chains encoded by DQ on the antigen-presenting cell surface, there is a strong biological basis supporting the role played by structural changes produced by DQ polymorphisms in the pathogenesis of type 1 diabetes.

Siblings of patients with type 1 diabetes are more likely to develop diabetes if they are HLA identical than those who share no haplotypes. The absolute risk for such an individual may be up to 20% by age 30, whereas those who share no haplotypes may have approximately a 1% risk.

B. The Role of Viruses

An infectious etiology for type 1 diabetes has been suspected because of the seasonal variation that has been observed. The highest incidence occurs in the winter and the lowest in the warmer summer months. Multiple viruses have been implicated in the pathogenesis of type 1 diabetes, and their role has been supported by laboratory and epidemiological data. Viral agents such as coxsackievirus B4, cytomegalovirus (CMV), mumps, and rubella have been studied most intensively as etiological agents in type 1 diabetes. Circulating antibodies to coxsackievirus B4 are found in a high percentage of new-onset type 1 diabetes, and a diabetic syndrome similar to type 1 diabetes can be produced in laboratory animals infected with the encephalomyocarditis virus, which along with the coxsackievirus is a member of the picornavirus family. Persistent CMV infections have been associated with the incorporation of viral DNA into host cells, which could change beta-cell antigenicity and lead to an autoimmune process. Approximately 20% of those with the congenital rubella syndrome (CRS) develop type 1 diabetes, and studies have also shown increased rates of type 1 diabetes 4 years after an epidemic of mumps virus. A role for possible host–viral interactions has come from data showing that coxsackievirus B infections are more common in association with HLA DR3, and that the highest frequency of diabetes occurred in the CRS with DR3 or DR4.

Some have questioned that an etiological relation exists between viral infections and type 1 diabetes, suggesting instead that the nonspecific increase in insulin requirements associated with acute infections precipitates overt diabetes in a group of patients who already have significant beta-cell damage. It has also been postulated that interferon or other cytokines associated with viral infections may trigger an incipient autoimmune process.

C. The Role of Autoimmunity

There is a significant body of data currently available supporting an autoimmune etiology for type 1 diabetes.

1. Humoral Markers

There are a number of humoral immune markers of islet cell inflammation associated with type 1 diabetes (3). These are particularly useful to the clinician because they can be used as markers for incipient beta-cell damage. A high prevalence of circulating anti-islet antibodies has been found in patients with newly discovered type 1 diabetes (anticytoplasmic and cell surface antibodies), and the presence of these antibodies seems to be predictive for the eventual onset of type 1 diabetes. Anti-insulin antibodies are also found in 30% of patients with new-onset type 1 diabetes and an increased prevalence of IA-2 autoantibodies against a beta–cell-associated enzyme (tyrosine phosphatase) has also been observed. Although increased titers of these IgG antibodies can be demonstrated in type 1 diabetes, it appears that they are not directly involved in the pathobiology of islet cell damage, although they serve as important clinical markers of an ongoing autoimmune process.

2. T–Cell Mediated Beta-Cell Damage

Activated CD4 and CD8 T cells produce cell-mediated cytotoxicity against insulin-secreting cells, and they inhibit insulin release from beta cells in vitro. These T cells also constitute most mononuclear cells that infiltrate the islet and are beta-cytotoxic producing the characteristic insulitis seen in type 1 diabetes. Activated T cells and macrophages also release cytokines, such as tumor necrosis factor (TNF), interleukin-1 (IL-1), or toxic free radicals (superoxide) and nitric oxide (NO) that may be important mediators of beta cell damage.

3. Beta-Cell Antigens That Trigger the Immune Process

There has been intense interest in the putative islet antigen or antigens that may initiate the autoimmune process that eventually leads to beta-cell destruction. One recent candidate has been a 64-kDa antigen that has been identified as glutamic acid decarboxylase (GAD), and antibodies to this islet protein may be more predictive for susceptibility to diabetes than other measurable antibodies (4). Two recent studies have shown that loss of tolerance and the appearance of sensitized T cells and antibodies to GAD occur early in genetically diabetic (NOD) mice and precedes loss of tolerance to most other beta-cell antigens. These studies suggest that autoimmunity directed against GAD on the islet surface is the initial step in the destruction of the beta cells in this important model of type 1 diabetes. Recent data has also indicated that the important beta-cell insulin precursor, proinsulin, may also be an antigenic trigger for type 1 diabetes. Adoptive transfer of proinsulin reactive T cells can rapidly produce insulitis and diabetes, and 100% of new-onset type 1 diabetes patients have T cells that are reactive with proinsulin.

4. Association with Other Autoimmune Endocrine Diseases

An increased incidence of endocrine diseases, characterized by autoimmune destruction of specific endocrine tissues (Hashimoto's thyroiditis, adrenal insufficiency, vitiligo, pernicious anemia, and others) has also been found in association with type 1 diabetes, which further supports the role of autoimmunity in the pathogenesis of type 1 diabetes.

D. Environmental Factors

Several studies have suggested that children fed cows milk at a young age are more likely to develop type 1 diabetes than those who were breastfed. Increased titers of antibodies to a specific antigenic segment of cows milk protein (bovine serum albumin; BSA) have also been demonstrated in subjects with type 1 diabetes, and these antibodies cross-react with p69, a beta-cell surface protein (5). Work in this area is ongoing, and the nutritional and practical implications of this data have yet to be addressed.

IV. CLINICAL PRESENTATION

A. Presentation with Diabetic Ketoacidosis

Clinically, approximately 20–30% of those who present with type 1 diabetes do so with virtually complete lack of insulin effect, manifested as a severe metabolic syndrome, such as diabetic ketoacidosis. When a child or teenager presents with polyuria, polydipsia, nausea, vomiting, weight loss, and breathlessness and when hyperglycemia (> 200 mg/dL) and strong serum ketones are found, there is little doubt that one is dealing with type 1 diabetes. The clinical manifestations of severe insulin deficiency are primarily related to hyperglycemia and metabolic acidosis resulting from high levels of strongly acidic ketoacids.

1. Hyperglycemia

Elevated serum glucose concentrations (> 200 mg/dL) can result in an osmotic diuresis and lead to the symptoms of polyuria and polydipsia that are characteristic of diabetes. This diuresis leads to excessive urinary loss of sodium and results in varying degrees of sodium depletion and dehydration. Other salts, such as potassium, phosphate, and magnesium, are also lost, resulting in total body depletion. These losses may be less obvious at the time of diagnosis owing to intracellular–extracellular shifts from concurrent acid–base disturbances and that these salts are primarily found intracellularly. The major symptoms resulting from hyperglycemia and dehydration are fatigue and reduced stamina, weight loss, postural lightheadedness, visual blurring, and genital yeast infections. As progressive dehydration occurs, more marked degrees of hyperglycemia may be seen, leading to a hyperosmolar state and mental status changes.

2. Ketosis

If severe insulin deficiency is present, ketosis or ketoacidosis is likely to occur. Insulin deficiency results in a massive mobilization of fatty acids from adipose tissue that are converted to ketones (acetoacetate and β-hydroxybutyrate) which, in turn, produce metabolic acidosis. The major symptoms resulting from diabetic ketoacidosis (DKA) include nausea and vomiting, breathlessness, and abdominal pain.

3. Laboratory Confirmation

It requires only two blood tests that quantify pathologically elevated levels of plasma glucose and serum ketones to confirm the diagnosis of DKA. Ketoacidosis is associated with blood sugar levels higher than 200 mg/dL although it is more common to see values in the 500–600 range, and glucose concentrations can run up to more than 1000 mg/dL in severe cases. Elevated levels of ketoacids are generally established by measuring acetoacetate in plasma by the nitroprusside reaction (Acetest). Observing a strong purple color when one places a drop of serum or plasma on a crushed nitroprusside tablet is diagnostic of pathological levels of ketoacids and when found with hyperglycemia, is diagnostic of diabetic ketoacidosis. Other laboratory tests are used to confirm the diagnosis, including a reduced level of bicarbonate, an increased anion gap, hyperkalemia, a low pH and P_{CO_2} concentration on arterial blood gas determination.

B. Other Causes of Ketoacidosis

There are relatively few other disease states that can be confused with DKA. Alcoholic ketoacidosis presents with metabolic acidosis and elevated levels of ketoacids in plasma, following heavy ethanol intake (6). It can be differentiated from DKA, however, by measuring blood glucose levels, which are generally either normal or low. Prolonged fasting also leads to increased breakdown of fat, resulting in increased ketone production. Although some ketonuria can be seen with fasting, the slight increase in plasma ketones that accompanies it does not result in a positive plasma nitroprusside test, and should not be confused with ketoacidosis.

C. Treatment

The treatment of DKA will be discussed in Chap. 40, thus, it will not be discussed in detail here. It basically involves the intravenous infusion of insulin and the replacement of lost fluid and electrolytes. Replacement of depleted levels of potassium, and in some patients, phosphate and magnesium, is also required.

D. Differentiating Type 1 from Type 2 Diabetes

Although the diagnosis is not difficult to make when a young person presents with DKA, distinguishing type 1 from type 2 diabetes is less obvious when a slightly overweight, middle-aged individual presents with hyperglycemia and negative ketones test results. It is not unusual for a person with type 1 diabetes to retain residual beta-cell function and present with nonketotic hyperglycemia, a picture that can be easily confused with new-onset type 2 diabetes. Under these circumstances, there are certain points in the history and physical examination as well as laboratory tests that can be helpful in differentiating type 1 from type 2 diabetes.

1. Clinical Factors

A person presenting with type 1 diabetes is more likely to be lean or have a normal body weight, and his or her family history will reveal that fewer than 20% will have a first-degree relative (parent, sibling, or child) with diabetes. Most patients have also experienced significant weight loss just before diagnosis. Age is also helpful, in that type 1 diabetes is more likely to be present in younger persons, particularly in those whose age is less than 20 years. Another characteristic suggestive of type 1 diabetes is the presence of another autoimmune endocrine disease, such as primary hypothyroidism (Hashimoto's thyroiditis), hyperthyroidism (Graves disease), vitiligo, or less commonly, addisonian adrenal insufficiency and pernicious anemia. A strong family history of such conditions, and perhaps of autoimmune disease, such as rheumatoid arthritis, is also seen more commonly in association with type 1 diabetes.

2. Glycemic Patterns

The glycemic patterns and response to exogenous insulin may also be helpful in determining if one is dealing with type 1 or type 2 diabetes. Individuals with type 1 diabetes owe their diabetic state to beta-cell failure and an inability to increase insulin secretion. The insulin response to meals and stress is more severely impaired in type 1 diabetes, resulting in greater elevation of glucose levels in the postprandial period and greater fluctuations from day to day. Individuals with type 1 diabetes are also likely to show more dramatic increases in glycemia with stress caused by intercurrent illnesses and emotional stressors.

3. Insulin Sensitivity

Another characteristic associated with type 1 diabetes is relatively normal tissue sensitivity to insulin when compared with most individuals with type 2 diabetes.

Although DKA and chronic hyperglycemia secondary to type 1 diabetes may be associated with substantial and reversible insulin resistance, an individual with type 1 diabetes and sporadic elevations of blood glucose will generally respond promptly to relatively small doses (< 10 U) of rapid-acting insulin.

4. Response to Oral Agents

Some patients with type 1 diabetes and persistent beta-cell function may initially respond to enhances of insulin secretion, such as sulfonylureas and repaglanide, if sufficient beta-cell reserve exists. Conversely, their response to these agents may be slight if beta-cell damage is more advanced, and no response will occur once the disease is fully established. Insulin sensitizers, such as metformin and troglitazone, are generally ineffective because inherent insulin resistance plays a relatively minor role in the pathogenesis of type 1 diabetes.

5. Laboratory Tests

In selected patients, the use of laboratory tests that quantify autoimmunity or insulin secretion may be useful in differentiating type 1 from type 2 diabetes. The presence of a positive test for islet cell antibodies (ICAs) in plasma is virtually diagnostic for type 1 diabetes in the setting of hyperglycemia (3). Approximately 80% of individuals with type 1 diabetes will have detectable titers of ICAs at the onset, whereas the titers fall off substantially over the next 5–10 years. To have confidence that you are obtaining an accurate ICA measurement, it is important that the performing laboratory have a test standardized to the Juvenile Diabetes Foundation (JDF) standards. Tests for anti-insulin antibodies are less useful owing to the lower incidence of diagnostic titers. Anti-GAD antibodies have promise as a diagnostic test in the future, but are currently less useful owing to the lack of availability and standardization (3).

Measurement of plasma insulin or C peptide levels may also be useful in deciding whether one is dealing with type 1 or type 2 diabetes. Demonstrating low basal levels of insulin ($< 5 \mu$ U/mL) before treatment is highly suggestive of the diagnosis of type 1 diabetes for most persons with type 2 diabetes have higher fasting levels (15–20μ U/mL), secondary to insulin resistance, and greater degrees of residual beta-cell function. If the patient has already been started on a therapeutic insulin regimen, one can take advantage of the fact that equivalent amounts of connecting peptide (C peptide) are secreted for each mole of insulin secreted by the beta cell, although C peptide remains elevated because of its longer half-life. Measurement of C peptide, therefore, will reveal the degree of persistent insulin secretion and, if low, is also suggestive of type 1 diabetes. A low level within 1 or 2 h of a meal or following the administration of glucagon is even more specific for low beta-cell reserve.

6. Less Common Diabetes Types with a Similar Clinical Picture

Discrimination of several other types of diabetes from type 1 diabetes may be particularly difficult. One obvious type is diabetes secondary to pancreatic disease, such as chronic pancreatitis or following pancreatectomy. This type of diabetes may appear quite similar to type 1 diabetes, except for a tendency to greater glycemic fluctuations and insulin sensitivity owing to concurrent glucagon deficiency. Pancreatic diabetes may require management strategies similar to type 1 and can usually be identified by the medical history. Another type of diabetes that may resemble type 1 in its initial stages is a group of diabetes types that involve genetically programmed beta-cell dysfunction (7). This syndrome previously called maturity-onset diabetes in the young (MODY), is characterized by autosomal dominant inheritance, and it may be diagnosed before the age of 20. It is not associated with obesity, tends to present with only mild to moderate hyperglycemia, is ICA-negative, and does not tend to show progression over time. The chromosomal location of the genes responsible for each type (MODY 1–3) has been identified, as have the downstream consequences manifested by specific types of beta-cell insensitivity to glucose-stimulated insulin release.

Another possible type of diabetes that can be confused with type 1 diabetes is one seen in young African American patients who can present with acute symptoms of hyperglycemia and initially require insulin. Months to years later, however, a more typical non–insulin-dependent picture ensues, when the insulin is discontinued, and a more typical type 2 diabetes pattern is seen (8). This may be similar to a syndrome called J-type diabetes that has been observed in young black Jamaican patients.

V. TREATMENT OF TYPE 1 DIABETES

A. Dietary Treatment

The patient with full-blown type 1 diabetes is absolutely dependent on insulin, but a nutritious, balanced diet, with the appropriate caloric distribution to balance the administered insulin, is important to maintain glycemic control. There are more or less rigid approaches to dietary therapy, but most subscribe to the recommendations of the ADA on dietary principles. The calories should be distributed to avoid excessive excursions in blood sugar and to prevent hypoglycemia while maintaining nutrition and body weight. A common pattern includes three meals, combined with midmorning, midafternoon, and bedtime snacks. Exchange lists, which provide lists of foods with similar content of carbohydrate, protein, or fat, are also commonly used, allowing meals to be planned using foods within each group interchangeably. Because carbohydrates (including sugars and starches) are the major cause of postprandial glycemic excursions, a method of counting the amount of carbohydrate (carbohydrate counting) in each meal and covering it with rapid-acting insulin in a ratio of 1 U/10–20 g, has been used with considerable success. Dietary composition should also be modified for other commonly associated risk factors, such as hyperlipidemia, hypertension, and such. Only 10% of fat is generally given as saturated fat. The more traditional approach to achieve balance between administered insulin and caloric intake has been to design an insulin schedule and to have the patient ''eat up'' to the insulin dose administered. With the advent of carbohydrate counting and rapid-onset insulins, it is now possible to selectively cover each meal with the appropriate amount of insulin. This allows one to achieve optimal control while avoiding weight gain and reducing the frequency of hypoglycemia.

B. Insulin Therapy

1. Introduction

Because patients with type 1 diabetes are insulinopenic, the major goal of insulin therapy is to provide full 24-h replacement of the patient's insulin needs. The normal pattern of beta-cell function in nondiabetic individuals is to constantly secrete small quantities of basal insulin in the fasting state and to provide immediate, quantitative intraportal boluses of insulin in response to food ingestion. Modern insulin therapy attempts to deliver exogenous subcutaneous insulin in patterns that mimic normal endogenous secretion. To achieve currently acceptable goals for glycemic control in type 1 diabetes, intensive insulin regimens are generally required. These employ multiple injections of insulin or the use of devices (insulin pumps) that can be programmed to continuously deliver basal and intermittent boluses of rapid-acting insulin.

2. Multiple (Split)-Dose Insulin Injections

This pattern of insulin administration is necessary in most patients with type 1 diabetes. Generally, combinations of short (regular or lispro), intermediate (NPH or Lente), and long-acting (Ultralente) insulins are used to provide optimal insulinization in the fasted, fed, and postabsorptive (4- to 5-h postprandial) states. Understanding the idealized time course of the currently available injectable insulins is necessary to use them successfully in the clinical setting.

Automated insulin delivery devices (insulin pumps) that can be programmed to infuse variable basal rates of short-acting insulin as well as preprandial boluses of insulin subcutaneously are now available. These or multiple insulin injections can be used as part of an intensive therapeutic regimen. More detailed information on the use of insulin pumps and multiple injections are discussed in Chap. 19 on insulin therapy.

3. Complications Involved in Intensive Insulin Regimens

Achieving optimal glycemic control in type 1 diabetes involves a trade-off between the glucose-lowering effects of insulin and the increasing risk of hypoglycemia that occurs as tighter glycemic control ensues.

a. Hypoglycemia

Hypoglycemia (9) is common during intensive insulin therapy of type 1 diabetes and can present as shakiness, hunger, anxiety, sweating, tachycardia, confusion, and behavioral change, or with other more atypical patterns. In a given patient the symptom complex associated with hypoglycemia may be quite reproducible. In its most severe form hypoglycemia can result in coma, seizures, or central nervous system (CNS) damage, secondary to prolonged neuroglycopenia. Hypoglycemic unawareness, the loss the adrenergic warning signs of hypoglycemia, may occur following 5 or more years of type 1 diabetes, and is particularly common in patients with autonomic neuropathy. In persons with hypoglycemic unawareness, the first symptoms of hypoglycemia generally relate to neuroglycopenia, and can rapidly lead to confusion or more severe manifestations if not promptly treated. The loss of counterregulation, or the ability to spontaneously raise the blood sugars in response to hypoglycemia, can accompany hypoglycemic unawareness and can further increase the risk of prolonged hypoglycemia. Both of these problems are exacerbated by tighter glycemic control (10), and a hypoglycemic event increases the risk of hypoglycemic unawareness and poor counterregulation during the next event (11). In patients who lack adequate early-warning signs, the danger of severe hypoglycemic reactions is increased; under these circumstances, it may become necessary to compromise on the treatment goals for tight glycemic control. For suggestions on methods of managing this difficult problem in the clinical setting refer to Chap. 31 on the management of hypoglycemia.

b. Somogyi Effect and Dawn Phenomenon

Glycemic control during the night, when prolonged fasting and less frequent blood glucose testing occur, can be particularly difficult. Nocturnal control is also more complicated because it includes the juxtapositioning of a time characterized by the greatest insulin sensitivity (midnight to 4 AM), with the period of greatest insulin resistance (4–8 AM) of the 24-h day.

The greater insulin sensitivity occurring from bedtime to 4 AM increases the risk of hypoglycemia during this time, which may awaken the patient with typical symptoms or may occur silently. Nocturnal hypoglycemia can also result in a glycemic rebound (the Somogyi effect), leading to morning hyperglycemia. The situation is further complicated in patients with poor counterregulation because nocturnal hypoglycemia can persist until the prebreakfast period, rather than leading to the classic rebound hyperglycemia. Another pattern that can be observed is a spontaneous morning rise in blood sugar levels (dawn phenomenon) following normal blood sugar levels in the middle of the night. Both this and the Somogyi phenomenon can be confused with nocturnal underinsulinization and lead to inappropriate increases in the evening insulin dose. One should consider these potential nocturnal glycemic patterns when deciding on the patient's evening insulin dose and insulin type. For example, one should avoid giving insulins that peak between midnight and 4 AM (NPH or Lente before supper, or excessive doses of rapid-acting insulins at bedtime) and consider using NPH or Lente HS, or a nonpeaking, longer-acting insulin before supper (Ultralente) instead. If you are unable to solve the problem with intuitive insulin adjustments, it may be necessary to have the patient repeatedly check their blood sugar in the middle of the night to resolve the issue.

c.   Insulin Allergy and Immune Insulin Resistance

Administering insulin can also result in a wide spectrum of immune reactions, including cutaneous and systemic hypersensitivity reactions, and insulin resistance, secondary to circulating IgG anti-insulin antibodies. Insulin lipoatrophy at the injection site can also be seen, as can lipohypertrophy (deposition of subcutaneous fat at the injection site). Although these reactions are less common than in the past now that highly purified pork and biosynthetic human insulins are available, they can still be a significant cause of morbidity in type 1 diabetes, particularly in the atopic patient.

Desensitization with highly purified insulins and occasionally glucocorticoid therapy may be required. Some resistance (insensitivity) to insulin action can also occur with persistent hyperglycemia and may be partially reversible with good control (so-called glucose toxicity).

d.   Other Potentially Correctable Factors That May Impair Glycemic Control

Several other possible causes for the clinically observed variation in response to insulin may exist. An understanding and correction of these problems may lead to better glycemic control and avoidance of hypoglycemia.

Injection Sites.   Although it is commonly taught that insulin injection sites can be randomly rotated, there is substantial data showing more rapid insulin absorption from abdominal sites and slower absorption from the leg. Areas of subcutaneous scarring or lipohypertrophy resulting from repeatedly injecting the same site can also lead to decreased absorption of injected insulin.

Activity.   It has long been recognized that physical activity enhances insulin action. This is partly due to exercise-induced tissue glucose utilization, but can also result from increased rates of insulin absorption from subcutaneous sites in an exercised limb.

Intermuscular Versus Subcutaneous Insulin Injection. The inadvertent intramuscular injection of insulin can cause more rapid and intense insulin action than that experienced with subcutaneous injection.

Temperature. Higher skin temperatures caused by a hot bath, can increase the rapidity of insulin absorption.

Mixing Insulin. Mixing regular insulin with either NPH or Lente/Ultralente insulins, and letting the mixture dwell in the syringe for more than a few minutes, can result in reduced availability and antihyperglycemic effect of regular insulin. This effect does not appear to occur when LisPro insulin is mixed with NPH, however.

Circulating Antibodies to Insulin. The time course of insulin absorption may vary considerably, owing to variable absorption of insulin from the injection site and to modification of insulin bioavailability caused by binding with endogenous IgG anti-insulin antibodies. These variations appear to be less striking in recent-onset type 1 diabetes or with the use of highly purified insulins.

e. Brittle Diabetes

Some patients show wide swings in glycemic control in spite of our best efforts (brittle diabetes). In these patients, tight control is particularly difficult to achieve, although careful investigation in a controlled setting usually will reveal significant, potentially correctable, deficiencies in their treatment regimen.

f. Insulin Coverage of Stress and Illness

Specific regimens must be used to provide the increased dosage of insulin needed for hyperglycemia associated with *acute stress* (infections, emotional, or other). It is virtually never appropriate to stop insulin in type 1 diabetes, and most acute illnesses lead to increased insulin requirements even with decreased food intake.

VI. MONITORING GLYCEMIC CONTROL

A. Self-Monitoring of Blood Glucose

Frequent and consistent monitoring of blood glucose levels is critical if one is to achieve glycemic goals in type 1 diabetes. Determining glucose levels in the pre- and postprandial state is necessary in determining the appropriate insulin dosage and achieving balance between this and other factors, such as meals and exercise, on a day-by-day basis. Most intensive treatment regimens for type 1 diabetes require at least three to four glucose determinations each day. There are many accurate, compact, and user-friendly glucose meters available for this purpose. All still require obtaining a drop of blood from a fingerstick, although there are several noninvasive meters under development.

There are many advantages of blood glucose monitoring in type 1 diabetes, including the following: This method documents blood glucose levels achieved in ordinary life and is the only effective method to safely achieve blood glucose levels of less than 150 mg/dL. Regular monitoring gives warning of hypoglycemia and helps in solving specific problems with control. It also reduces the frequency of hospital admissions and increases the rapport between physicians and patients, while increasing the patient's understanding of treatment goals. Urinary glucose determination is inaccurate and is no longer used, owing to the poor correlation with blood glucose levels.

B. Glycated Hemoglobin or Hemoglobin A_{1c} Determination

The glycated hemoglobin (HbA_{1c}) laboratory assay provides a single number that reflects average glycemic control over the preceding 2–3 months and is widely used as the method to monitor long-term glycemic control (12). It takes advantage of a spontaneous nonenzymatic chemical reaction between a protein (hemoglobin) and glucose, resulting in a stable ketoamine product. The level of this product reflects the exposure of hemoglobin to glucose levels over time and provides a clinical measurement of the average glucose concentration. The reaction of glucose with hemoglobin is part of generalized protein–sugar reaction, which occurs with virtually all of the proteins in the body.

Various methods are used to measure glycated hemoglobin, some of which measure the specific A_{1c} fraction, and some of which measure total glycated hemoglobin. The best-characterized and most-useful method in accurately predicting glycemic control and propensity to complications is the chromatographic assay by high performance liquid chromatography (HPLC). Other tests include ion-exchange and affinity minicolumns, immunoassays, electrophoretic methods, and others. Because there is considerable variation in the ability of these tests to determine the level of glycemic control, it is reasonable to ask your laboratory to justify the use of the assay that they have chosen and to provide you with data supporting its accuracy and normal range relative to the HPLC assay. The HbA_{1c} is actually relatively insensitive for the diagnosis of the diabetic state, because the levels can remain normal or only slightly elevated in the face of postprandial glucose concentrations higher than 200 mg/dL (13). Tests, such as fructosamine and glycated albumin, are also available to measure glycation of other circulating proteins (14). These tests are less widely used than the HbA_{1c} and reflect glycemic control over a shorter 3–4 week time period. They can be particularly useful when spurious HbA_{1c} values occur secondary to hemolytic anemia or hemoglobinopathies.

C. Glycemic Control and Complications

The long-standing debate over the effect of diabetic control on the development of diabetic complications has finally been resolved for type 1 diabetes, with the completion of the Diabetes Control and Complications Trial (DCCT; 15). This historic multicenter study prospectively compared 1440 subjects with IDDM who maintained good or poor glycemic control for 9 years for the development of diabetic microvascular and neuropathic complications. It unequivocally showed the benefit of tight glycemic control on the development of retinopathy (76% reduction), nephropathy (54% reduction), and neuropathy (60% reduction) in the intensive-control group and achieved these goals with an acceptable frequency of severe hypoglycemia.

VII. TREATMENT GOALS

It is critically important to set individual treatment goals for your patient with type 1 diabetes based on self-monitoring of blood glucose (SMBG) and hemoglobin A_{1c} levels. The reduction in microvascular and neuropathic complications in the DCCT were observed with an average HbA_{1c} of 7.2% in the intensively treated patients, compared with 9.0% in those treated by conventional methods. Because the reduction in risk of complications correlated continuously with the reduction in HbA_{1c} produced by intensive treatment, the results suggest that normalization may prevent complications altogether. The SMBG goals in the DCCT were 70–120 mg/dL before meals and at bedtime and less than 180 mg/dL 1.5–2 h postprandially. Achieving these goals, however, was associated with a threefold increase in the risk of severe hypoglycemia. Therefore the SMBG goals suggested by the ADA for type 1 diabetes are 80–120 mg/dL before meals and 100–140 at bedtime. The desired goal for HbA_{1c} is less than 7.0% (normal 4.0–6.0%), although this may have to be modified relative to the patients ability to learn an intensive regimen and risk of hypoglycemia (hypoglycemic awareness), as well as their age, degree of existing complications (end-stage renal disease or advanced cardiovascular–cerebrovascular disease), or the presence of coexisting diseases that might shorten their life expectancy.

VIII. STANDARDS OF CARE FOR TYPE 1 DIABETES

Standards of care have been formulated for patients with type 1 diabetes by an expert panel convened by the ADA (16). These standards provide clear and rational guidelines to assist the practicing physician in caring for their patient with type 1 diabetes, and are detailed in the reference provided as well as in publications provided by state and local diabetes groups.

A. Comprehensive Medical History

The initial visit includes a comprehensive medical history that will help in establishing the diagnosis or that confirms the diagnosis, as well as reviewing the current treatment plan, the degree of glycemic control, and the presence or absence of chronic complications. An accurate family history of diabetes or cardiovascular risk factors is important, as are the details of prior nutritional or diabetes education. It of particular importance to determine how the patient spends his or her day, including the degree and consistency of exercise, eating patterns, and determination of the degree of stress.

B. Physical Examination

The patient with type 1 diabetes is at high risk of developing eye, kidney, foot, nerve, cardiac, and vascular complications. A physical examination focused on the detection of pathological changes in these systems should be performed at the initial visit. Because persons with type 1 diabetes are at increased risk of other autoimmune endocrine diseases, a thyroid examination should also be performed, and because poor glycemic control can lead to delayed growth and maturation, children should be carefully evaluated for these factors.

C. Laboratory Examination

The laboratory examination should include tests that evaluate glycemic control (glucose and HbA_{1c}) as well as those that define associated complications, such as hyperlipidemia, renal function, albuminuria (routine urinalysis and albumin/creatinine ratio), and thyroid function.

D. Management Plan

Given these factors a management plan should be formulated for both short-term and long-term treatment goals. An optimal treatment plan should also include individualized nutritional recommendation, preferably by a registered dietitian familiar with diabetes, and patient and family education for self-management by a certified diabetes educator (CDE).

Continuing care is essential to the successful management of every patient with type 1 diabetes. At each visit the patient's progress in achieving treatment goals should be evaluated, and problems that have occurred should be reviewed and corrected. The frequency of visits will vary, depending on the needs of the patient. Those initiating therapy with insulin or starting intensive insulin regimens may have to be contacted daily during the initial stages. Weekly visits or contact may be needed in patients who are not meeting glycemic or blood pressure goals, or in those with progressive and unstable microvascular or macrovascular complications. Generally, it is advised that patients with type 1 diabetes should be seen at least quarterly for evaluation of their success at meeting treatment goals and for monitoring blood pressure, weight, foot care, and unstable eye or renal disease.

It is also recommended that quarterly determinations of HbA_{1c} be performed to monitor glycemic control.

Regular screening for progression of retinopathy, nephropathy, and neuropathy is also important to perform. After 3–5 years of type 1 diabetes it is recommended that yearly dilated retinal examinations be performed by an ophthalmologist or optometrist experienced in the management of diabetic retinopathy. Beginning at puberty or 5 years after the onset of type 1 diabetes, it is also recommended that yearly screening for albuminuria be performed. If an initial routine urinalysis is negative for protein, yearly screening for microalbuminuria with an overnight collection or with an albumin/creatinine ratio on a spot urine should be performed. Adult patients with type 1 diabetes should also be checked yearly with a fasting lipid profile to be sure that they meet the standards set forth by the National Cholesterol Education Program.

Knowledge of diabetes and self-management skills should also be assessed annually, and continuing education should be encouraged. Greater detail on standards of care for type 1 diabetes are reviewed in a later chapter in this text.

IX. CONCLUSIONS

Treating type 1 diabetes provides a significant challenge for the physician, the entire health care team, and most of all for the patient. Our role as health care providers is to understand this disease and its treatment and to provide the long-term medical and emotional support required. Because living with type 1 diabetes affects all aspects of your patient's life, it is best treated by a team approach. This team, which includes you, should also be composed of diabetes educators, dietitians, and optimally an endocrinologist who has a special interest in the treatment of diabetes. As for all chronic diseases, you must be there for the patient over the long-run, employing all of the skills that best exemplify the science and the art of medicine.

REFERENCES

1.   G Eisenbarth, A Ziegler, P Colman. Pathogenesis of insulin-dependent (type I) diabetes mellitus. In: GC, CR Kahn Weir, eds. Joslin's Diabetes Mellitus. Philadelphia: Lea & Febiger, 1994.
2.   MA Atkinson, NK McLaren. The pathogenesis of insulin-dependent diabetes mellitus. N Engl J Med 331:1428–1436, 1994.
3.   JP Palmer. Predicting IDDM: use of humoral immune markers. Diabetes Rev 1: 104–115, 1993.

4. TM Ellis, MA Atkinson. The clinical significance of an autoimmune response against glutamic acid decarboxylase. Nature Med 2:148–153, 1996.

5. J Karjalainen, JM Martin, M Knip, J Ilonen, BH Robinson, E Savilahti, HK Akerblom, H Dosch. A bovine albumin peptide as a possible trigger of insulin-dependent diabetes mellitus. N Engl J Med 327:302–307, 1992.

6. KD Wrenn, CM Slovis, GE Minion, R Rutkowski. The syndrome of alcoholic ketoacidosis. Am J Med 91:119–127, 1991.

7. SS Fajans, GI Bell, DW Bowden, JB Halter, KS Polonsky. Maturity onset diabetes of the young (MODY). Diabetic Med 13(suppl 6):90–95, 1996.

8. WE Winter, NK Maclaren, WJ Riley. Maturity-onset diabetes of youth in black Americans. N Engl J Med 316:285–291, 1987.

9. PE Cryer, J Gerich. Glucose counterregulation, hypoglycemia, and intensive insulin therapy in diabetes mellitus. N Engl J Med 313:232–241, 1985.

10. SA Amiel, WV Tamborlane, DC Simonson, DC Sherwin. Defective glucose counterregulation after strict glycemic control of insulin dependent diabetes mellitus. N Engl J Med 316:1376–1383, 1987.

11. PE Cryer. Iatrogenic hypoglycemia as a cause of hypoglycemic-associated autonomic failure in IDDM: a vicious cycle. Diabetes 41:255–260, 1992.

12. DE Goldstein, RR Little, RA Lorenz, JI Malone, DM Nathan, CM Peterson. Tests of glycemia in diabetes. Diabetes Care 18:896–909, 1995.

13. AL Peters, MB Davidson, DL Schriger, V Hasselblad. A clinical approach for the diagnosis of diabetes mellitus: an analysis using glycosylated hemoglobin levels. JAMA 276:1246–1252, 1996.

14. PH Winocour, D Bhatnager, P Kalsi, V Hillier, DC Anderson. Relative clinical usefulness of glycosylated serum albumin and fructosamine during short-term changes in glycemic control in IDDM. Diabetes Care 12:665–672, 1989.

9
Type 2 Diabetes Mellitus

Jack L. Leahy
University of Vermont College of Medicine, Burlington, Vermont

I. INTRODUCTION

Type 2 diabetes mellitus is a common metabolic disorder that is characterized by hyperglycemia without absolute insulin deficiency, and the triad of impaired glucose uptake into insulin-sensitive tissues, with skeletal muscle most affected, increased glucose production by the liver, and impaired insulin secretion. It is typically accompanied by other metabolic disorders that share defective insulin action as part of their pathogenesis (*metabolic syndrome* or *syndrome X*), such as central obesity, hypertriglyceridemia, atherosclerosis, hypertension, and hyper-androgenism in women secondary to polycystic ovaries (PCO). In the past, type 2 diabetes was often portrayed as the "mild" form of diabetes, with little prognostic significance. We now know that nothing could be farther from the truth. Diabetes has the dubious distinction of being the number 1 cause of adult blindness, kidney failure, and nontraumatic limb amputation in much of the industrialized world; type 2 diabetes makes up the majority of these statistics because of the 10:1 ratio of affected persons versus type 1 diabetes. Moreover, the worldwide incidence of type 2 diabetes and associated illnesses is skyrocketing, which has led the World Health Organization (WHO) to designate diabetes as a health crisis. A positive development is the availability of antidiabetic drugs that act at many different sites in the glucose homeostasis system. Thus, we now have the ability to use multidrug regimens that allow most patients to attain their target goal for glycemia, and the onus is on practicing physicians to be familiar with their use.

II. DIAGNOSIS

The report from the U.S. Expert Committee on the Diagnosis and Classification of Diabetes Mellitus (discussed in Chap. 4) published in 1997–1998 redefined

115

Table 1   Criteria[a] for the Diagnosis of Diabetes Mellitus

1. Symptoms of diabetes plus casual plasma glucose concentration $\geq$ 200 mg/dL (11.1 mmol/L). *Casual* is defined as any time of the day without regard to time since last meal. The classic symptoms of diabetes include polyuria, polydipsia, and unexplained weight loss.
2. FPG $\geq$ 126 mg/dL (7.0 mmol/L). Fasting is defined as no caloric intake for at least 8 h.
3. 2-h PG $\geq$ 200 mg/dL (11.1 mmol/L) during an OGTT. The test should be performed as described by WHO, using a glucose load containing the equivalent of 75 g of anhydrous glucose dissolved in water.

[a] These criteria are currently under review by the World Health Organization for worldwide adoption. *Source:* U.S. Expert Committee, 1998.

the biochemical criteria for the diagnosis of diabetes mellitus because the previous criterion of fasting plasma glucose higher than 140 mg/dL (7.8 mmol/L) did not identify all persons with microvascular complication-susceptible glucose intolerance, which is the phenotypic definition of diabetes. The revised criteria are shown in Table 1: fasting plasma glucose 126 mg/dL (7.0 mmol/L) or higher, 2-h plasma glucose during a 75-g oral glucose tolerance test (OGTT) of 200 mg/dL (11.1 mmol/L) or higher, random plasma glucose 200 mg/dL (11.1 mmol/L) or higher, *in combination* with symptoms of diabetes, such as polyuria, polydipsia, and unexplained weight loss. Confirmation of the diagnosis is required by repeat testing on a different day or by another of the diagnostic criteria. Note, glycated hemoglobin is not a diagnostic criteria because of concern over the lack of world-wide standardization for this test.

The Expert Committee also clarified criteria for the intermediate stage between normal glucose tolerance and diabetes. *Impaired fasting glucose* (IFG) is defined as 110–125 mg/dL (6.1–7.0 mmol/L) and *impaired glucose tolerance* (IGT) is defined as a 2-h OGTT plasma glucose 140–199 mg/dL (7.8–11.1 mmol/L). These categories have taken on increased significance of late. Although not typically associated with the microvascular complications of diabetes, they manifest increased cardiovascular risk factors, and several prevention trials against progression to full-blown diabetes or cardiovascular disease are planned or underway, including the National Institutes of Health-sponsored Diabetes Prevention Program (DPP).

Thus, the diagnosis of diabetes or an intermediate stage is rigidly defined. Once established, the next step is to identify the etiology from the classification shown in Table 2. Type 1 diabetes (approximately 10% of U.S. patients) entails autoimmune beta-cell destruction that usually results in absolute insulinopenia. The diagnosis is relatively easily made based on a typical presentation or the use

Table 2 Etiological Classification of Diabetes Mellitus

I. Type 1 diabetes (beta-cell destruction, usually leading to absolute insulin deficiency)
   A. Immune mediated
   B. Idiopathic
II. Type 2 diabetes (may range from predominately insulin resistance with relative insulin deficiency to a predominately secretory defect with insulin resistance).
III. Other specific types

Genetic defects of beta-cell function
　　Chromosome 12, HNF-1α (MODY3)
　　Chromosome 7, glucokinase (MODY2)
　　Chromosome 20, HNF-4α (MODY1)
　　Mitochondrial DNA
　　Others
Genetic defects in insulin action
　　Type A insulin resistance
　　Leprechaunism
　　Rabson–Mendenhall syndrome
　　Lipoatrophic diabetes
　　Others
Diseases of the endocrine pancreas
　　Pancreatitis
　　Trauma/pancreatectomy
　　Neoplasia
　　Cystic fibrosis
　　Hemochromatosis
　　Fibrocalculous pancreatopathy
　　Others
Endocrinopathies
　　Acromegaly
　　Cushing's syndrome
　　Glucagonoma
　　Pheochromocytoma
　　Hyperthyroidism
　　Somatostatinoma
　　Aldosteronoma
　　Others

Drug- or chemical-induced
　　Vacor
　　Pentamidine
　　Nicotinic acid
　　Glucocorticoids
　　Thyroid hormone
　　Diazoxide
　　β-adrenergic agonists
　　Thiazides
　　Phenytoin (Dilantin)
　　α-interferon
　　Others
Infections
　　Congenital rubella
　　Cytomegalovirus
　　Others
Uncommon forms of immune-mediated diabetes
　　"Stiff-man" syndrome
　　Anti-insulin receptor antibodies
　　Others
Other genetic syndromes sometimes associated with diabetes
　　Down's syndrome
　　Klinefelter's syndrome
　　Turner's syndrome
　　Wolfram's syndrome
　　Friedreich's ataxia
　　Huntington's chorea
　　Laurence-Moon-Biedl syndrome
　　Myotonic dystrophy
　　Porphyria
　　Prader-Willi syndrome
　　Others

IV. Gestational diabetes mellitus

Source: U.S. Expert Committee, 1998.

of specific immune markers, such as islet cell or anti-glutamic acid decarboxylase (GAD) antibodies. In contrast, type 2 diabetes has no specific diagnostic test and, instead, is a grouping of diseases with widely varying etiologies that share an ability to predispose to hyperglycemia. The diagnosis is made by a typical presentation and course, plus exclusion of as many of the other types of diabetes in Table 2 as seems relevant.

The terms *type 1* and *type 2 diabetes* were coined by the U.S. National Diabetes Data Group and the World Health Organizations in 1979–1980 to clarify the inexact terminology at the time, such as juvenile-onset, maturity-onset, ketosis-prone, and others. Also, *insulin-dependent diabetes* (IDDM) and *non–insulin-dependent diabetes* (NIDDM) were sanctioned to be synonymous terms for type 1 and 2 diabetes, respectively. However, these last terms have proved problematic, as IDDM is often incorrectly applied to patients with type 2 diabetes who take insulin. Subsequent attempts to clarify the confusion with terms, such as insulin-requiring non–insulin-dependent diabetes are unwieldy. Thus, the Expert Committee from 1997–1998 affirmed type 1 and 2 diabetes (using arabic numerals) as the only proper terms.

III. PATHOGENESIS

A. Genetic Basis

The pathogenesis of type 2 diabetes has been the subject of intense investigation. Figure 1 shows a general schema for the current understanding. It is clearly a genetic disease, as shown by how it runs through families. Many physicians consider the presence of a family history so central to the diagnosis that its absence mandates consideration of other etiologies.

Little information is known about the genetic defect(s). It is generally presumed that multiple gene defects exist (termed *heterogeneity*) in different patients and ethnic populations who share the ability to predispose to glucose intolerance. Inheritance fits no classic mendelian pattern, which has suggested that more than one gene defect is present in each patient (*polygenic*). Specific mutations are not yet identified. However, the last few years have seen the discovery of genetic etiologies for multiple rare diabetes syndromes, and one can assume the answers for type 2 diabetes will not be long in coming. Once mutations are identified, the door will open for screening high-risk persons before the onset of disease, development of targeted therapies, and a clearer understanding of the pathogenesis of the disease by studying animals with the same defects created by molecular techniques that "knockout" or disrupt that gene.

B. Environmental Factors

Affected persons inherit a predisposition for hyperglycemia, rather than an absolute process whereby hyperglycemia invariably occurs. This is evident from the

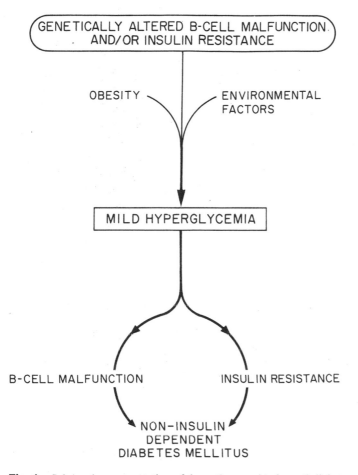

Fig. 1 Schematic representation of the pathogenesis of type 2 diabetes showing the three stages: genetic predisposition; environmental factors, including obesity, that determine whether the diabetes phenotype is expressed; and acquired (nongenetic) defects in insulin secretion and sensitivity that occur following onset of mild hyperglycemia.

rising incidence of diabetes in third-world populations who are undergoing urbanization and the well-known association between type 2 diabetes and its many exacerbating factors, such as obesity, aging, high fat diets, inactivity, hypertension, steroids, and pregnancy, all of which are associated with insulin resistance. Factors that impair insulin secretion, such as certain drugs, hypokalemia and hypocalcemia, and poor nutrition, are also linked to a higher incidence of diabetes. These factors are collectively referred to as environmental influences in type 2 diabetes. One understands the associations if glycemia is viewed as a balance between insulin secretion and tissue insulin sensitivity. When a genetic predisposition for hyperglycemia is present, anything that impairs the insulin sensitivity or insulin secretory capacity will cause a greater risk of glucose intolerance.

This concept provides a framework for prevention strategies. Multiple studies have shown a lowered conversion rate of IGT to frank diabetes using diet and weight loss programs. Even better-documented is the protective effect of regular exercise. Both strategies promote insulin sensitivity, or more accurately reduce insulin resistance. Insulin-sensitizing drugs may be equally effective, which underlies the drug treatment arm of the NIH-sponsored Diabetes Prevention Program. Persons with a family history of type 2 diabetes should be counseled that regular exercise and avoidance of obesity are proved ways to lower the risk of diabetes in themselves and their children. Prevention goals are not established, but general guidelines are to avoid obesity (within 10–20% of ideal body weight, or a body mass index [BMI] of ≤ 25) and perform every-other-day 30-min aerobic exercise.

C. Glucose Toxicity and Lipotoxicity

The third element is acquired defects in insulin secretion and sensitivity that appear coincident with the onset of mild hyperglycemia. These were recognized in the late 1970s, when studies reported improvements in insulin secretory capacity and sensitivity after intensive blood glucose control. The 1980s focused on hyperglycemia as the detrimental factor—the term *glucose toxicity* is used for this condition. A recent concept is that excessive blood and tissue levels of free fatty acids (FFA), which are metabolic breakdown products of triglycerides, may be causative of the defective insulin secretion and impaired insulin sensitivity (*lipotoxicity*).

Whether glucose toxicity, lipotoxicity, or another factor, such as beta-cell exhaustion is proved to cause the acquired defects in type 2 diabetes, this area of investigation holds promise for yielding novel pharmacological agents. Moreover, the concept is seen in the relatively easy hyperglycemic control that is observed in new-onset patients with type 2 diabetes after restoration of normoglycemia. Many experts recommend intensive blood glucose control early in the course of type 2 diabetes for this reason. No target range for HgA$_{1c}$ is established, but experience has suggested that near-normoglycemia is needed to reverse the acquired defects, and no higher than 7% is recommended.

IV. NATURAL HISTORY OF INSULIN RESISTANCE AND BETA-CELL DYSFUNCTION

Figure 2 shows the pathogenesis of type 2 diabetes in terms of the metabolic derangements of insulin resistance and impaired insulin secretion. *Insulin resis-*

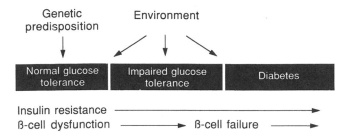

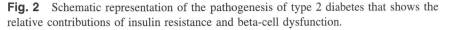

Fig. 2 Schematic representation of the pathogenesis of type 2 diabetes that shows the relative contributions of insulin resistance and beta-cell dysfunction.

tance is a commonly used term that confuses students and physicians who are new to the field of type 2 diabetes. Most tissues are insulin-sensitive, and there are multiple tissue-specific pathways and signaling systems. Type 2 diabetes is a complex syndrome, with some insulin-mediated effects being impaired and others spared, so that the typical usage of "insulin resistance" represents the two defective insulin-mediated processes that characterize type 2 diabetes—impaired glucose clearance or metabolism into insulin-sensitive tissues, and lowered effectiveness of insulin to suppress glucose production by the liver (see Chap. 6 for in-depth discussion)—as opposed to a global defect in insulin action.

Prospective studies of persons at risk for type 2 diabetes have shown that insulin resistance, in terms of impaired glucose clearance to skeletal muscle, predates the hyperglycemia. This finding is so well known that most physicians consider type 2 diabetes to be a disease of insulin resistance. However, the situation is more complex. Methods to quantify beta-cell function have been crude, until recently. Newly described methods have found that beta-cell dysfunction also is evident before hyperglycemia. The last two decades saw great disagreement over what constitutes the primary defect in type 2 diabetes—insulin resistance or beta-cell dysfunction? There is now a consensus that *both* pathogenic elements are active in the vast majority of affected persons.

The important concept from Fig. 1 and 2 is that persons with type 2 diabetes have insulin resistance and beta-cell dysfunction through genetic or acquired mechanisms. This explains why virtually all persons with this disease show the characteristic triad of elements for hyperglycemia, despite presumed diverse genetic etiologies. Stated another way, evolving diabetes *causes* part of the diabetes phenotype so that everyone would be expected to present with similar clinical characteristics. It also underlies why we treat virtually all populations with the same drugs.

V. ORGAN DYSFUNCTION CAUSING HYPERGLYCEMIA

Many reviews have been written about the triad of organ dysfunction that characterizes type 2 diabetes: beta-cell dysfunction, impaired glucose uptake and metabolism into insulin-sensitive tissues, and increased glucose production by the liver. An in-depth analysis is beyond the scope of this volume but some familiarity is necessary because it underlies the commonly used drug therapy.

A. Beta-Cell Dysfunction

Insulin secretion is highly regulated, reflecting its crucial role to regulate the storage, release, and metabolism of cellular fuels. Islet beta-cells respond to changes in glycemia and food intake in a complex fashion that maintains normoglycemia throughout the day. Beta-cell function is impaired in multiple ways in type 2 diabetes so that pharmacological augmentation of insulin secretion is one approach to treatment. Sulfonylureas act through this mechanism by binding to a protein on the beta-cell membrane that associates with the ATP-sensitive K^+ channel causing beta-cell depolarization and insulin secretion. The effect is sustained over the 24-h period, as opposed to a new class of drugs, meglitinides, that act in a comparable fashion, but have a very fast on–off insulinotropic effect and are taken premeals to selectively promote meal-induced insulin secretion.

B. Impaired Glucose Uptake and Metabolism Into Tissues

Insulin-mediated glucose disposal is mostly to skeletal muscle, with brain, splanchnic tissues, and adipocytes less important. Countless studies have shown impaired skeletal muscle glucose disposal or metabolism in type 2 diabetes. Troglitazone (thiazolidinedione class of drugs) promotes glucose uptake into muscle through its interaction with transcription factors, called peroxisome proliferator-activated receptors (PPARs), although other potential mechanisms have also been reported.

C. Increased Hepatic Production and Release of Glucose

The liver is the factory that transforms breakdown products of nutrient stores (amino acids, fatty acids, lactate) into glucose to prevent hypoglycemia between meals and overnight. It also stores glucose as glycogen for rapid delivery during emergent situations, such as acute hypoglycemia. Type 2 diabetes entails enhanced glucose production by the liver, and this mechanism mediates the fasting hyperglycemia. In other words, the normal nighttime production of glucose by the liver that prevents us from becoming hypoglycemic is exaggerated because of augmented gluconeogenesis. Metformin lowers hepatic glucose production in type 2 diabetes through an unknown cellular mechanism.

D. Postprandial Hyperglycemia

An increasingly used term is postprandial hyperglycemia, which refers to excessive rises in glycemia after meals, as opposed to premeal glycemia, which is less affected—it provides a physiological explanation for the prediabetes stage of impaired glucose tolerance (IGT). Postprandial hyperglycemia also accounts for the failed glycemic control in treated patients with full-blown diabetes who have acceptable fasting and premeal blood glucose levels, but have an unacceptable glycohemoglobin level. The most physiological approach to this problem is to replace dietary sugar and fat with complex carbohydrates and fiber, but that is not easily attained in many patients. α-Glucosidase inhibitors are competitive inhibitors of small-intestine disaccharidases, thus causing slowed carbohydrate absorption. Alternatively, meglitinides have a fast on–off insulinotropic effect and are used to selectively promote meal-induced insulin secretion.

VI. CLINICAL PRESENTATION

A. History

Most patients report no symptoms at presentation, which explains why the disease is discovered in most on a routine physical, during insurance screening, or as an unrelated finding when they go to the doctor for another reason. This concept also explains why so many cases remain undiagnosed, and why screening of high-risk persons is the cornerstone for finding those with this disorder. Symptoms, when present, are often insidious and may stem from a diabetes complication that is bringing them to medical attention (visual trouble, pain in the feet or a foot ulcer, impotence, cardiovascular or macrovascular disease) or a coexisting illness that exacerbates the hyperglycemia to symptomatic levels, such as dentition problems or an acute or chronic infection. Many physicians are unaware that the classic symptoms of diabetes (polyuria, polydipsia, weight loss) are rarely found in type 2 diabetes. In fact, the latter is so unusual that it suggests some other process, such as adult-onset type 1 diabetes, underlying malignancy, hyperthyroidism, or pancreatic disease and malabsorption. The one diabetes symptom that may be evident is nocturia, although it is rarely a complaint of the patient, and may stem from other causes, including prostatic hypertrophy, diuretic use, caffeine, alcohol, and such.

    Particularly troubling for physicians is nonspecific complaints, such as not feeling well or a lack of energy, when patients are found to be diabetic. The tendency is to identify these symptoms as being related to the diabetes when nothing else is found, and to use that to induce the patient to control their glycemia. Patients then expect reversal of their complaints when the target blood sugar is attained, which rarely occurs. The reality is that patients often feel poorly for a host of nonmedical reasons, and medical management of the diabetes does not solve those issues.

Thus, the principles are to screen for diabetes in high-risk individuals and in everyone older than 45 years of age using the recommendations in Table 3, and there are typically few or no symptoms so that new-onset diabetes with profound symptoms of whatever type warrants evaluation for alternative causes of that complaint.

The history serves other purposes. A general review of systems is performed to elicit findings that suggest a diabetic etiology other than type 2 diabetes. Factors that may have caused a recent onset or exacerbation of hyperglycemia are sought with weight gain, a lowered physical activity (work-related injury, job change, season change, recent stroke), and new medications (see Chap. 13), or illnesses most common. A complete medical and surgical history and medication list are crucial, as virtually any major illness is associated with a raised incidence of type 2 diabetes. Symptoms of other aspects of the metabolic syndrome are screened for including chest pain, shortness of breath, changed exercise capacity, ankle edema, or heart failure symptoms (coronary disease), claudication (peripheral vascular disease), and menstrual or fertility complaints (PCO).

Table 3 Screening in Asymptomatic, Undiagnosed Individuals

---

1. All individuals at 45 years of age and older. If normal, then at 3-year intervals.
2. Younger age (arbitrarily > 25 years of age) in high-risk individuals to be performed yearly:

        Obese (≥ 120% desired body weight or a BMI ≥ 27 kg/m^2)

        First-degree relative with diabetes of any type

        Member of a high-risk ethnic population (e.g. African American, Hispanic or Latino–American, Native American, Asian American, Pacific Islander)

        Delivered a baby weighing > 9 lb or have been diagnosed with gestational diabetes

        Hypertensive (≥ 140/90 mmHg)

        HDL cholesterol level ≤ 35 mg/dL (0.90 mmol/L) and/or a triglyceride level ≥ 250 mg/dL (2.82 mmol/L)

        On previous testing, impaired glucose tolerance (IGT) or impaired fasting glucose (IFG)

Source: U.S. Expert Committee, 1998

B. Physical Examination

There are no physical findings that diagnose type 2 diabetes. Instead, the examination is targeted to look for complications (retinopathy, neuropathy, carpel tunnel syndrome, cranial nerve palsies, peripheral vascular disease, foot examination), associated illnesses (central obesity, hypertension, and xanthomas), and findings for diabetes syndromes other than type 2 diabetes (Cushing's, acromegaly, hyperthyroidism, lipodystrophies). Acanthosis nigricans (see Chap. 32) is a dermatological manifestation of insulin resistance that is most often found at the base of the back of the neck. It has a black granular appearance that is velvety to touch, and is often described by patients as looking like dirt they cannot wash off. It is best known for its association with syndromes of extreme insulin resistance. However, given their rarity, it is most often found with milder forms of insulin resistance, such as obesity or PCO, with or without diabetes, and also in states that are not associated with insulin resistance, such as some cancers, or as an isolated finding. Other parts of the examination are to check injection sites for bruising in persons who are taking insulin suggesting poor technique or lipohypertrophy in patients who are not rotating their sites enough. The blood pressure and a careful thyroid examination are performed.

The foot examination holds particular significance, as no other aspect of the physical is so overlooked. Feet should be carefully inspected for altered anatomy, skin dryness, poor hygiene, and callouses, all of which may imply the need for more careful attention by the patient to routine foot care or the need for different shoes or inserts to counterbalance anatomical changes that promote abnormal pressure distribution. Any ulcer or other skin breakdown should be aggressively treated, usually in tandem with a podiatrist or vascular surgeon. Web spaces should be carefully inspected, as patients often do not dry adequately between their toes after washing their feet or when they use moisturizing cream, which over time macerates that area. Nails are carefully inspected with ingrown and pinched nails often needing removal. Chronic fungal nail infections are common, and well tolerated by most patients; it is up to the discretion of the physician whom to treat. Evidence for peripheral vascular disease is sought by palpation of pulses and feeling the warmth of the foot, although the latter can be misleading if neuropathy is present because blood can be shunted from the interior of the foot to the skin. The traditional screening method for neuropathy is a low-frequency tuning fork, which is subjective on the part of the patient and not quantitative. Newer methods use filaments. The testing of light touch or pain has little role in screening because both disappear when neuropathy is far advanced (see Chaps. 28 and 29 for detailed information on foot care and screening). Also, absence of the ankle reflex is a nonspecific finding that holds little import.

C. Laboratory Testing

Laboratory testing serves three main goals: (a) it eliminates causes of diabetes other than type 2 diabetes; (b) it screens for complications; and (c) it establishes the degree of hyperglycemic control.

By this point, the diagnosis of diabetes should be made. Because there is no specific diagnostic test for type 2 diabetes, the next step is to eliminate as much of Table 2 as seems pertinent for that patient. No routine screening is recommended, although frequently obtained tests are thyroid-stimulating hormone (TSH) reflecting the high frequency of hypothyroidism in the general population plus the occasional patient who has diabetes secondary to hyperthyroidism; ratio of iron to iron-binding capacity (hemochromatosis); and routine blood chemistry and hematology profiles, looking for undiagnosed systemic diseases. Targeted screening is done for conditions that are suggested by the history or physical examination. It is recommended that physicians search diligently and have a high suspicion level for another diabetic etiology for many of the illnesses associated with diabetes are insidious and subtle in presentation. Stated another way, if anything makes you consider another illness, screen for it. Relatively common reasons are weight loss or otherwise an atypical presentation for type 2 diabetes (type 1 diabetes); excessive alcohol use, weight loss, diarrhea or steatorrhea, hyperlipidemia history or xanthomas on examination (chronic pancreatitis); unusual facial, hand, or feet features, cardiomegaly, thyromegaly, sleep apnea (acromegaly); unexplained cardiac, neurological, pituitary, or hepatic disease (hemochromatosis); central obesity and hypertension, proximal muscle weakness or atrophy, striae, hirsutism, bruising (Cushing's); weight loss, atrial fibrillation, hypermetabolic state, thyromegaly (hyperthyroidism); difficult-to-control hypertension (pheochromocytoma); unusual appearance, altered physical or mental development (variety of genetic syndromes).

The second step is to screen for diabetes complications and other illnesses in the metabolic syndrome. Physicians are often surprised that type 2 diabetes can have established complications at diagnosis—one recent study noted a 25% incidence of retinopathy—which presumably reflects many patients going for years before the diagnosis is made. Moreover, visual loss, kidney failure, foot ulcer, or major vascular insufficiency event in the leg, impotence, or myocardial infarction may be what brings the patient to medical attention. *Thus, patients need to be screened carefully for complications at diagnosis.* Nephropathy is screened for by an assessment of urine protein; the current recommendation is to perform a routine urinalysis, and if positive for protein, to quantify albuminuria. However, many experts recommend going directly to quantify urine microalbumin using a laboratory-based measure, or the new high-sensitivity dipsticks. Blood lipid levels are assessed by total cholesterol, HDL cholesterol, LDL cholesterol, and triglycerides. Triglycerides are best measured fasting (which is the recommendation), although many physicians for convenience obtain a nonfasting lipid profile when the patient is first seen, and a fasting sample only if the triglyceride level is more than 200 mg/dL. Other diabetes complications are screened for by history (impotence, gastroparesis, coronary disease), examination (hypertension), or both (macrovascular disease and peripheral neuropathy).

The third step is to establish the degree of blood glucose control by a measure of glycated hemoglobin or another marker, such as fructosamine. Testing by glycated hemoglobin is familiar to most physicians. The principle is that most proteins undergo nonenzymatic glycosylation, with the proportion that is glycosylated at any time depending on its avidity for glucose, its turnover rate, and the blood/tissue glucose level. Hemoglobin is glycosylated at several sites. Modern methods reliably quantify the proportion of hemoglobin that is glycosylated with some methods identifying multiple peaks. Hemoglobin A_{1c} (HbA_{1c}) is the largest glycosylated peak and has been validated to be an accurate reflector of glycemia over the preceding 6–8 weeks, which reflects the long life span of red cells (the normal value is about 6% of the hemoglobin being HbA_{1c}). The test is particularly useful because virtually all of the studies that have determined current practice guidelines used this measure, and state and national guidelines are generally based on it. Furthermore, office-based relatively inexpensive machines are available that measure HbA_{1c} within a few minutes. A related test is total glycosylated hemoglobin, which combines the other minor peaks of glycated hemoglobin with HbA_{1c} (normal is generally 7.5–8%). It is comparable with HbA_{1c} in terms of quantifying glycemia, although there is a major risk that unknowing physicians will misinterpret the value as HbA_{1c}—*always know the normal values for results that come from unfamiliar laboratories or referring doctors.* Also, there are not the same national guidelines for this test as for HbA_{1c}, although many assays report an extrapolated HbA_{1c} value along with the glycohemoglobin value.

There are important subtleties to the interpretation of these tests in selected patients. There are multiple commercial assays for HbA_{1c} and total glycosylated hemoglobin, which use different techniques and have small differences in cross-reacting substances, and how they are affected by hemoglobinopathies, altering the avidity for glycosylation. You must know your assay. Also, anything that affects the life span of the red cell will alter the result. Best known are its being lowered by hemolytic anemias, sickle crisis, hypersplenism, recent transfusion, or hemorrhage. Finally, the long time to attain steady-state for this test has positive and negative effects; it allows an assessment of glycemia that is minimally influenced by a few days of nonrepresentative blood sugars because of illness or dietary issues, but also mandates waiting 1–2 months after a treatment change before requantifying the level. In that respect, fructosamine is preferable, as the equilibration time to steady-state measure is 7–10 days.

VII. ESTABLISHED TYPE 2 DIABETES

The prior discussion focused on the diagnosis and evaluation of persons with newly identified type 2 diabetes. Evaluation of a patient with established type 2 diabetes, who you are seeing for the first time, follows similar principles by assessing the following questions.

1. Is this typical type 2 diabetes using the history, physical examination, and available laboratory data? Is the course to date including response to therapy as expected? Are there historical or physical findings that suggest another etiology? Prior laboratory findings that are unexplained? The principle behind these questions is that the nonavailability of specific laboratory tests for type 2 diabetes means that physicians must constantly question the diagnosis, and be on the lookout for another etiology that is masquerading as type 2 diabetes.

2. What is the diabetes complication profile of your patient? This question requires knowing the current status, documented history, and prior and current therapy for established complications plus screening for nonidentified complications:

   Retinopathy as determined during a dilated examination by a qualified eye professional.

   Nephropathy by urine protein screening and quantification of albuminuria plus an assessment of creatinine clearance when indicated.

   Cardiovascular disease by history in terms of complaints related to chest pain, shortness of breath, especially during exercise or at night, altered exercise tolerance, or general nonspecific complaints of episodic not feeling well. An important parallel evaluation is the lipid status for HDL, LDL, and triglycerides, the smoking history, and whether the patient is taking aspirin for cardioprotection as is generally recommended.

   Lower extremity vascular insufficiency by physical examination and noninvasive or arteriogram studies indicated for complaints of claudication or physical findings that suggest vascular insufficiency.

   Neurological examination for cranial nerve palsies, mononeuropathies, carpel tunnel compression, and polyneuropathies. Also included is a careful examination of the feet for hygiene, calluses, and the shoes that are commonly worn to construct a risk profile for foot ulcers.

   Gastroparesis as suggested by early satiety or postmeal nausea and vomiting.

   Impotence in males or *dyspareunia or orgasmic dysfunction* in women.

   Blood pressure measurement for diagnosis or adequacy of treatment for hypertension.

Table 4 Complication Screening Guidelines

Every visit
    Measure weight and blood pressure
    Foot examination (high-risk)
    Counsel smoking cessation
Two to four times annually
    HbA$_{1c}$ twice yearly if meeting treatment goals and quarterly if not
Annually
    Fasting lipid profile
    Urine protein excretion with microalbumin and serum creatinine quantification as
        appropriate
    Dilated eye examination by qualified professional
    Dental examination by qualified professional
    Foot examination (low risk)

Source: Diabetes Care 22(Suppl1):S32–S41, 1999.

    An important difference from the newly diagnosed patient is the need to determine if the patient has been getting regular screening for complications, according to current guidelines (Table 4). Has the patient had a yearly dilated eye examination? Why not—what are the barriers? The same question can be asked for a yearly lipid profile, urinary protein, and regular blood pressure measurements and foot examinations. A flowsheet that tracks these parameters is extremely useful at making sure that guidelines are followed.

    The physician cannot depend on the patient to provide correct information on screening in terms of has it been performed, when, and what were the results? Pertinent studies that have been performed elsewhere *require written documentation of the findings.* It is extremely important when referring a patient to a specialist or to another physician that actual copies of laboratory and consultation reports be sent.

3. What is the glycemic control of your patient on their current therapy regimen? Home blood glucose measurements are very useful here, but the final answer requires a glycated hemoglobin measurement, which will also serve to confirm the accuracy of the patient's home blood glucose measurements. One caveat is that it may be prudent to wait 1 or 2 months before obtaining the baseline glycated hemoglobin if the patient's home blood glucose measurements suggest a change in the glycemia level within the last 4 weeks.

    The physician needs to develop a profile of previous glycemic control, based on glycohemoglobin measures, often with the help of the patient to interpret what might have been happening at those times. What is the weight and exercise history? Family or job stresses? Complicating medical issues such as surgeries or periods of lowered activity because of back or joint pain? A critical issue is to establish an accurate profile of prior oral hypoglycemic use. What drugs have been tried, at what doses, under what conditions, singly or in combination, with what effect? A common complaint from patients is physicians who try them on a drug (without effect) that had been used without success by another physician.

A critical part of the evaluation is to enlist the patient's insight into what has or has not worked for them. What is the biggest difficulty they have with blood sugars? Weight? Better exercise habits? What has been the most effective approach in the past? What has not worked and why? Patients should be included in developing the goals for therapy in terms of glycohemoglobin and others that may be pertinent such as blood pressure, weight loss, lipid values, exercise habits, and such. They need to understand what they are trying to do and why. Make the goals realistic. At times, a reduction of glycated hemoglobin to a level that is well above the national guideline is a triumph that has required great effort on the part of the patient, and needs to be acknowledged and celebrated. Too many patients feel alienated from their doctors because the message they get (real or imagined) is that it is never good enough.

VIII. THERAPY

Physicians are generally familiar with the stepped approach to the treatment of type 2 diabetes (Table 5; another version of the same concept is shown in Fig. 3 from the American Diabetes Association, although it was published before troglitazone and repaglinide became available), because that principle has been around for decades. However, its application is becoming increasingly difficult as the number of available oral hypoglycemic agents increases. Also, the sad fact is that having more drugs has not resulted in better diabetes control for everyone,

Table 5   Stepped Therapy for Type 2 Diabetes

Step 1:	Nutritional therapy, exercise, lifestyle changes
	Training in self management and survival skills
Step 2:	Add oral agents
	Monotherapy
	Combination therapy
Step 3:	Add or change to insulin
Step 4:	Intensive insulin therapy program

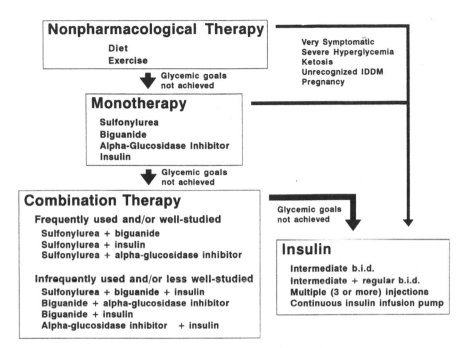

Fig. 3 Stepped approach to the therapy of type 2 diabetes. Note the schema was developed before troglitazone and repaglinide's availability. (From ADA, 1995.)

and that optimal control remains elusive for many patients despite complex multidrug regimens. Complicating the issue is the high price of many of the drugs, and patients are frequently receiving medication lists that defy their ability to keep everything straight. Add to that a disease that takes away freedoms that we take for granted, and too many patients feel disenfranchised and defeated by life.

Physicians must counter these feelings by instilling a belief that the diabetes is controllable. Patients want to view their physicians as advocates and confessors, not as detached or critical. Be flexible; different treatment approaches work for different people. Celebrate successes, even when small. A 5-lb weight loss in a grossly overweight patient may be of little practical significance, but may motivate them to go farther. Enlist the help of the patient's family and friends. Patients need to know they are not alone. Emphasize positives about the treatment program, such as the diet having health benefits for the whole family. Family-based walking or exercise programs can make patients feel their diabetes has brought the family closer together. A fear of many patients is that the diabetes will be passed down to their children. Empowering the patient to achieve control of their own lifestyle so that positive habits can be instilled in their children can have emotional and practical benefits. The summary of all these comments is: Know your patient. Approach their diabetes as a joint effort between you, them, and their family. Advise and guide, do not demand or dictate. Define treatment goals clearly. Do not be satisfied until they are met, but understand the process takes time. Be positive. Celebrate success.

A. Treatment Goals

Perhaps the most critical element of a treatment program is to define the goals. Treatment must be based on results. Even when patients feel well and there has been a lowering of glyccmia, blood pressure, or lipemia with a particular medication, if the treatment goal is unmet then a change must be made. This can be difficult, as improvements of any magnitude often leave patients energized, and being told that it is not enough can be deflating. That is why patients need to be aware of the goals from the beginning—what has to be done and why. Well-known guidelines for blood glucose control and associated parameters, such as blood pressure and lipemia exist; Table 6 shows those from the American Diabetes Association (see Chap. 4). Although these goals are appropriate for many if not most patients, each patient must be assessed individually.

B. United Kingdom Prospective Diabetes Study

Any discussion of treatment goals for type 2 diabetes must consider the U.K. Prospective Diabetes Study (UKPDS; published in September 1998), as it will

Table 6 Treatment Goals

	Goal	Action required
Glycemic indices		
Preprandial (mg/dL)	80–120	$< 80, > 140$
Bedtime (mg/dL)	100–140	$< 100, > 160$
HbA$_{1c}$ (%)	< 7	> 8
Lipids		
Total cholesterol (mg/dL)	< 200	
HDL cholesterol (mg/dL)	> 45	
LDL cholesterol (mg/dL)	Acceptable < 130 Optimal < 100	
Triglycerides (mg/dL)	Acceptable < 200 Optimal < 150	
Blood pressure	$< 130/85$	140/90

Source: ADA, 1998.

predictably influence future guidelines. Nearly 4000 persons in the United Kingdom with new-onset type 2 diabetes (mostly whites) received 3 months of intensive diet. If glycemic control was inadequate, they were randomized to intensive treatment using metformin, a sulfonylurea, or insulin, and compared with conventional therapy using continued diet alone (for the most part, although there was some overlap in groups if hyperglycemia in the conventional group became severe) over 10 years. The major findings were: HbA_{1c} 7.0% in the intensive groups versus 7.9% in the conventional group, with no clear superiority of any of the intensive treatment regimens; this difference in glycemic control was associated with a 25% lowered incidence of microvascular complications with a minimal increase of hypoglycemia and some mild weight gain. Importantly, cardiovascular events were not increased in any intensive-treated group, which puts to rest the concern that sulfonylureas or insulin may induce coronary disease through their effects to promote hyperinsulinemia.

There was a subarm of the study that examined intensive (starting with atenolol or captopril, although many patients required two or three agents) versus conventional blood pressure control in 1148 hypertensive patients. The intensive group blood pressure averaged 144/82 mmHg, with no major difference in the effectiveness of atenolol or captopril, versus 154/87 mmHg in the conventional group. Macrovascular endpoints of death and stroke were lowered 32–44%. Unexpectedly, microvascular endpoints (primarily retinal photocoagulation) were also lowered, independently of any change in glycemia. Finally, poor glycemic and blood pressure control produced a "double jeopardy," with clear additive consequences on long-term outcome.

The major messages for practicing physicians are (a) subtle changes in glycemia and blood pressure are associated with major microvascular and macrovascular risks, and those effects are highly additive. Prevention requires very tight goals for HbA_{1c} (7.0%) and blood pressure (144/82 or less); (b) no treatment regimen is clearly superior in either endeavor—attaining the goal is the key, not the drug(s) used. Having said that, patients often require combination therapy with multiple agents for both blood pressure and glycemic control; (c) the whole patient must be treated—glycemia, blood pressure, and lipemia independently influence the outcome of our patients, and aggressively treating one without the others fails to meet our full responsibility to the patient.

C. Diet

Diet therapy is a cornerstone of treatment for type 2 diabetes. This does not mean that the diet needs to be changed in every patient when first seen. They should be evaluated by a dietitian; if good practices are found, then the patient already is performing dietary therapy. Diet is generally viewed as a "good news–bad news story"; countless studies have shown glycemic improvement or reversal of

Table 7 Nutrition Recommendations for Patients with Diabetes Mellitus

1. Aid in the maintenance of as near-normal blood glucose levels as possible
2. Achieve optimal serum lipid levels
3. Provide adequate calories to attain and maintain a reasonable weight in adults, and for normal growth and development of children and during states of high metabolic needs such as pregnancy and lactation
4. Prevention and treatment of hypoglycemia
5. Improve overall health through optimal nutrition

Source: Diabetes Care 22(Suppl1):S42–S45, 1999.

type 2 diabetes with diet alone, but they have also pointed out the inability that most patients have in staying with the diet (on average, less than 10% of patients lose more than a few pounds and keep them off). Glycemic levels for the most part mirror those statistics, although there are patients who attain normoglycemia with no weight loss. This finding illustrates a key principle; the diet promotes calorie restriction when appropriate, but also alters dietary components to less-saturated fat and more complex carbohydrate, which can improve glycemia through an attenuation of fat-induced insulin resistance, slowed gastrointestinal absorption because of the higher fiber content with complex carbohydrate, and less gorging of high-fat, calorically dense foods. Moreover, lowering of fat intake is a key principle behind prevention of heart disease and treatment of hyperlipidemias. Thus, meeting glycemic or lipemic targets is the main goal of diet therapy, even if body weight is unchanged. One proviso is that diet is most effective in obese subjects. Although seemingly obvious, I have seen elderly patients who were undernourished, or even cachectic when diabetes was diagnosed, who were placed on a calorie-controlled diet. Those patients instead need caloric supplementation, and control of their diabetes invariably requires rapid institution of drugs or insulin. The goals of nutrition therapy as outlined by the American Diabetes Association are shown in Table 7, and specifics of the diabetes diet are discussed in Chap. 15. Useful clinical guidelines are the following:

1. Limit the Trial of Diet Alone to a 1 to 3 Month Time Period

The onus is on the physician to provide adequate time for patients to attempt diet treatment, but he or she must also know when to go to drug therapy. A common occurrence is patients who report they have not worked as hard at diet as they could have because of a wedding, vacation, under a lot of stress, or other. They request another chance to try diet alone, but then return is rarely different. Most patients who are going to respond to diet in terms of glycemic control do so within the first month; few take longer. Moreover, if there is not substantial improvement in glycemia within 3 months, it rarely happens thereafter. I give patients a 1-month trial, followed by reassessment by myself and the dietitian, for whom they collect a 3-day food record. If glycemia is unchanged, no weight loss has occurred, and the dietitian reports ongoing dietary problems, we proceed to drug therapy. Alternatively, if desired glycemic control is attained, as determined by preprandial blood glucose levels being mostly less than 140 mg/dL (7.4 mmol/L), the diet is maintained, and the patient is again seen for a glycated hemoglobin measurement 1–2 months later. A third scenario is that food records show better eating habits, and the weight is down some, but there is little improvement in glycemia. Patients are congratulated but counseled that glycemic control is the necessary endpoint. They are maintained on diet therapy alone and reevaluated in another 2 months; failure to meet target glycemia at that time results in adding drug therapy. The one exception is sustained weight loss and an improvement in blood glucose level that has not yet reached target. Diet alone is continued for an additional 2–3 months.

2. Dieting Must Be Continued to Be Successful

In diet-controlled patients, the diet must be maintained to prevent return of the diabetes. Dieting is unpleasant and patients easily slip back into bad habits. Even a few-pound weight gain can reverse all of the benefits. Patients must know the diet is focused on the retraining of dietary habits, not simply to diet to a target weight.

3. Weight Loss Is Greatest in the First Month of a Diet

The initial stage of a diet causes a diuresis in many patients, with a weight loss often of 10 lb or more. This effect occurs with only modest reductions in calorie intake. Many patients are lulled into thinking that this modest dieting will result in an ongoing monthly weight loss of 10 lb. In fact, additional weight loss is slow (1–3 lb/month) and requires sizeable reductions in intake. The latter point is crucial. Patients who tell you after the first month that it has not been overly hard to follow the diet often return a few pounds heavier the next month. Alternatively, patients who tell you that their diet is the most difficult thing they have ever tried to do, and they are hungry a lot of the time, are often those who enter a period of sustained weight loss.

4. Diets Must Reflect the Patient's Cultural and Ethnic Background

Food goes far beyond simply how humans replenish nutrient stores. It has cultural and ethnic significance; tastes differ, as do likes and dislikes. Patients need dietary instruction from professionals who are sensitive to their cultural issues and can design a diet around food preferences of that patient. Language can also be a barrier. Physicians should identify dietitians in their communities who work with or, better still, come from the major ethnic groups in the population they serve.

5. Use Registered Dietitians and Other Trained Professionals to Evaluate and Train Your Patients

Tear-off diet sheets are a thing of the past. Dietitians are trained to evaluate dietary habits and teach the intricacies of the diabetic diet in a fashion that few physicians can match. It is usually the dietitian who identifies problem food practices, such as a substantial intake of fruits, juices, milk, alcohol, or other high-calorie foods, or alternatively high use of "light" cookies, muffins, pastries, that are mistaken to be calorically free foods. The dietitian is trained to evaluate what a particular patient's food habits are, and how they can be changed in a fashion that holds the greatest potential to work.

D. Exercise

Step 1 therapy also entails regular exercise, which has multiple benefits, although its use is often complex (see Chap. 16 for a detailed discussion). The term *exercise* is unclear to many patients, especially those who have been sedentary and suffered from obesity for much of their lives and who often do not know how or where to exercise. It must be recommended with caution in persons who may be at risk for undiagnosed coronary disease. Certain forms of exercise are prohibited when proliferative retinopathy (so that intra-abdominal pressure is not raised), or peripheral neuropathy (to avoid structural damage to the foot or a fall) is present. Exercise-induced hypoglycemia is troubling for some patients. Finally, there is minimal to no improvement in glycemia from an exercise program in persons with type 2 diabetes. This seems counterintuitive, but a study some years ago may provide insight: careful evaluation of the dietary practices of subjects in a rigorous exercise program for type 2 diabetes showed an increased caloric intake that exactly matched what was expended by the exercise, despite being instructed at the beginning of the study to maintain their diet exactly as it was. Stated another way, patients often reward themselves for the exercise, or they drink juice or snack to prevent hypoglycemia, which cancels out the caloric usage.

Regardless, the positives for regular exercise outweigh the negatives in most patients. It is additive with diet therapy in terms of promoting weight loss in some patients. Also, regular exercise improves the cardiovascular risk profile by lowering blood pressure, increasing cardiac contractility and mechanics, altering lipid profiles, and raising tissue insulin sensitivity so that circulating insulin levels or insulin doses fall. These effects are well known in persons without diabetes—they constitute the cardioprotective effect of exercise that is so highly touted for the general population. The same benefits are generally found in type 1 and type 2 diabetes subjects and also in the elderly. It is the cardiac benefits that are most frequently cited as the main benefit of exercise in type 2 diabetes. Of crucial importance, these benefits require *regular* exercise (every-other-day) and take about a month to develop; the term *training* is used to differentiate these prolonged effects from the brief metabolic changes of a single bout of exercise. Furthermore, it takes 30 min of aerobic exercise per session to gain the training effect with the degree of benefit graded for the duration and strenuousness of the exercise. Depressingly, the metabolic benefits are quickly lost after exercise ceases—within a few days—which underlies some of the worsening glycemia that is seen when patients are bedridden. Thus, the message to give patients is to perform regular exercise (a 2-h bout of tennis on the weekend does not equate to an every-other-day 30-min workout), and it must be continued lifelong. Useful clinical guidelines are the following:

1. Define What You Mean by Exercise

It is preferable to talk about "physical activity" because everyday nonrecreational activities, such as physical jobs, going up and down steps, housework, gardening, walking to work, have the desired physiological benefits.

2. Age Is Rarely a Contraindication for Exercise

There are a host of benefits from even modest exercise in the elderly, including psychological benefits, some prevention of osteoporosis, and overall improved muscle strength.

3. There Are No Required Activities in an Exercise Program

Encourage patients to partake in whatever interests them, as that is most likely to be followed long-term. Patients should begin slowly. Many patients have not exercised before in a regular fashion, and if they begin with activities that they cannot perform, the tendency is to give up.

4. Screen for Undiagnosed Cardiovascular Disease

The risk of nondiagnosed cardiovascular disease remains a difficult issue, and there are few guidelines for who and how to screen. The safest approach is to screen, by a standard graded stress test virtually all persons with type 2 diabetes who are embarking on an exercise program.

E. Oral Hypoglycemic Drugs

Many patients proceed to adding a pharmacological agent to the diet and exercise. The conundrum faced by physicians is what exactly should be done. Common questions asked of experts are: Which drug is best? What persons should be given which drug? These are not easy questions, and experts give varying answers. Moreover, the literature does not show that one class of drugs is superior to the others. On the contrary, one is struck that the different oral agents as monotherapy produce a fairly consistent reduction of glycated hemoglobin of about 1–1.5%. An issue when trying to compare different drugs is that new-onset patients generally respond better to drugs than those with long-standing diabetes, presumably reflecting the natural history of the disease. Viewed another way, drugs, as second- or third-line agents, always produce a lower success rate of glycemic management than when used as first-line agents. As such, one must be careful when reviewing product literature to make sure the patient populations are similar.

A commonly recommended approach for drug therapy is to target mechanisms of action to physiological defects—metformin for patients with fasting hyperglycemia because its dominant effect is to suppress hepatic glucose production; troglitazone for obese, insulin-resistant patients; and sulfonylureas in relatively normal-weight patients because of presumed insulin secretory defects.

Although making theoretical sense, the clinical usefulness is unproved. On the contrary, in studies that have compared antidiabetic drugs head-to-head in the same population, little to no difference in effectiveness is observed; most recent, the UKPDS failed to identify a "best" drug for treatment of type 2 diabetes. I recommend that physicians begin therapy with whichever drugs they are familiar with in terms of the effective-dosing range and side effects. More important than which drug is chosen is to define and maintain a goal for glycemic control so that failure to attain it leads to rapid institution of a multidrug regimen.

In patients with established hyperglycemia, the major choices for monotherapy are a sulfonylurea, metformin, or a thiazolidinedione. Combination therapy entails all permutations of these three, including patients increasingly being placed on a triple therapy regimen. For patients with primarily postprandial hyperglycemia, acarbose or repaglinide are used. The important principle is there is no best drug in either situation. A detailed discussion of oral hypoglycemics is found in Chap. 17.

1. Sulfonylureas

Sulfonylureas have been used as antidiabetic agents since the 1950s, and were the only available oral agents in the United States for much of the past four decades. They promote insulin secretion through binding to a subunit of the ATP-sensitive K^+ channel on the beta-cell membrane causing beta-cell depolarization. Some years ago, it was postulated they also increased tissue insulin sensitivity, although this idea was countered by studies that failed to show a glucose-lowering effect in persons with type 1 diabetes. The newest member of this group (glimepiride) is touted to have this hybrid effect, although clinically there is no clear clinical difference in this drug's effectiveness versus the other available sulfonylureas.

A major change occurred in the 1980s when the second-generation sulfonylureas glyburide and glipizide appeared. They rapidly took over the market from the first-generation drugs because of more hepatic and less renal metabolism that lessened hypoglycemia, especially in the elderly (for the first-generation drugs were cleared by the kidneys combined with the aging-induced lowering of glomerular filtration), elimination of protein displacement problems with drugs such as warfarin, and few side effects, as opposed to the alcohol flushing, and the syndrome of inappropriate antidiuretic hormone (SIADH) effects of chlorpropamide. In contrast, effectiveness was not better—patients who failed to respond to the first-generation drugs also were unresponsive to the newer compounds.

The dosing range for glyburide and glipizide (GITS) is up to 20 mg/day, and for glimepiride, up to 8 mg/day. However, a characteristic of sulfonylureas is that the effective dosing range is steep; consequently, most patients who are going to respond do so with no more than half the maximal dose; it is generally recommended that higher doses be tried for a short time (no more than a month) before going to a multidrug regimen. A second issue is the time to response. Maximal drops in glycemia generally occur within a week of starting a sulfonylurea regimen or going to a higher dose, so that dose adjustments can be made biweekly by phone using the at-home patient's blood glucose values.

A well-known problem with sulfonylureas is secondary failures, or persons who respond initially, but then again become hyperglycemic. This problem was presumed to be unique for sulfonylureas until the recent UKPDS study, which noted an identical deterioration of glycemic control over time in persons treated with sulfonylureas, metformin, or insulin, suggesting it reflects the natural history of the disease.

The profile of the typically recommended patient for sulfonylureas is one who does not have much obesity, and who has a fasting plasma glucose value less than 250 mg/dL (13.9 mmol/L); one for whom beta-cell dysfunction, rather than insulin resistance, is presumed dominant but one with sufficient remaining beta-cell function to undergo pharmacological stimulation. However, on average 50–70% of obese new-onset diabetic patients respond to these drugs, and only 15% show no response, which is as good or better than the drugs that are typically recommended for obese patients; therefore, it is reasonable to try them in virtually any patient. One area of concern is the elderly (arbitrarily those older than 70 years of age) and persons with underlying cardiac or cerebral ischemia in whom hypoglycemia might be dangerous, sulfonylureas are not appropriate in this setting. Otherwise, side effects are few, with skin rashes most common. Hypoglycemia is not much of a problem with the second-generation compounds when they are used carefully, including avoiding excessive alcohol, which suppresses hepatic glucose production. A theoretical concern is whether these drugs promote atherosclerosis, as they act by stimulating insulin secretion and thus raise insulinemia. There remains no solid evidence supporting that concern, including the UKPDS study, which found no increased cardiac disease or death in sulfonylurea-treated patients.

In summary, sulfonylureas are reasonably effective, relatively inexpensive, safe drugs. Although many experts argue against their use because newer more exciting drugs in terms of mechanistic action have appeared during the last 2 years, clinical experience has proved them to be at least as good in terms of glycemic control as the newer drugs, making them an acceptable choice for mono-therapy in the average patient.

2. Biguanides

The biguanide drug class has been used as antidiabetic agents since the 1950s. Phenformin was available in the United States until 1977, when it was withdrawn because of fatal lactic acidosis. Metformin has been used in most of the world for 40 years, without major incidence of lactic acidosis. It did not become available in the United States until 1995, but rapidly became the most prescribed antidiabetic agent in terms of individual compounds, although sulfonylureas, as a class, still dominate. Biguanides act through an unknown cellular mechanism to lower hepatic glucose output in type 2 diabetes. Glucose uptake into skeletal muscle also increases slightly, but its primary effect is on the liver.

On average, 30–50% of patients attain glycemic control with metformin as monotherapy (somewhat less than with sulfonylureas). However, several additional clinical effects account for its heavy use. The insulin-sensitizing effect leads to lower insulinemia; hence hypoglycemia is less frequent than with sulfonylureas. Triglyceride levels are lowered (on average 15%), which has significance because hypertriglyceridemia is common in these patients, although many still require an antilipidal agent. Of most interest, studies over many years have reported less weight gain with metformin than other treatments, although, in real terms, that effect is not large, for studies generally show less than a 10-lb difference between metformin-treated and other patients. Recent information has suggested the weight-control benefit may be of particular importance in terms of promoting better glycemic control in patients who receive metformin with bedtime insulin. Additional benefits that have been touted include a restoration of cycling and fertility in women who have polycystic ovaries (insulin resistance is a key pathogenic element of PCO) and interruption of nonenzymatic protein glycosylation through an effect related to the metformin structure, rather than insulin sensitizing per se.

The dosing range for metformin is up to 2.5 g/day (850-mg tablet with each meal), but equal effectiveness has recently been shown with two 500-mg tablets at breakfast and supper so that it is a twice-a-day drug. The starting dose is 500 mg at breakfast and supper, which is increased over 4 weeks to minimize gastrointestinal side effects, typically diarrhea. Patients should be instructed to take the pill immediately before beginning a meal, which reduces gastrointestinal intolerance. Unlike sulfonylureas, the glucose-lowering effect increases over the complete dosage range, and many patients require the maximal dose. The time required for response also differs, in that the maximal effect accrues over a few weeks. Although, classically, secondary failure is not associated with metformin, the UKPDS noted the same waning of its effect as sulfonylureas in some successfully treated patients.

The profile of the typical patient who is recommended for metformin is one who has marked obesity and manifestations of insulin resistance, such as hypertension, hypertriglyceridemia, and PCO, along with the diabetes. There are several relative or absolute contraindications to minimize any risk of lactic acidosis. Absolute contraindications are renal dysfunction, as reflected in creatinine values of 1.4 or higher in females or 1.5 or higher in males, or a creatinine clearance of less than 60 mL/min in the elderly, for metformin levels correlate with the risk of lactic acidosis, and metformin is cleared by the kidney. For similar reasons, it is held during states of dehydration such as a febrile or viral illness, and following an iodinated contrast dye study. Relative to the latter, when released in the United States the package insert mandated that it be stopped for 2 days before dye studies and held until 2 days after. The recommendation now is to begin holding the medicine at the time of the study for 2 days. Additional contraindications are states of increased lactate production, such as congestive heart failure requiring pharmacologic therapy, severe infections, hypoxemic states, and states of impaired lactate clearance, such as known hepatic disease or an increased risk for hepatic disease (excessive alcohol intake). Finally, it is usually discontinued during hospitalizations of any kind because the risks generally outweigh problems with hyperglycemia.

In summary, metformin when used as recommended is a safe, effective drug. Its lipid-lowering and weight-sparing effects make it an attractive monotherapy in many patients.

3. Thiazolidinediones

Troglitazone was released in the United States and the rest of the world in 1997. Others such as rosiglitazone and pioglitazone may have some differences from troglitazone, including less hepatotoxicity. Thiazolidinediones promote glucose clearance into muscle (i.e., they are insulin sensitizers). The postulated mechanism is through their interaction with transcription factors called peroxisome proliferator-activated receptors (PPARs), although other effects have been reported; hence, the exact molecular action is under investigation.

The effectiveness and clinical use of troglitazone-type agents are less well known than other antidiabetic agents because of their newness. Studies to date have suggested the percentage of patients who respond is equal to metformin (30–50%), but the overall effectiveness at lowering glycated hemoglobin may be minimally less. As such, many physicians consider them more of a second- or third-line agent. One caveat is that they are targeted at markedly insulin-resistant patients, which usually entails marked obesity: anecdotal experience has shown success with troglitazone as monotherapy in these patients, although whether it is superior to other drugs is unknown. Despite its insulin-sensitizing effect, there are minimal effects on lipemia or blood pressure.

The recommended starting dose for troglitazone is 400 mg with breakfast or supper, and the maximal dose is 600 mg (two 300-mg tablets, usually taken at one time). A characteristic feature that differentiates troglitazone from other antidiabetic agents is that several weeks are required for the full effect, so that 400 mg is tried for 6 weeks and 600 mg for another 6 weeks before concluding that it is ineffective. Troglitazone is well tolerated, with few side effects, but two exceptions. The first is weight gain. Although not typically found, weight gain is marked in a few patients and exceeds that from sulfonylureas or insulin, suggesting that a mechanism other than reversal of glycosuria is operative. One possibility is that troglitazone promotes adipocyte genesis under in vitro conditions. The second issue is hepatotoxicity that was discovered after the drug was released. Subsequent experiences have suggested this effect is uncommon and is mostly reversible by discontinuing the drug, and most experts consider it safe *if used as recommended,* which mandates liver blood testing before beginning therapy with the drug, and then monthly for the first year and quarterly therafter. The newer agents are said not to be hepatotoxic although more experience is needed. Renal dysfunction is not a contraindication, although hepatic disease obviously is. Also, because they work peripherally and not through insulin secretion, there is minimal to no hypoglycemia when used as monotherapy. On the other hand, the insulin-sensitizing effect *requires adequate insulinemia.* This is important because these drugs have not been useful as adjunctive therapy in patients with type 1 diabetes.

In summary, thiazolidinediones provide another option for oral therapy in type 2 diabetes, often in combination with metformin or sulfonylureas.

4.   α-Glucosidase Inhibitors

Acarbose competitively inhibits gut wall disaccharidases, which slows carbohydrate absorption because only monosaccharides are transported across the gut mucosa (sugar is a disaccharide). Disaccharidases are concentrated in the jejunum; thus, carbohydrate processing and absorption occur mostly in the proximal small intestine. They are also located in the ileal wall, but are normally minimally active at this site because little unprocessed carbohydrate passes to the distal small bowel. Acarbose's effect is dose-dependent and rapidly reversible. The intent is to give the dose that exactly lowers jejunal processing and absorption, while allowing sufficient activity within the ileum such that the supernormal level of carbohydrate that escapes to the distal small bowel is processed and absorbed. The result would be a blunted rise in postprandial glycemia, with no flatulence or bloating, for no unprocessed carbohydrate makes it to the large bowel for colonic metabolism and gas formation. Attaining that goal is difficult and many patients complain of excessive gastrointestinal gas production, especially when the drug is first introduced. This problem is circumvented somewhat by beginning with small doses and going slowly, for distal small bowel enzyme activity seems to compensate over time; the current dosing protocol entails starting with a half tablet (25 mg) at supper and, over 12 weeks, working up to the standard dose of 1–2 tablets (50–100 mg) with each meal.

Acarbose physically associates with the disaccharidases in the gut mucosa to competitively impair their activity. The effect rapidly reverses as the drug disengages and escapes into the stool. Virtually none is absorbed, which makes it safe in patients with kidney or hepatic diseases, although it is generally not recommended if the serum creatinine value is higher than 2 mg/dL. Additional contraindications are inflammatory bowel disease or bowel obstructive problems. Because of the rapid reversibility, the timing of when it is taken is critical. Patients are instructed to wait until immediately before starting the meal and, in some patients, taking it during the meal before a high carbohydrate load of pasta or potatoes is most effective. Except for gastrointestinal side effects of flatulence, bloating, and mild diarrhea, there are few other side effects, although early reports of increased hepatic transaminases initially caused some concern. However, the incidence is now believed to be minimal, although it is recommended that serum liver function tests be measured every 3 months for the first year and administration of drug stopped if a doubling is seen. It is not associated with any significant risk of hypoglycemia.

Several issues should be discussed with patients when acarbose is being considered to avoid common misconceptions. It slows carbohydrate absorption by spreading it over more of the small bowel, thereby blunting postprandial glycemia. Carbohydrate absorption is not reduced overall, which is a key misunderstanding for patients who often expect to lose weight because they have been told it "prevents carbohydrate absorption": typically, weight loss does not occur. Physicians should also anticipate that patients who measure only premeal glycemia at home may be skeptical about starting therapy with such a drug, especially one with troubling gastrointestinal side effects, when their blood glucose values may be very favorable and often within standard treatment guidelines; by definition, postprandial hyperglycemia in patients who progress from IGT to mild type

2 diabetes entails relatively normal premeal glycemic levels. The same concern exists for patients taking acarbose who measure only premeal glycemia because the treatment effect may be hidden. Before starting a treatment regimen with acarbose, patients should perform 2-h postmeal glycemia testing to document the extent of the hyperglycemia—how far above the goal of less than 140 mg/dL (7.8 mM) are they? Continued postmeal testing after acarbose is begun is used to monitor the treatment benefits.

The profile of the typical patient for acarbose is a newly diagnosed patient with significantly raised postmeal glycemia (2-h value > 140 mg/dL), as opposed to premeal glycemia that is close to the desired range (< 140 mg/dL). Moreover, patients whom consume large amounts of carbohydrate are good candidates. When acarbose is tolerated, studies have shown glycemic control as dependable as that of sulfonylureas or metformin in these groups. By the same reasoning, it should theoretically be an effective preventative treatment to slow the progression of IGT to frank hyperglycemia, and a large international trial is underway to test that possibility.

5. Meglitinides

Repaglinide stimulates insulin secretion through a molecular effect similar to that of sulfonylureas by interacting with the ATP-sensitive K^+ channel on the beta-cell. The major difference is a fast on–off insulinotropic effect; therefore, it is administered for postprandial hyperglycemia. The starting dose is 0.5 mg 0–30 min before meals to a maximum of 16 mg daily, with the major caution being liver disease. The recommended patient is the same as the one for acarbose. Because of its newness, the relative effectiveness of repaglinide versus acarbose is unknown, as is the potential for combination repaglinide–acarbose therapy.

F. Combination Orals

Most patients will end up on more than one oral agent. Several important principles apply. First, as detailed in the foregoing, the available classes of drugs work at different sites in the glucose homeostasis system so that any combination is theoretically possible and effective. A favored one is a sulfonylurea and metformin (insulin secretagogue and sensitizer). Moreover, recent information has shown additive effects of metformin and troglitazone (two insulin sensitizers), which is not a surprise, as the former targets the liver and the latter skeletal muscle. No study has shown that one combination is clearly superior to another, or that one is clearly inferior to another. Second, side effect profiles do not prevent combining one drug with another (i.e., even though troglitazone and acarbose rarely elevate transaminases, there is no undue concern in using them together in the average patient). The same can be said for the intestinal side effects of acarbose and metformin. Third, maximal dosages of the individual drugs are unchanged when they are used in combination. To summarize, as patients progress to multidrug therapy, it makes sense to chose as the second drug one that best fits the glycemic and physiological profile of that patient—metformin for patients with high fasting glycemia, obesity or hypertriglyceridemia; thiazolidinediones for sustained hyperglycemia and presumed marked insulin resistance; acarbose or repaglinide for postprandial hyperglycemia. The key is not which drugs are used, but that enough drugs are used to attain the target glycemic control.

G. Insulin

Step 3 entails addition of insulin with, or instead of, oral medications, and step 4 is intensification of the insulin treatment program. There is no more difficult and emotional time for the patient then when insulin is first discussed. Fears include pain from the injections, hypoglycemia, weight gain, employment barriers, and loss of independence. Additionally, patients often worry that their diabetes has become so serious that blindness, kidney failure, or amputation is inevitable. Physicians must approach this time empathetically, but firmly. Do not be talked out of an insulin program. Moreover, recognize that our responsibility goes beyond simply choosing a program and doses, to ensure that the transition to insulin is a positive experience for the patient. A distressingly common story is patients who are told they need insulin, given prescriptions, and shown the basics of mixing and injecting by the office nurse, all over no more than 30 min so they leave confused and in a panic. Patient's fears must be attacked head on. Never raise the topic of insulin and then put off the discussion until the next visit. Be sensitive that patients are skeptical when physicians say "it won't hurt." Insulin must be discussed carefully and completely in terms of why it is needed, what implication it holds for the seriousness and long-term outcome of the diabetes, what effect there will be on the patient's lifestyle and job, identify misconceptions and fears the patient may have ("my mother went on insulin and had a heart attack 6 months later"), followed by injecting them with saline to show that the injections really are painless. By using this approach, insulin is introduced relatively easily in most patients. However, reimbursement issues and the busyness of many doctors' practices often preclude this relaxed approach. In that case, patients should be referred to a diabetes center or specialty practice.

Type 2 diabetes usually entails substantial endogenous insulin secretion, which has important implications for how to use an insulin program in type 2 diabetes and the potential problems that typically differ from type 1 diabetes. The preciseness of the timing and dosing of the insulin are less critical than with type 1 diabetes. Hypoglycemia is less frequent because endogenous insulin can shut off as glycemia falls and the counterregulatory system is largely unimpaired in type 2 diabetes. Problems with fluctuating glycemia throughout the day are fewer. Instead, the major difficulties are the large insulin doses that are often needed because of the insulin resistance (frequently more than 100 U/day), and patients often gain weight, resulting in a cycle whereby glycemia rises and the insulin dose is increased to compensate. The weight gain is distressing to patients, but should not be blamed on the insulin per se; stopping glycosuria is an important element so that the patient retains more calories despite no change in their intake. Thus, when beginning an insulin program, there should always be a review by the dietitian of current food practices, with a reduction of daily intake by 200–400 calories if appropriate. The exception to this scenario is patients with impaired beta-cell function, as is thought to occur in relatively thin elderly patients.

1. Combined Insulin and Oral Hypoglycemics

The transition to insulin in many patients is performed by adding it to their oral drugs. When only sulfonylureas were available in the United States, patients with inadequate glycemic control had NPH insulin added at bedtime (BIDS; bedtime insulin daytime sulfonylurea). A well-known paper from Yki-Järvinen in 1992 compared insulin programs in persons with type 2 diabetes and showed that BIDS produced glycemic control equal to multishot insulin regimens with less weight gain. The BIDS regimen fell out of favor as new oral agents became available so that multidrug regimens took over. However, for patients who fail to obtain adequate glycemic control with orals, adding a bedtime dose of NPH remains a useful next step.

A confusion for many physicians is what drugs should the patient continue to take. Only a sulfonylurea? Others? How many? No study has critically addressed this question, but it seems reasonable to assume that bedtime insulin should be additive to any oral agent. My own practice adds NPH insulin at bedtime (9–11 PM) to their regimen irrespective of how many drugs they are taking; when acceptable control is attained, individual drugs are weaned as appropriate. The starting NPH dose is 10–20 U based on the presumed insulin sensitivity of the patient, with older or mildly obese patients receiving the lower figure and obese patients receiving the higher. Patients perform daily fasting blood glucose measurements and are instructed to adjust the dose upward 2–3 U every 4–7 days until a FBS of 90–120 mg/dL (5.0–6.7 mmol/L) is consistently attained. In contrast, fasting glycemia levels below the target range are handled by the physician who differentiates overinsulinization (consistently below the target range) from variable eating or exercise habits (some mornings too low and others normal to high). The tight target glycemia level is crucial; part of how bedtime insulin is thought to work entails reversal of the glucose toxicity effect on beta-cells or insulin sensitivity which requires near-normoglycemia. Once the correct insulin dose is identified, the patient maintains the program for 2 months and performs glucose measurements throughout the day. Also, a weekly 2–3 AM glucose value is obtained to ensure that asymptomatic nocturnal hypoglycemia is not occurring (defined as glycemia < 65 mg/dL or 3.6 mmol/L). After the 2 months, a glycated hemoglobin test determines whether acceptable glycemic control has been attained, with the target HbA_{1c} for most patients of close to 7%. A common scenario is patients who have acceptable glycemia up to late afternoon, but then break through postdinner. Those patients can often be switched to NPH/lispro or NPH/regular presupper, with the proviso that nocturnal hypoglycemia must be carefully excluded.

2. Insulin Only

Once the decision is made to go to a multishot insulin program, oral antidiabetic drugs are usually stopped; they are expensive and carry side effects, and there is no clear reason to believe that their use with insulin brings any benefit over insulin alone. The one exception is troglitazone, which was originally released for insulin-treated type 2 diabetic patients. The original hope that troglitazone would replace insulin in many patients was wishful thinking—perhaps 15% of insulin-treated patients discontinue that therapy—but it does lower insulin doses while improving overall glycemia in many patients. As such, troglitazone and insulin are a useful combination for many patients as long as liver function blood tests are carefully monitored and weight gain is not excessive.

A common confusion is what insulin program to use: traditional NPH and regular regimens or the newer Ultralente–lispro or multishot insulin pen regimens. There is no "best" regimen. In particular, the endogenous insulin production in type 2 diabetes means that many patients can attain glycemic control with virtually any regimen. Having said that, my own practice uses almost exclusively Ultralente and lispro (Ultralente–lispro prebreakfast, lispro prelunch, Ultralente–lispro presupper) or insulin pens (regular prebreakfast, regular prelunch, regular presupper, NPH at bedtime). Daytime use of NPH is saved mostly for the elderly or others who need premixed insulin preparations. This practice is not based on the presumption that metabolic control will be better with the three- or four-shot regimens, but purely for lifestyle reasons, as they provide maximal flexibility for the varying eating and exercise habits that are increasingly demanded by the hectic and unpredictable job and personal lifestyles of our patients.

IX. WHO AND WHEN TO REFER?

An ongoing issue is who should be providing diabetes care? The answer varies, depending on with whom you talk. There are increasingly highly charged debates at national meetings and a flood of recent (often poorly balanced) articles in the literature that are struggling with this issue. The sad fact is that patients are often forgotten in these "turf" discussions. More than 90% of diabetes care in the United States is delivered by generalists; this is appropriate and will not change. Balancing that, we have national guidelines that cover almost all aspects of diabetes care, and studies of compliance always find dismal results. Several conclusions seem obvious. Training programs for primary care physicians need to emphasize diabetes, so that generalists develop confidence and expertise in its management. National guidelines need to be known and aggressively followed. However, if guidelines cannot be met despite best efforts, or if the patient has specialized needs that exceed the physician's expertise (intensive insulin treatment, insulin pump, pregnant diabetics, complex lifestyle or job schedules, hypoglycemic unawareness, complications), they should be referred to a diabetes center or a specialty practice. Stated another way, if the treatment program works for you and your patient, why refer? If not, seek help. The ideal situation is to have primary physicians and diabetologists working as a team in the best interests of patients, not arguing over theoretical issues. Diabetes care must be goal-driven. Are the goals met? If not, then a referral is warranted.

CURRENT REVIEWS

American Diabetes Association (ADA). Clinical Practice Recommendations 1999. Diabetes Care 1999; 22 (suppl 1).

American Diabetes Association (ADA). Diabetes Care 1995; 18:1510–1518.

Alberti KG. The clinical implications of impaired glucose tolerance. Diabetic Med 1996; 13:927–937.

Assal JP, Jacquemet S, Morel Y. The added value of therapy in diabetes: the education of patients for self-management of their disease. Metab Clin Exp 1997; 46(suppl 1):61–64.

Cefalu WT. Treatment of type II diabetes: what options have been added to traditional methods? Postgrad Med 1996; 99:109–119.

Dagogo-Jack S, Santiago JV. Pathophysiology of type 2 diabetes and modes of action of therapeutic interventions. Arch Intern Med 1997; 157:1802–1817.

DeFronzo RA. Pathogenesis of type 2 diabetes: metabolic and molecular implications for identifying diabetic genes. Diabetes Rev 1997; 5:177–269.

Dunaif A. Insulin resistance and the polycystic ovary syndrome: mechanism and implications for pathogenesis. Endocr Rev 1997; 18:774–800.

Edelman SV. Type II diabetes mellitus. Adv Intern Med 1998; 43:449–500.

Fore WW. Noninsulin-dependent diabetes mellitus. The prevention of complications. Med Clin North Am 1995; 79:287–298.

Franz MJ. Lifestyle modifications for diabetes management. Endocrinol Metab Clin North Am 1997; 26:499–510.

Garg A, Grundy SM. Diabetic Dyslipidemia and its therapy. Diabetic Rev 1997; 5: 425–433.

General review of therapies. Endocrinol Metab Clin North Am 1997; 26:3.

Gerich JE. Pathogenesis and treatment of type 2 (noninsulin-dependent) diabetes mellitus (NIDDM) Horm Metab Res 1996; 28:404–412.

Groop LC, Tuomi T. Non-insulin-dependent diabetes mellitus—a collision between thrifty genes and an affluent society. Ann Intern Med 1997; 29:37–53.

Heine RJ, Mooy JM. Impaired glucose tolerance and unidentified diabetes. Postgrad Med J 1996; 72:67–71.

Henry RR. Glucose control and insulin resistance in non-insulin-dependent diabetes mellitus. Ann Intern Med 1996; 124:97–103.

Leahy JL. β-Cell dysfunction in type II diabetes mellitus. Curr Opin Endocrinol Diabetes 1995; 2:300–306.

Leahy JL. β-Cell dysfunction with chronic hyperglycemia: the "overworked β-cell" hypothesis. Diabetes Rev 1996; 4:298–319.

Riddle MC. Tactics for type II diabetes. Endocrinol Metab Clin North Am 1997; 26: 659–677.

Sheen AJ. Non–insulin-dependent diabetes mellitus in the elderly. Baillieres Clin Endocrinol Metab 1997; 11:389–406.

United Kingdom Prospective Diabetes Study (UKPDS). Glycemia control final results. Lancet 1998; 352(Sept 12): Blood pressure control final results. Br Med J 1998; 317(Sept 12).

U.S. Expert Committee on the Diagnosis and Classification of Diabetes Mellitus, 1997–1998. Diabetes Care 1998; 21(suppl 1):S5–S19.

Yji-Järvinen H, et al. Comparison of insulin regimens in patients with non–insulin-dependent diabetes mellitus. N Engl J Med 1992; 327:1426–1433.

10
Diabetes in Children

Joseph I. Wolfsdorf
Children's Hospital, Boston, Massachusetts

Daniel J. Nigrin
*Children's Hospital and Harvard Medical School,
Boston, Massachusetts*

I. EPIDEMIOLOGY

The prevalence of type I diabetes mellitus (type 1 DM) in children in the United States is approximately 1.7 cases per 1000 or 1:600 children and adolescents younger than 20 years of age. It is estimated that there are approximately 125,000 children and teenagers with diabetes mellitus. The frequency varies with age, from approximately 1:1430 children at age 5 years to 1:360 at age 16 years. The prevalence of type 1 DM appears to vary slightly according to race. Rates are lower among African Americans, Hispanic Americans, and Asian Americans compared with whites. It is rare in Native Americans. There is no apparent correlation with socioeconomic status; boys and girls are equally affected.

There is seasonal variation in the incidence of type 1 DM, with a slight decline in cases during the summer months and an increased incidence in temperate climates during late winter and early spring. The worldwide incidence of type 1 DM varies enormously from 0.7:100,000 in Shanghai, China to 35:100,000 in Finland (a 50 times greater incidence). The annual incidence in the United States falls between these extremes—approximately 18 new cases per 100,000 or 13,200 new cases each year in children younger than 20 years of age. In some parts of the world, particularly Europe, Asia, and the Western Pacific, the incidence of type 1 DM appears to be increasing. In Allegheny County, Pennsylvania, the incidence of type 1 DM increased markedly in males but not in females during 1985–1989 compared with 5-year intervals over the previous 20 years.

The overall risk of a child developing diabetes before the age of 20 is approximately 0.5%. It is rare in the first year of life. Thereafter, the incidence increases with age until puberty; the peak incidence is at age 10–12 years in girls and 12–14 years in boys.

II. INITIAL MANAGEMENT OF NEWLY DIAGNOSED DIABETES MELLITUS

The initial goals of therapy are threefold: (a) to stabilize the metabolic state with insulin; (b) to restore fluid and electrolyte balance; and (c) to provide basic diabetes education and self-care training for parents (and child when appropriate) and other important caregivers (e.g., grandparents, older siblings, daycare providers, babysitters, and such).

At the time of diagnosis, the educational program in diabetes self-management should begin in a safe and supportive environment, either in a hospital or in an ambulatory setting suitable for the purpose. It is currently our practice to admit most children with a new diagnosis of type 1 DM to the hospital for initial treatment. The diagnosis of diabetes in a child usually is a major crisis for the family, who require emotional support and time for adjustment and healing. Shocked, grieving, and overwhelmed parents usually take 2–3 days to acquire ''survival'' skills while they are coping with the emotional upheaval that inevitably follows the diagnosis of diabetes.

A suitable alternative to hospitalization for many children who are not in diabetic ketoacidosis is a comprehensive day-treatment center staffed by a multidisciplinary diabetes team. The decision concerning whether or not a child with newly diagnosed diabetes should be admitted to hospital depends on several factors. Of these, the most important is the severity of the metabolic derangement, the psychosocial assessment of the family, and the resources available at the treatment center.

The initial management of the child who presents with newly diagnosed diabetes mellitus also varies depending on the clinical presentation. A relatively high proportion (from 20 to 50%) of infants, toddlers, and young children with newly diagnosed diabetes mellitus are in diabetic ketoacidosis (DKA) by the time they come to medical attention. An overview of the clinical manifestations, pathophysiology, and treatment protocol for DKA used at this institution (Children's Hospital, Boston) is presented in the following. For initial management of patients who do not present in DKA see Sec. V.A.

III. DIABETIC KETOACIDOSIS

A. Definition of DKA

Hyperglycemia with plasma glucose concentration usually higher than 300 mg/dL

Ketonemia, with total serum ketone (β-hydroxybutyrate and acetoacetate) concentration higher than 3 mmol/L and ketonuria

Acidosis with a venous pH value of less than 7.30 and a serum bicarbonate concentration of 15 mmol/L, or less

B. Clinical Manifestations of DKA

Rapid, deep, sighing (Kussmaul) respiration.

Signs of dehydration varying from mild dehydration to shock.

Nausea, vomiting, abdominal pain that can mimic an acute surgical abdomen.

Increased leukocyte count with a left shift.

Nonspecific elevation of serum amylase.

Fever only when there is associated infection.

Obtundation and loss of consciousness related to the degree of hyperosmolality. Serum osmolality can be calculated as [serum sodium (mmol/L) $\times$ 2] + [plasma glucose (mg/dL) $\div$ 18] + [BUN (mg/dL) $\div$ 2.8].

C. Pathophysiology

The metabolic derangements of DKA result from a combination of either absolute or relative insulin deficiency and the effects of increased plasma concentrations of the counterregulatory hormones, catecholamines, glucagon, cortisol, and growth hormone. Absolute insulin deficiency occurs in previously undiagnosed type 1 DM and when established patients already receiving treatment deliberately or inadvertently omit insulin. Relative insulin deficiency occurs when the concentrations of the counterregulatory hormones (that oppose the effects of insulin) increase under conditions of stress—infection, surgery, trauma, gastrointestinal illness with diarrhea and vomiting, and severe emotional stress.

The combination of low serum insulin levels and high counterregulatory hormone concentrations results in an accelerated catabolic state characterized by increased glucose production and impaired glucose utilization; increased serum free fatty acid and glycerol levels; increased formation of ketoacids (β-hydroxybutyrate and acetoacetate). Excessive production and diminished utilization of glucose leads to hyperglycemia. Polyuria is caused by the osmotic diuresis that occurs when the renal threshold for glucose (approximately 180 mg/dL) is exceeded. Osmotic diuresis and urinary excretion of keto-anions is associated with the loss of large quantities of electrolytes. Vomiting often augments the loss of fluid and electrolytes.

Despite dehydration (usually 5–10%), patients continue to have a large urine output unless they are extremely volume depleted and on the verge of circulatory collapse. Accumulation of ketoacids leads to a metabolic acidosis, which may be aggravated by lactic acidosis from poor tissue perfusion. The net effect is severe depletion of water and electrolytes. The plasma glucose concentration and the magnitude of specific deficits vary among patients. Factors that influence the biochemical profile at the time of presentation are the duration of illness and the type and amount of food and fluid consumed in the days before presentation.

D. Management of DKA

Specific details of the management of DKA vary among physicians. The treatment protocol used at this center is presented in the following.

1. Initial Evaluation

1. Perform a clinical evaluation to establish the diagnosis and determine its cause (especially any evidence of infection) and to assess the patient's degree of dehydration. Weigh the patient and measure height or length.
2. Determine the blood glucose concentration at the bedside with a glucose meter.
3. Obtain a blood sample for measurement of plasma glucose, electrolytes, and total CO_2 (bicarbonate), blood urea nitrogen, creatinine, serum osmolality, venous pH, P_{CO_2}, P_{O_2} (if patient is in coma or is hemodynamically unstable arterial pH is preferable), complete blood cell count and differential white cell count, calcium, magnesium, and phosphorus, levels.
4. Calculate the anion gap, $Na^+ - [Cl^- + T_{CO_2}]$; normal is 12 ± 2.
5. Perform a urinalysis and obtain appropriate specimens for culture (blood, urine, throat) even if the patient is afebrile.
6. Perform an electrocardiogram (ECG) for baseline evaluation of potassium status.
7. Determine the patient's baseline neurological status (Glasgow coma scale).

2. Supportive Measures

1. In semiconscious or unconscious patients, secure the airway and empty the stomach by nasogastric suction to prevent aspiration.
2. Give supplementary oxygen to patients who are cyanosed, in shock, and when the Pa_{O_2} is < 80 mmHg.
3. Accurately measure urine output; use bladder catheterization or condom drainage if necessary.

4. Use a flowchart to record the patient's clinical and laboratory data, details of fluid and electrolyte therapy, administered insulin, and urine output. Successful management of DKA requires meticulous monitoring of the patient's clinical and biochemical response to treatment so that timely adjustments in the treatment regimen can be made when necessary.

5. Measure levels of plasma glucose, serum electrolytes (and corrected sodium), pH, Pco_2, Tco_2, anion gap, calcium, and phosphorus, every 2 h for the first 8 h, and then every 4 h until they are normal. The corrected sodium is calculated: Na^+ + (1.6 × [plasma glucose mg/dL − 100] ÷ 100).

6. Infants, toddlers, and severely ill older children with DKA, especially those with central nervous system obtundation or cardiovascular instability, should be admitted to an intensive care unit or comparable facility where intensive clinical and metabolic monitoring can be carried out.

7. Broad-spectrum antibiotics should be given to febrile patients after appropriate cultures of body fluids have been obtained.

3. Fluid and Electrolyte Treatment

1. All patients with DKA are dehydrated and have total body depletion of sodium, potassium, chloride, phosphate, and magnesium. Patients with mild to moderate DKA are usually about 3–5% (50 mL/kg) dehydrated, and those with severe DKA are up to 10% (100 mL/kg) dehydrated.

2. Infuse 10 mL/kg isotonic saline intravenously (IV) over 60 min to correct hypovolemia. The severely dehydrated patient or patient in shock, initially, should receive 20 mL/kg. If hypotension or shock persists, an additional 10 mL/kg isotonic saline (or an equal amount of fresh-frozen plasma) should be given.

3. Once the circulation has been stabilized, change to half-normal saline and replace the balance of the estimated fluid deficit at an even rate over 24–48 h. If osmolality is less than 320 mOsm/L, replenish the fluid deficit in 36 h, and if higher than 340 mOsm/L, correct in 48 h. Aim to achieve *slow* correction of serum hyperosmolality and to avoid a rapid shift of water from the extracellular to the intracellular compartment. The sodium concentration of the solution should be increased to 100–154 mEq/L if the corrected serum sodium concentration falls or fails to rise as the plasma glucose concentration decreases.

4. Maintenance fluid is given as half isotonic saline at a rate of 1500 mL/m^2 per day.

5. Add 5% dextrose to the infusion fluid when the plasma glucose concentration reaches 300 mg/dL, and attempt to maintain the plasma glucose concentration at or above approximately 200 mg/dL for the first 36–48 h. To avert hypoglycemia while continuing to infuse insulin to correct acidosis, it may be necessary to use 7.5 or 10% dextrose.

6. Early in the course of therapy, continued osmotic diuresis contributes significantly to ongoing fluid losses. To stabilize the circulation and achieve positive fluid balance, the rate of fluid administration may have to be temporarily increased.

7. Intravenous fluid administration is continued until acidosis is corrected and the patient can eat and drink without vomiting. Persistent tachycardia in the absence of fever is a sign of inadequate fluid administration.

4. Insulin

1. Regular insulin is diluted in saline (50 U regular insulin in 50 mL saline). After an initial IV bolus of 0.1 U/kg, insulin is given IV at a rate of 0.1 U/kg per hour, controlled by an infusion pump. Insulin has a serum half-life of approximately 5 min. If the insulin infusion is interrupted, insulin deficiency develops rapidly. Therefore, low-dose insulin therapy must be closely supervised to ensure no interruption of the infusion.

2. During initial fluid expansion, the blood glucose level may decrease 150–300 mg/dL before any insulin has been given.

3. When DKA has resolved (venous pH higher than 7.32, Tco_2 higher than 18 mmol/L), insulin is administered subcutaneously (SC) and the insulin infusion is discontinued.

4. The first SC injection of regular insulin should be given 60–120 min before stopping the infusion to allow sufficient time for the injected insulin to be absorbed. If lispro insulin is used instead of regular insulin, the insulin infusion can be stopped 15 min after the first SC injection.

5. Potassium Replacement

1. All patients with DKA are potassium depleted (4–6 mEq/kg) despite an initial serum potassium concentration that may be normal or high. With the administration of fluid and insulin, serum potassium concentration may decrease abruptly, predisposing the patient to cardiac arrhythmia. Patients whose initial serum potassium level is low are the most severely depleted.

2. The addition of potassium should begin after insulin has been given (provided the patient has urinated, serum potassium level is less than 6 mEq/L, and the ECG shows no evidence of hyperkalemia). The serum

potassium concentration should be measured hourly and maintained in the normal range.

3. Half the potassium is given as potassium acetate and the other half as potassium phosphate. This reduces the total amount of chloride administered and partially replaces the phosphate deficit, but is unlikely to induce hypocalcemia.

6. Acidosis

1. Routine administration of bicarbonate neither hastens resolution of acidosis nor improves survival and may impair tissue oxygenation and cause hypokalemia. Its routine use, therefore, is not recommended.
2. However, when acidosis is severe (arterial pH < 7.0) or there is hypotension, shock, or an arrhythmia, sodium bicarbonate 1–2 mEq/kg or 40–80 mEq/m^2, should be infused slowly over 2 h.

7. Cerebral Edema

As an uncommon complication of DKA, cerebral edema can cause acute brain stem herniation and death. It typically develops abruptly within 2–12 h of starting treatment and manifests as severe headache, vomiting, altered level of consciousness, agitation, delirium, combativeness, restlessness, incontinence, changes in vital signs (bradycardia, increased blood pressure, hypothermia), pupillary changes, papilledema, respiratory arrest, or sudden onset of polyuria from acute diabetes insipidus. Computed tomography (CT) of the brain confirms brain swelling. The decision to intervene should not depend on the results of a CT scan; it should be made on clinical grounds. When cerebral edema is suspected, the following steps should be taken immediately:

1. Administer mannitol 1 g/kg IV over 15 min and repeat as necessary.
2. Reduce the rate of fluid administration.
3. Insert an endotracheal tube and hyperventilate the patient.
4. Intracranial pressure monitoring should be performed in an intensive care unit.

IV. DIABETES CARE IN THE OUT-PATIENT SETTING

A. The Diabetes Team

Optimal care of children with type 1 DM is complex and time-consuming and requires the integrated efforts of several disciplines—the diabetes team. Few general practitioners or pediatricians have the expertise and resources, nor can they devote the time required to provide all of the various components of an optimal treatment program. We believe, therefore, that treatment of children with diabetes, ideally, should be by a diabetes treatment team working closely with the child's primary care physician.

The team should include a pediatric endocrinologist, a pediatric diabetes nurse specialist/educator, a dietitian, and a mental health professional, either a social worker or clinical psychologist. The most important members of the team, however, are the patient and his or her family, whose goals and concerns should receive priority in planning and implementing the treatment program.

B.   Initial Diabetes Education

All members of the diabetes team participate in the educational process. Learning about diabetes management of children is based on a structured diabetes education curriculum adapted to the individual child and family. The process of educating parents and children in diabetes care begins at the time of diagnosis. Initially, most parents and children are too anxious and overwhelmed to be able to assimilate an extensive body of abstract information. Therefore, the education program is staged. Initial goals are limited to ensure that the essential "survival skills" are acquired so that the child can be safely cared for at home and return to his or her daily routine. The essential elements of initial diabetes self-management training are an understanding of what causes diabetes, how it is managed, how to administer insulin, basic meal planning, self-monitoring of blood glucose (SMBG), urine ketone measurement, and recognition and treatment of hypoglycemia.

Once the grief reaction subsides, most families are more prepared to learn the intricate details of diabetes management. It is at this stage that one begins to provide parents with the knowledge and skills they need to maintain optimal glycemic control while coping with the challenges imposed by variable exercise, fickle appetite and varying food intake, intercurrent illnesses, and the other normal variations that occur in a child's daily routine.

In addition to teaching facts and practical skills, the education program should promote desirable health beliefs and attitudes in the young person who has to live with a chronic and as yet incurable disease. For some children, this may best be accomplished in a nontraditional educational setting, such as summer camp for children with diabetes. The educational curriculum must be concordant with the child's level of cognitive development and has to be adapted to the learning style and intellectual ability of the individual child and family. We urge all parents, grandparents, older siblings, and other important people in the child's life to participate in the diabetes education program so that they can share in the diabetes care and help to enable the child continue to do the things she or he did before diabetes was diagnosed.

C. Continuing Diabetes Education and Long-Term Supervision of Diabetes Care

When the child is medically stable and parents (and other care providers) have mastered survival skills, the child is discharged from the hospital or ambulatory treatment center. In the first few weeks after diagnosis, frequent, often daily, telephone contact provides emotional support, helps parents interpret the results of SMBG, and provides an opportunity to adjust the dose(s) of insulin, if necessary. Within a few weeks of diagnosis, many children enter a partial remission, evidenced by normal or near-normal blood glucose levels on a low-dose (< 0.25 U/kg per day) of insulin.

In the first month after diagnosis, the patient is seen frequently by members of the diabetes care team, primarily by the nurse specialist/diabetes educator, to review and consolidate the diabetes education and practical skills learned in the first few days and to extend the scope of diabetes self-care training. Thereafter, follow-up visits with members of the diabetes team occur with a minimum frequency of every 3 months. Regular clinic visits are to ensure that the child's diabetes is being appropriately managed at home and the goals of therapy are being met. A focused history should obtain information about self-care behaviors; the child's daily routines; the frequency, severity, and circumstances surrounding hypoglycemic events; and symptoms of hyperglycemia. At every visit, height and weight are measured and plotted on a growth chart. The weight curve is especially helpful in assessing adequacy of therapy. Significant weight loss usually indicates that the prescribed dose is insufficient, or the patient is not receiving all the prescribed doses of insulin. A complete physical examination should be performed at least twice per year, focusing on blood pressure, signs of puberty, evidence of thyroid disease, and examination of the skin at the injection sites for evidence of lipohypertrophy resulting from overuse of the site.

Insulin therapy must be dynamic and take into account growth and development, changes in lifestyle and physical activity, intercurrent illness, and other factors that influence insulin requirements. Doses are adjusted to maintain blood glucose levels within or near the target range as much as possible. The target range (Table 1) varies with the age of the patient, motivation of the parents and patient, support of the family system, and willingness to monitor blood glucose levels frequently. For infants and toddlers unable to recognize or treat hypoglycemia themselves, the target range is higher and broader to minimize the risk of severe hypoglycemia.

Regular clinic visits also provide an opportunity to review, reinforce, and expand on the diabetes self-care training begun at the time of diagnosis. The goal at each visit is to increase the patient's and family's understanding of diabetes management, the interplay of insulin, food, and exercise, and their influence on blood glucose levels. As the child's cognitive development progresses, she or he

Table 1 Target Blood Glucose Levels[a] for Children

Age group	Fasting (mg/dL)	Premeal (mg/dL)	2–4 AM (mg/dL)
Infant or toddler	80–180	100–200	80–180
School age	70–150	70–180	80–150

[a] Target blood glucose levels for patients who practice intensive diabetes management and have normal counterregulatory mechanisms are: 70–120 mg/dL fasting and before meals, < 180 mg/dL 90–120 min after meals, and 70–100 mg/dL at 2–4 AM.

should become more involved in diabetes management and assume increasing age-appropriate responsibility for daily self-care.

Parents are encouraged to call for advice if the pattern of blood glucose levels changes between routine visits, suggesting the need to adjust the insulin dose. Eventually, when parents have gained enough knowledge and experience, they are encouraged to independently make minor adjustments.

D. Psychosocial Issues

A medical social worker should perform an initial psychosocial assessment of all patients with newly diagnosed disease, to identify families at high risk who need additional services. Thereafter, patients are referred to the mental health specialist (social worker or clinical psychologist) when emotional, social, environmental, or financial concerns are suspected or identified that interfere with the ability to maintain acceptable diabetes control. Some of the more common problems in families that have a child with diabetes are parental guilt, resulting in poor adherence to the treatment regimen; inability to cope with the child's rebellion against treatment; anxiety or depression; missed appointments and financial hardship; loss of health insurance, affecting the ability to attend scheduled clinic appointments or purchase supplies necessary for diabetes care. Recurrent ketoacidosis is the most extreme indicator of psychosocial stress; evaluation of such patients is incomplete without a comprehensive psychosocial assessment.

V. INSULIN THERAPY

The aim of insulin therapy is to simulate as closely as possible the fluctuations in plasma insulin levels that normally occur in nondiabetic individuals. In children with severe insulin deficiency, practical considerations of acceptability and adherence make it extremely difficult, if not impossible, to simulate normal physiology.

A. Standard Insulin Therapy

The initial route of insulin administration is determined by the severity of the child's condition. As described earlier (see Sec. III.D4), insulin is given IV for the management of DKA. However, if the newly diagnosed child is not vomiting, is not dehydrated, does not have ketosis, or DKA is mild (arterial pH > 7.25, venous pH > 7.20), insulin may be started SC. In the child who has recently recovered from DKA, we usually begin SC insulin treatment with a total dose of 0.5 U/kg per day using either a two-dose per day ''split-mixed'' regimen—a mixture of human intermediate-acting (NPH or Lente) and short-acting (regular or lispro) insulin or a three-dose regimen described below. The child's age and weight guide the initial insulin dose selection. When the diagnosis has been made early, before significant metabolic decompensation has occurred, we start at a dose of 0.25 U/kg per day. A useful ''rule of thumb'' is 1 U/year of age per day. When metabolic decompensation is more severe (e.g., ketonuria, but no acidosis nor dehydration) the initial dose is 0.5 U/kg. We aim for premeal blood glucose levels less than 200 mg/dL and supplement, if necessary, with 0.1 U/kg regular insulin SC at 4 to 6-h intervals.

Three major categories of insulin preparations are available, which differ in their absorption kinetics (Table 2). Several insulin regimens can be used (Table 3). Each has the same goal: to provide basal insulin throughout the day and night and more insulin with meals. The regimen most commonly used in children consists of a mixture of rapid-acting (either regular or lispro) and an intermediate-acting (NPH or Lente) insulin preparation given twice daily, before breakfast and before the evening meal. The total daily dose is divided so that two-thirds is given before breakfast and one-third is given before the evening meal. For older children and adolescents we recommend a modification of this regimen that involves three doses per day. The second dose of intermediate-acting insulin is

Table 2 Insulin Preparations[a]

Action	Type	Onset of Action (h)	Peak action (h)	Duration of action (h)
Short-acting	Lispro	< 0.25	0.5–1.5	3–4
	Regular	0.5	2–4	6–8
Intermediate-acting	NPH (isophane)	1–3	6–12	18–24
	Lente	1–3	6–12	18–24
Long-acting	Ultralente	4–6	8–20	24–28

[a] These figures are for human insulin and are approximations from laboratory studies in test subjects. The times of onset, peak, and duration of action vary greatly within and between patients and are affected by many factors, including the size of the dose, site and depth of injection, exercise, temperature, and insulin antibodies.

Table 3   Insulin Regimens[a,b]

Doses	Breakfast	Lunch	Dinner	Bedtime
Two	R + NPH/L		R + NPH/L	
	R + NPH/L		R + UL	
	R + UL		R + UL	
Three	R + NPH/L		R	R + NPH/L
	R + NPH/L	R	R + NPH/L	
	R + NPH/L	R	R + UL	
	R + UL	R	R + UL	
Four	R	R	R	R + NPH/L
	R + NPH/L	R	R	R + NPH/L

[a] R, regular (or lispro) insulin; NPH, neutral protamine Hagedorn insulin; L, Lente insulin; UL, Ultralente; NPH/L, either intermediate-acting insulin may be selected for use with this regimen.
[b] Intensified insulin therapy is defined as three or more doses of insulin daily.

given at bedtime, rather than before supper (see Sec. V.B). If one chooses a three-dose regimen from the outset, the evening dose is divided between rapid-acting insulin before supper and intermediate-acting insulin at bedtime. The initial ratio of rapid- to intermediate-acting insulin at both times is 1:2. For example, a 10-year-old prepubertal boy who weighs 30 kg and presents without ketonuria and a venous pH of 7.35, would receive an initial dose of 0.25 U/kg per day (7.5 U) distributed: a mixture of 1.5 U regular and 3.5 U NPH before breakfast, and 1 U regular and 1.5 U NPH before dinner, or 1 U regular before dinner and 1.5 U NPH at bedtime. Toddlers and young children typically require a smaller fraction of rapid-acting insulin (10–20% of the total dose) and proportionately more intermediate-acting insulin.

Target blood glucose goals (see Table 1) vary according to the age of the patient and the psychosocial circumstances of the individual patient and family. Blood glucose targets and the intensity of treatment should be individualized. The insulin dose is adjusted until satisfactory blood glucose (BG) control is achieved with most BG values in or near the target range. Injections of regular insulin are given 30 min before eating; lispro insulin is given no more than 5–15 min before eating.

The optimal ratio of rapid-acting to intermediate-acting insulin for each patient is determined empirically, guided by the results of frequent blood glucose measurements. Five daily measurements are initially required to determine the effects of each component of the insulin regimen. Blood glucose concentrations are measured before each meal, before the bedtime snack, and at 2–4 AM. Day-to-day adjustments of insulin doses are of two types. In patients receiving two injections per day, small compensatory adjustments in the prebreakfast and pre-dinner doses of rapid-acting insulin can be made if blood glucose values are outside the target range. Parents are taught to look for patterns of hyperglycemia or hypoglycemia that indicate the need for an adjustment in the usual dose. Adjust-ments are made to individual components of the insulin regimen, usually in 5–10% increments or decrements, in response to patterns of consistently elevated (above the target range for at least 3–5 days) or low blood glucose levels, respec-tively (referred to as pattern adjustment).

At the time of diagnosis, most children have some residual beta cells and enter a period of partial remission ("honeymoon"), during which normal or nearly normal glycemic control is relatively easily achieved with a low dose of insulin, usually less than 0.25 U/kg per day. The honeymoon manifests with recurrent biochemical or symptomatic hypoglycemia. At this stage, the second dose of intermediate-acting insulin should be reduced if nocturnal hypoglycemia occurs because residual endogenous insulin secretion helps control the fasting blood glucose (FBG) concentration. Most patients also require a reduction in their morning mixture and in the predinner dose of rapid-acting insulin. After destruction of the remaining beta cells has occurred, the insulin dose gradually increases until the full replacement dose is reached. In children with long-standing diabetes, the average daily insulin dose is approximately 0.8 U/kg per day.

B. Intensified Insulin Therapy in Children

Insulin replacement therapy with three or more injections per day or with continu-ous subcutaneous insulin infusion (CSII) by a portable pump can more closely simulate normal insulin profiles and avoid some of the limitations inherent in a two-dose regimen. A major problem of the two dose "split-mixed" regimen is that the peak effect of the predinner intermediate-acting insulin tends to coincide with the time of minimal insulin requirement (midnight to 4 AM). Thereafter, serum insulin levels decline from 4 to 8 AM, when basal insulin requirements normally increase. Consequently, the tendency for blood glucose levels to rise before breakfast (dawn phenomenon) may be aggravated by the secretion of counterregulatory (anti-insulin) hormones in response to a fall in blood glucose levels during sleep (Somogyi phenomenon). A three-dose insulin regi-men—mixed rapid- and intermediate-acting insulins before breakfast, only rapid-acting insulin before dinner, and intermediate-acting insulin at bedtime—may remedy these problems. Alternatively, Ultralente, a long-acting insulin, can be used to provide basal insulin and rapid-acting insulin is injected before each meal (the basal-bolus regimen). Several widely used insulin regimens are shown in Table 2. Adherence and compliance issues are the major obstacles that have limited the use of complex, multiple dose regimens in children. The care provider should frankly discuss treatment options with parents and child, and explain the advantages and disadvantages of each in attempting to meet the overall goals of treatment. The most suitable regimen for a given child and family should be determined by mutual consent and not by coercion.

The use of CSII in children has been quite limited. The most obvious disadvantage is the presence of the pump itself because children do not wish to appear different from their peers. Only short-acting insulin is used with CSII; therefore, any interruption in the delivery of insulin rapidly leads to metabolic decompensation. To reduce this risk, meticulous care must be devoted to the infusion system, and blood glucose levels must be measured frequently. The added responsibility of caring for the pump may be more than many children can manage.

Intensified insulin therapy requires more time, effort, and thought on the part of patients and parents, and considerable education and support from the diabetes team. The DCCT showed that this investment is worthwhile in reducing the risk of microvascular complications in adults and adolescents (13–18 years old at entry into the study). The risk/benefit ratio may not be as favorable in younger children with type 1 diabetes, especially in infants, toddlers, and preschool age children who may not be able to identify and treat hypoglycemia themselves. In prescribing insulin for this age group, the diabetes treatment team must weigh the perceived benefits against the risk of severe hypoglycemia and potential cerebral injury from recurrent hypoglycemia. Several studies have shown that severe hypoglycemia may have more profound adverse effects on the brain development of very young children.

C. Technical Details of Insulin Therapy

Caring for young children with diabetes is challenging for many reasons, not least of which is the need to accurately and reproducibly measure and inject tiny doses of insulin that is supplied in a concentration of 100 U/mL. To administer a dose of 1 U (0.1 U/kg in a 10-kg child) requires the ability to accurately measure 10 μL (1/100 mL) of insulin. A dose change of 0.25 U translates into a volume difference of 2.5 μL in a 300-μL syringe. Measurement of such small volumes is inaccurate using a standard commercial 30-U (300-μL) syringe. When parents attempt to measure a dose of 0.25 U of insulin, they consistently measure more than the prescribed amount. Therefore, to enhance accuracy and reproducibility of measuring small doses, insulin should be diluted to U 25 or U 10. Then, each unit measured on the syringe is actually 0.25 or 0.1 U. This also allows greater flexibility when the child's insulin dose has to be adjusted. Diluted insulin is essential if doses need to be changed in fractions of a unit. Some pharmacists will provide this service. Alternatively, parents can be taught to make diluted insulin using a sterile vial and specific diluent available from the insulin manufacturers.

To avoid painful intramuscular injections, syringes with 30-gauge 8-mm (short) needles should be used to administer insulin to infants and young children with little subcutaneous fat. These syringes are also suitable for use in older nonobese children.

VI. MEDICAL NUTRITIONAL THERAPY

The nutritional needs of children with diabetes do not differ from those of healthy children. Children in whom the disease is newly diagnosed are often underweight; therefore, the initial diet prescription aims to restore a desirable weight/height ratio. Once this has been achieved, the total intake of calories and nutrients should be sufficient to balance the daily expenditure of energy and satisfy the child's requirements for normal growth and development. A method commonly used to estimate energy requirements is based on age and provides a crude approximation for children up to 12 years of age. For all children, basal calorie needs equal 1000 kcal, to which is added ($125 \times$ age in years) for boys and ($100 \times$ age) for girls. For example, a 7-year-old girl requires 1700 kcals/day.

The American Diabetes Association recommends that carbohydrate provide 50–60% of the total calories, with protein and fat making up 15 and 30%, respectively. The diet prescription has to be adjusted periodically to achieve an ideal or desirable body weight and to maintain a normal rate of physical growth and maturation. The same principles apply to the overweight or obese patient, with the added goal of achieving optimal or desirable body weight.

Meals and snacks should be eaten at approximately the same times each day. The total consumption of calories and the proportions of carbohydrate, protein, and fat in each meal and snack should be consistent from day-to-day. Because insulin is continuously absorbed from the injection site, hypoglycemia may occur if snacks are not eaten between the main meals. Most children who receive twice-daily injections of insulin (split-mixed insulin regimen) have a snack between each meal and at bedtime.

The meal plan is formulated using the system of food exchanges, which is individualized to meet the ethnic, religious, and economic circumstances of each family and the food preferences of the child. The diet prescription must take into account the child's school schedule, times of physical education classes, and after-school and weekend sports programs. The exchange system is based on six food groups: milk, fruit, vegetable, bread (starch), meat (protein), and fat. The individual food items included in each exchange list contain approximately the same amount of carbohydrate, protein, and fat. Within the six food groups, the portion size of each item is listed by weight or volume. Thus, the meal plan or diet prescription is prescribed in terms of the number of items (exchanges) from each food group to be included in each meal and snack. Parents and children, also, must be taught how to read and interpret nutrition information on food labels.

Ingested carbohydrate is nearly all converted to glucose within about 90 min of consuming a meal. Therefore, of the various nutrients contained in a given meal, the carbohydrate content is the principal determinant of the amount of insulin needed before that meal. Carbohydrate counting is a method used to assist patients to include a consistent amount of carbohydrate in their meals and snacks. It is also a valuable tool for patients using intensified insulin therapy regimens. An insulin algorithm is devised to match a dose of rapid-acting insulin to a specific amount of dietary carbohydrate. Many families use a combination of the exchange system and carbohydrate counting to allow greater flexibility with the planning of meals and snacks.

Because individuals with diabetes are predisposed to atherosclerosis, they should follow a prudent fat diet. The amount of fat should not exceed 30% of the total daily calories. Dietary cholesterol should be reduced to 300 mg/day. The amount of polyunsaturated and monounsaturated fatty acids is increased, whereas the consumption of saturated fat is reduced to less than 10% of calories by consuming less red meat, choosing lean cuts of meat, and including more chicken, turkey, fish, low-fat milk, and vegetable proteins in the diet.

Dietary fiber may benefit the patient with diabetes by blunting the rise in blood glucose after meals and helping with satiety. Unrefined or minimally processed foods, such as grains, legumes, and vegetables, should replace highly refined carbohydrates. Children should be encouraged to eat fresh fruit and limit their consumption of fruit juices.

VII. EXERCISE

Physical exercise is complicated for the child with diabetes by the need to prevent hypoglycemia. This requires planning. However, with proper guidance and preparation, participation in exercise should usually be a safe and enjoyable experience. Children with diabetes are encouraged to participate in sports and make regular exercise a part of their daily lives. It normalizes the child's life, enhances self-esteem, improves physical fitness, helps control weight, and can improve glycemic control. Over the course of a lifetime, regular exercise improves insulin sensitivity, cardiovascular fitness, blood lipid profiles, and lowers blood pressure.

Exercise lowers the blood glucose concentration by increasing utilization of glucose to a variable degree that depends on the intensity and duration of physical activity and the concurrent level of insulin in the blood. Hypoglycemia can be prevented by supplemental snacks before, during, and after activity, depending on the intensity and duration of the physical activity and its timing relative to the child's dietary and insulin schedule. Consideration is given to several factors when selecting the content and size of the snack. Among these are the current blood glucose level, the amount of insulin acting during and after the period of anticipated exercise, the interval since the last meal, and the duration and intensity of physical activity.

A useful guide is to provide an additional 15 g of carbohydrate (one bread or fruit exchange) per 60 min of vigorous physical activity. Prolonged and strenuous exercise in the afternoon or evening should be followed by a 10–20% reduction in the presupper or bedtime dose of intermediate-acting insulin. In addition, the bedtime snack should be larger than usual to reduce the risk of nocturnal or early-morning hypoglycemia caused by the lag effect of exercise. Parents should be encouraged to monitor the blood glucose concentration in the middle of the night until they are experienced in modifying the evening dose of insulin.

Exercising the limb into which insulin has been injected accelerates the rate of insulin absorption. If possible, the insulin injection preceding exercise should be given in a site least likely to be affected by exercise. Because physical training increases tissue sensitivity to insulin, children who participate in organized sports are advised to reduce the dose of the insulin preparation that is predominantly active during the period of sustained physical activity. The size of such reductions is determined by measuring blood glucose levels before and after exercise and is generally on the order of 10–30% of the usual dose.

Vigorous exercise in the child with poorly controlled diabetes can aggravate hyperglycemia and ketoacid production. Therefore, a child with ketonuria should not exercise until satisfactory biochemical control has been restored.

VIII. MONITORING DIABETES CONTROL

A. Self-Monitoring of Blood Glucose

The cornerstone of diabetes care is SMBG. Patients and parents should be taught how to use the data to adjust the components of their diabetes treatment regimen to achieve specific blood glucose goals (see Table 3). For most patients with type 1 DM, SMBG should be performed, ideally, at least four times daily: before each meal and at bedtime. At a minimum, patients should measure their blood glucose levels before each dose of insulin and perform additional tests before lunch and at bedtime at least twice each week. To minimize the risk of nocturnal hypoglycemia, blood glucose measurements between midnight and 4 AM should be performed once every week or every-other-week, and whenever the evening dose of insulin is adjusted.

If children are not properly supervised, it is not unusual for them to fabricate the results recorded in the logbook to please their parents and physician and avoid criticism.

B. Urine Ketone Testing

The presence of urine ketones may indicate impending or established ketoacidosis. Urine should routinely be tested for ketones during acute illness or stress, when blood glucose levels are persistently elevated (e.g., > 300 mg/dL), or when the patient feels unwell.

C. Glycosylated Hemoglobin, Glycated Hemoglobin, Hemoglobin A_{1c}

Hemoglobin A_{1c} (HbA_{1c}) is a minor fraction of adult hemoglobin, which is formed slowly and nonenzymatically from hemoglobin and glucose. Because erythrocytes are freely permeable to glucose, HbA_{1c} is formed throughout the lifespan of the erythrocyte and its rate of formation is directly proportional to the ambient glucose concentration. The concentration of HbA_{1c}, therefore, provides a glycemic history of the previous 120 days (i.e., the average lifespan of erythrocytes). Quarterly determinations of the HbA_{1c} concentration are used to provide an objective measure of average glycemia in the intervals between office visits. The normal upper limit of HbA_{1c} in most laboratories is 4–6%. Modern management of diabetes aims to maintain the HbA_{1c} concentration as near normal as possible. We advise parents of children with diabetes to attempt to maintain a HbA_{1c} of 8.0%, or less.

X. HYPOGLYCEMIA

Because insulin replacement therapy is unphysiological, occasional episodes of hypoglycemia are unavoidable if one aims to maintain blood glucose levels near normal. The goal is to minimize the frequency and severity of hypoglycemia while maintaining blood glucose levels as near normal as possible. The most common reasons for hypoglycemia are meals or snacks that are delayed, omitted, or incompletely consumed; physical activity without a preceding snack; prolonged or strenuous exercise without a reduction of insulin dose; inadvertent errors in insulin dosage; and inappropriate insulin regimens.

Neurogenic symptoms of hypoglycemia result from the perception of physiological changes caused by the autonomic nervous system discharge triggered by hypoglycemia. Children are taught to recognize the early symptoms of hypoglycemia and what to do when they have the symptoms. Family members, teachers, and daycare providers must learn to recognize the signs of hypoglycemia (pallor, sweating), its characteristic neuroglycopenic manifestations (weakness, inability to stand or walk, drowsiness, inability to think clearly, confusion, dysarthria, bizarre behavior), and to promptly treat the child with a suitable form of concentrated carbohydrate. Because infants and toddlers are unable to interpret and verbalize their symptoms, the responsible adult should measure the blood glucose concentration whenever the child's behavior is unusual or in any way suggestive of hypoglycemia.

Most episodes of hypoglycemia in infants and toddlers can be satisfactorily treated with 5 g of glucose; older children require 10–15 g. Suitable forms of rapidly absorbed carbohydrate for treatment of hypoglycemia are glucose tablets (each contains 5 g of glucose), Lifesavers (3 g sugar), granulated table sugar (4 g of sucrose per teaspoon), fruit juice (10–12 g/120 mL). The blood glucose concentration should be measured 20 mins after treatment to ensure that it has been restored to normal. Family members and daycare providers are taught to use glucagon to treat an episode of severe hypoglycemia in which the child is unconscious or unable to swallow or retain ingested carbohydrate. A glucagon emergency kit should be available at home and at school or daycare center. Glucagon (0.02–0.03 mg/kg, maximum dose 1.0 mg) is injected IM or SC and raises the blood glucose level within 5–15 min. Nausea and vomiting frequently follow the administration of glucagon. Oral carbohydrate to prevent further hypoglycemia should be given when consciousness has been regained after an episode of severe hypoglycemia. If the patient cannot swallow or retain sugar-containing solutions, glucose, 0.5 g/kg is injected IV followed by a continuous IV glucose infusion at a rate of 10 mg/kg per minute. Blood glucose is monitored frequently to determine the appropriate rate of glucose infusion. After the occurrence of an episode of severe hypoglycemia, the possible reason(s) should be carefully explored and, if necessary, the treatment regimen should be modified to minimize the risk of subsequent episodes.

A Medic Alert bracelet or necklace should always be worn to identify the patient as having diabetes mellitus.

X. SPECIAL CIRCUMSTANCES

A. Management of Sick Days

Even a relatively minor illness in a child with diabetes can cause rapid deterioration in metabolic control. The stress of infection, surgery, injury, or severe emotional disturbance increases secretion of the stress or counterregulatory hormones: glucagon, epinephrine, growth hormone, and cortisol. These hormones cause insulin resistance and tend to raise the blood glucose level. Despite reduced intake of carbohydrate associated with the underlying illness, blood glucose levels typically increase, and enhanced ketoacid production results in ketonuria. Unchecked, these metabolic disturbances can rapidly progress to DKA. The aim of sick day management, therefore, is to minimize deterioration of metabolic control and prevent DKA from developing. In addition to managing the diabetes, the underlying illness should be treated appropriately.

The major principles of treatment are

Never omit administration of insulin
Prevent dehydration
Monitor levels of blood glucose and urine ketones frequently
Give supplemental insulin according to the accompanying guidelines
Monitor the child's condition for signs and symptoms that demand immediate attention of a physician

1. Never Omit Insulin Injections

Patients with type 1 DM always need insulin and the child's schedule of insulin injections should not be changed. If the blood glucose concentration is low, the dose of insulin may have to be reduced (Table 4). More often, supplemental injections of rapid-acting insulin are required because blood glucose levels are high during intercurrent illness, despite reduced calorie consumption, and ketonuria is frequently present.

2. Prevent Dehydration

The child should be encouraged to drink at least 1–2 mL/lb pound of body weight per hour (or 1.5–3 L/m² per 24 h). The fluids should contain salt and potassium to replace the losses of these electrolytes that occur with metabolic decompensation. A combination of fluids is recommended to ensure that the child receives salt, glucose, and potassium. Fluids suitable for sick days are broth or bouillon, water, carbonated beverages, and fruit juices. Sugar-free fluids are recommended if the child is able to follow his or her meal plan. However, if the child is unable to eat solid foods, the liquids chosen should contain a source of glucose; for example, fruit juices, popsicles, regular jello, or sweetened carbonated beverages (e.g., cola, lemonade, ginger ale).

3. Monitor Blood Glucose and Urine Ketones at Least Every 4 Hours

Weight loss is a reliable sign of dehydration. The child should be carefully weighed several times each day. Blood glucose and urine ketones should be measured every 3–4 h around-the-clock.

4. Give Supplemental Insulin

Depending on the blood glucose levels and whether there is ketonuria additional rapid-acting insulin may be necessary every 3–4 h until blood glucose is less than 200 mg/dL. An empirical guide to how much and when supplemental rapid-acting insulin should be given is shown in Table 4.

Table 4 A Guide to Supplemental Rapid-Acting Insulin When the Child is Sick[a]

Blood glucose (mg/dL)	< 80	80–200	201–300	301–400	> 400
Urine ketones > trace positive	Yes or no	Yes or no	Yes or no	Yes or no	Yes or no
Amount of extra insulin needed	Omit rapid-acting insulin; decrease NPH/Lente by 1/2; test again in 1–4 h, notify MD	No extra insulin; test again in 3–4 h	Give 5–10% of usual total daily dose; test again in 3–4 h; repeat if no improvement	Give 10–15% of usual total daily dose; test again in 3–4 h; repeat if no improvement	Give 20% of usual total daily dose; test again in 3–4 h, repeat if no improvement

[a] Aim to maintain blood glucose 80–200 mg/dL and urine with no ketones or trace ketones. Supplemental insulin is given exclusively as rapid-acting (regular or lispro) insulin. The dose of supplemental insulin is calculated as a percentage of the usual total daily dose of insulin (the sum of both regular and intermediate-acting insulin, NPH or Lente). For example, for a child whose usual total daily insulin dose is 30 Units, a 10% supplemental or booster dose would be 3 U, and a 20% supplemental dose would be 6 U. When there is anorexia, vomiting, or diarrhea, and the child's ability to tolerate fluids or food is uncertain, in addition to omitting rapid-acting insulin, the dose of intermediate-acting insulin should, initially be reduced to half the usual dose.

5. Signs and Symptoms That Demand Medical Attention

In any of the following circumstances, the child must be seen immediately by a physician because continued attempts to manage the diabetes at home may not be safe.

1. If the child exhibits any signs of dehydration: dry mouth or tongue, cracked lips, sunken eyes, dry flushed skin, weight loss.
2. If the child is unable to consume the recommended amount of fluid or carbohydrate, or if vomiting persists for more than an hour or two.
3. If the child develops symptoms of DKA, such as nausea, abdominal pain, vomiting, hyperventilation, drowsiness.
4. If blood glucose exceeds 250 mg/dL and ketonuria persists for more than 12 h.

By assiduously following the guidelines outlined in this protocol, most intercurrent illnesses in children can be managed successfully at home.

B. Minor Surgery

Few children with diabetes ever require surgery. Occasionally, the child with diabetes has to undergo either minor or major surgery or a diagnostic procedure that requires the child to fast for several hours. A safe and simple regimen for managing these situations should aim to maintain "reasonable" blood glucose levels and avoid hypoglycemia.

On the day before the procedure, the child should receive his usual dose of insulin. For minor day surgery, the child is admitted on the day of the procedure. Ideally, she or he should be the first case of the day. On the morning of surgery, no rapid-acting insulin (regular or lispro) is given unless the blood glucose level is higher than 200 mg/dL. The child should receive half the usual morning dose of intermediate-acting insulin (NPH or Lente). If the procedure is likely to last only 1 or 2 h and one anticipates that the child will be able to drink after the procedure, it is usually unnecessary to start an intravenous infusion. However, if the duration of fast is likely to be more prolonged, an intravenous infusion of 5% dextrose in 1/4 or 1/2 normal saline should be given at the maintenance rate. After the procedure, a "sliding scale" is used to determine the need for additional rapid-acting insulin (see Table 4). If the child is able to resume a normal diet later in the day, the usual insulin regimen is reinstituted.

XI. SCREENING FOR LONG-TERM COMPLICATIONS

Diabetes affects the eyes, kidneys, peripheral nervous system, and circulatory system. Development of diabetic complications is insidious, but can usually be detected years before the patient has symptoms or organ function is impaired. Systematic screening can detect abnormality at an early stage when intervention to arrest, reverse, or retard the disease process will have the most beneficial effect.

Diabetic retinopathy is rare before the onset of puberty or in patients who have had diabetes for fewer than 5 years. Therefore, beginning 5 years after diagnosis, patients should have an annual dilated retinal examination. Renal disease is first detected by persistent albuminuria. Similarly, after 5 years of diabetes, an annual screening measurement of urine albumin and creatinine concentrations should be performed to detect microalbuminuria. Circulatory and neurological complications of diabetes are seldom clinically significant in the pediatric and adolescent population.

XII. CONCLUSION

In the past two decades, considerable progress has been made in the treatment of diabetes in children. It is now possible to ensure normal growth and development and safely achieve a level of blood glucose control previously unattainable. It is reasonable to expect that the benefits of sustained improvement in glycemic control will prevent or, at least, delay the appearance of the chronic complications of diabetes. It is important, however, to remember that the arduous and unending task of controlling blood glucose in a child is difficult and frustrating. Members of the diabetes team must set realistic and attainable goals for each patient, while constantly providing encouragement and support. The resources of a multidisciplinary health care team—physician, nurse educator, dietitian, mental health specialist, and ophthalmologist—are essential for the successful management of childhood diabetes.

BIBLIOGRAPHY

American Diabetes Associates. Intensive Diabetes Management, 2nd edition. Alexandria, VA: American Diabetes Association, 1998.

American Diabetes Association. Diabetes 1996: Vital Statistics. Alexandria, VA: American Diabetes Association, 1996.

Cryer PE. Hypoglycemia: the limiting factor in the management of IDDM. Diabetes 1994; 43:1378–1389.

Davis EA, Keating B, Byrne GC, Russell M, Jones TW. Hypoglycemia: incidence and clinical predictors in a large population-based sample of children and adolescents with IDDM. Diabetes Care 1997; 20:22–25.

Diabetes Control and Complications Trial Research Group. The effect of intensive treatment of diabetes on the development and progression of long-term complications in insulin-dependent diabetes mellitus. N Engl J Med 1993; 329:977–986.

Diabetes Control and Complications Trial Research Group. Effect of intensive diabetes treatment on the development and progression of long-term complications in adolescents with insulin-dependent diabetes mellitus: Diabetes Control and Complications Trial. J Pediatr 1994; 125:177–188.

Goldstein DE, Little RR, Lorenz RA, Malone JI, Nathan D, Peterson CM. Tests of glycemia in diabetes [technical review]. Diabetes Care 1995; 18:896–909.

Holleman F, Hoekstra J. Insulin lispro. N Engl J Med 1997; 337:176–183.

Kistler J. Children and adolescents. In: Ruderman N, Devlin JT, ed. The Health Professional's Guide to Diabetes and Exercise. Alexandria, VA: American Diabetes Association, 1995:217–222.

Rosenbloom AL, Hanas R. Diabetic ketoacidosis (DKA): treatment guidelines. Clin Pediatr 1996; 35:261–266.

Santiago J. Insulin therapy in the last decade: a pediatric perspective. Diabetes Care 1993; 16(suppl 3):143–154.

Silva S, Clark L, Goodman S, Plotnick L. Can caretakers of children with IDDM accurately measure small insulin doses and dose changes? Diabetes Care 1996; 19:56–59.

Wolfsdorf JI, Anderson BJ, Pasquarello C. Treatment of the child with diabetes. In: Kahn CR, Weir GC, eds. Joslin's Diabetes Mellitus. 13th ed. Philadelphia: Lea & Febiger, 1994:530–552.

Wolfsdorf JI, Quinn M. Diabetes mellitus. In: Walker WA, Watkins JB, eds. Nutrition in Pediatrics: Basic Science and Clinical Applications. 2nd ed. Hamilton, Ontario: BC Decker, 1996:583–593.

11
Diabetes Care in the Adolescent

Nathaniel G. Clark
University of Vermont College of Medicine, Burlington, Vermont

Paul B. Madden
Joslin Diabetes Center, Boston, Massachusetts

I. INTRODUCTION

This chapter will serve as a companion to the Chap. 10 on diabetes in children. The adolescent, while often seen as a child in the eyes of physicians who care for adults, has characteristics that make their management more similar to adults. It is true that as the child moves farther into the adolescent age range he or she wishes to be seen and treated more like an adult than like a child. This confusion in the way in which the adolescent patient is viewed by medical specialists mirrors very closely the conflict within the adolescent over how they see themselves. This chapter focuses on issues specific to the adolescent with diabetes.

During adolescence, tremendous changes occur in many areas of development. It is a period of rapid physical growth and maturity that may or may not be pleasing to the patient. Puberty itself can be traumatic for many individuals. Puberty also has a major effect on diabetes, as insulin requirements increase secondary to the insulin resistance that occurs during puberty. Issues surrounding weight and perceived body image can become very complicated, particularly in the adolescent girl. The adolescent is changing intellectually as well, and with this increase in knowledge and maturity can come new understanding and fears about the realities of having diabetes. On the other hand, with the changes in intellect and maturity comes an opportunity to help adolescents take increasing responsibility for the management of his or her diabetes, as they now have the capacity to understand the theoretical basis and importance of healthy behaviors.

There are also very dramatic changes during adolescence both within the family and school. Adolescence is a time when most young persons want to be part of a group and to have as few distinguishing characteristics as possible that prevent them from blending in with their peers. Diabetes presents an enormous challenge in this area and often results in reluctance on the part of the adolescent with diabetes to have teachers and peers know about their disorder. On the other hand, in the interest of safety, it is clearly best if those around the person with diabetes know of their disease so that if assistance is needed, for example, during a hypoglycemic episode (e.g., an accident), appropriate help could be provided.

II. THE INSULIN RESISTANCE OF PUBERTY

Doses of insulin may increase significantly as the patient enters puberty. Multiple studies have demonstrated that puberty is characterized by insulin resistance, necessitating higher doses than before puberty. During the Diabetes Control and Complications Trial (DCCT), adolescents required approximately 30% more insulin per kilogram than their adult counterparts. Whereas the mean insulin dose in the "intensive" group for adults was 0.75 U/kg, in the adolescent group it was 1.0 U/kg. Adolescents in the midst of puberty often require as much as 1.5 U/kg to achieve optimal control. These increased doses may necessitate changing to larger syringes. In adjusting the insulin dose, the blood glucose record is still the most important piece of data; the dosage is increased as needed to achieve adequate control, regardless of how many units of insulin are required.

III. THE IMPORTANCE OF BLOOD GLUCOSE CONTROL

Two issues that have been raised for the adolescent with diabetes are (a) to what extent do the years of prepubertal diabetes matter relative to the risk of long-term complications of diabetes given that the onset of long-term complications are rarely noted in prepubertal children; and (b) to what extent are the findings of the landmark DCCT applicable to adolescent patients? For the first question, there is no clear and widely accepted answer. Studies have been performed suggesting that the years of prepubertal diabetes may have little influence on the overall risk of complications, and they postulate that the prepubertal state provides some protection from the long-term risks of ongoing hyperglycemia. This impression has led many practitioners to believe that blood glucose control need not be maximized before puberty and also has caused some to believe, and the ADA to recommend that screening for complications (i.e., retinopathy and nephropathy) does not need to begin until puberty, even in those children in whom the disease was diagnosed in infancy. More recent studies have concluded that there is clearly a risk associated with poorly controlled diabetes, even in the prepubertal years, and that the two major determinants of the risk of long-term complications of diabetes are overall blood glucose control and the number of years of diabetes. Clearly, formation of positive health practices in diabetes management during adolescence is a key to future success.

A very reasonable approach is to understand that blood glucose control should be individualized and that, in each patient, the relative benefits and risks of intensive management should be considered. In all children and adolescents, one worries more about the risks of hypoglycemia than in the adult, because the child is still developing mentally as well as physically. This may cause us to accept higher hemoglobin (Hb) A_{1c} levels in the adolescent patient. In the patient who over time has not had significant difficulties with hypoglycemia, more aggressive attempts to maximize control are warranted; in the patient with frequent episodes of significant hypoglycemia, one needs to keep this in mind when setting HbA_{1c} goals.

For the second issue, the relative benefits and risks of intensive therapy in the adolescent were examined in the DCCT. Of those in the trial, 14% were between the age of 13 and 17 years. When the data on this age group were analyzed, it was clear that adolescents showed benefits from intensified treatment similar to their adult counterparts. In the adolescent group, there was a 30% decreased risk of the development of retinopathy and a 61% decrease in the risk of progression of baseline retinopathy in the group receiving intensive management. There was also a significant decrease in the development of microalbuminuria, similar to that seen in the overall study. Notable, however, was that the occurrence of severe hypoglycemia in adolescents was significantly higher when compared with the adults in the trial, although the relative risk was not statistically different between the adolescent and adult groups. Lastly, intensive blood glucose control can lead to weight gain, which is particularly problematic for many adolescent girls.

Many leaders in the field of diabetology have commented on what lessons have been learned from the DCCT relative to the treatment of adolescents with diabetes. In summary, the data from the DCCT demonstrated that good control of blood glucose levels significantly reduces the risk of long-term complications in adolescents as well as in adults. The importance of a multi-disciplinary approach to the treatment of diabetes was clearly demonstrated as the "intensive group" received far more than simply more injections of insulin or the use of insulin pumps. These patients were in regular contact with a member of "the team" on almost a daily basis. Finally, the risks of hypoglycemia need to be considered carefully when setting blood glucose goals for each patient. In the adolescent age group where there can be tremendous variability in carbohydrate intake, meal times, and levels of physical activity, the risks of hypoglycemia can be far greater than in adults. Of note, since the advent of Humalog (lispro) insulin, many patients have been able to reduce their HbA_{1c}s without any increase (or a decrease) in hypoglycemic events.

IV. "ACCENTUATE THE POSITIVE"

In dealing with the adolescent, one of the most important precepts is to be as positive as possible in helping the patient deal with the demands of diabetes. When one thinks of all the changes that an adolescent is going through during this critical time in their development, it is certainly true that diabetes is a confounding and complicating factor. Although it would be easy to list a multitude of ways on how having diabetes can makes life more difficult, adolescents do not see having diabetes as entirely negative. When asked, adolescents often state that having diabetes has been a positive aspect in their lives. (a) They may believe that they have done better academically because of the need to be more organized; (b) they are often considered more mature and, thereby, given greater responsibility; (c) they have greater knowledge of health issues, their bodies, and specifically issues of nutrition; and (d) they tend to be more active physically and, therefore, to be in better physical condition. These positive notions on diabetes may be even more appreciated in those adolescents who have had "positive group experiences" (camps, support groups) with other young people who have diabetes and with adult role models who are doing well with their diabetes.

As the patient moves farther into adolescence, the realities of having diabetes can be overwhelming at times. When expressions of frustration, anger, and fear over the possible long-term complications of diabetes are expressed, they should be discussed openly with the patient. On the other hand, attempting to scare the patient into better control of his or her diabetes by citing the long-term complications (or taking the patient to see a person who has suffered severe complications) has little value in changing behavior and may have a detrimental effect on the adolescent.

Nothing can substitute for the support that patients can give each other. Setting up a regularly scheduled opportunity for adolescents to meet and interact is invaluable. These groups are best facilitated by a responsible adult who is viewed as a neutral party. Typically, a psychologist or social worker is very effective in this role. Parents also should meet (separately) and often wish to have caregivers update them on "new developments" in addition to listening to their concerns and giving suggestions. Diabetes camps play a very important role in the care of children with diabetes, including adolescents, for all the foregoing reasons.

When the patient comes in for office visits, we must strive to be as positive as we can to acknowledge and reinforce any good behavior(s). If a patient comes in having missed previous appointments, it is far better to express how happy you are that he or she is here today, that you were worried when he or she did not come in for the previous appointments, and that you want to work closely with him or her now and in the future in managing the diabetes, rather than to scold the patient for the missed appointments. If you have asked that such patients check their blood glucose level four times per day and they bring in records indicating that they have only checked two times per day, it is best to express how happy you are that they have been checking *at least* two times per day and then to explain to them how much more information could be gleaned from checking more frequently. If the patient's HbA$_{1c}$ level is still significantly higher than target, it is best to comment that although the number is too high, it still reflects the tremendous amount of good work that the patient is doing relative to his or her diabetes. If he or she was not doing this positive work, the number would be even higher.

V. WHO'S IN CHARGE

One of the most frequently discussed issues relative to diabetes and the adolescent has to do with when and how the responsibility for the diabetes shifts from the parent to the adolescent. Just as the goals for diabetes management need to be individualized, so must this transfer of responsibility. There are clearly children who enter adolescence and are already taking significant responsibility for the testing of blood glucose levels, the injection of insulin, and even determination of insulin doses. On the other hand, others, even in late adolescence, still are allowing the parent to take responsibility for keeping the blood glucose records and performing most of the injections. There is no right or wrong in this area. The adolescent takes more responsibility for his or her diabetes in a gradual matter that is appropriate for that patient and the parent(s). Some parents seem only too happy to give up their responsibility, having carried this burden for many years, and may allow their child too much responsibility too early. Others find it difficult to give up any of the responsibility owing to concern for their child, but also because over a the years they have developed a system that they feel is successful and, therefore, is difficult to abandon. Trust and open communication must be the foundation for the transfer of responsibility. All parents need to maintain some level of involvement with what is being done for their child's diabetes. Exercising this involvement should always be explained openly to the child and a dialogue about ''how things are going'' should be encouraged. Parents reviewing blood glucose logs when their child is out of the home or downloading the meter to check the accuracy of the log book is clearly discouraged, unless the adolescent has ''ok'd'' this. The adolescent continues to require the support of his or her parents, whether this is acknowledged openly or not by the patient. During office visits it is best to see the patient both with the parent(s) present and also alone. Discussions on smoking, alcohol or drugs, and sexuality are best discussed without the parent(s) present. The adolescent patient needs to understand that you are his or her doctor and that these discussions will not be shared with parents without the patient's consent.

VI. PREGNANCY AND CONTRACEPTION

Pregnancy demands excellent blood glucose control both before conception and throughout pregnancy. A pregnancy in a woman with diabetes should be planned well in advance. If the adolescent patient is sexually active, issues of contraception should be discussed openly.

VII. TOBACCO, ALCOHOL, AND DRUGS

Issues of smoking should be discussed openly with the adolescent. Smoking has a multitude of health risks associated with it as well as having additional specific risks for the person with diabetes. The effects of smoking on the vascular system and those of diabetes are additive; thus, persons with diabetes who smoke are at significantly increased risk of complications. Patients should be advised and encouraged to quit smoking at every visit. Referral of the patient to smoking cessation programs or the use of nicotine withdrawal medications, or both is encouraged.

The consumption of alcohol is a more complicated issue because the use of this drug is so widely accepted in our society and because its use is considered a "rite of passage" by some. Adolescents are encouraged not to drink alcohol for a wide variety of reasons, which will not be reviewed here. If the older adolescent is going to consume alcohol, this should be discussed openly, and advice should be given on how this can be done safely. The effects of alcohol on inhibiting gluconeogenesis and, thereby, increasing the risk for hypoglycemia, the importance of consuming food while consuming alcohol, and how one can responsibly include limited amounts of alcohol into the meal plan should be discussed openly. The dietitian can be very helpful in explaining how to figure both alcohol itself as well as various "mixers" into the diet program.

The use of recreational drugs other than alcohol is less complicated for most practitioners. Each of the various drugs brings with it a specific list of risks, and these risks are greater in those with diabetes. Good diabetes care requires paying attention to a wide variety of factors and the ability to recognize specific signs of hypoglycemia so that significant episodes can be avoided. The adolescent who is impaired by the use of excessive amounts of alcohol or the use of other drugs is far less likely to respond appropriately and therefore, is at far higher risk for either significant hypoglycemia or for ongoing hyperglycemia, potentially leading to diabetic ketoacidosis.

VIII. WEIGHT, WEIGHT LOSS, AND BODY IMAGE

There can be major issues relative to weight and body image, particularly in adolescent girls. There are substantial health risks of anorexia nervosa or bulimia in the patient who does not have diabetes. In the patient with diabetes, these diagnoses can pose tremendous problems. Having a counselor (psychiatrist, psychologist, or social worker) on the diabetes care team is imperative in managing these patients. One specific disorder that occurs not uncommonly in patients (usually women) with diabetes is the withholding of insulin for weight control. Insulin is an anabolic hormone that is normally high in the fed state and leads to the storage of carbohydrates as glycogen or fat. During puberty, when insulin doses are increased, weight gain often ensues. When this weight gain is not welcomed, it is often learned that by omitting or reducing insulin doses weight loss occurs owing to the catabolism in general and the loss of calories by glucosuria. However, when insulin is withheld, these patients are at a tremendous risk for recurrent diabetic ketoacidosis. Although this practice of insulin withholding is not technically an eating disorder, it is managed in much the same way with direct involvement of a counselor and focusing on issues of weight and body image. The involvement of a dietitian can also be extremely helpful to titrate caloric (carbohydrate) intake with insulin therapy to minimize weight gain and maximize blood glucose control. An exercise physiologist or sports coach can also be very helpful focusing on the energy expenditure side of weight control.

IX. SUMMARY

The adolescent with diabetes presents enormous challenges, but also the potential for great rewards. As with all patients with diabetes, one strives to find a balance that promotes maximum blood glucose control while minimizing the burden of diabetes. The benefits of good blood glucose control are as great for the adolescent as for any other patient, and these goals are best achieved using a multidisciplinary approach to care. The lifestyle modifications that we suggest, however, when viewed through the eyes of the adolescent, can be "huge." At all times remain positive in your approach and counsel your patients that diabetes is neither a disability nor a barrier. Urge your patients to state their goals followed by "*and* I have diabetes" and not "*but* I have diabetes." Encourage your patient to take as much responsibility for his or her diabetes as appropriate while involving the parents extensively in the process. Be open in your discussions on all aspects of diabetes care, including smoking, drugs (including alcohol), and body weight. Try at all times to lessen your patient's burden of diabetes not add to it. Enjoy your adolescent patients, they are a gift and have a great deal to teach us all.

BIBLIOGRAPHY

American Diabetes Association. Care of children with diabetes in the school and day care setting. Diabetes Care 1999; 22:S94–S97.

American Diabetes Association. Management of diabetes at diabetes camps. Diabetes Care 1999; 22:S98–S101.

Diabetes Control and Complications Trial Research Group. Effect of intensive diabetes treatment on the development and progression of long-term complications in adolescents with insulin-dependent diabetes mellitus: Diabetes Control and Complications Trial. J Pediatr 1994; 125:177–188.

Tamborlane WV, Ahern J. Implications and results of the diabetes control and complications trial. In: Styne DM, ed. Pediatric Clinics of North America. Philadelphia: WB Saunders, 1997:285–300.

Wolfsdorf JI, Anderson BJ, Pasquarello C. Treatment of the child with diabetes. In: Kahn CR, Weir GC, eds. Joslin's Diabetes Mellitus. Baltimore; Williams & Wilkins, 1994:530–551.

12

Diabetes in Pregnancy

Karen Hugo and Lois Jovanović

Sansum Medical Research Institute, Santa Barbara, California

I. INTRODUCTION

Before the discovery of insulin and its appropriate implementation, pregnancy complicated by diabetes was associated with significant maternal and fetal morbidity and mortality. With improvements in care, the fetal and neonatal mortality has dropped from 60% in the preinsulin era to 2–4% (1). Diabetes is present in 4% of all pregnancies in the United States. Gestational diabetes accounts for approximately 88%, or 135,000 of such pregnancies, whereas pregestational diabetes, both type 1 and 2, account for the remainder (2). *Gestational diabetes mellitus* (GDM) is defined as any degree of glucose intolerance with its onset occurring during pregnancy (3). Pregestational diabetes mellitus encompasses both type 1 diabetes mellitus, a state of absolute insulin deficiency most frequently immune-mediated, and type 2 diabetes mellitus, a state of relative insulin deficiency, often associated with insulin resistance and secretory defects. Because poor glycemic control at conception and during the period of organogenesis is associated with an increased risk of spontaneous abortion and a high incidence of major congenital anomalies, it is imperative that the woman with preexisting diabetes plan her pregnancy achieving satisfactory metabolic control before conception.

II. PREPREGNANCY COUNSELING

In the woman with preexisting diabetes, pregnancy should be deferred until the patient is under good glycemic control and has been thoroughly evaluated for complications of diabetes. Prepregnancy counseling for the young woman with diabetes should begin at the onset of puberty, with the need for abstinence or effective contraception clearly explained and understood. There is no single contraceptive agent that is appropriate for all women with diabetes. Progestin-only compounds, including the Norplant system, may be associated with worsening lipids and glucose intolerance. The rhythm method is not sufficiently reliable to recommend for women with preexisting diabetes. Barrier methods can generally be recommended as good choices. Oral contraceptives with the new formulations of synthetic progestins, such as norgestimate, have less androgenic properties, a reduced influence on lipid levels, and lower anti-insulin activity, making them an attractive choice for contraception in the pregestational diabetic. Ideally, preconception care should involve a team approach, including the patient foremost, a physician with diabetes expertise, a nutritionist, and a nurse educator. Unfortunately, women with type 2 diabetes are less likely to receive preconception care, often because the diagnosis has not yet been made, and access to adequate medical care is lacking for those of lower socioeconomic status in whom type 2 diabetes is more common.

Glycosylated hemoglobin or HbA_{1c} provides an excellent starting point in the initial evaluation. It accurately represents the previous several weeks of glycemic control. There is a substantial increase in both major malformations and spontaneous abortions in women who enter pregnancy in poor metabolic control, as reflected by an elevated HbA_{1c} (Fig. 1). The congenital malformations observed in these infants of diabetic mothers are described in Table 1. Although most pregestational studies have been performed in type 1 diabetes, the same risks of hyperglycemia apply to type 2 diabetic mothers and infants (5,6). Interestingly,

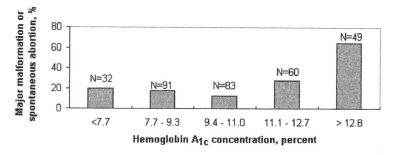

Fig. 1   Deleterious effect of poor glycemic control on fetal outcome. Combined incidence of major malformation and spontaneous abortion according to the hemoglobin A_{1c} concentration during the first trimester of pregnancy in 315 women with insulin-dependent diabetes mellitus. The risk rose markedly at HbA_{1c} concentrations above 11%; other studies have found an increase in risk at levels above 9.5%. (Data from Ref. 7.)

Table 1 Congenital Malformations in Infants of Diabetic Mothers

Anomaly	Ratios of incidence compared with control population
Caudal regression	252
Spina bifida, hydrocephalus, or other CNS defect	2
Anencephalus	3
Heart anomalies (includes VSD, ASD, and transposition of the great vessels)	4
Anal/rectal atresia	3
Renal anomalies	5
Agenesis	6
Cystic kidney	4
Ureter duplex	23
Situs inversus	84

Source: Ref. 4.

the risk of congenital malformations in type 2 pregnancies is related chiefly to maternal metabolic control and not to the mode of antidiabetic therapy in early pregnancy, including oral sulfonylureas. However, because the safety of currently available oral antidiabetic agents has not been firmly established, the type 2 diabetic woman seeking pregnancy should be switched to an insulin regimen. Fortunately, normalizing blood glucose before and early in pregnancy can reduce the risk of spontaneous abortions and malformations to nearly that of the general population (7–10). A glycosylated hemoglobin value within or near the upper limit of normal for the laboratory should be strived for preconceptionally. Reaching this goal entails the use of frequent home blood glucose monitor checks with the following targets:

Preprandial	70–100mg/dL (3.9–5.6 mmol/L)
Postprandial 1-h	< 140 mg/dL (< 7.8 mmol/L)
Postprandial 2-h	< 120 mg/dL (< 6.7 mmol/L)

Maintaining these goals necessitates an intensive regimen of usually three to four insulin injections daily. A combination of a short-acting and intermediate-acting insulin is ideal to provide both meal and basal coverage. A premixed insulin, such as 70/30, likely will not provide the necessary flexibility. Insulin pumps can provide exquisite control and may be continued or initiated in this period. Inherent in the implementation of tight glycemic control is the risk of hypoglycemia. The patient and her family should be educated in how to manage this, including the use of glucagon. Prepregnancy assessment of the diabetic woman should include a thorough evaluation for the complications of diabetes, a careful obstetric history, and a close look at concomitant medical conditions. A possible concomitant medical condition in patients with type 1 diabetes is thyroid disease; therefore, free-thyroxine and thyroid-stimulating hormone (TSH) values should be obtained to rule out coinciding autoimmune thyroid disease. Hypertension is a frequent finding in pregestational diabetes and may potentially be aggravated in pregnancy. Angiotensin-converting enzyme inhibitors (ACEIs) are associated with appreciable risk to the fetus and should be discontinued in the patient contemplating pregnancy. Alternatively, ACEIs have been used to decrease significant proteinuria and then discontinued before conception with excellent results. Other acceptable agents include α-methyldopa, α-adrenergic receptor blockers (prazosin), and calcium channel blockers. Diabetic retinopathy progresses in some women during pregnancy, although it is unlikely to appear de novo in women without preexisting retinopathy (11). Retinopathy is primarily related to the duration of diabetes and the degree of control. In those with diabetes for longer than 15 years duration, nearly 98% demonstrate background retinopathy, whereas 20–25% display more severe proliferative changes (12). Unfortunately, the strict glycemic control so critical for the developing fetus has been associated with worsening maternal retinopathy (13). As the degree to which this occurs during pregnancy is related to the baseline level of retinal disease, the diabetic woman planning a pregnancy should be evaluated and monitored by an ophthalmologist. Proliferative retinopathy should be treated with laser, diminishing the risk of worsening neovascularization, hemorrhage, detachment, and macular edema. Normalization of glycemic control before pregnancy appears to be the best strategy with control attained more gradually over 3–6 months in the diabetic woman with proliferative retinopathy.

Renal function must also be assessed, including 24-h urine for creatinine clearance, protein, and microalbuminuria. The hypertension and preeclampsia frequently associated with nephropathy can have devastating implications for the fetus, including growth retardation, fetal distress, premature labor, and possibly death. Although pregnancy does not appear to increase the risk of future diabetic nephropathy (14), the physiological changes accompanying pregnancy, such as hyperfiltration and increased protein excretion may aggravate preexisting diabetic nephropathy. Fortunately, pregnancy is not associated with permanent worsening of renal function in the majority of diabetic patients in the absence of uncontrolled hypertension or a baseline creatinine value higher than 1.5 mg/dL (130 μmol/L; 24,25). In the latter group, however, permanent worsening of renal disease can be expected to occur in up to one-third of patients. A creatinine value of less than 50 mL/min is associated with a high prevalence of hypertension and fetal wastage. (15) Additionally, those with incipient renal failure, serum values of 3 mg/dL or more, or creatinine clearance of less than 50 mL/min should be counseled to avoid pregnancy unless the renal function can be stabilized with transplantation (16). Control of hypertension and blood glucose is paramount in the diabetic woman with milder renal disease to ensure a good outcome for both mother and fetus. Women currently taking an ACEI for either proteinuria or hypertension, should be switched to another agent before conception, as discussed previously.

Neuropathy is a frequent finding among longstanding diabetics. Although there is little information about the influence of neuropathy on pregnancy available, severe neuropathy often reflects a long history of poor metabolic control. Evaluation for autonomic and peripheral neuropathy should be undertaken. Diminished hypoglycemic awareness and gastroparesis may occur greatly impairing efforts at glycemic control and should be clearly and effectively addressed before recommending pregnancy. Fortunately, coronary artery disease is rare in young diabetic women; however, cardiac disease should be sought in the woman who has had diabetes for 10 years or longer, or has other vascular complications of diabetes.

Atherosclerotic heart disease carries a high risk and has been associaed with a maternal mortality rate exceeding 50% in some series. A baseline electrocardiogram (ECG) should be obtained with further cardiac testing if clinical suspicion is high or the patient has other risk factors, including cigarette smoking, hypertension, or hyperlipidemia.

A certified nutritionist is an integral part of the preconception team. Good habits are best acquired before pregnancy. The optimal goals are to achieve ideal body weight and provide the best possible nutrition for mother and child-to-be. A caloric intake of approximately 30 kcal/kg will maintain an average woman at her weight. To gain or lose approximately 1 lb/week, the woman may subtract or add 500 kcal from her daily caloric intake and alter her exercise level accordingly. Ideally, the daily carbohydrate intake should be consistent, to allow appropriate adjustment of insulin. A prenatal vitamin supplement, with a minimum of 400 μg of folate, should be started in the preconception period to decrease the risk of neural tube defects should pregnancy occur. General principles of good health, including cessation of smoking and alcohol, are always advisable (Table 2).

III. PREGNANCY AND THE PANCREAS

Simply put, pregnancy increases the demand for fuel. The hormones of pregnancy, estradiol, prolactin, human placental lactogen, cortisol, and progesterone, create a diabetogenic state where glucose is reserved for the fetus, and alternative fuels

Table 2 Preconception Control Protocol in Preexisting Diabetes

Effective contraception until glycemic goals met and evaluation of diabetic complications
  complete
History and physical examination
  Hypertension
    Blood pressure ideally < 130/80 mmHg
    Stop smoking, discontinue illicit drugs
    Discontinue ACEI change to other antihypertensive if indicated
  Retinopathy
    Ophthalmological consult
    Fundus photography
    Untreated active proliferative retinopathy is a potential contraindication
  Cardiac
    Rule out ischemic disease
    ECG, exercise test, if indicated
  Renal
    24-h urine for C_{CL}, protein, microalbuminuria
    Urinalysis and culture
    Plasma creatinine concentration > 3 mg/dL is a contraindication for pregnancy
  Thyroid
    Free T_4, TSH, antithyroid peroxidase antibodies
Diabetes
  Achieve diabetic control before conception including nutrition consult
  If glycosylated hemoglobin greater than 4 standard deviations above a normal mean
    glycosylated hemoglobin for women without diabetes, intensive insulin delivery
    program warranted, or "permission granted" if HbA_{1c} at or near upper limit of
    normal (e.g., if laboratory normal range is 5.7–6.1%, then HbA_{1c} should be less
    than 6.1% to safely proceed with pregnancy)
  Normalization programs require 3–4 injections per day of subcutaneously injected
    insulin (NPH and regular) or insulin infusion pump
  Self-blood glucose monitoring at least six times a day (before and 1 h after each
    meal)
  Preconception goals include premeal glucose levels of 70–100 mg/dL and 1-h post-
    meal levels below 140 mg/dL
  Repeat HbA_{1c} measurement 1 month after initiation of program
  Retest every month until target HbA_{1c} achieved—once in target range, permission
    granted to become pregnant on the next cycle
  A pregnancy test 1 day after missed period will confirm pregnancy
  Each cycle should have a repeat HbA_{1c} performed by day 5 to allow the woman to
    receive permission to become pregnant
Psychosocial
  Assess mental, emotional, and financial "readiness" of patient
  Obtain maximal commitment and cooperation from patient, partner, and family

such as lipids maintain the mother. The normal pancreas can compensate for the diabetogenic stresses with hyperinsulinemia and pancreatic islet cell hypertophy. The woman with pregestational diabetes cannot combat these forces either because of the absolute insulin deficiency of type 1 diabetes or the relative insulin deficiency and insulin resistance of type 2 diabetes. Her insulin requirements will continue to increase as the pregnancy progresses. The most common form of diabetes complicating pregnancy, GDM, does not occur until the diabetogenic forces overwhelm the maternal pancreas, which has limited insulin secretory capacity. GDM, thus, is usually detected in the second half of pregnancy when placental synthesis of peptide and steroid hormones peak.

IV. GESTATIONAL DIABETES MELLITUS

The prevalence of GDM varies worldwide and among racial and ethnic groups. It is higher among African Americans, Hispanics, Native Americans, and Asians (17). Different studies have shown a relatively wide range in the prevalence rate from approximately 1 to 12% (18–22). Factors placing a woman at higher risk for GDM are the following (23):

> Family history of diabetes
> Prepregnancy obesity
> Advanced maternal age
> Previous large baby
> Nonwhite ethnicity
> Previous unexplained loss or birth of malformed child
> Mother was a large infant (> 9 lb)

Universal screening of all pregnant women between the 24th and 28th weeks of gestation has been the standard of practice. Currently, selective screening is advocated as being more cost effective. This entails screening women between the 24th and 28th week if they meet one or more of the following criteria (16).

> 25 years of age or older
> Less than 25 years of age and obese (≥ 20% of ideal body weight or a body mass index [BMI] ≥ 27 kg/m^2)
> Family history of diabetes in first-degree relatives
> Member of ethnic or racial group with high prevalence of diabetes (e.g., Latino, Native American, Asian American, African American, or Pacific Islander)

The selective screening approach was supported by a study of over 3000 pregnant women, although the Canadian population studied may not be representative of the U.S. pregnant population (24). The investigators found that increasing age, BMI, and race were independent predictors of an increased risk for GDM. These characteristics could then be used to selectively screen women, resulting in a reduction of the false-positive rate and potential cost savings. These criteria, however, may be difficult to properly implement in the busy obstetrician's or family practitioner's office and the suggested algorithm may actually be more complicated than universal screening. As the population becomes more heterogeneous, lines of ethnicity become more difficult to define. We still favor universal screening for all pregnant women between the 24th and 28th week of gestation, because in our state of California, the substantial Hispanic population is at considerable risk for GDM. Additionally, it is not uncommon to first detect previously undiagnosed type 2 diabetes in our California population with universal screening and this allows earlier and critical intervention. We believe that screening should be performed before the 24th week of gestation if there is a high degree of suspicion that the woman has GDM, such as having a previous GDM pregnancy, and that screening be performed at the first visit if the physician strongly suspects the patient may have type 2 diabetes.

As GDM does not appear until the second or third trimester, organogenesis has been completed in a euglycemic milieu, making major congenital anomalies uncommon. Also, women with GDM do not have the vasculopathy that often accompanies those with pregestational diabetes, and so surveillance for retinopathy, nephropathy, and neuropathy is generally not necessary. Macrosomia with potential shoulder dystocia and birth injury, metabolic derangements, including neonatal hypoglycemia, are real dangers and provide the rationale for intensive glycemic control in the mother with GDM. Maternal complications include an increased rate of cesarean delivery and hypertensive disorders.

V. SCREENING AND DIAGNOSIS

The screening test for GDM consists of a 50-g oral glucose load followed by a plasma glucose assay 1 h later. The patient need not be fasting for the screening test. A value of 140 mg/dL (7.8 mmol/L) or more, is considered abnormal and the patient should go on to complete a 100-g 3-h oral glucose tolerance test (OGTT). Further evaluation of any random plasma glucose of 200 mg/dL (11.1 mmol/L) or higher, or any fasting plasma glucose level higher than 126 mg/dL (7.0 mmol/L) is also recommended because these findings alone are strongly suggestive of diabetes (25).

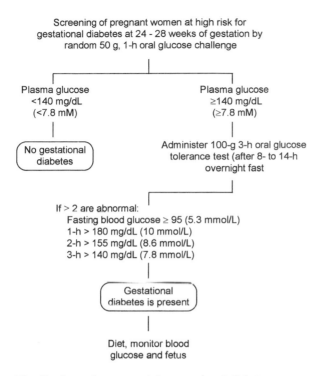

Screening of pregnant women at high risk for
gestational diabetes at 24 - 28 weeks of gestation by
random 50 g, 1-h oral glucose challenge

Plasma glucose
<140 mg/dL
(<7.8 mM)

Plasma glucose
≥140 mg/dL
(≥7.8 mM)

No gestational
diabetes

Administer 100-g 3-h oral glucose
tolerance test (after 8- to 14-h
overnight fast

If > 2 are abnormal:
  Fasting blood glucose ≥ 95 (5.3 mmol/L)
  1-h > 180 mg/dL (10 mmol/L)
  2-h > 155 mg/dL (8.6 mmol/L)
  3-h > 140 mg/dL (7.8 mmol/L)

Gestational
diabetes is present

Diet, monitor blood
glucose and fetus

Fig. 2   Screening protocol for gestational diabetes.

According to the Fourth International Workshop, the diagnosis of GDM is
made if two or more of the following plasma glucose levels are exceeded.

Fasting plasma glucose concentration	> 95 mg/dL (5.3 mmol/L)
1-h glucose value	> 180 mg/dL (10 mmol/L)
2-h glucose value	> 155 mg/dL (8.6 mmol/L)
3-h glucose value	> 140 mg/dL (7.8 mmol/L)

Once the diagnosis is secured, a strategy composed of diet, insulin, and
exercise is planned (Fig. 2).

VI. GDM MANAGEMENT

An effective treatment regimen consists of dietary management, self-monitoring
of blood glucose (SMBG), and the administration of insulin if the glucose targets

are not met with diet alone. Self-monitoring of blood glucose and HbA_{1c} measurements are necessary to demonstrate glycemic control. The patient is asked to check the blood sugar levels fasting, preprandial, and 1 h postprandial, bedtime, and sometimes a 3 AM blood sugar value if the fasting blood sugar value is problematic. Two criteria should be met to assure that the degree of glycemic control is adequate to prevent macrosomia (26):

1. The fasting capillary glucose level should be less than 90 mg/dL (5 mmol/L), equivalent to a plasma whole blood determination of 105 mg/dL (5.8 mmol/L).
2. The 1-h capillary glucose level after beginning the meal should be < 120 mg/dL (6.6 mmol/L) equivalent to a plasma whole blood of 140 mg/dL (7.8 mmol/L).

If these criteria cannot be met after 1–2 weeks of appropriate dietary implementation, or if the woman can meet this goal, but only at the expense of severe caloric restriction and weight loss, insulin treatment needs to be instituted. Although HbA_{1c} levels are not sufficiently sensitive to aid in screening for GDM, they are helpful in assessing glycemic control throughout pregnancy. The average plasma glucose value is about 20% lower in the nondiabetic pregnancy, leading to a similar reduction in the HbA_{1c} levels which should be approximated in the diabetic pregnancy. HbA_{1c} levels should be measured every 4–6 weeks, although more frequent measurements may provide the patient much needed positive feedback and help demonstrate that SMBG is accurately reflecting maternal glycemic control.

Nutritional counseling is the cornerstone of the management of all women with GDM. An effective diet should provide the necessary nutrients, maintain normoglycemia, prevent ketosis, and result in the appropriate weight gain. Caloric allotment is based on ideal body weight. The recommended caloric intake is approximately (27)

1. 30 kcal per present pregnant weight in kilograms per day in a woman who is 80–120% of ideal body weight.
2. 24 kcal per present pregnant weight in kilograms per day in overweight women (120–150% of ideal body weight).
3. 12–15 kcal per present pregnant weight in kilograms per day for morbidly obese women (> 150% of ideal body weight).
4. 40 kcal per present pregnant weight in kilograms per day in women who are underweight, weighing less than 80% of ideal body weight.

The optimal weight gain during pregnancy should be a gradual process, with only 2–5 lb gained during the first trimester and a 0.5- to 1-lb/week gain during the second and third. Weight gains between 25 and 35 lb are associated with the best outcomes; however, overweight women, who make up a significant proportion of those with GDM, benefit from a more modest weight gain of less than 15 lb.

Current recommendations for caloric distribution are 40% of calories coming from carbohydrate, 20% from protein, and 40% from fat (27–29). This caloric distribution allows 75–80% of gestational diabetic women to achieve normoglycemia.

Postprandial blood sugar levels are directly related to the carbohydrate content of a meal, with more complex carbohydrates less likely to cause significant blood glucose excursions. Postprandial blood sugar levels play a major role in neonatal macrosomia (30).

Most programs recommend three meals and three snacks. Snacks often need to be eliminated in the overweight individual to avoid excessive weight gain. As insulin resistance is greatest in the morning, calories and carbohydrates often need to be restricted in the morning. The breakfast meal should consist of approximately 10% of the days total calories, with the remainder divided among lunch, dinner, and snacks.

By helping overcome peripheral insulin resistance, exercise can be a useful adjunct to diet in GDM. The safest form of exercise for both mother and fetus is one that does not cause fetal distress, low birth weight, uterine contractions, or maternal hypertension (31). Appropriate exercises use the upper body muscles placing little stress on the trunk region, such as the arm ergometry and the recumbent bicycle. However, active women may be encouraged to continue their moderate exercise program safely. Women should be taught how to palpate their own uterus for contractions and cease exercising should contractions occur. Contraindications to exercise include vaginal bleeding, placenta previa, cardiac disease, severe hypertension, malpresentation, intrauterine growth retardation, and morbid obesity.

If diet and exercise are not successful in bringing at least 70% of the patient's capillary glucose levels to within the target range of below 90 mg/dL fasting and less than 120 mg/dL postprandially, within 1–2 weeks, insulin therapy needs to be started.

VII. INSULIN THERAPY FOR THE DIABETIC PREGNANCY

Approximately 15% of women with GDM and all women with pregestational diabetes, type 1 and type 2, will require insulin treatment. Ideally, the pregestational diabetic woman will have entered her planned pregnancy in good glycemic control. The average requirement in type 1 diabetes is 0.7 U/kg per day early in the first trimester. The first trimester often is rocky in the type 1 diabetic with frequent episodes of problematic nocturnal hypoglycemia. Potential contributors to this "brittleness" include hypertrophy of existing beta cells, morning sickness, and possibly impairment of counterregulatory hormone responses (32–33). Other causes of hypoglycemia should also be considered, such as fetal death or hypothyroidism. A high protein, complex carbohydrate snack at bedtime may help alleviate episodes of nocturnal hypoglycemia. At 18–24 weeks of gestation, the diabetogenic stress of pregnancy begins, and women often find that their insulin requirements increase.

Requirements typically increase to 0.8 U/kg for weeks 18–26, 0.9 U/kg for weeks 26–36, and 1.0 U/kg for 36 to term. During the first trimester, insulin requirements are similar between type 1 and type 2 diabetes or about 0.8 U/kg daily, unless obesity increases insulin resistance. However, as pregnancy proceeds into the third trimester, insulin requirements increase proportionately more in type 2 than in type 1, and can rise to doses between 1.6 and 2.2 U/kg per day. Women with gestational diabetes frequently need more insulin than their type 1 counterparts reflecting their insulin resistance and close association with type 2 diabetes.

Regimens that achieve tight glycemic control usually require three to four injections per day of a combination of an intermediate-acting insulin such as NPH and a short-acting regular insulin. Ultralente insulin is discouraged, as its longtime course does not allow for the rapid changes often necessary in managing diabetes in pregnancy. Likewise, premixed 70/30 insulin lacks the flexibility needed. A safety and efficacy trial of Humalog (lispro insulin) is currently underway at our center. With its unique rapid onset of action, Humalog (lispro insulin) may be especially useful in the pregnant diabetic women with problematic postprandial blood sugar levels. If the patient currently in good control with an insulin pump, she may continue. However, we recommend that the pump insulin be switched to regular insulin rather than lispro insulin so that should the pump malfunction or be dislodged, the patient may have a little added protection against entering ketosis.

We have found the regimen described in Table 3 useful. First, the day's total insulin dose is calculated based on the patient's weight and gestational week. Approximately 4/9 of the total insulin is given as NPH and 2/9 is given as regular at breakfast. Before dinner 1/6 of total insulin is given as regular while the remaining 1/6 is given as bedtime NPH. Lunch may be covered by a modest sliding scale if needed. Blood sugars are adjusted accordingly to meet goals of a fingerstick fasting blood sugar less than 90 mg/dL and 1-h postprandial less than 120 mg/dL. Increased insulin requirements are often seen during infections and should prompt the physician to actively find a source, such as urinary tract infection. Increased insulin needs are also seen in betamethasone therapy given for lung maturation and terbutaline tocolytic treatment. Both often require a doubling of the insulin dose to maintain euglycemia.

Intrapartum glycemic control plays a major role in the well-being of the neonate. Maternal hyperglycemia is the major cause of neonatal hypoglycemia.

Table 3 Insulin Dosage Regimen for Diabetic Pregnancy

☐ 1. Pregnancy NPH plus Regular Insulin schedule.   Patient Weight in Kg=

DATE & TIME Nursing will calculate and administer the starting dose of insulin as outlined below: "Big I" = Total daily units of insulin.

"BIG I"

Date: Circle One: Gestational Weeks = | 0-12 | 13-28 | 29-34 | 35-40 | OTHER
Units of insulin = | 0.7 | 0.8 | 0.9 | 1.0

Calculate desired units of insulin from above line.
"Big I" = _____ (units X weight KG/24 hours) divide so that 4/9 of "Big I" is NPH given before Breakfast, and 1/6 of "Big I" is NPH given before bedtime.
Regular insulin is given before Breakfast as 2/9 of "Big I", and before Dinner as 1/6 of "Big I". The regular insulin is titrated based on the blood glucose.

BREAKFAST

DO NOT FEED THE PATIENT UNTIL THE BLOOD SUGAR IS BELOW 120 mg/dl.

0730 Pre-Breakfast: NPH = 4/9 "Big I" = _____ .

Check yesterday's pre Dinner BS:

If yesterday's pre Dinner BS is < 60, then decrease today's AM NPH by 2 units.
If yesterday's pre Dinner BS is 60 - 90, then no change in today's AM NPH.
If yesterday's pre Dinner BS is > 90, then increase today's AM NPH by 2 units.

Regular = 2/9 Insulin "Big I" = _____ to be adjusted according to the following scale:

BS < 60 = _____ = (2/9 "Big I" dose) - 3% of the "Big I".

60 - 90 = _____ = 2/9 "Big I" dose.

91 - 120 = _____ = (2/9 "Big I" dose) + 3% of "Big I".

> 121 = _____ = (2/9 "Big I" dose) + 6% of "Big I".

If today's BS 1 hour after Breakfast < 110, then decrease tomorrow's Pre-Breakfast regular insulin by 2 units.
If today's BS 1 hour after Breakfast is 110 - 120, no change in tomorrow's Pre-Breakfast regular insulin.
If today's BS 1 hour after Breakfast is > 120, then increase tomorrow's Pre-Breakfast regular insulin by 2 units.

LUNCH

DO NOT FEED THE PATIENT UNTIL THE BLOOD SUGAR IS BELOW 120 mg/dl.

1130 Pre lunch. Regular insulin is given based on the following scale:
BS < 90 = 0 insulin.

91 - 120 = (1/18 "Big I") = _____ .

121 - 140 = 1/18 "Big I" + 2 units) = _____ .

> 141 = 1/18 "Big I") + 4 units = _____ .

DINNER

DO NOT FEED THE PATIENT UNTIL THE BLOOD SUGAR IS BELOW 120 mg/dl.

1700 Pre dinner: Regular Insulin is 1/6 "Big I" = _____ and based on the following scale.

BS < 60 = _____ = (1/6 "Big I" dose) - 3% of "Big I".

60 - 90 = _____ = 1/6 "Big I" dose.

91 - 120 = _____ = (1/6 "Big I" dose) + 3% of "Big I".

> 121 = _____ = (1/6 "Big I" dose) + 6% of "Big I".

If today's BS 1 hour after Dinner is < 110, then decrease tomorrow's Dinner regular insulin by 2 units.
If today's BS 1 hour after Dinner is 110 - 120, no change in tomorrow's Dinner regular insulin.
If today's BS 1 hour after Dinner is > 120, then increase tomorrow's Dinner regular insulin by 2 units.

BEDTIME

2330 Bedtime NPH: Give 1/6 "Big I" = _____ .

If today's pre Breakfast BS is < 60, then decrease today's Bedtime NPH by 2 units.

If today's pre Breakfast BS is 60 - 90, then no change in today's Bedtime NPH.

If today's pre Breakfast BS is > 90, then check the 3AM BS and, if it is < 70 (regardless of today's pre Breakfast BS), decrease today's Bedtime NPH by 2 units.
If today's pre Breakfast is > 90, and the 3AM BS > 70, increase today's Bedtime NPH by 2 units.
Also, if the 3AM is > 90, then call the doctor for 3AM regular insulin scale equal to the pre-Lunch regular insulin scale.

NOTE: ALL ORDERS CHECKED OR HAND WRITTEN WILL BE FOLLOWED

M.D. _____   Date _____   Time _____

Table 4 Insulin Management for Labor and Delivery

Blood glucose (mg/dL)	Adjustment[a]
< 60	D10NS at 100 mL/h (recheck in 15 min; once > 60, start D5NS or D5LR
60–90	D5NS or D5LR at 100 mL/h
91–120	NS or LR at 100 mL/h
121–140	NS or LR at 100 mL/h and 4 U regular insulin IV
141–180	NS or LR at 100 mL/h and 5 U regular insulin IV
> 180	NS or LR at 100 mL/h and 6 U regular insulin IV

[a] D, dextrose; NS, normal saline; LR, lactated Ringers.

When active labor commences, insulin requirements decrease to zero and glucose requirements are relatively constant at 2.5 mg/kg per minute (34). If induction or cesarean is elective, the patient may take her usual bedtime dose of intermediate-acting insulin. On the morning of induction, subcutaneous insulin should be withheld. Blood sugar levels should be monitored hourly once active labor commences. A protocol used at our institution is given in Table 4. Blood glucose targets for labor and delivery are generally in the range of 70–100 mg/dL. The infant of the diabetic mother is at increased risk for neonatal complications if he or she was born prematurely and if glycemic control was poor during the pregnancy and the intrapartum period. Macrosomia (> 90th percentile in weight adjusted for gestational age and gender) is common in the poorly controlled diabetic pregnancy and a difficult vaginal delivery may result in shoulder dystocia, with brachial plexus or phrenic nerve injury, resulting in respiratory failure. Hypoglycemia in the neonate may result if the fetal pancreas has been overstimulated by maternal hyperglycemia. Vigilance must be high for other metabolic disturbances, including hypocalcemia, hypomagnesemia, erythremia, and hyperbilirubinemia.

After delivery, insulin requirements diminish precipitously in the pregestational diabetic. Often, there is no requirement for insulin for 24–48 h. Insulin requirements are generally recalculated at 0.6 U/kg per day based on postpartum weights and should be instituted when fasting or postprandial blood sugar levels are higher than 150 mg/dL. Women with true gestational diabetes do not need insulin after delivery, but do require appropriate follow-up for the potential development of type 2 diabetes.

Breastfeeding is generally recommended for women with diabetes. Oral hypoglycemics may be secreted in breast milk and should be avoided. There is some evidence that lactation may provide protection against future development of type 1 diabetes in the child, as cows milk may elicit a strong humoral response to bovine proteins and trigger the autoimmune process of type 1 diabetes. Breastfeeding, however, may accelerate retinopathy in a woman with proliferative retinopathy and is wisely avoided in these diabetic women. Additionally, lactation may lead to erratic episodes of hypoglycemia. This often requires having a small snack before breastfeeding and checking blood sugar levels approximately 1 h after breastfeeding, the time hypoglycemia is most likely.

VIII. POSTPARTUM FOLLOW-UP

About two-thirds of mothers with GDM will have GDM in a subsequent pregnancy (35). The women with recurrences tend to be older, more parous, and have increased weight gain between the pregnancies. Risk factors for future impaired glucose tolerance and overt diabetes include increased gestational insulin requirements, obesity, elevated fasting glucose levels during pregnancy, and early postpartum, and an early gestational age at the time of diagnosis (36–40). A 5-year incidence up to 50% for type 2 diabetes has been found in two studies of women with GDM (41,42). Although women with GDM who develop diabetes after pregnancy usually develop type 2 diabetes, a smaller subset may develop type 1. The presence of autoantibodies to pancreatic beta-cell antigens is highly predictive of the development of type 1 diabetes in this group (43). In the postpartum period, the woman with previous GDM should monitor her blood sugars to ensure a return to normal. Additionally, diagnostic testing should be performed at 6 weeks postpartum with appropriate reclassification (Table 5; 16). Lifestyle changes including exercise, diet, and maintenance of ideal body weight are essential. Again, pregestational diabetic women should receive appropriate and effec-

Table 5 Criteria for the Diagnosis of Diabetes Mellitus

Normoglycemia	Impaired glucose metabolism	Diabetes mellitus
FPG < 110 mg/dL	FPG ≥ 110 mg/dL and < 126 mg/dL	FPG ≥ 126 mg/dL
2-h PG < 140 mg/dL	2-h PG ≥ 140 mg/dL and < 200 mg/dL	2-h PG ≥ 200 mg/dL
		Symptoms of diabetes mellitus and casual plasma glucose concentration ≥ 200 mg/dL

FPG, fasting plasma glucose; 2-h PG, 2-h 75 g postload glucose.

tive contraception counsel. Good glycemic control will allow the new mother to have a long and healthy life to enjoy her child.

REFERENCES

1. BE Metzger. Overview of GDM: accomplishments of the last decade, challenges for the future. Lancet 1993; 341:1306–1309.
2. MM Engelgau, WH Herman, PJ Smith. The epidemiology of diabetes and pregnancy in the U.S., 1988. Diabetes Care 1995; 18:1029–1033.
3. BE Metzger, ed. Proceedings of the Third International Workshop—Conference on Gestational Diabetes Mellitus. Diabetes 1991; 40 (suppl. 2):1–201.
4. JL Mills, L Baker, AS Goldman. Malformations in IDM occur before the seventh gestational week: implications for treatment. Diabetes 1979; 28:292–293.
5. JE Becerra, MJ Khoury, JF Cordero. Diabetes mellitus during pregnancy and risks for specific birth defects: a population based case control study. Pediatrics 1990; 85:1.
6. D Towner, SL Kjos, B Leung. Congenital malformations in pregnancies complicated by NIDDM. Diabetes Care 1995; 18:1446.
7. MF Greene, JW Hare, JP Clohert. First trimester hemoglobin A_1 and risk for major malformation and spontaneous abortion in diabetic pregnancy. Teratology 1989; 39:225–231.
8. JL Kitzmiller, LA Gavin, GD Gin. Preconception care of diabetes: glycemic control prevents congenital anomalies. JAMA 1991; 265:731.
9. K Fuhrmann, H Reiher, K Semnler. The effect of intensified conventional insulin treatment before and during pregnancy on the malformation rate in offspring of diabetic mothers. Exp Clin Endocrinol 1984; 83:173.
10. JM Steel, FD Johnstone, DA Hepburn. Can prepregnancy care reduce the risk of abnormal babies? Br J Med 1990; 301:1070.
11. KD Elman, RA Welch, RN Frank. Diabetic retinopathy in pregnancy: a review. Obstet Gynecol 1990; 75:119.
12. R Klein, BEK Klein, S Moss. The Wisconsin epidemiologic study of diabetic retinopathy. Prevalence and risks of diabetic retinopathy when age at diagnosis is less than 30 years. Arch Ophthalmol 1984; 102:520.
13. EY Chew, JL Mills, BE Metzger. Metabolic control and progression of retinopathy: The diabetes in early pregnancy study. Diabetes Care 1995; 18:631.
14. M Miodovnik, BM Rosenn, JC Khoury. Does pregnancy increase the risk for development and progression of diabetic nephropathy? Am J Obstet Gynecol 1996; 174:1180.
15. L Jovanovic, CM Peterson. Is pregnancy contraindicated in women with diabetes mellitus? Diabetic Nephropathy 1984; 3:36.
16. Position Statement on Preconception Care of Women with Diabetes. ADA: Clinical Practice Recommendations. 1998.
17. Centers for Disease Control. Prenatal care and pregnancies complicated by diabetes, US reporting area 1989. MMWR CDC Surveill Summ 1993; 42:119.

18. JB O'Sullivan, CB Mahan. Criteria for oral glucose tolerance test in pregnancy. Diabetes 1964; 13:278.
19. JH Mestman. Outcome of diabetes screening in pregnancy and perinatal morbidity in infants of mothers with mild impairment in glucose tolerance. Diabetes Care 1980; 3:447.
20. KS Amanhwah, RL Prentice, RJ Fleury. The incidence of gestational diabetes. Obstet Gynecol 1977; 49:497.
21. MW Carpenter, DR Coustan. Criteria for screening test for gestational diabetes. Am J Obstet Gynecol 1982; 144:768.
22. DR Haddin. Geographic, ethnic and racial variations in the incidence of gestational diabetic patients. Diabetes 1985; 34(suppl 2):8.
23. CG Solomon, WC Willett, VJ Carey. A prospective study of pregravid determinants of gestational diabetes mellitus. JAMA 1997; 278:1078.
24. CD Naylor, N Sermen, E Chen. Selective screening for gestational diabetes mellitus. N Engl J Med 1997; 337:1591.
25. Report of the Expert Committee on the Diagnosis and Classification of Diabetes Mellitus. Diabetes Care 1997; 20:1183.
26. L Jovanovic, CM Peterson. The Diabetes in Early Pregnancy Study. Postprandial blood glucose levels predict birth weight. Am J Obstet Gynecol 1991; 164:103.
27. L Jovanovic, CM Peterson. Guest editorial: nutritional management of the obese gestational diabetic woman. J Am Coll Nutr 1992; 11:246.
28. CM Peterson, L Jovanovic. Percentage of carbohydrate and glycemic response to breakfast, lunch, and dinner in women with gestational diabetes. Diabetes 1991; 40(suppl 2):172.
29. L Jovanovic, CM Peterson. Dietary manipulation as a primary treatment strategy for pregnancies complicated by diabetes. J Am Coll Nutr 1990; 9:320.
30. L Jovanovic, CM Peterson, G Reed. NICHD-DIEP: maternal postprandial glucose levels predict birth weight. Am J Obstet Gynecol 1991; 164:103–111.
31. EP Durak, L Jovanovic, CM Peterson. Comparative evaluation of uterine response to exercise on 5 aerobic machines. Am J Obstet Gynecol 1990; 162:754.
32. MP Diamond, EA Reece, S Caprio. Impairment of counterregulatory hormonal responses to hypoglycemia during pregnancy. Am J Obstet Gynecol 1992; 166:70–77.
33. BM Rosenn, M Miodovnik, JC Khoury. Counterregulatory hormonal responses to hypoglycemia. Obstet Gynecol 1996; 87:568–573.
34. L Jovanovic, CM Peterson. Insulin and glucose requirements during the first stage of labor in insulin-dependent diabetic women. Am J Med 1983; 75:607–612.
35. EH Phillipson, DM Super. Gestational diabetes mellitus: does it reoccur in subsequent pregnancy? Am J Obstet Gynecol 1989; 160:1324.
36. PM Catalano, KM Vargo, IM Bernstein. Incidence and risk factors associated with abnormal postpartum glucose tolerance in women with gestational diabetes. Am J Obstet Gynecol 1991; 165:914.
37. SL Kjos, TA Buchanan, JS Greenspoon. Gestational diabetes intolerance and diabetes mellitus in the first two months postpartum. Am J Obstet Gynecol 1990; 163:453.
38. M Stangenberg, N Agarwal, F Rahman. Frequency of HLA genes and islet cell antibodies and result of postpartum oral glucose tolerance test (OGTT) in Saudi

Arabian women with abnormal oral glucose tolerance test (OGTT) during pregnancy. Diabetes Res 1990; 14:9.

39. A Dornhorst. Abnormalities of glucose tolerance following gestational diabetes. Q J Med 1990; 77:1219.

40. P Damm, PC Bailey, V Anyaoku. Predictive factors for development of diabetes in women with previous gestational diabetes mellitus. Am J Obstet Gynecol 1992; 167: 607.

41. BE Metzger, NH Cho, SM Roston. Prepregnancy weight and antepartum insulin secretion predict glucose tolerance 5 years after gestational diabetes mellitus. Diabetes Care 1993; 16:1598.

42. SL Kjos, RK Peters, A Xiang. Predicting future diabetes in Latino women with gestational diabetes: utility of early postpartum glucose tolerance testing. Diabetes 1995; 44:586.

43. M Fuchtenbusch, K Ferber, E Stanl. Prediction of type 1 diabetes postpartum in patients with GDM by combined islet cell autoantibody screening: a prospective multicenter study. Diabetes 1997; 46:1459–1467.

13
Drug-Induced Disorders of Glucose Metabolism

Sri Prakash L. Mokshagundam
University of Louisville, Louisville, Kentucky

Alan N. Peiris
East Tennessee State University, Johnson City, Tennessee

I. DRUG-INDUCED HYPERGLYCEMIA

Drug-related illness is a major cause of morbidity and mortality in the United States; the annual cost is estimated to be close to $136 billion. The aging of the population, increasing use of multiple medications, and a general lack of understanding of drug interactions are some of the reasons for the increasing number of drug-related illnesses. Disorders of glucose metabolism are induced by many drugs, or preexisting diabetes mellitus can be worsened. During the initial evaluation of patients with diabetes mellitus, it is important to review the drug history and determine if the diabetes could be medication-related. The history should include a thorough assessment of all prescription drugs, over-the-counter medications, herbal preparations, and supplements that the individual is taking. Complicating a full understanding of this issue, few studies have comprehensively evaluated the frequency of drug effects on carbohydrate metabolism. Drug-induced diabetes holds no distinguishing clinical features from the naturally occurring disease, and the risk of diabetes mellitus from a particular drug in any individual is unpredictable. Thus, the practicing physician needs to be familiar with the drugs that affect glucose metabolism and hold a high index of suspicion, particularly in high-risk situations in which monitoring for diabetes becomes critical. This chapter provides an overview of the major drugs that impair glucose metabolism, either alone or in combination with other medications, and suggests ways

Table 1   Drugs Causing Hyperglycemia

Antihypertensives
    Thiazide diuretics
    Diazoxide
    Furosemide
    Indapamide
    Verapamil
    Diltiazem
    Nicardipine
    Propranolol
    Minoxidil
Lipid-lowering agent
    Niacin
Drugs used in HIV infection
    Pentamidine
    Protease inhibitors
    Megesterol acetate
β-Sympathomimetic Agents
    Albuterol
    Terbutaline
Antipsychotics
    Phenothiazines
    Lithium
Antituberculosis medications
    Rifampin
    Isomazid
Miscellaneous
    Somatostatin and its analogues
    Recombinant human growth hormone
    Theophylline
    Dilantin (phenytoin)
Other
    L-dopa, asparaginase, encainide, acetazolamide, nalidixic acid, amiodarone, strepto-
    zotocin

for their recognition, treatment, and prevention Table 1 shows the drugs that are linked to precipitating and/or worsening hyperglycemia, and Table 2 shows those linked with hypoglycemia.

A.   Antihypertensives

Several drugs that are used in the management of hypertension can affect glucose metabolism. Some cause glucose intolerance and can cause diabetes, whereas

Table 2 Drugs Causing Hypoglycemia

Drugs used in diabetes management
    Insulins
    Sulfonylureas
    Repaglinide
    Metformin
    Acarbose
Antihypertensives
    β-Adrenergic-blockers
    Angiotensin-converting enzyme inhibitors
    α-Adrenergic
Antimicrobials
    Pentamidine
    Quinine
    Mefloquine
    Quinolones
    Tetracyclines
    Sulfonamides
    Cibenzoline
    Gancyclovir
Antidepressants
    MAO inhibitors
    Doxepin
    Tricyclics
Antiarrhythmics
    Quinidine
    Diisopyramide
Analgesics
    Acetaminophen
    Propoxyphene
Miscellaneous
    Ethanol
    Fibrates
    Streptozotcin
    β-Sympathomimetics
    Salicylates
    Stanazolol

others enhance the action of insulin and can cause hypoglycemia. However, the enhanced risk of diabetes mellitus in subjects with hypertension makes it difficult to establish a causal relation with a particular drug and the development of diabetes; often, stopping the drug is the only way to determine its importance.

1. Diuretics

Hypokalemia, hyperlipidemia, and impaired glucose tolerance are well-known effects of thiazide diuretics. In the Framingham study, the relative risk of developing type 2 diabetes mellitus in persons taking thiazides, adjusted for covariant risks, such as the body mass index (BMI), lipid profile, and such, was 1.2 for men and 1.6 for women. These metabolic effects are partly dependent on the type and dosage of the medication. Several mechanisms are responsible: hypokalemia leads to decreased insulin secretion and correlates with the degree of hyperglycemia; there is a direct inhibitory effect of thiazides on insulin secretion, which is independent of hypokalemia; large thiazide doses impair insulin action, although there appears to be little effect of low-dose thiazides. Thiazide-induced diabetes mellitus typically resolves when the drug is withdrawn. Moreover, potassium supplementation in hypokalemic subjects often improves and sometimes reverses the glucose intolerance. It is recommended that blood glucose levels be periodically monitored in subjects receiving thiazide diuretics.

Other diuretics can impair glucose tolerance. The incidence with furosemide is uncommon and is likely related to hypokalemia, as correction of hypokalemia typically restores normoglycemia. Long-term use of indapamide has also been reported to cause glucose intolerance. Potassium-sparing diuretics have the least effect on glucose metabolism.

2. Beta-Adrenergic Blockers

The adrenergic β-blockers have been reported to impair glucose tolerance in diabetic and nondiabetic subjects through multiple mechanisms: decreased peripheral tissue insulin sensitivity, inhibited insulin secretion, and impaired β-adrenergic stimulation of glycogenolysis in muscle. These effects vary with the dosage and selectivity of the agent that is used. Generally, nonselective β-blockers have the greatest effects on glucose metabolism, although nonselective agents that possess α-blocking activity (carvedilol) appear to have minimal to no effect. β-Blockers used in combination with thiazide diuretics can potentiate the diabetogenic effects, making this a poor combination for hypertension control. Furthermore, β-blockers are generally not recommended as antihypertensive agents in persons with preexisting diabetes or in high-risk individuals, such as those with a family history of type 2 diabetes or previous gestational diabetes. However, in view of the known benefits of these agents in established coronary artery disease, the benefits tend to outweigh the risks in these patients.

3. Alpha-Adrenergic Blocking Agents

α_1-adrenergic blocking agents are increasingly being used for the management of hypertension, plus their beneficial effects in subjects with benign prostatic hyperplasia (BPH) may make them the preferred agent in subjects with hypertension and BPH. Recent studies have shown an effect of terazosin to enhance insulin sensitivity in subjects with diabetes mellitus and impaired glucose tolerance. More information is needed on other α-blockers, such as prazosin and doxazosin.

4. Calcium Channel Blockers

Insulin release from pancreatic islets is dependent on an increased cytosolic calcium level within the β-cell, and when calcium channel blockers first appeared it was feared a failure to appropriately raise the β-cell intracellular calcium concentration would impair insulin secretion. Instead, there are few reports of hyperglycemia attributable to calcium channel blockers in otherwise healthy subjects with or without diabetes, and their clinical effects on glucose metabolism are generally minor.

5. Minoxidil

Increased plasma glucose values have been reported with the use of minoxidil in subjects with type 2 diabetes mellitus.

B. Glucocorticoids

Glucocorticoids elevate plasma glucose levels, and are the most commonly encountered cause of drug-induced diabetes mellitus. Several mechanisms are responsible that reflect the pleotrophic effects of glucocorticoids on multiple tissues: increased hepatic glucose production, decreased peripheral insulin sensitivity, and inhibited insulin production and secretion from pancreatic β cells. The risk of developing glucose intolerance from glucocorticoids varies with the dose of steroid and somewhat with the preparation used; diabetes from topical steroids is uncommon. Although steroid-induced diabetes is most often found with pharmacological doses of steroid, recent reports have suggested that hyperglycemia is occasionally found with physiological steroid replacement in subjects with pituitary insufficiency, which may reflect the difficulty in accurately defining the physiological dose of steroid replacement in any individual patient.

It is generally assumed that persons who develop diabetes with steroid use are genetically predisposed to type 2 diabetes, and that the steroid-induced insulin resistance brings out the diabetes. Supporting this idea, first-degree relatives of individuals with type 2 diabetes have an enhanced risk of developing diabetes mellitus when given steroids. Thus, a family history of diabetes or history of gestational diabetes should be carefully sought in all patients before beginning steroid administration, and those persons should be carefully monitored for glucose intolerance during therapy. Glucocorticoid-induced diabetes often, but not always, resolves after withdrawal of the steroids.

The clinical manifestations of steroid-induced diabetes are similar to spontaneous type 2 diabetes mellitus. Especially when a high dose of steroid is used, the elevation of blood glucose values can be very marked, including the development of a hyperosmolar nonketotic state. Hence, all subjects on high-dose steroid therapy should be monitored for development of diabetes mellitus. Furthermore, in subjects with established diabetes, blood glucose levels must be closely monitored following the introduction of steroids, and diabetes medications should be adjusted as needed. In persons with steroid-induced diabetes, careful attention to dietary measures should be initiated, but most patients rapidly progress to oral agents or insulin therapy. Subjects receiving alternate-day steroid therapy might notice an increased blood glucose level only on the day they take the steroid; intermittent use of hypoglycemic therapy on those days is often successful. Also, subjects receiving a large dose of steroid once daily sometimes notice elevations in blood glucose values that are most pronounced following administration of the steroid, which then abate through the rest of the day. In such individuals, it is helpful to administer hypoglycemic medications to parallel using short-acting oral medications or insulin. When steroids are tapered, it is essential to closely monitor blood glucose levels in diabetic patients and to make changes in the diabetes therapy to *prevent* significant hypoglycemia, rather than responding after hypoglycemic reactions have occurred.

C. Estrogens and Oral Contraceptive Agents

The interaction between female sex steroids and carbohydrate metabolism is complex. The effects of estrogen and progestational agents vary, and depend on the dose and type of medication used. Estrogen deficiency induces impaired insulin secretion and a progressive increase in insulin resistance that are improved by physiological estrogen replacement. However, paradoxically, large doses of estrogens can worsen insulin resistance and occasionally lead to increased plasma glucose levels. Progestational agents more consistently cause insulin resistance and lead to glucose intolerance, although this effect varies with the type of agent used. A key factor, here, is the androgenic potency, as reflected by the direct relation with the development of diabetes.

There have been significant changes in oral contraceptive agents over the last 25 years, with a fivefold decrease in estrogenic potency and a 25-fold decrease in progestational activity of the commonly used preparations. Hence, reports in the past noted a relatively high incidence of impaired glucose intolerance among pill users (16% vs. 8% among nonusers in one study), but recent studies have demonstrated no effect on glucose tolerance. An exception is the progestin-only contraceptive pill, which is associated with a threefold increased risk of type 2 diabetes, such that blood glucose should be periodically monitored in subjects using these agents, and progestin-only contraceptives should be avoided in subjects with diabetes mellitus or a history of gestational diabetes. Furthermore, during lactation there is a high risk of developing diabetes mellitus with the use of progestational agents, and progestin-only contraceptives should be avoided. In terms of postmenopausal hormone use, there is a growing literature of beneficial effects in terms of decreasing the incidence of glucose intolerance and diabetes mellitus. Thus, it may be concluded that hormone replacement therapy postmenopause is not associated with an increased risk of diabetes mellitus in most women, and it may even be beneficial. One note of caution is that women with a history of gestational diabetes mellitus and those with hyperandrogenism appear at increased risk of developing diabetes mellitus with hormone therapy. In women with a history of gestational diabetes, low-dose estrogen–progesterone combinations are the preferred choice for oral contraceptive, and blood glucose levels should be monitored closely. Ovarian hyperandrogenism is associated with insulin resistance, hyperinsulinemia, and glucose intolerance, and oral contraceptives are typically used in the management of these individuals. Despite favorable changes in the androgen/estrogen ratio, the insulin resistance can increase, and glucose intolerance occasionally appears or worsens. Pills that contain progestational agents with high androgenicity are most likely to cause this problem and should be avoided. Careful monitoring of blood glucose levels is necessary in these subjects.

In women with preexisting type 1 or type 2 diabetes, the use of low-dose contraceptive pills has not worsened metabolic control and may have some beneficial effect. Again, it must be emphasized that progestin-only contraceptives, especially those with progestational agents that have high androgenic potency, are most likely to cause problems.

D. Anabolic Steroids

Anabolic steroids are used therapeutically in several disorders and are misused by athletes and others to augment strength and enhance athletic performance. Use of these agents can lead to several side effects, including glucose intolerance, insulin resistance, and increased cardiovascular risk. Powerlifters who use anabolic steroids have been noted to have diminished glucose tolerance, whereas endurance athletes who take these drugs appear less affected. Blood glucose levels should be carefully monitored in anabolic steroid users.

E. Niacin

Niacin causes deterioration in glucose tolerance because of decreased insulin sensitivity. Although new-onset diabetes is uncommon with low doses, worsening hyperglycemia in persons with preexisting glucose intolerance is the norm, and diabetes in previously unaffected persons is frequently seen when doses exceed 2 g/day. Withdrawal of the drug typically reverses the glucose intolerance. Moreover, the use of sustained-release and extended-release niacins allows administration of smaller dose of niacin and is less likely to induce glucose intolerance. Persons taking niacin, especially those with preexisting glucose intolerance, should have glycemia carefully monitored.

F. Pentamidine

Hypo- and hyperglycemia are both reported with the use of pentamidine. Also, permanent diabetes of an insulin-dependent type (including overt diabetic ketoacidosis in some patients) can occur 2–3 months after pentamidine therapy. The mechanism is a cytotoxic effect of pentamidine on the pancreas and β-cells causing pancreatitis and insulinopenia. Higher doses of pentamidine, renal insufficiency, and a poor initial clinical status of the patient, such as the presence of hypoxia, cardiovascular collapse, or the need for corticosteroids, increase the likelihood of diabetes mellitus after using pentamidine. Pentamidine-induced pancreatic damage and diabetes mellitus have been reported after the use of aerosolized pentamidine. Diabetes mellitus from pentamidine typically requires insulin therapy.

G. Protease Inhibitors

Several reports of diabetes mellitus caused by protease inhibitors have appeared. One study reported five patients who developed diabetes mellitus shortly after initiation of therapy with protease inhibitors; none required insulin therapy. Others have reported diabetes mellitus that required insulin therapy. The mechanism of the glucose intolerance has not been well studied, and some have questioned the causal association between protease inhibitors and diabetes because of the concomitant use of pentamidine, megestrol acetate, or glucocorticoids in many of these patients. An additional issue is that protease inhibitors have recently been linked in selected patients with lipodystrophy-like changes in fat distribution and higher triglyceride levels and insulin resistance. However, the incidence of diabetes in this group appears to be low.

H. Megestrol Acetate (Megace)

Megestrol acetate, an oral progestational agent, is being used more commonly in the treatment of breast and endometrial carcinoma and in the management of cachexia associated with acquired immunodeficiency syndrome (AIDS). Several cases of diabetes have been reported with this medication. One mechanism is insulin resistance, which reverses after discontinuation of the drug. In addition, megestrol acetate has glucocorticoid-like activity; Cushing's syndrome and adrenal insufficiency secondary to suppression of hypothalamopituitary–adrenal axis have been observed with this medication. The diabetes is dose-dependent, and the hyperglycemia usually is noted within the first 2 months of treatment and resolves after discontinuing the drug.

I. Immunosuppressants

Diabetes mellitus often develops after transplantation of a kidney, liver, or heart, with an overall incidence of 4–20%. Antirejection medications are a major factor in the posttransplant diabetes; glucocorticoids, cyclosporine, and tacrolimus, all have diabetogenic tendencies, plus these drugs are often used in combination. These drugs have various effects that impair insulin secretion and worsen insulin resistance.

Cyclosporine-related diabetes mellitus has been reported since 1984, with the major mechanism being inhibition of insulin production and secretion. Cyclosporine-induced diabetes occurs mostly within the first weeks after transplantation, and up to 40% of subjects need insulin for blood glucose management. Tacrolimus (FK 506) has been used over the last few years, particularly in cardiac and liver transplant recipients, with up to a 30% incidence of diabetes mellitus, mainly owing to impaired insulin secretion through a mechanism that closely resembles the β-cell inhibitory effect of cyclosporine. Mycophenolate mofetil, desoxyspergualin, sirolimus, and leflunomide, which are under development for use in organ transplantation, are thought to have little or no effect on islet function. However, clinical experience with these drugs is too limited to allow firm conclusions in terms of diabetes risk.

J. Interferons (Alfa and Gamma)

Interferon alfa is being increasingly used for the treatment of chronic hepatitis and other disorders. There have been several reports of diabetes mellitus following the use of interferon alfa, although overall, the frequency of diabetes is low. The clinical picture of the diabetes can be either type 1 on type 2. Subjects who develop insulinopenic diabetes (type 1 diabetes picture) after interferon alfa treatment have autoimmune islet markers, including islet cell and glutamic acid decarboxylase (GAD) antibodies. The onset of the diabetes can vary from 10 days to 4 years following administration of interferon-alfa. Hence, blood glucose levels should be monitored periodically after a patient has received interferon alfa therapy. Interferon gamma induces marked insulin resistance when used in the treatment of renal carcinoma and has been reported to cause hyperglycemia, in rare patients, that resolves after discontinuation of interferon.

K. Phenytoin (Dilantin)

Diabetes mellitus including diabetic ketoacidosis and hyperglycemic nonketotic coma has been described in rare subjects after starting phenytoin (Dilantin) therapy. The mechanism is mainly decreased insulin release, although minor inhibitory effects of phenytoin on insulin sensitivity are also reported. A reduction in the dosage or discontinuation of the phenytoin usually results in improved carbohydrate tolerance.

L. Somatostatin Analogue

Somatostatin suppresses insulin and glucagon secretion from the islet along with hormones from many other organs. In contrast, its analogue (octreotide) has relatively negligible effects on insulin secretion, so hyperglycemia is an uncommon side effect. Octreotide has been used in a variety of clinical situations in which diabetes mellitus may be present, including management of acromegaly, diabetic diarrhea, orthostatic hypotension associated with diabetes mellitus, and diabetic neuropathy. In the latter, a lowering of glycemia may be seen through an effect of the somatostatin analogue to suppress growth hormone secretion and, thereby, increase insulin sensitivity.

M. Growth Hormone and Insulin-like Growth Factor-I

With the increasing use of recombinant human growth hormone therapy in children and adults, diabetes mellitus from this therapy has been reported owing to the inhibitory effect of growth hormone on insulin sensitivity. This is particularly common in children with chronic renal failure and those with Turner's syndrome. Glucose intolerance reverses after discontinuation of the growth hormone therapy, and permanent diabetes mellitus has not been reported. Many of the biological actions of growth hormone are mediated through insulin-like growth factor-I (IGF-1). Paradoxically, the administration of IGF-1 increases insulin sensitivity in nondiabetic subjects and in those with type 1 and type 2 diabetes, perhaps through cross-activation of insulin receptors by IGF-1, and IGF-1 remains an investigational therapeutic agent in syndromes of extreme insulin resistance.

N. Antituberculosis Medications

Rifampin has been reported to increase insulin requirements in type 1 diabetes. Rifampin is also a potent inducer of hepatic microsomal enzyme systems and can enhance the metabolism of several drugs, including glyburide (and presumably other sulfonylureas), such that a worsening of glucose tolerance has been reported with rifampin in subjects with type 2 diabetes mellitus who are taking glyburide. Isoniazid has also been reported to impair glucose tolerance.

O. β-Sympathomimetic Agents

Activation of the β-adrenergic system increases insulin resistance and decreases insulin secretion. Large doses of intravenous albuterol have been reported to induce diabetic ketoacidosis, whereas smaller doses have minimal to no effect on glucose metabolism. Diabetic ketoacidosis and insulin resistance were also reported after subcutaneous injection of terbutaline in a diabetic patient. Oral terbutaline and ritodrine have been reported to cause hyperglycemia, as have large doses of inhaled salbutamol in children. Finally, very high doses of theophylline, from overmedication or intentional overdose, have induced hyperglycemia, with its β-sympathomimetic and hypokalemic effects presumed to be responsible. The adverse effects of these agents on glucose metabolism typically reverse following discontinuation of the drug.

P. Others

There have been anecdotal reports of several other drugs leading to hyperglycemia, including streptozcin, L-dopa, asparaginase, phenothiazines, lithium, cncainide, acetazolamide, morphine, dapsone, nalidixic acid, dopamine and its analogues, amiodarone, droperidol, amoxapine, doxapram, and chlordiazepoxide.

II. DRUG-INDUCED HYPOGLYCEMIA

Several drugs can induce hypoglycemia, alone or in combination. The most common offending drugs are the oral agents used for the management of diabetes mellitus. A review of the Swedish Drug Registry revealed that sulfonylurea use accounted for 63% of all episodes of hypoglycemia, and ethanol, propranolol, and salicylates are the next most common offenders. Factors that predispose to drug-induced hypoglycemia include poor nutritional status, advanced age, hepatic disease, and renal failure. In addition to hypoglycemia from a prescribed drug, reports of hypoglycemia because of a drug dispensing error have also been published. It is thus occasionally necessary to confirm by pill appearance what drugs a patient actually is taking.

A. Antidiabetic Agents

Sulfonylureas act by directly stimulating insulin secretion, and one side effect is hypoglycemia. However, the annual incidence of hypoglycemic episodes among subjects using sulfonylureas is only approximately 1.8%, and severe hypoglycemia is rare. Concomitant use of insulin, a β-adrenergic blocker, or other sulfonylurea-potentiating agents holds the greatest risk for hypoglycemia and, at times, can be very severe. Hypoglycemia caused by overdose of these medicines may be prolonged (can last up days), especially with long-acting preparations, such as chlorpropamide and renal insufficiency. Antidiabetic agents that enhance insulin action (metformin or troglitazone) or impair carbohydrate absorption (acarbose or miglitol) are rarely associated with hypoglycemia when used as single agents. However, when used in combination with insulin or a sulfonylurea, the risk of hypoglycemia markedly increases. The recently introduced sulfonylurea-like agent, repaglinide (Prandin), likely causes less hypoglycemia than sulfonylureas because of its short duration of action.

B.   Pentamidine

Hypoglycemia caused by pentamidine is well documented on the basis of cytotoxic damage to beta cells and release of their intracellular stores of insulin. This can result in transient hypoglycemia, which at times is severe. Pentamidine may cause a triphasic response in terms of glycemia: initial β-cell destruction, leading to hypoglycemia, followed by insulinopenia from the β-cell destruction, and hyperglycemia, with the final stage being recovery of islet mass and function so that blood glucose levels normalize. A significant precipitating factor for hypoglycemia with pentamidine in AIDS patients is nephrotoxicity. Other associated factors include the cumulative dosage of the drug, concurrent use of other nephrotoxic drugs, and nonwhite ethnicity. Diazoxide may be useful for treating hypoglycemia induced by pentamidine. The availability of other agents with greater potency and less toxicity has resulted in a decreased use of pentamidine.

C. β-Adrenergic Blockers

The β-adrenergic system plays a key role in the counterregulatory response to hypoglycemia, especially in diabetics in whom the glucagon response to hypoglycemia is often impaired. β-Blockers occasionally impair glucose recovery from insulin-induced hypoglycemia in type 1 diabetes, and these agents have been implicated in potentiating hypoglycemic unawareness or loss of the ability to perceive hypoglycemia by blocking the adrenergic manifestations. However, the risk of severe hypoglycemia with these agents in persons with type 1 diabetes may have been overemphasized, particularly when selective β-blockers are used. In one study, labetalol (combined $\alpha-\beta$-blocker) and metoprolol (selective β-blocker) did not impair the awareness of hypoglycemia, nor alter the metabolic response to hypoglycemia. Moreover, a study of 50 subjects with type 1 diabetes mellitus taking β-blockers showed no increased frequency of hypoglycemic unawareness nor hypoglycemic episodes. Thus, β-blockers are well tolerated by many subjects with diabetes mellitus, although it seems prudent to choose selective β-blockers and avoid their use in persons with a history of severe hypoglycemia, excess alcohol use, or heavy exercise.

D. Quinine, Mefloquine, Quinidine, Diisopyramide

Quinine and its isomer quinidine occasionally cause severe hypoglycemia by increasing insulin secretion; the effect is most pronounced with renal insufficiency. Severe hypoglycemia in patients with malaria is clearly more often related to the use of antimalarial medication than to the underlying disease. Quinine-induced hypoglycemia is reversed by the use of the somatostatin analogue octreotide. The related drugs chloroquine, mefloquine, amodiaquine, and halofantrine have little effect on insulin secretion and are not likely to cause hypoglycemia when used for malarial treatment, although mefloquine has been linked to severe hypoglycemia in patients with AIDS when used for the management of cachexia and intractable diarrhea associated with the disease.

There are several reports of diisopyramide, a related drug to quinine, causing severe hypoglycemia, mainly by increasing insulin secretion. The effect is predominantly in elderly subjects, and in those with hepatic or renal disease. Blood glucose levels usually normalize rapidly after the agent is withdrawn.

E. Angiotensin-Converting Enzyme Inhibitors

Angiotensin-converting enzyme (ACE) inhibitors enhance peripheral insulin action. Concurrent use of an ACE inhibitor and a sulfonylurea or insulin rarely leads to severe hypoglycemia. The Diabetes Audit Research Study in Tayside, Scotland (DARTS) confirmed an association between the use of an ACE inhibitor and hospital admissions for hypoglycemia, although the authors cautioned against overinterpretation of that result. In contrast, studies in nondiabetic users have generally failed to see any major hypoglycemic effect with ACE inhibitors. Thus, a potentiating effect of ACE inhibitors on the hypoglycemic risk of other drugs, such as insulin or sulfonylureas, is most important, and patients should monitor glycemia carefully when an ACE inhibitor is added to hypoglycemic therapy.

F. Ethanol

Ethanol is believed to be one of the more common causes of hypoglycemia in the United States, although a retrospective survey in an urban emergency department revealed the frequency of ethanol-induced hypoglycemia was less than commonly believed, and was most likely to occur in subjects who repeatedly abused alcohol, rather than occasional bingers. Alcohol suppresses hepatic glucose production from gluconeogenesis, with the greatest risk for hypoglycemia being the fasting state. Decreased food intake during or after alcohol consumption potentiates the risk, as does concomitant use of hypoglycemic agents. Accidental ingestion of alcohol by children has been reported to cause severe hypoglycemia.

G. Antidepressants

Depression has been reported in 8.5–27.3% of subjects with diabetes mellitus. Several antidepressants including monoamine oxidase inhibitors (MAOI), tricyclic antidepressants, and serotonin-selective reuptake inhibitors (SSRI) can affect glycemia, although the exact mechanisms are not well understood. Tricyclic antidepressants such amitryptiline, imipramine, and others, have been reported to cause hypoglycemia alone or in combination with antidiabetic drugs; these agents are frequently used in the management of painful diabetic peripheral neuropathy. Severe hypoglycemia has been reported with addition of a tricyclic antidepressant to sulfonylurea therapy, mandating careful monitoring of glycemia when a tricyclic agent is started.

H. Analgesics (Acetaminophen, Propoxyphene)

Hypoglycemia and lactic acidosis has been reported with acetaminophen-induced hepatotoxicity. Hypoglycemia from propoxyphene has been reported particularly in patients with renal failure.

I. Fibric Acid Derivatives

Gemfibrozil is reported to enhance the hypoglycemic effect of oral hypoglycemic agents. Clofibrate was noted to increase insulin sensitivity and decrease glucagon secretion. Benzafibrate and fenofibrate perhaps have similar actions and can potentially lead to hypoglycemia. However, the clinical significance of this effect is unclear.

J. Sulfonamides

Sulfonylureas are structurally related to the sulfonamide class of antimicrobials. Indeed, sulfonylureas were serendipitously discovered while studying sulfonamides for the treatment of bacterial infections. However, sulfonamides are not potent hypoglycemic agents, and they do not cause hypoglycemia when used in standard doses to treat bacterial infection. The hypoglycemic effect of these agents is due to increased insulin secretion, and it is mostly seen in patients with renal failure. Alternatively, high-dose intravenous cotrimoxazole–sulfametaxazole combination for the treatment of *Pseudomonas carinii* infection in patients with AIDS and those with renal transplantation is reported to cause hypoglycemia.

K. Salicylates

Acute salicylate intoxication, particularly in children, can lead to severe hypoglycemia. The exact mechanism is unclear, but increased insulin secretion and decreased insulin clearance are both reported. Aspirin can enhance the hypoglycemic effect of other hypoglycemic agents, particularly in the presence of liver or renal dysfunction. One mechanism is the effect of aspirin to alter the pharmacokinetics of glyburide, resulting in an increased plasma glyburide free fraction. Other nonsteroidal anti-inflammatory drugs, such as ibuprofen have a smaller effect.

L. Miscellaneous

A variety of other drugs have been reported to cause hypoglycemia, including quinolone antibiotics, tetracycline, mebendazole, cibenzoline, stanazolol, and gancyclovir. The exact mechanisms and clinical significance are unclear.

BIBLIOGRAPHY

Bressler P, De Fronzo RA. Drugs and diabetes. Diabetes Rev 1994; 2:53–84.

Chan JCN, Cockram CS. Drug induced disturbances of carbohydrate metabolism. Adv Drug React Toxicol Rev 1991; 10:1–29.

Chan JC, Cockram CS, Critchley JA. Drug-induced disorders of glucose metabolism. Mechanisms and management. Drug Safety 1996; 15:135–157.

Ferner RE. Drug-induced diabetes. Baillieres Clin Endocrinol Metab 1992; 6:849–866.

Pandit MK, Burke J, Gustafson AB, Minocha A, Peiris AN. Drug-induced disorders of glucose tolerance. Ann Intern Med 1993; 118:529–539.

Seltzer HS. Drug-induced hypoglycemia: a review of 1418 cases. Endocrinol Metab Clin North Am 1989; 18:163–183.

14

Secondary Forms and Genetic Syndromes of Diabetes Mellitus

Shirwan A. Mirza and Jack L. Leahy
University of Vermont College of Medicine, Burlington, Vermont

I. INTRODUCTION

Diabetes mellitus is an etiologically and clinically heterogeneous group of disorders with hyperglycemia as the shared feature. Type 1 and type 2 diabetes make up the vast majority of cases seen by primary physicians. However, hyperglycemia or impaired glucose tolerance is a feature of a large number of illnesses and genetic syndromes that are collectively termed *secondary forms of diabetes* (classification from the American Diabetes Association is shown in Table 1). Although many are rare, each has characteristic clinical features that are of diagnostic value, and the onus is on practicing physicians to have some familiarity and a high index of suspicion. A useful rule is if a patient presents with features in the history, physical examination, or laboratory evaluation that seem atypical for type 1 or type 2 diabetes, then a careful evaluation of secondary forms of diabetes is warranted. This chapter provides an overview of the more common types following the format of Table 1.

II. GENETIC DEFECTS OF BETA-CELL FUNCTION

A. Maturity-Onset Diabetes of the Young (MODY Syndromes)

Maturity-onset diabetes of the young, which is defined as nonketotic diabetes before age 25, is a group of genetically diverse abnormalities that share this common phenotype. Mutations in four genes have been described to date; how-

Table 1 Etiologic Classification of Diabetes Mellitus

I. Type 1 diabetes (β-cell destruction, usually leading to absolute insulin deficiency)
    A. Immune-mediated
    B. Idiopathic
II. Type 2 diabetes (may range from predominately insulin resistance with relative insulin deficiency to a predominately secretory defect with insulin resistance).
III. Other specific types

Genetic defects of β-cell function
   Chromosome 12, HNF-1α (MODY3)
   Chromosome 7, glucokinase (MODY2)
   Chromosome 20, HNF-4α (MODY1)
   Mitochondrial DNA
   Others

Genetic defects in insulin action
   Type A insulin resistance
   Leprechaunism
   Rabson-Mendenhall syndrome
   Lipoatrophic diabetes
   Others

Diseases of the endocrine pancreas
   Pancreatitis
   Trauma/pancreatectomy
   Neoplasia
   Cystic fibrosis
   Hemochromatosis
   Fibrocalculous pancreatopathy
   Others

Endocrinopathies
   Acromegaly
   Cushing's syndrome
   Glucagonoma
   Pheochromocytoma
   Hyperthyroidism
   Somatostatinoma
   Aldosteronoma
   Others

Drug- or chemical-induced
   N-3-pyridylmethyl-N-p-nitrophenylurea
   (Vacor)
   Pentamidine
   Nicotinic acid
   Glucocorticoids
   Thyroid hormone
   Diazoxide
   β-Adrenergic agonists
   Thiazides
   Phenytoin (Dilantin)
   Interferon-alfa
   Others

Infections
   Congenital rubella
   Cytomegalovirus
   Others

Uncommon forms of immune-mediated diabetes
   "Stiff-man" syndrome
   Anti-insulin receptor antibodies
   Others

Other genetic syndromes sometimes associated with diabetes
   Down syndrome
   Klinefelter's syndrome
   Turner's syndrome
   Wolfram syndrome
   Friedreich's ataxia
   Huntington's chorea
   Laurence-Moon-Biedl syndrome
   Myotonic dystrophy
   Porphyria
   Prader-Willi syndrome
   Others

IV. Gestational diabetes mellitus

Source: U.S. Expert Committee, 1998.

ever, there are patients with the clinical syndrome who do not have mutations in these genes, so that additional causes presumably exist. The relative frequencies of the genetic subtypes vary regionally and by ethnic population, plus there are differences in the clinical course and response to therapy. *Clinical clues:* Diabetes in the proband or a family member before age 25 with features of nonketotic diabetes including correction of the hyperglycemia without insulin for at least 2 years. Obesity is uncommon, markers of islet autoimmunity are absent, and there is no association with HLA antigens. A hallmark feature is autosomal dominant inheritance; patients typically provide a family history of multigenerational young-onset diabetes. However, some forms entail mild hyperglycemia that may be asymptomatic at young ages so the diabetes goes unrecognized until middle or late adult life and is mistaken for type 2 diabetes.

1. MODY 1

The first MODY family to be extensively studied was the famous RW pedigree from the University of Michigan. The locus is on the long arm of chromosome 20 and was recently identified to be a mutation in the hepatic nuclear factor-4α (HNF-4α) gene, which is a beta-cell and liver transcription factor. MODY 1 is an uncommon form of MODY, which is characterized by severe insulin secretory dysfunction, so that patients typically end up taking insulin and may develop neuropathic and vascular diabetes complications.

2. MODY 2

This form stems from mutations in the glucokinase gene on chromosome 7p and has been described mostly in Japanese and European kindreds (accounts for 60% of MODY in France), as opposed to the United States where it is less common. Glucokinase is a key glucoregulatory enzyme in beta-cells and the liver, so that MODY 2 is characterized by impaired glucose sensing for insulin secretion and hepatic glucose production. The diabetes is typically mild and is often treatable with sulfonylureas; hence, few require insulin. Vascular complications are uncommon.

3. MODY 3

The MODY 3 form stems from a recently described locus on chromosome 12q that has been mapped to the hepatic nuclear factor-1α (HNF-1α) gene, which is another beta-cell transcription factor. MODY 3 has been described mostly in Europe, Japan, and North America (mostly white). Patients are similar to MODY 1 in terms of marked hyperglycemia and a tendency for complications, although the course evolves more slowly; glucose tolerance is often normal in childhood, with diabetes occurring in the teens or early adulthood followed by progression over several years to eventual beta-cell failure.

4. MODY 4

Insulin promoter factor 1 (IPF-1; also called PDX-1) is a pancreas developmental factor; "knockout" mice for IPF-1 show total pancreatic agenesis. A child with pancreatic agenesis was recently described with homozygous mutations in this gene. Early-onset diabetes was subsequently identified in heterozygous family members. Little clinical information is otherwise known, and it is expected this will be a rare cause of MODY.

5. MODY in African American and Latino Populations

A clinical subtype of MODY that lacks a genetic or pathophysiological etiology is teenagers who present with severe impairment of insulin secretion, often with diabetic ketoacidosis, but with no evidence of pancreatic autoimmunity. The disease is autosomal dominant. Patients require insulin initially, but many discontinue insulin later without redeveloping ketosis. Although first described in African Americans, a similar syndrome has been noted in Latino Americans; it is relatively common in these populations and makes the diagnosis of type 1 diabetes complex. The presence of islet cell immune markers is helpful, although their absence does not exclude type 1 diabetes.

B. Mitochondrial DNA Mutations

Insulin secretion entails high-energy utilization in beta-cells, so that mitochondrial metabolism plays a crucial role in that cell's function. Cells according to their various levels of energy demand have hundreds to thousands of mitochondria, each containing two to ten copies of mitochondrial DNA (mtDNA), which is a double-stranded, circular DNA that is inherited exclusively from the mother, for mitochondria of the sperm do not remain in the oocyte during fertilization. The mtDNA has a high rate of mutations that underlie several clinical syndromes, with the tissues that are affected presumed to reflect tissue heterogeneity of the mtDNA mutations.

  Maternally Inherited Diabetes and Deafness (MIDD) is characterized by the triad of diabetes, deafness, and maternal inheritance, and results from a point mutation (A→G) at position 3243 of the mitochondrial gene for leucine tRNA. A variation is the mitochondrial myopathy, encephalopathy, lactic acidosis, and stroke-like episodes (MELAS) syndrome, which shares the same genetic mutation, but has muscular and neurological abnormalities without diabetes. Japan has the highest incidence of mitochondrial genome defects causing diabetes, with approximately 1% of the diabetes population affected; prospective studies have provided important clinical details about the syndrome. Affected persons can present with either phenotypic type 1 or 2 diabetes. Further confounding the diagnosis versus type 1 diabetes, islet cell antibodies can be found, suggesting that beta cells with these mutations are at risk for autoimmune attacks. A sizeable fraction of the patients with diabetes, on the basis of a mitochondrial mutation, have subclinical hearing loss so profound deafness is typical. *Clinical clues:* Maternal inheritance of diabetes (type 1 or 2 in appearance) in a young or middle-aged adult in tandem with sensorineural hearing loss and a thin body habitus should prompt one to suspect a mitochondrial genome mutation. Associated findings are stunted growth and neurological symptoms, such as encephalopathy, dementia, seizures, stroke-like episodes, or episodic vomiting. A blood test for A 3243 MELAS mutation makes the diagnosis, although a negative test does not exclude it if heteroplasmy (coexistence of mutant and wild-type mtDNA in one cell) is present.

III. DEFECTS IN INSULIN ACTION

Over 60 inherited or acquired syndromes of extreme insulin resistance have been described that are associated with glucose intolerance, and in some case, diabetes. The distinctive features result from the impaired insulin action, such as growth retardation in leprechaunism, or as a consequence of the compensatory hyperinsulinemia, such as acanthosis nigricans or hyperandrogenism in females. Affected persons are often first recognized when very high doses of insulin are required for glycemic control (sometimes thousands of units) or occasionally in nondiabetic persons because of typical physical findings and unusually high plasma insulin levels (10–100 times normal). The syndromes are rare and complex to diagnose and treat, and if suspected should be evaluated by specialized centers.

A. Type A Insulin Resistance

The type A syndrome is typically secondary to defective insulin receptors—either reduced affinity for insulin binding or impaired receptor function—as a result of a point mutation in the insulin receptor gene, although patients have been described with the clinical syndrome, but with normal receptors, who presumably have mutations in postreceptor steps in the insulin action cascade (for a short while, type C syndrome was applied to persons without receptor mutations, although that terminology is no longer used). *Clinical clues:* Very high insulin requirements in relatively young individuals who range from thin to minimally obese, with normal growth and development. A common finding is acanthosis nigricans, which is hyperpigmented hyperkeratotic skin plaques that have a velvety texture, and typically occur at the back of the neck, axillae, anticubital and popliteal fossae (see Chap. 32); it stems from a direct growth-promoting effect of hyperinsulinemia on skin pigment cells so that it is associated with insulin resistance in general, rather than being unique to any syndrome. Acromegaloid features are sometimes found in the type A syndrome, but growth hormone and insulin-like growth factor-1 (IGF-1) levels are normal so that the acromegalic features are thought secondary to cross-reactivity of the high plasma insulin levels with IGF-1 receptors. *Diagnosis:* The diagnosis is clinical, based on marked insulin resistance, as suggested by very high insulin requirements and the other typical features; specific mutations within the insulin receptor are sought only for research purposes, because multiple sites throughout the gene have been described in different families, making identification very complex. *Treatment:* Very high doses of insulin are typically required; U500 insulin is available by special request. Recombinant human IGF-1 is an effective hypoglycemic agent in some patients, although its use is investigational.

B. Type A Syndrome Subtypes

A subtype of the type A syndrome is obese female adolescents with ovarian hyperandrogenism and signs of virilization, insulin resistance, and acanthosis nigricans (HAIR-AN). They are phenotypically similar to the type A syndrome, but the insulin resistance is milder and is often improved by caloric restriction. These patients are sometimes identified because of oligomenorrhea or amenorrhea, hirsutism, or acne, rather than diabetes. Another subtype is the Rabson-Mendenhall syndrome, which entails the features of the type A syndrome plus precocious puberty, hyperplasia of the pineal body, and dystrophic nails and teeth.

C. Variant of Type A Syndrome

Some years ago, women with obesity, acanthosis nigricans, and hyperandrogenism (typically PCO that are being evaluated for infertility or hirsutism) were described who had more insulin resistance and hyperinsulinemia than a weight-matched cohort of hyperandrogenic women with simple obesity. Diabetes or IGT was also frequent. The pathogenesis is not fully known, but importantly, a few days of fasting reversed the glucose intolerance (the same effect occurs in typical type 2 diabetes), in contrast to the syndromes of extreme insulin resistance, which are generally unaffected. Thus, an acquired cause of insulin resistance, such as down-regulation of insulin receptors from the obesity-induced hyperinsulinemia is operative in these women, rather than a genetic defect in insulin action. Stated another way, acanthosis nigricans and hyperandrogenism are relatively common in the diabetic population as manifestations of hyperinsulinism from insulin resistance (of whatever type) in contrast with syndromes of extreme insulin resistance, which are extremely rare. The importance for practicing physicians is to recognize that the vast majority of patients who present with acanthosis nigricans do not have one of the extreme insulin resistance syndromes.

D. Lipoatrophic Diabetes

The lipoatrophy–dystrophy syndromes are a heterogeneous group of rare disorders that are typified by regional or global absences of subcutaneous adipose tissue in combination with moderate to severe insulin resistance, with or without diabetes mellitus. Multiple subtypes (congenital and acquired, partial and complete) are known. Also, lipodystrophy has recently been described in human immunodeficiency virus type 1 (HIV-1) seropositive patients taking protease inhibitors. The pathogenesis is not fully defined, but a regional variation in sympathetic nervous tone may promote accelerated regional lipolysis. The resulting augmented release of free fatty acids may promote insulin resistance by competition with glucose for metabolism (so-called Randle effect), or there may be undefined postreceptor defects in insulin action.

1. Congenital Partial Lipodystrophy—Kobberling-Dunningan Syndrome

Onset is in childhood or early adolescence. Two subtypes are described: the type 1 syndrome involves absence of subcutaneous fat only on the limbs, and the type 2 syndrome involves the limbs and trunk, whereas the vulva is spared. A characteristic feature is the absence of subcutaneous fat in the affected areas, with sparing of the cheeks, palms, and soles, and intrathoracic, bone marrow, and intra-abdominal fat.

2. Congenital Generalized Lipodystrophy—Seip-Berardinelli Syndrome

A characteristic feature is a generalized absence of subcutaneous, intracavity, buccal, and mammary fat that is usually noticed in infancy. Associated features are prominent muscles, veins, and thyroid; hepatomegaly owing to massive glycogen deposits; severe hypertriglyceridemia, with eruptive xanthomas, lipemia retinalis, and episodic pancreatitis. Diabetes usually develops in the second decade.

3. Acquired Generalized Lipodystrophy—Lawrence Syndrome

Normal fat distribution at birth, but subsequent generalized absence of fat. This syndrome is sporadic without familial aggregation. In half the cases, there is a preceding viral syndrome that may be important in the pathogenesis. The onset is usually in childhood or postpuberty. Clinical diabetes follows the lipoatrophy an average of 4 years later. Patients have hyperhidrosis, hyperlipidemia, and hepatosplenomegaly, cirrhosis, and premature atherosclerosis.

E. Type B Insulin Resistance—Anti-insulin Receptor Antibodies

The type B syndrome is an acquired form of insulin resistance that stems from polyclonal autoantibodies against insulin receptors (located in Table 1 under "uncommon forms of immune-mediated diabetes"). This syndrome occurs mostly (80%) in women in their 40s, with an autoimmune disorder such as systemic lupus erythematosus, Sjogren's syndrome, idiopathic thrombocytopenic purpura, or primary biliary cirrhosis. The diagnosis is made using readily available assays for insulin receptor antibodies (usually of IgG type) in serum. In some patients, the autoantibodies activate the insulin receptor, causing paradoxical hypoglycemia; fluctuating periods of hypo- and hyperglycemia also can be found. A characteristic feature is spontaneous remission of the antibody production, and thus the insulin resistance and hyperglycemia, after months to a year or two. *Clinical clues:* Very large doses of insulin for glycemic control in combination with clinical evidence of systemic autoimmunity, such as an elevated sedimentation rate, decreased complement, positive antinuclear antibodies, pancytopenia, or proteinuria. These patients often have features that mimic the type A syndrome, including acanthosis nigricans and hyperandrogenism. *Treatment:* Steroids, cytotoxic drugs, and plasmapheresis or immunosuppression to reduce the autoantibody titer; high-dose prednisone or cyclophosphamide are preferred agents.

IV. DISEASES OF THE EXOCRINE PANCREAS

Diabetes secondary to pancreatic disease represents approximately 0.5% of all cases of diabetes, which increases to 1% in alcoholic populations and to 10–20% of cases in the tropics. Multiple exocrine pancreatic illnesses are described with the common pathogenic element being an infectious, chemical, or infiltrative process that also destroys the islet tissue. Several characteristic clinical elements then result. Hyperglycemia stems from the loss of endogenous insulin; hence, many patients eventually end up taking insulin. However, absolute insulinopenia leading to insulin treatment requires profound pancreatic damage, which is unusual for most of these illnesses, except for a surgical pancreas removal or calamitous pancreas damage, such as occurs with hemorrhagic pancreatitis. The natural history of the others is a slow progression to diabetes, often with a prolonged period of oral agent responsiveness. Furthermore, islets contain not only insulin-secreting beta cells, but also alpha cells which secrete glucagon; thus, pancreatic diabetes is a state of relative glucagon deficiency. Diabetic ketoacidosis requires not only insulinopenia to promote fatty acid mobilization from adipose tissue, but also glucagon to make the liver ketogenic. As such, diabetic ketoacidosis (DKA) is rare in pancreatic forms of diabetes. Glucagon is also a potent counter-regulatory hormone that exacerbates acute and chronic hyperglycemic states, so hyperglycemia is often relatively mild in pancreatic forms of diabetes. An additional factor sometimes is subclinical malabsorption caused by exocrine insufficiency. Finally, micro- and macrovascular complications are relatively uncommon for most of these forms of diabetes, presumably because of their relatively mild hyperglycemia. As such, neuropathy in patients with chronic pancreatitis from alcohol use is more commonly alcohol related.

A. Acute and Chronic Pancreatitis

Transient hyperglycemia is seen in about 50% of patients during an acute episode of pancreatitis, although it is rarely severe. In contrast, diabetes persisting after a single episode of uncomplicated pancreatitis is unusual, although 5% of such patients eventually become diabetic because of ongoing chronic painless pancreatitis. Diabetes following acute fulminant pancreatitis, with multiorgan failure, occurs in up to 26% of patients. Chronic pancreatitis results in diabetes in about 10–30% of patients.

B. Cystic Fibrosis

Cystic fibrosis (CF) is an autosomal recessive disorder that results from a mutation of a chloride channel protein that causes thickening of secretions with ductular plugging and pneumonias culminating in fibrosis of the lungs and exocrine pancreas. CF is present in 1:3000 whites, and the incidence of cystic fibrosis-related diabetes (CFRD) is increasing as the life expectancy improves; the risk of diabetes currently is 20 times higher in CF patients than in the general population, with up to 25% developing overt diabetes. CFRD typically occurs between 15 and 25 years of age, although it can develop earlier, and there is no correlation between severity of the disease and the presence or severity of glucose intolerance. In many patients, it is preceded by a gradual deterioration of glucose intolerance as insulin secretion declines over time, presumably because of slow pancreatic fibrosis and beta-cell destruction. Patients typically respond to oral agents early in the course of the disease, although most progress to insulin. Some patients instead have a precipitous course, with rapid progression to absolute insulinopenia and insulin use, often in the presence of islet cell antibodies. The incidence of HLA-DR4 and HLA-DR3 antigens (the high-risk HLA antigens for type 1 diabetes) is increased in CF patients, and some authors have hypothesized that in genetically predisposed individuals for type 1 diabetes, the CF pancreas damage may initiate autoimmune beta-cell destruction.

C. Hemochromatosis

Hereditary hemochromatosis is an HLA-linked autosomal recessive disorder of iron overload and deposition that leads to tissue fibrosis and organ failure. It is mostly due to the C282Y mutation of the recently identified HFE gene although some cases are not HFE related. One in ten persons in the white population are carriers (heterozygous) and 0.3% are affected (homozygous). Secondary forms also occur, with the most common causes being thalassemia major, chronic hemolytic anemias, multiple blood transfusions, porphyria cutanea tarda, and dietary or medical iron overload. The main affected organs are liver, skin, heart, and brain, along with multiple endocrine organs, including pancreatic islets, testicles, and anterior pituitary. The constellation of clinical findings stem from dysfunction of the infiltrated organs, including cirrhosis, cardiac failure, arthropathy, and nonspecific brain dysfunction, along with hypoendocrine states of hypoandrogenism with or without hypopituitarism and diabetes. Importantly, males are clinically affected at ten times more frequently than females, because menstrual blood loss is presumed somewhat protective.

The pathogenesis of glucose intolerance in hemochromatosis is multifactorial. Pancreatic iron deposition is well known to medical students from slides of the classic "blue" pancreas that are shown during their gross pathology lectures. However, insulin resistance caused by hepatic and extrahepatic iron deposition is also described in the prediabetic stage when insulin secretion is relatively intact. As such, islet iron deposits and the resulting toxic damage impairing insulin synthesis and secretion is a relatively late event. *Clinical clues:* Triad of diabetes mellitus, hepatomegaly, and skin pigmentation ("bronzed diabetes"), although in reality, few patients present with the full-blown picture. Instead, the presentation is usually insidious without organ failure, although subtle evidence of multiorgan dysfunction is often found (abnormal liver function tests, mild congestive heart failure, glucose intolerance, impotence) in tandem with the diabetes. As such, the important feature that suggests this diagnosis is multiorgan dysfunction. A useful rule is that any patient with diabetes who also has undiagnosed cardiac, hepatic, arthritic, or neurological dysfunction should be screened for hemochromatosis. *Diagnosis:* Screening is performed by the ratio of serum iron to ironbinding capacity (saturation ratio)—a value above 50% (normal < 30%) suggests hemochromatosis. Serum ferritin concentration is also often used for screening; the one confusion is that ferritin is an acute-phase reactant that is often raised in stressed hypoinsulinemic states, such as out of control type 1 diabetes or inflammatory conditions. Although these patients are rarely confused with hemochromatosis, many authors advocate screening in terms of diabetes etiology, using the iron saturation ratio rather than ferritin. If screening is positive, definitive diagnosis is made by computed tomography (CT) densitometry or magnetic resonance imaging (MRI) of the liver for iron overload, and usually liver biopsy. A genetic diagnostic test for the C282Y mutation in the HFE gene is also available.

D. Malnutrition-Related Diabetes: Fibrocalculous Pancreatopathy

Fibrocalculous pancreatopathy is a common cause of diabetes in developing countries (particularly within the tropical belt) and is thought to be malnutrition-related. Two main subgroups are recognized by the World Health Organization: fibrocalculous pancreatic diabetes (FCPD) and protein-deficient pancreatic diabetes (PDPD). Clinical features of FCPD stem from chronic calcific pancreatitis of poorly defined etiology, although protein–calorie malnutrition is thought an important factor. Affected persons are generally young and lean, with the triad of abdominal pain that can be severe, pancreatic calculi, and diabetes that requires insulin, but is ketosis resistant if insulin is withdrawn. Specialized testing shows the presence of pancreatic exocrine deficiency, although malabsorption or steatorrhea is uncommon, presumably because of a low dietary fat intake in this part of the world. *Diagnosis:* Pancreatic calculi are easily visualized by a plain x-ray film or with more specialized imaging techniques.

Less understood is the PDPD form of diabetes that was referred to as the "J type" of diabetes in the past. Several clinical features are shared with FCPD including its presence in developing nations and association with protein–calorie malnutrition, young-onset diabetes, insulin-requiring and ketosis resistance, with the key difference being lack of pancreatic calcifications. However, none of these features are specific, and there are no unique diagnostic markers or test for this form of diabetes, making its diagnosis often by intuition.

V. ENDOCRINOPATHIES

Endocrinopathies precipitate diabetes through many mechanisms (it is important to differ diabetes *caused* by an endocrine process, as opposed to occurring in tandem with endocrinopathies in the polyglandular syndromes that are discussed in Chap. 42). Best known are the counterregulatory hormone hypersecretion syndromes of growth hormone (acromegaly), cortisol (Cushing's), glucagon (glucagonoma), and catecholamines (pheochromocytoma) which cause insulin resistance; pheochromocytoma has an additional mechanism whereby insulin secretion is inhibited by a direct suppressive effect of epinephrine on insulin secretion. Hyperthyroidism causes insulin resistance and also lowers endogenous insulinemia by speeding up its metabolic clearance rate.

Somatostatinomas inhibit insulin secretion. These syndromes are rare and insidious in presentation plus diabetes is found in fewer than 30% of affected individuals, which is presumed to reflect a need for a genetic predisposition to type 2 diabetes that is unmasked by the hormonal hypersecretion. An exception is hyperthyroidism, which is common; however, diabetes from thyrotoxicosis is very uncommon, as opposed to IGT which is frequently seen if tested for. Taken together, it is rare for even diabetes specialists to encounter an endocrinopathy causing diabetes. Regardless, they carry a multitude of health consequences, depending on the hormone involved, and treatment of the diabetes is best focused on reversing the hormone hypersecretion. Thus, primary physicians need to be familiar with the typical clinical features and screening methods, and to have a high index of suspicion.

A. Acromegaly

Acromegaly stems from chronic excess of growth hormone (GH), with the clinical features being mostly secondary to the effect of GH to accelerate the production of insulin-like growth factor-I (IGF-1; also called somatomedin C) as opposed to the elevated level of GH per se. The usual cause is a GH-secreting tumor of the anterior pituitary, although ectopic secretion of its tropic hormone (growth hormone-releasing hormone; GHRH) from diverse neoplasms is rarely found. Acromegaly is an insidious process that evolves over years to the characteristic acral and soft tissue growth that is familiar to most physicians: broad hands and feet with sausage-like fingers and a shoe size that slowly increases over the years; coarse facial features with frontal bossing, thick skin folds, and a prominent jaw, with an overbite and wide spacing between the teeth; generalized organomegaly, including thyroid, sweat glands, liver, kidney, spleen, and heart; osteoarthrities, sleep apnea, and carpel tunnel syndrome also occur. Linear height is unaffected unless the GH excess begins in childhood (before the bone epiphyses close) when gigantism occurs. Diabetes is found in 13–32% of patients and IGT in another 60% because of the effects of growth hormone–IGF-1 to inhibit glucose uptake into skeletal muscle and adipose tissue, stimulate lipolysis, and increase hepatic glucose production, thereby causing insulin resistance. *Diagnosis:* Screening is performed by a random somatomedin-C blood level; a normal value eliminates the diagnosis unless the clinical suspicion is high, then a formal glucose tolerance test may be warranted. In contrast, random growth hormone levels are not sufficiently discriminatory for screening, especially when diabetes is present. The diagnosis is confirmed by failure of growth hormone to suppress below 2.5 ng/mL during a 75-g oral glucose tolerance test although renal failure, malnutrition–starvation, and poorly controlled diabetes can cause a false lack of appropriate suppression. As such, the test is best performed when glycemic control is relatively good.

B. Cushing's Syndrome

Glucocorticoids antagonize insulin action at liver, adipose tissue, and muscle, causing insulin resistance. Chronic hypercortisolemia (Cushing's syndrome) occurs through several mechanisms, with diabetes occurring in approximately 30% of cases: exogenous steroid use is most common, with 60% of remaining cases stemming from an corticotropin (adrenocorticotropic hormone; ACTH) secreting anterior pituitary tumor (so-called Cushing's disease), 20% a benign or malignant adrenal neoplasm, and 20% from ectopic secretion of ACTH from multiple benign and malignant tumors. The typical physical features stem from the diverse cellular actions of cortisol to promote lipogenesis, but otherwise to be catabolic for many tissues, plus the concomitant adrenal hypersecretion of androgens: central obesity with prominent supraclavicular fat pads, dorsal hump, and moon face; thin extremities and proximal muscular atrophy and weakness; thin skin, easy bruisability, and violaceous striae on the abdomen and often the folds of the knees, elbows, and axillae; osteoporosis causing back pain, compression fractures, and a dowager hump; hypertension; menstrual irregularity, acne, and hirsutism. In reality, few patients present with the complete picture, and the diagnosis is more often questioned in patients with obesity, hypertension, and diabetes that comprise a sizable portion of any diabetes practice. A useful clue is muscle strength and bulk in the upper leg and buttocks—carrying around the weight of simple obesity promotes prominent thigh musculature as opposed to Cushing's in which the musculature is often thin and flabby and has almost no tone. However, physical findings are not adequate to rule in or out the diagnosis, and given the seriousness of Cushing's syndrome, if the diagnosis crosses your mind, then appropriate screening should be performed. *Diagnosis:* Morning and afternoon cortisol levels are frequently obtained when Cushing's syndrome is considered, but they are inadequate to eliminate or make the diagnosis. Instead, one of two screening tests must be performed. The most frequent is to give 1 mg of dexamethasone at 11 PM and to obtain an 8 AM serum cortisol level (overnight dexamethasone suppression test)—appropriate suppression is a cortisol level lower than 5 μg/mL, which effectively eliminates Cushing's. This test is complicated by a high false-positive rate (failure to get full suppression) in 30% or more of obese, hypertensive, otherwise healthy individuals. Additional issues that raise the false-positive rate are estrogen use or pregnancy, which raises cortisol-binding globulin, and drugs (typically anticonvulsants) that accelerate hepatic metabolism of dexamethasone. Incomplete suppression mandates additional investigation, typically a 24-h urine for cortisol (and creatinine to ensure adequacy of the urine collection), which has a lower incidence of false-positives. Given the high rate of false-positives with overnight dexamethasone, many authors advocate using 24-h urine cortisol assay as the primary screen. If the screening tests are positive, the workup proceeds, with imaging and additional blood and urine suppression testing to rule in or out Cushing's syndrome, followed by identifying the specific etiology; the workup is complex and is recommended to be done in tandem with endocrinology consultation.

C. Glucagonoma

Glucagon-secreting islet tumors are very rare. They are characterized by the triad of diabetes, anemia, and a characteristic migratory necrolytic erythematous rash on the back and trunk that is secondary to hypoproteinemia and hypoaminoacidemia as a result of the intense gluconeogenesis. Other features include weight loss, thromboembolism, stomatitis, and diarrhea. It is typically seen in postmenopausal women, and most tumors are malignant. *Diagnosis:* Very high glucagon level (typically 1000–7000 pg/mL when the normal is 50–100 pg/mL). However, marked insulinopenia, such as is seen in decompensated type 1 diabetes, also coexists with high circulating glucagon levels, although not to the level seen with a glucagonoma, so a glucagon value is best obtained when glycemia is reasonably well controlled. Importantly, these tumors often secrete other islet cell hormones such as insulin, ACTH, panathormone (PTH), vasoactive intestinal polypeptide (VIP), or pancreatic polypeptide (PP) that can confuse the clinical presentation.

D. Pheochromocytoma

Pheochromocytoma stems from excess catecholamine secretion (norepinephrine with or without epinephrine) from tumors of chromaffin tissue that are typically of the adrenal medulla, although extra-adrenal sites are occasionally found, with the key clinical features being hypertension and headaches. Additional features, especially with increased epinephrine secretion, are sweating, palpitations, and nervousness. The hypertension is usually sustained, although paroxysms of worsening symptoms, severe hypertension, and skin blanching are frequent. Pheochromocytoma promotes glucose intolerance through the complex multiorgan effects of catecholamines on the glucose homeostasis system, although diabetes is unusual: α_2-adrenergic receptor activation inhibits insulin secretion (beta-cell receptors) and stimulates glycogenolysis, lipolysis, and gluconeogenesis; β-adrenergic stimulation impairs glucose utilization in muscle; catechols directly stimulate glucagon secretion. *Diagnosis:* Screening is based on showing excess production of catecholamines by measuring total or fractionated (epinephrine and norepinephrine) catechols or their metabolites metanephrines and vanillylmandelic acid (VMA) in a 24-h urine. Unfortunately, none of these measurements is perfect, with VMA having a false-negative rate of 20% and catecholamines having a false-positive rate of at least that—remember stress appropriately raises catecholamine secretion so that urine determinations are not performed in hospitalized patients and are often high in patients with chronic illness. Thus, at least two urine parameters should be measured in the 24-h urine, and many authors recommend all three. If screening is positive, the workup proceeds to establish a positive diagnosis and localization with suppression tests, MRI, and radiolabel scans.

E. Thyrotoxicosis

Hyperthyroidism stems from excess circulating thyroid hormone, with the most common causes being taking too much exogenous hormone, Graves' disease which stems from an autoantibody that activates the thyrotropin (also called thyroid hormone stimulating hormone; TSH) receptor on the thyroid, hyperactive single or multiple thyroid nodules, and thyroiditis, which is a self-limited process that results in lysis of thyroid cells and release of their stored hormone. Typical symptoms and signs stem from thyroid hormone-activating sympathomimetic, catabolic, and hypermetabolic activity: weight loss, heat intolerance, irritability, and emotional lability, sweating, palpitations, hyperdefecation, fatigue, weakness, and menstrual irregularity. Classic physical findings are tachycardia, sometimes with atrial fibrillation, fever, tremor, lid lag, and stare. Insight into the etiology is often obtained from the thyroid examination: the diffusely enlarged goiter, with bruit which is characteristic for Graves' disease, a uninodular or multinodular thyroid gland, or a thyroid examination that is often perfectly normal, except occasionally for some tenderness with thyroiditis. When present, the symptoms and signs are strong indicators of hyperthyroidism, although their absence does not exclude the diagnosis. In particular, the elderly can present with few specific complaints or physical findings, sometimes just a failure to thrive, worsening congestive heart failure, or new-onset atrial fibrillation.

Excess thyroid hormone has multiple metabolic effects that promote hyperglycemia although overt diabetes is uncommon: rapid gastric emptying and enhanced glucose absorption from the gut; increased sympathetic activity, with enhanced gluconeogenesis, glycogenolysis, lipolysis, and proteolysis, causing insulin resistance; the clearance rate of insulin is increased on average 40%. *Diagnosis:* Standard testing of TSH and thyroid levels—the diagnostic pattern is elevated thyroid levels in combination with a TSH below the measurable range. There are occasional patients with only the T_3 level being increased as opposed to normal T_4 levels (T_3 thyrotoxicosis) so that a total T_3 should be obtained with T_4 testing.

F. Somatostatinoma

Somatostatin-secreting tumors are extremely rare. They usually originate from the islet cells of the pancreas, although tumors from the gut, paraganglia, and thyroid have been described. Typically, they are malignant and may be identified only after metastatic spread. Somatostatin suppresses both insulin and glucagon secretion so that the diabetes is usually mild. Symptoms are nonspecific and include diarrhea, gallstones, anemia, hypochlorhydria–dyspepsia, and abdominal pain.

G. Aldosteronoma (Conn's Syndrome)

Hyperaldosteroism is characterized by the triad of hypertension, hypokalemia, and glucose intolerance. The latter occurs in about 50% of patients with Conn's syndrome, although overt diabetes is unusual. The hypertension and hypokalemia reflect volume expansion and the action of aldosterone to promote urinary potassium excretion. Insulin secretion is a potassium-regulated process, and the glucose intolerance is believed to stem from a delayed and subnormal secretion of insulin, although other unknown factors may also contribute. *Clinical clue and diagnosis:* Any patient with hypertension and hypokalemia who is not taking diuretics should be considered for hyperaldosteronism. In most laboratories, the normal range for serum potassium is 3.5–5.0 mEq/L, but studies some years ago showed about 20% of these patients have a potassium between 3.5–4.0 mEq/L, so that persistent low normal values should raise your suspicion. Screening entails confirmation of renal urinary potassium-wasting by 24-h urine; if higher than 30 mEq, the next step is to show that aldosterone production is increased plus the renin–angiotensin system is suppressed to exclude secondary hyperaldosteroism (from diuretics, hepatic insufficiency, congestive heart failure, hypoalbuminemia, and nephrotic syndrome) by obtaining a plasma renin and 24-h urine for aldosterone. If these confirm the presence of primary hyperaldosteronism, the workup proceeds to differentiate adrenal adenoma from bilateral hyperplasia by CT scan and other provocative testing.

VI. DRUG-INDUCED DIABETES

Drug-induced diabetes is discussed in Chap. 13.

BIBLIOGRAPHY

Bacon BR. Diagnosis and management of hemochromatosis. Gastroenterology 1997; 113: 995–999.

Baynes KC, Whitehead J, Krook A, O'Rahilly S. Molecular mechanisms of inherited insulin resistance. Q J Med 1997; 90:557–562.

Dabon-Almirante CL, Surks MI. Clinical and laboratory diagnosis of thyrotoxicosis. Endocrinol Metab Clin North Am 1998; 27:25–35. [The cited volume of this journal (March 1998) is a complete overview of thyrotoxicosis.]

Edwards CQ, Kushner JP. Screening for hemochromatosis. N Engl J Med 1993; 328: 1616–1620.

Ganda OP. Secondary forms of diabetes. In: Kahn CR, Weir GC, eds. Joslin's Diabetes Mellitus. 13th ed. Malvern, PA: Lea & Febiger, 1994:300–316.

Goldstein BJ. Syndromes of extreme insulin resistance. In: Kahn CR, Weir GC, eds. Joslin's Diabetes Mellitus, 13th ed. Malvern, PA: Lea & Febiger, 1994:282–299.

Hattersley AT. Maturity-onset diabetes of the young: clinical heterogeneity explained by genetic heterogeneity. Diabetic Med 1998; 15:15–24.

Lanng S. Glucose intolerance in cystic fibrosis. Dan Med Bull 1997; 44:23–39.

Maassen, JA, Kadowaki T. Maternally inherited diabetes and deafness: a new diabetes subtype. Diabetologia 1996; 39:375–382.

Maugans TA, Coates ML. Diagnosis and treatment of acromegaly. Am Fam Physician 1995; 52:207–213.

Mohan V, Nagalotimath SJ, Yajnik CS, Tripathy BB. Fibrocalculous pancreatic diabetes. Diabetes Metab Rev 1998; 14:153–170.

Moran A, Doherty L, Wang X, Thomas W. Abnormal glucose metabolism in cystic fibrosis. J Pediatr 1998; 133:10–17.

Newell-Price J, Trainer P, Besser M, Grossman A. The diagnosis and differential diagnosis of Cushing's syndrome and pseudo-Cushing's states. Endocr Rev 1998; 19: 647–672.

Tripathy BB, Samal KC. Overview and consensus statement on diabetes in tropical areas. Diabetes Metab Rev 1997; 13:63–76.

U.S. Expert Committee on Diagnosis and Classification of Diabetes Mellitus, 1997–8. Diabetes Care 1998; 21(suppl 1):S5–S19.

Velho G, Froguel P. Genetic, metabolic and clinical characteristics of maturity onset diabetes of the young. Eur J Endocrinol 1998; 138:233–239.

Werbel SS, Ober KP. Pheochromocytoma. Update on diagnosis, localization, and management. Med Clin North Am 1995; 79:131–153.

Wermers RA, Fatourechi V, Wynne AG, Kvois LK, Lloyd RV. The glucagonoma syndrome. Clinical and pathologic features in 21 patients. Medicine 1996; 75:53–63.

Yaouanq, JM. Diabetes and haemochromatosis: current concepts, management and prevention. Diabetes Metab 1995; 21:319–329.

15

Medical Nutrition Therapy in Diabetes: Clinical Guidelines for Primary Care Physicians

Melinda Downie Maryniuk

Joslin Diabetes Center, Boston, Massachusetts

I. INTRODUCTION

Medical nutrition therapy is commonly described as the ''cornerstone'' of diabetes treatment. The effectiveness of nutrition to improve diabetes control and reduce glycosylated hemoglobin has been demonstrated in several research studies. However, it is also frequently acknowledged that patients find following a diet the most challenging part of the diabetes regimen. Also, physicians are often poorly trained in nutrition and do not have the time to provide patients with an individualized meal plan. What usually results is that patients are handed a preprinted diet tear-off sheet and told to ''watch what you eat'' or ''lose some weight.'' This advice inevitably results in poor compliance and ''diet failure.'' Therefore, given the importance of nutrition therapy, what can a busy physician do to enhance its effectiveness?

This chapter is divided into two main sections: Sec. II addresses five practical guidelines for physicians related to nutrition therapy (Table 1). It offers a variety of tools and guidelines to help ensure that patients are provided with realistic nutrition recommendations. Section III includes specific information related to developing and implementing a nutrition prescription. This is particularly helpful for providers who may not have easy access to a registered dietitian.

Table 1   Recommendations to Enhance Medical Nutrition Therapy

A.   Address the importance of nutrition therapy
B.   Dispel nutrition myths and provide facts
C.   Assess lifestyle first, then determine prescriptions
D.   Evaluate the therapy and adjust to meet goals
E.   Team up with a registered dietitian

II. RECOMMENDATIONS TO ENHANCE MEDICAL NUTRITION THERAPY

A.   Address the Importance of Nutrition Therapy

Patients will have more success following nutritional recommendations if the physician supports the importance and effectiveness of this therapy. Each person with diabetes should have an individualized meal plan. As part of an annual review, the physician should assess the patient's need for additional nutrition intervention. Guidelines for when additional nutrition instruction or a revised meal plan may be warranted are listed in Table 2.

However, stressing the importance is not enough. Be convinced that effective nutritional therapy yields results. Research has shown in both type 1 and type 2 diabetes, patients who receive nutritional intervention by a registered dietitian who follows practice guidelines, as published by the American Dietetic Association, have significant improvements in glycohemoglobin (HbA$_{1c}$). Studies from the Diabetes Control and Complications Trial (DCCT) have identified key nutritional behaviors that are also associated with significantly improved blood

Table 2   Referral Guidelines for Nutrition Therapy

Newly diagnosed
New on insulin
Unexplained, recurrent hypoglycemia
Unexplained, recurrent hyperglycemia
Risk factor modification: hyperlipidemia, hypertension, or nephropathy
Weight loss or gain
Pre- or postconception
Elevated glycohemoglobin (> 8)
At patient's request
Ideally, once a year

glucose control. These behaviors include following the recommended meal and snack plan, adjustment of insulin dose in response to meal size, prompt treatment of hyperglycemia (less food or more insulin) and avoidance of overtreatment of hypoglycemia. Nutrition counseling, therefore, should emphasize these effective behaviors.

B. Dispel Nutrition's Myths and Provide the Facts

The American public has been flooded with messages about diets, food, and nutrition. If, in fact, 70% of the adult population finds nutrition "confusing" then it is likely that an even a greater percentage of the population of adults with diabetes is confused by what to eat. Many of the traditional dietary recommendations are based on minimal scientific research.

1.   Myth 1: A Diabetic Diet for Women Is 1200 Calories and for Men Is 1400 Calories

There is no such thing as a "diabetic diet." There are as many different approaches to meal planning as there are people with diabetes. Unfortunately, for many years, a diabetic diet was defined by a restricted calorie level, distributing the calories according to a standard prescription (50% carbohydrate, 20% protein, and 30% fat) and then spacing the calories in equal portions throughout the day (2/8 for breakfast, 2/8 for lunch, 1/8 for snack, 2/8 for supper, and 1/8 for bedtime snack). This method had little relevance for the way a person might usually eat. Today, with the wide variety of pharmaceutical regimens available for diabetes control, more flexibility in meal planning is possible.

The current recommendations from the American Diabetes Association (ADA) are that nutritional prescriptions must be tailored to the individual, based on usual habits and metabolic needs. Table 3 summarizes the ADA nutritional goals, principles, and recommendations.

Although the distribution of calories in a 50–20–30 pattern continues to be considered a healthy general recommendation for adults, needs of individuals may vary from a lower percentage of total fat (20–25%) for an individual with elevated low-density lipoprotein (LDL) cholesterol levels to a lower percentage of total carbohydrate (40–45%) for an individual with elevated triglyceride levels. The distribution of calories into meals and snacks should be based on the way the person usually eats, not on some fractionated formula. The caloric level should also be based on the usual intake and then adjusted if weight loss, maintenance, or gain is the objective. It typically takes up to 30 min to obtain the assessment information needed to develop an individualized meal plan, time usually best spent by a registered dietitian.

So, the "ADA diets" are a thing of the past, with the focus now being on developing a medical nutrition therapy plan specific for the individual. Also

Table 3 Diabetes Nutrition Goals, Principles, and Recommendations

Calories

    Sufficient to attain and/or maintain a reasonable body weight for adults, normal growth and development for children and adolescents, and adequate nutrition during pregnancy and lactation

Protein

    10–20% of daily calories

    No more than adult RDA (0.8 g/kg body weight per day) with evidence of nephropathy

Fat

    Saturated fat $<$ 10% of daily calories, $<$ 7% with elevated LDL cholesterol

    Polyunsaturated fat up to 10% of total calories

    Remaining total fat varies with treatment goals

    $\sim$ 30%—normal weight and lipids

    $<$ 30%—obese, elevated LDL cholesterol

    $\leq$ 40%—elevated triglycerides unresponsive to fat restriction and weight loss

    Predominately monounsaturated fat

Cholesterol

    $<$ 300 mg/day

Carbohydrate

    Difference after protein and fat goals have been met

    Percentage varies with treatment goals

Sweeteners

    Sucrose need not be restricted, must be substituted as carbohydrate

    Nutritive sweeteners have no advantage over sucrose and must be substituted as carbohydrate

    Nonnutritive sweeteners approved by the FDA are safe to consume

Fiber

    20–35 g/day

Sodium

    $<$ 3,000 mg/day

    $<$ 2,400 mg/day in mild to moderate hypertension

Alcohol

    Moderate usage, i.e., $<$ 2 alcoholic beverages daily

Vitamins and minerals

    Same as the general population

Goals must always be individualized. RDA, recommended dietary allowance.
Source: American Diabetes Assoc, 1998.

emphasized in nutrition therapy is the importance of understanding behavior change and incorporating these principles into counseling, as well as evaluating the meal plan at follow-up visits to assess its effect.

2. Myth 2: Sugar and Sweeteners Should Be Avoided

Scientific evidence does not support the common belief that sucrose should be restricted. The former view of looking at carbohydrates as "complex," or slower-acting, and "simple," or fast-acting, is not useful. Over a dozen studies in which sucrose was substituted for more complex carbohydrates found no adverse effect on glycemia. However, it is important to caution patients this does not mean that sugar is fine to eat as desired. Because the carbohydrate in foods is the major predictor of postprandial blood glucose levels, all carbohydrates should be controlled. A cup of rice will have three times the effect on blood glucose as a tablespoon of sugar. Therefore, emphasis should be placed on controlling the amount of carbohydrate foods in the meal plan. Patients need to learn which foods contain carbohydrate and to eat consistent, controlled amounts. Table 4 shows a variety of carbohydrate foods, in differing portion sizes, that all contain 15 g of carbohydrate. Notice that the serving size of the sweeter or sugary foods is smaller than their less sweet counterparts, reflecting the higher carbohydrate content.

Another related myth is "Don't drink fruit juice." Sometimes the opposite myth is heard, "Since fruit is healthy, fruit juice is a free food." Because fruit juice is often used for the treatment of hypoglycemia, it is considered by many as a food that will raise the blood glucose quickly. Although it is true that fruit juice will elevate glycemia, this is due to the quantity of juice consumed and not the type of carbohydrate. In fact, fruit juice may have less of a glycemic effect than other carbohydrates because of the lower glycemic index of fructose, a fruit sugar. As noted in Table 4, a 15-g serving of fruit juice is about ½cup (4 oz; 118 mL). So if a patient consumes large quantities of juice thinking that it is "healthy" or free, then an increase in blood glucose is to be expected.

Table 4 Carbohydrate Choices: 15 g/Serving

Bread/starch	Fruit	Milk	Other
1 slice bread	1 small apple	1 cup milk	½ cup ice
⅓ cup rice	½ cup fruit	⅓ cup regular	cream
¾ cup unsweetened	juice	fruit yogurt	¼ cup sherbet
cereal	2 tbsp raisins	1 cup aspartame	1 tbsp sugar,
½ cup sweetened cereal	1 ¼ cup	sweetened	honey or jam
½ cup corn or peas	strawberries	yogurt	

There are now four different types of nonnutritive or artificial sweeteners on the market: saccharin, aspartame, acesulfame K, and sucralose. All are U.S. Food and Drug Administration (FDA) approved and can be used safely for persons with diabetes, including during pregnancy.

3. Myth 3: The Diabetic Diet is Taught Using the ADA–ADA Exchange Lists

The exchange lists are one of many different, useful tools to teach diabetes meal planning. Unfortunately, because exchange lists had been so widely used in hospitals for diet instruction, they have almost become synonymous with the diabetic diet. Do not expect that every patient should or will receive a meal plan using this approach when they receive diet instruction. Instead, recognize that there are many different approaches to meal planning and tools to use when giving the patient guidelines for choosing foods. For some patients, a meal plan may not be based on a caloric level, but general guidelines for healthy eating based on the Food Guide Pyramid and USDA Guidelines for Healthy Americans. Others may receive a set of sample menus and recommendations for portion control, fat reduction, and regular exercise to promote moderate weight reduction. Still others may receive a gram allowance of fat or carbohydrate. For a list of suggested resources and publications for patient nutrition education, see Table 5.

Although the DCCT brought attention to carbohydrate counting, this is by no means a new approach. In 1935 Elliott Joslin, wrote, "In teaching patients their diet, I lay emphasis first on the carbohydrate values, and teach to a few only the values for protein and fat." Carbohydrate counting is a flexible approach that may be taught in a simplified version with a focus on blood glucose control or in a more detailed fashion for the patient managed by intensive insulin therapy. Patient using an insulin pump or receiving multiple injections of a fast-acting insulin may enjoy the flexibility of determining their premeal insulin dose based on their anticipated carbohydrate intake using a "insulin/carbohydrate ratio." From a detailed diet history and the patients metabolic goals, the patient is given guidelines for how much carbohydrate consumed will balance 1 U of insulin. An average ratio might be 1:15 or 1 U of insulin for every 15 g of carbohydrate eaten. Thus if a patient is planning to eat about 90 g of carbohydrate at supper, they would take 6 U of regular insulin if their premeal glucose was within target range.

Caution patients that carbohydrate counting alone can lead to unwanted weight gain and an increased fat intake if the patient is not conscientious of the hidden fats in their diet. A good general guideline is for adults to limit meat intake to 6–8 oz/day, and to limit added fat servings to two to three servings per meal.

Table 5 Resources and Publications for Patient Education

Several key organizations and diabetes centers publish material for diabetes patient education. Several sample titles are listed, along with the web site address and telephone number.

- American Diabetes Association
  Alexandria, VA
  www.diabetes.org / 800-232-3472
- American Dietetic Association
  Chicago, IL
  www.eatright.org / 800-366-1655
    The First Step in Diabetes Meal Planning
    Healthy Food Choices
    Exchange Lists for Meal Planning
    Carbohydrate Counting Series: Getting Started, Moving On, Carb-Insulin Ratios
    The Diabetes Carbohydrate and Fat Gram Guide
- National Institutes of Health/NIDDK
  Bethesda, MD
  www.niddk.nih.gov / 301-654-3327
  The NIH offers over 30 patient education publications
    I Have Diabetes: What Should I Eat?
    I Have Diabetes: How Much Should I Eat?
    I Have Diabetes: When Should I Eat?
- Joslin Diabetes Center
  Boston, MA
  www.joslin.org / 617-732-2695
    Menu Planning—Simple!
    Getting to the Heart of It
    The Joslin Diabetes Quick and Easy Cookbook
    Diabetes and You; An ''easy-to-read'' patient education series
- International Diabetes Center
  Minneapolis, MN
  www.idcpublishing.com / 612-993-3393
    Exchanges for All Occasions (4th ed)
    Fast Food Facts (5th ed)

When it is determined that prescribing an exchange list type of meal plan is the best approach, the physician should recognize that the following three elements of this food plan will make it easier for the patient and also make the plan metabolically more accurate. First, instead of working with six food groups (bread, fruit, vegetable, meat, milk, and fat), patients are generally taught using a three-group system: carbohydrate foods (breads, fruit, milk, and "other" carbohydrates), meats and meat substitutes, and fat. Unless three or more servings of vegetables are eaten at a meal, they are usually not "counted." Meats are divided into four subgroups, depending on their fat content. Patients should be guided to select from the very lean and lean groups as much as possible. Finally, the diet prescription (total calories, percentage distribution between nutrients, and specific numbers of servings from each group) is developed, based on an assessment of the way the patient usually eats, and the medication plan is adjusted accordingly. It is often easier to change a medication than a lifetime of eating habits.

4. Myth 4: Choosing Low Glycemic Index Foods or High-Fiber Foods Will Improve Glycemic Control

Research has been somewhat confusing and contradictory about the effects of particular foods on blood sugar. Although there was much attention given to the glycemic index of different carbohydrate foods during the 1980s, the unique glycemic effect of a particular food seems to be mitigated when eaten in combination with other foods. Therefore, there seems to be no rationale to discouraging the use of foods that have a high glycemic index, such as white or whole meal bread, cornflakes, mashed potato, or carrots, or encouraging use of only low glycemic index foods, such as milk, soybeans, fructose, barley, and apple juice.

    Dietary fiber is an important component of a healthy diet for all adults. Once again, research in the 1980s seemed to be pointing to a glycemic-lowering property of dietary fiber. These findings have not been borne out in multiple studies, however, so it is not accurate to encourage higher fiber intake on the basis that it will improve glycemic control. There is evidence however, that a high intake of soluble fibers (> 20 g/day) is associated with a reduction in serum cholesterol.

5. Myth 5: Weight Loss Diets Do Not Work

Nutrition therapy tends to be focused on weight reduction because 80–90% of adults with type 2 diabetes are obese. However, providers would do better to focus on specific steps to enhance blood glucose control, instead of continuously stressing weight loss, which tends to have a low success rate. If patients are truly ready to take steps toward weight loss, these are some approaches that can be taken to enhance the overall effectiveness of weight control:

a. Set Realistic Goals

Help the patient define a reasonable body weight, one that both patient and provider acknowledge is achievable and maintainable in the short and long term. This may not be the same as an ideal goal (body mass index [BMI] less than 25). Focus on the fact that just a moderate weight loss of 5–10% body weight or 10–15 lb (4.5–6.8 kg) can have a significant improvement on blood glucose control. This improvement comes from enhanced insulin sensitivity and glucose uptake, reduced insulin secretion and decreased hepatic glucose production. Guide the patient to measure success not in pounds lost, but in the improvement in glycohemoglobin and other medical parameters. In Table 6, note that a BMI ≥27 is associated with higher risk for diabetes and ≥30 is frank obesity.

b. Consider the Variety of Options Available for Obesity Treatment

The meal plan must be individualized; simply handing a patient a 1000 calorie diet plan will likely lead to diet failure. Weight reduction is best accomplished through modest caloric restriction, physical activity, behavior modification, and psychosocial support. Group support through programs such as Weight Watchers and Overeaters Anonymous can be very effective. Instead of telling the patient what to do, ask what changes they are willing to make. Focus on those changes that reduce fat and total caloric intake and increase caloric expenditure through exercise. A variety of high-protein, low-carbohydrate diets have returned to popularity. Known by various names (Atkins, Zone, Sugarbusters), these are all similar in that they push the intake of protein foods and severely limit carbohydrates. Despite much testimonial praise, these diets have not been proven effective for metabolic control or weight reduction. There is concern that the high-protein intake is often linked with high cholesterol and total fat intake. Thus, if a patient chooses to follow such a plan, the provider should monitor serum lipid levels and recommend vitamin and mineral supplements to compensate for the nutrients that may be missing from limited intakes of milk, dairy products, fruits, and vegetables. Surgical interventions have been successful in people with a BMI higher than 40, but should be only an adjunct to diet and exercise.

c. Recognize That Obesity Is a Chronic Disease

The new eating, exercise, and stress management behaviors that should be adopted for successful weight control should be adopted for life, and not just for a short-term "diet." Like diabetes, obesity is a chronic disease and requires lifelong treatment.

C. Assess Lifestyle First, Then Determine Prescriptions

Build your therapeutic plan around the patients usual habits and their readiness to change. In other words, to determine a suitable insulin prescription, the patients usual eating and exercise habits should be evaluated. It is much easier to design

Table 6 Body Mass Index (BMI) Values

BMI

	Good weights								▽						Increasing risk							
Height	19	20	21	22	23	24	25	26	27	28	29	30	31	32	33	34	35	36	37	38	39	40
	Weight (in pounds)																					
4'10"	91	96	100	105	110	115	119	124	129	134	138	143	148	153	158	162	167	172	177	181	186	191
4'11"	94	99	104	109	114	119	124	128	133	138	143	148	153	158	163	168	173	178	183	188	193	198
5'	97	102	107	112	118	123	128	133	138	143	148	153	158	163	168	174	179	184	189	194	199	204
5'1"	100	106	111	116	122	127	132	137	143	148	153	158	164	169	174	180	185	190	195	201	206	211
5'2"	104	109	115	120	126	131	136	142	147	153	158	164	169	175	180	186	191	196	202	207	213	218
5'3"	107	113	118	124	130	135	141	146	152	158	163	169	175	180	186	191	197	203	208	214	220	225
5'4"	110	116	122	128	134	140	145	151	157	163	169	174	180	186	192	197	204	209	215	221	227	232
5'5"	114	120	126	132	138	144	150	156	162	168	174	180	186	192	198	204	210	216	222	228	234	240
5'6"	118	124	130	136	142	148	155	161	167	173	179	186	192	198	204	210	216	223	229	235	241	247
5'7"	121	127	134	140	146	153	159	166	172	178	185	191	198	204	211	217	223	230	236	242	249	255
5'8"	125	131	138	144	151	158	164	171	177	184	190	197	203	210	216	223	230	236	243	249	256	262
5'9"	128	135	142	149	155	162	169	176	182	189	196	203	209	216	223	230	236	243	250	257	263	270
5'10"	132	139	146	153	160	167	174	181	188	195	202	209	216	222	229	236	243	250	257	264	271	278
5'11"	136	143	150	157	165	172	179	186	193	200	208	215	222	229	236	243	250	257	265	272	279	285
6'	140	147	154	162	169	177	184	191	199	206	213	221	228	235	242	250	258	265	272	279	287	294
6'1"	144	151	159	166	174	182	189	197	204	212	219	227	235	242	250	257	265	272	280	288	293	302
6'2"	148	155	163	171	179	186	194	202	210	218	225	233	241	249	256	264	272	280	287	295	303	311
6'3"	152	160	168	176	184	192	200	208	216	224	232	240	248	256	264	272	279	287	295	303	311	319
6'4"	156	164	172	180	189	197	205	213	221	230	238	246	254	263	271	279	287	295	304	312	320	328

a medication plan around typical lifestyle behaviors (which can be hard to change) than it is to change lifestyle behaviors to match an insulin regimen.

In general, small changes that the patient can make and adhere to, can make a big difference. Table 7 offers suggestions for assessing particular nutrition-related problem areas. Small changes in the timing of meals, maintaining consistency in the amount of food eaten, or in the types of foods selected when eating out frequently can have a significant influence on metabolic control. When a referral to a registered dietitian is not possible, focus your assessment on some of these key areas, which can make a difference.

When time is limited, help the patient identify a few key dietary changes that could be made that will affect metabolic control. Focusing on one to two specific changes will be more effective than telling the patient to "cut back on the fat" or to follow a diet sheet. Also recognize the nutritional priorities for the person taking insulin will be different from those of a person not taking insulin.

Although there are a variety of formulas to use to determine caloric needs, the caloric level for the person with diabetes should usually be based on the usual amount of calories eaten and adjusted accordingly for desired weight loss or gain (Table 8). Specific nutrient recommendations should not be set based solely on a formula, but on the usual eating habits, the patients willingness to change, and the metabolic goals. Table 9 outlines several typical patterns for guiding patients intake. These are not intended to be used as absolute criteria, but more as a reference to ensure that the individualized recommendations are close to target.

D. Evaluate the Therapy and Adjust to Meet Goals

Monitoring of blood glucose, lipids, weight, blood pressure, and renal status is the tool for evaluating the effectiveness of medical nutrition therapy. However, to see measurable change from use of nutrition therapy, the patient must be given time to incorporate the new eating habits into his or her lifestyle. Before moving the patient from diet as a monotherapy to diet and oral agents, ensure that the patient has had at least 6–8 weeks to implement recommend dietary changes. On the other hand, have realistic expectations for what nutritional therapy can accomplish. A low saturated fat (7–10% total calories from saturated fat) can reduce total serum cholesterol by only approximately 25 mg. If goals are not met, given an adequate trial, advance the therapy to the next level by adding or adjusting medication. This does not indicate the "failure" of the diet or of the patient, rather, it just profiles a fairly typical course of diabetes.

E. Team up with a Registered Dietitian

Although there are many important steps the primary care physician can take to provide medical nutritional therapy, every person with diabetes should receive a

Table 7 Tips for Conducting a Nutrition Assessment

Nutrition habits to evaluate	Ask	Rationale
Relations between food intake and home blood glucose results.	"Have you noticed any trends between what you eat and your blood sugar results?"	Determine if there is a pattern connecting food intake and glucose results. Target recommendations to address the problem; for example, do not skip breakfast if prelunch hypoglycemia has been occurring.
Usual eating and exercise habits—in terms of timing, quantity and consistency.	"What times are your meals and snacks eaten? Does that vary much from day to day? Describe two different typical lunches you might have."	The medical prescription should be based on a patient's usual lifestyle habits, and not the other way around. Sometimes dramatic improvements in glucose control can be realized if emphasis is placed on the importance of eating consistent amounts at consistent times.
Sources of fat in the diet.	"How do you prepare meats? Vegetables? What kind of fried foods do you eat regularly? What type of milk or cheese do you use? How often do you eat baked goods, desserts (sources of hidden fats)?"	Help the patient identify specific foods that contain fat and that can be limited or substituted for a lower-fat choice. Avoid general recommendations, such as "limit fried foods," but contract with the patient for a specific action to take.
Frequency of eating away from home.	"How many times each week do you eat a meal away from home?"	Frequent fast-food and restaurant meals can contribute a significant source of fat and calories. Help the patient identify ways to improve eating habits when on the go.
Past nutrition education and efforts to follow a diet.	"Tell me about any of the diets you have received in the past. What worked and what did not?"	Determine not only if the patient has ever received proper nutrition instruction, but also what experience, both positive and negative, they have with diets.
Use of vitamin and mineral supplements and botanical and herbal products.	"Tell me about any supplements that you take, such as vitamins."	A study showed that up to 33% adults practice some sort of alternative medicine, but few tell their physicians. It is important to encourage the patient to feel comfortable describing such practices.

Persons responsible for food purchasing and preparation.	"Who does the shopping and cooking at home?"	Whenever possible, nutrition education should include the person who obtains and prepares the food. Because food affects the whole family, the more the family is involved and understands, the better the compliance.
Overall nutritional balance.	"Tell me everything you ate over the past 24 hours."	A quick assessment of an adult's overall nutritional health should pay particular attention to the following: intake of 4–6 servings of fruit or vegetables; 2–3 servings of milk, yogurt, or sources of calcium; food choices low in saturated fat and high in fiber; moderate portion size of meat, fish, and poultry (generally not more than 6–8 oz/day); only moderate use of sodium, cholesterol, alcohol, and added sugars.
Frequency of skipping or missing an insulin dose.	"How many times a week might you forget to take your insulin?"	Asking in a nonjudgmental, nonthreatening way may foster honest dialogue about skipped insulin doses that may, in fact, be intentional. Women in particular recognize lipogenic properties of insulin and learn that skipping it can be a quick way to lose weight. This unhealthy route to weight control must be addressed.
Readiness to change (related to a particular behavior).	"Is starting a weight loss program something you are ready to do now? Within the next 3 months? Maybe sometime later?"	For a patient to adopt a new behavior, they must be ready to make the change. However, even if a patient may not be ready to take action, you can still help him or her progress along the stages of change and move from just thinking about it to preparing to take action.

Table 8 Estimating Daily Energy Needs for Adults

Basal calories	20–25 kcal/kg desirable body weight	
Add calories for activity	If sedentary	30% more calories
	If moderately active	50% more calories
	If strenuously active	100% more active
For weight loss	Subtract 500 kcal/day to lose 1 lb/wk	
For weight gain	Add 500 kcal/day to lose 1 lb/wk	
For pregnancy	Add 300 kcal/day during pregnancy; 500 kcal/day during lactation	

meal plan individualized for them by a registered dietitian. When possible, work collaboratively with the dietitian, discussing therapeutic goals and expectations of treatment interventions. Convey to the dietitian your therapeutic goals (target HbA_{1c}, target fasting blood glucose, target lipids), relevant laboratory data (HbA_{1c}, lipids, blood pressure, renal function tests), list of medications, and other medical problems. Mentor dietitians who are along the route to becoming a certified diabetes educator (CDE). Recognize that CDE dietitians generally have experience to serve expanded roles beyond just providing nutritional therapy, which can include providing training in blood glucose monitoring and interpretation, insulin adjustment guidelines, and risk factor reduction. Dietitians can be found in various settings, including hospitals, public health departments, managed care organizations, and private practice. The American Dietetic Association can provide information on dietitians in your area who accept referrals. [Contact the ADA at 1-800-877-1600 (then press 7)]. You can also find a diabetes educator in your area by calling the American Association of Diabetes Educators Access Hotline at 1-800-832-6874.

Table 9 Suggested Guidelines for Daily Intake

kcal	No. servings carbohydrate (15 g/serving)	Total grams fat	Servings lean meat (oz)	No. servings fat (5 g fat per serving)
1200	10	40	5–6	3–4
1400	12	47	6–8	3–4
1600	13	53	6–8	4–5
1800	15	60	6–8	5–6
2000	17	66	6–8	7–8

III. PROVIDING NUTRITIONAL GUIDANCE FOR YOUR PATIENTS

Although having access to a registered dietitian who is experienced in diabetes management is ideal, there may be times when the primary care provider will lay the basic groundwork. The provider needs to be able to develop and implement a basic nutrition prescription, and give guidance and recommendations related to the use of food and alcohol in special situations. The following section offers basic tools to complete these tasks.

A. Developing the Nutrition Prescription

An often asked question of dietitians is "how long does it take to teach a diet?" That is difficult to answer on two counts. Because of the wide variety of backgrounds and experiences each patient brings, the teaching time can vary greatly. Second, medical nutrition therapy is not as straightforward as just handing over a piece of paper with eating instructions on it. It is recommended that a four-step–counseling process be followed to ensure behavior change that will result in modified eating habits. The four steps include assessment, goal setting, implementation, and evaluation. In general, however, the dietitian will schedule a new patient assessment for 1 h, followed by at least one to two 30-min follow-up sessions within the first month. This is extremely important to assess the effectiveness of the therapy. After a trial period of at least 6–12 weeks, if the metabolic goals are not met as expected, medical therapy should be advanced.

Two of the most common meal-planning approaches are exchange lists and carbohydrate counting. The latter has received renewed attention over the past few years because its use is common by DCCT dietitians and patients enjoy the increased flexibility of this approach. It is suitable for almost all patients and the level of detail in the instruction can be adapted to match the patients interest, educational level, and desire for tight metabolic control. The complexity can range from giving guidelines for the number of carbohydrate servings to have at each meal, to calculating carbohydrate/insulin ratios for fine-tuned control. Table 10 illustrates the four-step medical nutrition therapy process and using carbohydrate-counting instruction as a model.

B. Special Topics

1. Protein

There is no demonstrated advantage to consuming higher or lower quantities of protein in the diet. With adequate insulin, protein has very little effect on blood glucose levels. A low-protein diet will not reduce risks for nephropathy, but if

Table 10   The Four-Step Process of Medical Nutrition Therapy: Illustration of
Carbohydrate Counting

Step 1: Assessment
    Calculate usual eating habits by evaluating 24-h recall and food history
    Determine usual carbohydrate intake for each meal and snack
    Evaluate other factors that may affect diabetes and nutritional health (timing of meals,
       timing and amount of exercise, frequency and treatments of hypoglycemia, dining
       out patterns, or others)
    Assess readiness to change
Step 2: Goal setting
    Determine the diet and lifestyle changes patient is willing to make
    Determine clinical or metabolic outcomes (target HbA_{1c}, fasting BG, target lipids)
Step 3: Intervention
Level 1
    Practice identifying carbohydrate foods (breads and starches, fruits, milk, sweets)
    Recognize 15-g carbohydrate portions of foods commonly eaten
    Demonstrate measuring skills using scale, measuring cups and spoons
    Discuss plan for keeping protein intake consistent and fat intake low to moderate
    Practice label-reading skills to obtain nutritional information
    Plan sample meals
Level 2
    Practice reading records of food intake, blood glucose, and physical activity to inter-
       pret blood glucose patterns
    Determine appropriate actions or strategies, including adjustment of carbohydrate
       level to achieve blood glucose goals
Level 3
    Calculate carbohydrate/insulin ratio by dividing the total grams of carbohydrate usu-
       ally consumed for each meal by the number of units of regular insulin taken before
       that meal.
    Demonstrate how both carbohydrate intake and insulin can be adjusted to fine-tune
       blood glucose levels.
Step 4: Evaluation
    Assess effect of intervention by conducting process, outcome, and impact evaluations
    Continuously collect data on progress towards behavioral goals and changes in medi-
       cal status (HbA_{1c}, weight, blood pressure, lipids), risk factor reduction (decrease
       in hypoglycemia, increase in exercise)

---

overt nephropathy exists, reducing fat to not less than 0.8 g/kg is advised. Once
the glomerular filtration rate begins to fall, further reduction to 0.6 g/kg per day
may prove useful in selected patients. However, a multisite, national clinical
trial—Modification of Diet in Renal Disease—failed to show a clear benefit of
protein restriction. If protein is reduced to levels of 0.6 g/kg, the provider should

watch for signs of malnutrition and muscle wasting which have been displayed in some patients.

2. Fiber

A healthy diet should include generous quantities of high-fiber, unprocessed foods (whole grains, dried beans, fruits, and vegetables). General guidelines are to consume 20–35 g dietary fiber per day from a wide variety of foods. There is little convincing evidence, however, that fiber diets have specific glycemic benefits, although there does appear to be a relations between increased soluble fiber (from oats and dried beans) and a reduction in serum lipids.

3. Alcohol

Because alcohol is not metabolized to glucose and it inhibits gluconeogenesis, it may have a hypoglycemic effect within 6–36 h after ingestion. Therefore, if patients choose to drink alcoholic beverages, they should drink with meals and not on an empty stomach. In addition, self-monitoring of blood glucose before and after alcohol intake enables the patient to predict potential hypoglycemia and to prevent it. The American Diabetes Association recommends not more than two drinks a day for men or one a day for women who choose to drink and have no other medical contraindications to alcohol.

Alcohol intake should be restricted in patients with elevated triglycerides. Alcohol also contributes significant calories and should be limited for weight control. If combined with sweet mixers, such as fruit juices or sodas, the carbohydrate content must be counted.

4. Vitamin and Mineral Supplements

Because nearly one-third of American adults take some type of nutritional supplement, it is important for providers to assess intake in an open, nonjudgmental way. Patients must be made to feel comfortable disclosing information about supplements. In general, the American Diabetes Association does not recommend supplements unless an individual has a specific deficiency. For example, in individuals who are magnesium deficient, an oral preparation of magnesium chloride may be recommended, or magnesium-containing antacids that provide 400 mg/dose. Low magnesium levels may be linked to poor diabetes control, reduced release of insulin, and hypertension. The recommended daily allowance (RDA) is 280 mg for women and 350 mg for men.

Chromium has been linked to diabetes for years, but with very little supporting research. It has been reported that this mineral helps keep blood glucose stable and reduce triglycerides; however, the limited research data have been collected from population groups around the world that may already be chromium-deficient. The recommended intake level is about 50–200 μg/day. Food sources include brewer's yeast, calves liver, wheat germ, and American cheese.

Much attention has been given to the category of supplements known as antioxidants. These include vitamin E, vitamin C, and β-carotene. There does appear to be accumulating evidence that there may be some benefits to these supplements. Research with vitamin E has linked it to decreased cardiovascular disease risk, decreased HbA_{1c}, increased insulin sensitivity, and decreased vascular changes that may lead to complications, such as retinopathy. Although the RDA for vitamin E is between 8 and 10 α-tocopherol equivalents (TE) daily for adult women and men, respectively, the usual supplement dose of 100–400 α-TE/day does not appear to be associated with any risks or side effects. Food sources of vitamin E, which is fat-soluble, include nuts, wheat germ, green vegetables, and oils.

Certain population groups who are likely to have marginal nutritional intakes may also be candidates for supplementation of certain nutrients, such as persons on weight-control diets, vegetarians, elderly with poor intakes, and pregnant women.

C. Hypoglycemia: Prevention and Treatment

Several new products referred to as ''medical foods'' or nutriceuticals have entered the market. These foods are made from natural food ingredients, but claim to have a use for medical purposes. There are several snack bars, referred to as timed-release glucose bars, that are being marketed for hypoglycemia prevention. These foods contain a resistant starch, such as uncooked cornstarch, which some research shows may delay the absorption of food and thus may be useful in the prevention of nocturnal hypoglycemia. These bars are not to be used for treating hypoglycemia because of their somewhat delayed absorption time. They typically contain approximately 100–150 calories. There is not enough research at this time to say if these snack bars have definite benefits over a the traditional bedtime snack.

The more common problem with hypoglycemia treatment is the tendency to give too many calories and too much carbohydrate. Patients should be given clear guidelines to take only 15 g of carbohydrate, and if after rechecking blood glucose 15 min later levels have not risen above 70, take another 15 g. Glucose, found in commercial tablets and gels specifically designed to treat hypoglycemia, is the most rapidly absorbed form.

IV. SUMMARY

Maximizing the role of medical nutrition therapy in diabetes care involves much more than developing a nutrition prescription and giving a diet. The complex food behaviors that many patients need to modify often require the expertise of someone skilled in understanding behavioral change. Nutritional interventions must be carefully tailored to what the patient is able and willing to do and then be revised, based on how the patient progresses towards metabolic and behavioral goals. Despite the many changes in the specifics of medical nutrition therapy, diet composition, and meal planning, one thing that has not changed is the importance of teamwork and empowering the patient to take control. It is the person with diabetes who is in the driver's seat—not the physician or the diabetes educator. As Joslin wrote in 1935:

> I look upon the diabetic as the charioteer and his chariot as drawn by three steeds named Diet, Insulin and Exercise. It takes will to drive one horse, intelligence to manage a team of two, but a man must be a very good teamster who can get all three to pull together.

BIBLIOGRAPHY

(Also note in Table 5 the list of patient education resources)

American Diabetes Association. Nutrition recommendations and principles for people with diabetes mellitus (position statement). Diabetes Care 21(suppl 1):S32–S35, 1998.

Delahanty LM, Halford BN. The role of diet behaviors in achieving improved glycemic control in intensively treated patients in the Diabetes Control and Complications Trial. Diabetes Care 16:1453–1458, 1993.

Franz MJ. Micronutrients, glucose metabolism, metabolic control and supplements. Diabetes Spectr 11:70–78, 1998.

Franz MJ, Bantle J, eds. American Diabetes Association Guide to Medical Nutrition Therapy for Diabetes. Alexandria, VA: American Diabetes Association, 1999.

Franz MJ, Horton ES, Bantle JP, Beebe CA, Brunzell JD, Coulston AM, Henry RR, Hoogwerf BJ, Stacpoole PW. Nutrition principles for the management of diabetes and related complications. Diabetes Care 17:490–518, 1994.

Franz MJ, Monk A, Barry B, McClain K, Weaver T, Cooper N, Upham P, Bergenstal R, Mazze R. Effectiveness of medical nutrition therapy provided by dietitians in the management of non–insulin-dependent diabetes: a randomized, controlled clinical trial. J Am Diet Assoc 95:1009–1017, 1995.

Gillespie SJ, Kulkarni KD, Daly AE. Using carbohydrate counting in diabetes clinical practice. J Am Dietet Assoc 98:897–905, 1998.

Kulkarni K, Castle G, Gregory R, Holmes A, Leontos C, Powers M, Snetselaar S, Splett P, Wylie-Rosett J. Diabetes Care and Education Practice Group. Nutrition practice guidelines for type 1 diabetes mellitus positively affect dietitian practices and outcomes. J Am Diet Assoc 98:62–70, 1998.

Nutrition Practice Guidelines for Type 1 and Type 2 Diabetes Mellitus. Chicago, IL: American Dietetic Association, 1996.

Powers MA. Handbook of Diabetes Medical Nutrition Therapy. 2nd ed. Gaithersberg, MD: Aspen Publishers, 1996.

Ruggerio L, Prochaska JO, eds. Readiness for change, application of the transtheoretical model to diabetes. Diabetes Spectr 61:21–60, 1993.

Scope of practice for qualified dietetics professionals in diabetes care and education. J Am Diet Assoc 95:607–607, 1995.

16

Exercise Therapy in Diabetes

John T. Devlin
Maine Center for Diabetes, Maine Medical Center, Portland, Maine

I. INTRODUCTION

Physical exercise plays an important role in the lives of all of us, whether or not we have diabetes. Not only does it provide the opportunity for recreation and improved quality of life, it is also one of the most important lifestyle variables affecting our longevity. Epidemiological studies have documented the strong relation between levels of physical activity and reduced rates of cardiovascular mortality in both type 1 and type 2 diabetes. Because macrovascular disease is the major cause of mortality in these individuals, exercise therapy plays a pivotal role in their health and well-being.

Exercise presents special challenges that differ considerably between type 1 and type 2 diabetic individuals. For the person with type 1 diabetes, appropriate insulin adjustments to avoid metabolic decompensation during and after exercise is of paramount importance. Taking into consideration the numerous variables that have an influence on the diet–exercise–insulin triad often presents a daunting task, but one that can be approached with useful guidelines, as will be outlined subsequently. For the person with type 2 diabetes, or the high-risk individual who is trying to prevent diabetes, the challenge is often one of initiating and maintaining an active lifestyle over the long term. Although there is a large body of literature documenting the numerous benefits of physical activity in preventing and treating both impaired glucose tolerance (IGT) and type 2 diabetes, there is a dearth of information on effective means of motivating long-term behavioral changes.

II. BENEFITS OF PHYSICAL EXERCISE IN DIABETES

A. Cardiovascular Mortality

One of the major anticipated benefits of an active lifestyle is a reduction in cardiovascular mortality. Epidemiological studies from the University of Pittsburgh have found that sedentary individuals with type 1 diabetes have as much as a threefold increase in mortality compared with those who regularly engage in physical activity that expends more than 2000 kcal/week.

B. Prevention of Type 2 Diabetes

In addition to reducing cardiovascular risk in subjects with already-diagnosed type 2 diabetes, increased levels of physical activity decrease the incidence of IGT and type 2 diabetes. In the University of Pennsylvania Alumni Health Study, leisure-time physical activity was inversely related to the development of type 2 diabetes. For each 2000-kcal increment in weekly energy expenditure, the risk of type 2 diabetes was reduced by 24%. This protective effect of physical activity was strongest in individuals at highest risk for type 2 diabetes.

In a recently published prospective trial of the effects of lifestyle changes in men and women identified with IGT in Da Qing, China, an exercise program was associated with a 46% reduction in the risk of developing diabetes over a 6-year period of follow-up. This compares to a 31% reduction in risk in those on diet therapy.

Recent studies by Perseghin et al. have elucidated some of the mechanisms whereby physical exercise may improve glucose metabolism in high-risk individuals. Using ^{13}C and ^{31}P NMR spectroscopy, they studied the effects of exercise training in adult children of parents with type 2 diabetes. After 6 weeks of aerobic training, the reduced rates of muscle glycogen synthesis found in these subjects at baseline had been increased by 69%. This improvement was due to an increase in insulin-stimulated glucose transport and phosphorylation.

C. Visceral Fat Stores, Serum Lipids, and Blood Pressure

There is a strong association between increases in visceral, or abdominal, fat stores and vascular disease risk. This type of "central obesity" is associated with insulin resistance, impaired glucose tolerance, dyslipidemia, and hypertension. Exercise training results in preferential loss of fat stores from these central regions of the body. Even short-term (7 days) aerobic exercise improves insulin sensitivity in obese, insulin-resistant and hypertensive subjects. The crucial role of visceral fat stores in promoting this "metabolic syndrome" may be highlighted by Sumo wrestlers. These physically active, obese individuals have low visceral fat stores, and do not demonstrate either hyperglycemia or dyslipidemia, despite subcutaneous obesity.

Aerobic exercise training improves serum lipid levels and blood pressure. In one recent study in type 2 diabetic subjects, a 3-month exercise training program (50–70% maximal effort) reduced serum triglycerides by 20%, and increased high-density lipoprotein (HDL) by 23%. In addition, both systolic and diastolic blood pressures decreased by 8 mmHg. These effects occurred independently of changes in body weight and glycemic control.

D. Effects of Exercise Training on Glycemic Control

Early observations by Bjorntorp et al. showed that increasing levels of physical activity resulted in improved insulin sensitivity, as indicated by lower serum insulin concentrations during an oral glucose tolerance test (OGTT). Subsequent studies examining the effects of physical training in type 2 diabetic subjects demonstrated that glycemic control (hemoglobin A_{1c}; HbA_{1c}) was improved by physical training. Although there are adaptations in skeletal muscle in response to physical training, the major glycemic benefits of exercise appear to be the result of the cumulative effects of single bouts of exercise to deplete muscle glycogen stores and to improve insulin-mediated glucose utilization for up to 48 h after each exercise session. There appears to be rapid attenuation of any "training effect" on insulin-mediated glucose uptake, with disappearance of the training-induced improvements by 72 h of the last bout of exercise. Fortunately, restoration of enhanced insulin sensitivity has been demonstrated within 1 week of starting a physical training program in type 2 diabetic subjects.

Although early studies have focused on the benefits of aerobic training, several recent reports have documented the benefits of circuit weight training. Strength training improved glucose tolerance to an extent comparable with aerobic training in subjects with type 2 diabetes or impaired glucose tolerance. The mechanisms appear to differ between the two types of physical training, with aerobic training increasing insulin-mediated glucose utilization per unit skeletal muscle mass, and weight training resulting in increased total muscle volume with largely unchanged insulin sensitivity per unit muscle mass.

Physical training has generally not resulted in improved glycemic control in type 1 diabetic subjects. Although insulin sensitivity may be increased, and other cardiovascular risk factors may be improved by physical training, these individuals generally must either increase their caloric intake or reduce their insulin does to accommodate the increase in physical activity. Exercise should certainly be encouraged in type 1 diabetic individuals, and appropriate advice given to prevent metabolic decompensation (Table 1), but improved glycemic control (i.e., lowering of HbA_{1c}) is not one of the anticipated benefits for most individuals.

III. RISKS OF EXERCISE IN DIABETES

A. Hypoglycemia

Since the early observations of Lawrence in the dawn of the insulin era, it has been well recognized that exercise potentiates the hypoglycemic action of insulin.

Table 1 Benefits of Exercise in Diabetes

Reduced cardiovascular mortality
Prevention of diabetes in high-risk groups
Improved insulin sensitivity
Improved glycemic control (in type 2 diabetes)
Improved lipid profile (reduced triglycerides and increased HDL-C)
Lowered blood pressure
Improved fibrinolysis
Potentiation of weight loss during hypocaloric dieting
Improved quality-of-life and self-efficacy

Exercise-induced hypoglycemia is a particular risk in insulin-treated subjects, although it may occur in those taking oral hypoglycemic agents. Although increased glucose utilization by exercising muscle is partly responsible, the major contributor is the failure of the normal suppression of insulin secretion and increased hepatic glucose production that occurs under sympathetic nervous system regulation during exercise in nondiabetic subjects. Strategies that mimic the normal exercise-induced suppression of insulin concentrations are needed to prevent hypoglycemia during and after exercise (see Table 2).

Studies by Schiffrin et al. have shown that a 33–50% reduction in dosage of the short-acting insulin preparation, which peaks during moderate-intensity aerobic exercise, is sufficient to prevent hypoglycemia and avoid hyperglycemia. This was reported to be the appropriate reduction in dosage of regular insulin

Table 2 Strategies to Avoid Exercise-Induced Hypoglycemia

Measure capillary blood glucose before, during, and after exercise.
For planned exercise, reduce the dose of short-acting insulin that is peaking during, and after, the exercise by 33–50% or more, depending on the individual's exercise routine and response.
For unplanned exercise, take additional carbohydrates (20–30 g for each 30 min of exercise) before starting the exercise; insulin doses may need to be reduced after exercise.
Avoid injecting insulin in an exercising limb if the exercise takes place within 30–60 min of the time of injection; take special care to avoid the inadvertent injection of insulin into skeletal muscle before exercise (this may require avoiding the thigh in certain individuals, or using a shorter needle).
If exercise takes place in the late afternoon or evening, make appropriate reductions in evening insulin doses; a larger bedtime snack including carbohydrate and protein should be taken.

for subjects on both multiple daily injections (MDI) of insulin, and in those using the continuous subcutaneous insulin infusion (CSII) pump method for attaining intensive management of type 1 diabetes. In the absence of specific data on the appropriate reductions in dosage of the insulin analogue lispro (Humalog) for planned exercise, similar reductions in the "peaking" dose of Humalog (33–50%) seem appropriate.

The greatest risk for hypoglycemia occurs when exercise is performed during the peak action of the insulin preparation. It is not surprising that hypoglycemia is approximately twice as likely to occur with lispro than with regular human insulin when exercise is conducted 40 min after injection, and twice as likely with regular than with lispro insulin when the exercise occurs 180 min after the injection.

It had formerly been thought that hypoglycemia was more likely to occur if short-acting insulin was injected into an exercising limb (e.g., into the thigh before running), although this has subsequently been shown to be a factor only if the exercise occurs within 30–60 min of the time of insulin injection. Probably more important clinically is the inadvertent injection of insulin into skeletal muscle. Studies using computed tomography (CT) scans suggest that this may be a common occurrence, especially in those individuals with decreased subcutaneous adipose tissue stores in the thigh region. Rates of insulin absorption after intramuscular injection are more than doubled when moderate-intensity cycle exercise takes place within 60–100 min of the time of injection, whereas the rate of absorption is not significantly altered by exercise after subcutaneous injection.

Clinicians are only too aware of the frequent occurrence of hypoglycemia several hours after the completion of exercise, with the most dramatic effects occurring during the night. MacDonald has reported its occurrence in 16% of adolescents followed over a 2-year period, with severe hypoglycemia (resulting in unconsciousness or seizures or requiring glucagon treatment) occurring in two-thirds of the cases. Most often the hypoglycemic event occurred during the night, 6–15 h after strenuous exercise that ended in the late afternoon or evening.

An insulin pump offers several advantages to type 1 diabetic individuals who are involved in vigorous sport activities. These include (a) the ability to use a temporary basal rate that delivers a constant low rate of insulin infusion (in 0.1-U/h increments), allowing the normal increase in hepatic glucose production during exercise; (b) the use of a single infusion site which is more likely to deliver insulin into the intended, subcutaneous tissue layer; (c) the absence of a large subcutaneous insulin reservoir, allows more rapid correction of hypoglycemia, should it occur; (d) the freedom from multiple insulin injections that would be required for an extended outing, such as hiking; and (e) the ability to place the pump in a waterproof housing while swimming. Potential disadvantages of the pump include the risk of needle dislodgment during vigorous activity, and the tendency to develop more rapid ketosis if insulin delivery is interrupted.

B. Metabolic Decompensation: Hyperglycemia and Ketosis

Two studies in the late 1970s demonstrated an exaggeration of ketosis, and an inability to lower plasma glucose concentrations, during exercise in insulin-withdrawn, hyperglycemic type 1 diabetic subjects. The proposed mechanism for this observation was the exercise-induced increases in counterregulatory hormone concentrations in the presence of severe insulinopenia. For this reason, insulin-deficient diabetic subjects are advised to test their urinary ketones before exercise whenever plasma glucose concentrations are higher than 250 mg/dL and, if ketonuria is present, avoid exercise until they are under improved glycemic control. Nonketosis prone, type 2 diabetic subjects may be able to exercise in the presence of hyperglycemia, but should also use caution if glucose level is higher than 300 mg/dL.

At times a patient will note a paradoxic increase in their blood glucose levels after exercise, even when they have been in good glycemic control. Sigal and colleagues have provided one mechanism that may explain this phenomenon in certain cases. During brief, very intense exercise ($> 90\%$ Vo_{2max}) the large increases in sympathetic nervous system activity, and plasma catecholamine concentrations, produce an abrupt increase in hepatic glucose production rates, before the exercising muscle is able to increase its uptake of glucose to match the increase in supply. This response might be seen in sprinters or other athletes engaging in brief bursts of near-maximal effort. Because the hyperglycemic effect is transient, and efforts to blunt the response may result in delayed hypoglycemia, one needs to be cautious about overaggressive attempts to prevent its occurrence.

C. Risks of Exercise in Those with Microvascular Complications

Diabetic subjects have unique risks when they exercise in the presence of the microvascular complications of diabetes. For a more thorough review of the recommended evaluation and appropriate restrictions on physical activity in those with complications, see the respective chapters in Ruderman and Devlin, *The Health Professional's Guide to Diabetes and Exercise.*

Those with diabetic retinopathy may need to limit the type and intensity of exercise, depending on their degree of retinopathy. If there is no retinopathy, or only mild nonproliferative diabetic retinopathy (NPDR), no limitations need be imposed. In the presence of moderate NPDR or more advanced stages of retinopathy, certain activities should be avoided to minimize the risk of hemorrhage. These activities include types of exercise that significantly elevate blood pressure, and those that result in a Valsalva maneuver, such as heavy weight lifting. Activities that result in head jarring, such as diving or boxing, should also be avoided with more advanced degrees of diabetic retinopathy.

Brief exercise increases rates of urinary albumin excretion, with the increase being proportional to elevations in blood pressure. However, no data are available that would indicate an increased risk for either the development or progression of early diabetic nephropathy owing to increased physical activity. Epidemiological data have not shown an increased prevalence of nephropathy in physically active diabetic individuals. Nevertheless, it is prudent to avoid strenuous exercise in the presence of significant nephropathy to prevent significant exercise-induced elevations in blood pressure.

If peripheral sensory testing (using a 10-g Semmes-Weinstein monofilament) demonstrates decreased or absent plantar sensation, running and other exercises resulting in foot pounding should be avoided. A list of recommended exercises includes swimming, cycling, rowing, and non–weight-bearing exercises.

Autonomic neuropathy presents special challenges for exercise. The presence of orthostatic hypotension usually indicates the need to avoid all but the mildest forms of exercise, to prevent significant hypotension, resulting from volume depletion and vasodilation in exercising muscles. Prevention of dehydration in hot weather needs to be emphasized. Cardiac autonomic neuropathy (CAN) may be indicated by the presence of resting tachycardia (caused by earlier involvement of the parasympathetic, versus the sympathetic, innervation) and absence of heart rate variation during a bedside Valsalva maneuver. If CAN is present, the heart rate response to exercise will be an unreliable indicator of the workload. In this setting, the Borg scale may be used to provide an appropriate workload target. This scale is also appropriate for individuals taking drugs such as β-adrenergic blockers, and in the elderly, in whom the heart rate response to exercise may be blunted. For aerobic training, workloads resulting in a Borg scale rating of 12–13 (''somewhat hard'') are appropriate. Because individuals with CAN may have ''silent'' coronary ischemia, from cardiac denervation, exercise stress testing is recommended before starting a new training program (Table 3). In

Table 3 The Borg Perceived Exertion Scale

Rating of perceived exertion (RPE)	Verbal description of RPE
7	Very, very light
9	Very light
11	Fairly light
13	Somewhat hard
15	Hard
17	Very hard
19	Very, very hard

Source: Borg, 1982.

Table 4   Indications for Cardiac Testing in Diabetic Individuals

Testing for CAD is warranted in patients with the following:
1. Typical or atypical cardiac symptoms
2. Resting ECG suggestive of ischemia or infarction
3. Peripheral or carotid occlusive arterial disease
4. Sedentary lifestyle, age ≥ 35 years, and plans to begin a vigorous exercise program
5. Two or more of the following risk factors in addition to diabetes
    a. Total cholesterol ≥ 240 mg/dL, LDL-C ≥ 160 mg/dL, or HDL-C ≤ 35 mg/dL
    b. Blood pressure > 140/90
    c. Smoking
    d. Family history of premature CAD
    e. Positive micro/macroalbuminuria test

addition to evaluating for possible coronary ischemia, the exercise test can be used to select an appropriate workload for the individual.

A careful medical history and physical examination, focusing on the symptoms and signs of macrovascular disease, need to be performed before the start of a new exercise program. From a recent Consensus Development Conference on the Diagnosis of Coronary Heart Disease in People With Diabetes, the American Diabetes Association has published recommendations for exercise stress testing in diabetic patients (Table 4).

The Consensus Development Conference stated that the "initiation of a graded walking exercise program can be accomplished without additional cardiac testing."

IV. THE EXERCISE PRESCRIPTION

Before embarking on a new exercise regimen, a thorough medical history and physical examination need to be done, with particular attention to the presence of the microvascular and macrovascular complications of diabetes. Discussion of appropriate types of exercise, with recommendations on the frequency, duration, and intensity of exercise sessions, can be made with the patient's preferences and goals in mind. Strategies to increase the likelihood of long-term adherence to the training program will need to consider the availability and cost of any specialized equipment or fitness center, and whether the patient is interested in exercising with their spouse or other individuals. There are advantages to providing more than one exercise option, to allow for changing weather and seasons, and to provide some variation and avoid "burnout" with one exercise routine.

Making use of local expertise, including physical therapists and exercise physiologists, is also important.

Table 5 shows the energy expenditure associated with various types of physical activity. This should be taken as a rough guide, with the possibility of wide interindividual variation. The estimate of caloric expenditure may be used

Table 5 Energy Expenditure Associated with Common Exercises

Activity	Calories burned per minute	Calories burned per hour
Light housework	2–2½	120–150
Polishing furniture		
Light handwashing		
Golf, using power cart	2½–4	150–240
Level walking 2 mph		
Cleaning windows, mopping or vacuuming	4–5	240–300
Golf, pulling cart		
Cycling 6 mph		
Bowling		
Scrubbing floors	5–6	300–360
Cycling 8 mph		
Walking 3½ mph		
Table tennis, badminton, and volleyball		
Doubles tennis		
Golf, carrying clubs		
Many calisthenics and ballet exercises		
Walking 4 mph	6–7	360–420
Ice or roller skating		
Cycling 10 mph		
Walking 5 mph	7–8	420–480
Cycling 11 mph		
Water skiing		
Singles tennis		
Jogging 5 mph	8–10	480–600
Cycling 12 mph		
Downhill skiing		
Paddleball		
Running 5 ½ mph	10–11	600–660
Cycling 13 mph		
Squash or handball (practice session)		
Running 6 mph or more	11 or more	660 or more
Competitive handball or squash		

Source: ADA, 1988.

to guide the carbohydrate requirement to prevent hypoglycemia during unplanned exercise, when insulin doses have not been decreased. Because approximately 50% of the calories burned come from carbohydrate sources during moderate-intensity exercise (with most of the remainder coming from fat sources), a rough estimate may be made as follows: for a 30-min exercise session, resulting in an excess caloric expenditure of 10 kcal/min above basal, the individual should ingest about 38 g of carbohydrate (50% $\times$ 300 kcal = 150 kcal, or 37.5 g of carbohydrate). Because much of the carbohydrate source for oxidation during exercise comes from endogenous glycogen stores, these must be taken as crude estimates.

Those who wish to begin an aerobic training program should begin slowly and allow sufficient time for a gradual buildup to the desired training level. After 8–12 weeks of adaptation, an appropriate exercise routine would include, at a minimum, 20–30 min of exercise at the target heart rate, 3–4 days/week. An estimate of the individual's age-predicted maximal heart rate is:

Age-predicted maximal heart rate = 220 − age (yr).

One way to estimate an appropriate aerobic training workload, in the absence of a treadmill exercise test, is to use the maximal heart rate reserve (max HRR) method. The max HRR is calculated as a percentage above the resting heart rate, based on the age-predicted maximal heart rate, as follows:

Max HRR = (age-predicted max heart rate) − (resting HR)

To achieve aerobic conditioning, one should try to maintain an exercise heart rate at 60–70% of the maximal heart rate reserve. As an example, a 45-year-old patient with a resting heart rate of 75 would have the following heart rate target:

Age-predicted max HR = 220 − 45 = 175
Max HRR = 175 − 75 = 100
Target (60–70% max HRR above resting) = (60–70% $\times$ 100) + 75 = 135–145.

Consideration of the possible presence of coronary artery disease needs to be given before embarking on a new exercise-training program, and cardiac stress testing performed following the guidelines outlined in Table 4. To minimize the potential for injury and to increase safety, each exercise session should be preceded with a 10- to 15-min period of stretching and warmup, and followed by a 10- to 15-min cooldown period.

V. GENERAL GUIDELINES FOR SAFE EXERCISE

The American Diabetes Association has made the following recommendations for safe exercise in all patients with diabetes:

Carry an identification card and wear a bracelet at all times that identifies one as having diabetes

Be alert for signs of hypoglycemia during and for several hours after exercise

Have immediate access to a source of readily available carbohydrate (such as glucose tablets) to treat hypoglycemia

Take sufficient fluids before, after, and if necessary, during exercise to prevent dehydration

Measure blood glucose, and take appropriate action if the reading is < 80 mg/dL or > 240 mg/dL.

VI. RESOURCES FOR THE DIABETIC INDIVIDUAL

Those interested in learning more about diabetes and exercise are referred to the following sources for additional information:

American Diabetes Association Council on Exercise; American Diabetes Association, Inc. 1660 Duke Street, Alexandria, VA 23314 (http//www.diabetes.org)

International Diabetic Athletes Association, 1647 West Bethany Home Road No. B Phoenix, AZ 85015-2507 Tel: 602-433-2113; Fax: 602-433-9331 (annual membership: $15.00; $20.00 outside the United States)

BIBLIOGRAPHY

American Diabetes Association (ADA). Physicians Guide to Non–Insulin-Dependent (Type 2) Diabetes (ADA Clinical Education Program). 2nd ed. ADA, 1988:36.

Borg GA. Psychophysical basis of perceived exertion. Med Sci Sports Exerc 14:377–387, 1982.

Consensus Development Conference on the Diagnosis of Coronary Heart Disease in People With Diabetes, American Diabetes Association. Diabetes Care 21:1551–1559, 1998.

Da Qing IGT and Diabetes Study. Effects of diet and exercise in preventing NIDDM in people with impaired glucose tolerance. Diabetes Care 20:537–544, 1997.

Devlin JT. Exercise in type 1 diabetes. Pract Diabetol 17:12–16, 1998.

MacDonald MJ. Postexercise late-onset hypoglycemia in insulin-dependent diabetic patients. Diabetes Care 10:584–588, 1987.

Perseghin G, Price TB, Petersen KF, Roden M, Cline GW, Gerow K, Rothman DL, Shulman GI. Increased glucose transport–phosphorylation and muscle glycogen synthesis after exercise training in insulin-resistant subjects. N Engl J Med 335: 1357–1362, 1996.

Position Statement: Diabetes Mellitus and Exercise, American Diabetes Association: Clinical Practice Recommendations 1998. Diabetes Care 21(suppl 1):S40–S44, 1998.

Ruderman N, Devlin JT, ed. The Health Professional's Guide to Diabetes and Exercise. Alexandria, VA: American Diabetes Association, 1995.

Schiffrin A, Parikh S. Accommodating planned exercise in type 1 diabetic individuals on intensive treatment. Diabetes Care 8:337–342, 1985.

Sigal RJ, Purdon C, Fisher SJ, et al. Hyperinsulinemia prevents prolonged hyperglycemia after intense exercise in insulin-dependent diabetic subjects. J Clin Endocrinol Metab 79:1049–1057, 1994.

17
Oral Pharmacological Agents

Andrew J. Ahmann and Matthew C. Riddle
Oregon Health Sciences University, Portland, Oregon

I. INTRODUCTION

In recent years oral agent therapy of diabetes has seen more therapeutic advancement than any other aspect of diabetes management. Because there are no oral agents available for treating type 1 diabetes, this topic clearly centers on the therapeutics of type 2 diabetes mellitus. A better understanding of the pathophysiology of type 2 diabetes, combined with the emergence of new agents having different pharmacological and pharmacokinetic profiles, have revolutionized the therapy of this increasingly common chronic disease. We see the opportunity for improved glucose control, reduced side effects, enhanced patient acceptance, and ultimately, reduced morbidity and mortality. However, with these new tools and the associated therapeutic options comes a new challenge for safe, effective, and cost-appropriate use by clinicians.

The significant progress over the past 5 years in development and clinical implementation of oral agents for treating type 2 diabetes comes at a propitious time. Many studies have now established the importance of blood glucose control as the central determinant in reducing the chronic complications of type 2 diabetes. Consequently, these agents have the potential to improve quality of life at a modest cost, compared with the costly outlay for managing those complications.

The reputation of oral agents as primary therapy for treating type 2 diabetes was tarnished by the 1970 report of the University Group Diabetes Program (UGDP) that suggested increased cardiovascular events in patients treated with the agents available at that time. Although these conclusions were highly controversial owing to a variety of potential flaws in the study design, the UGDP has caused concern, even to the present. The package insert for sulfonylureas continues to highlight this potential adverse effect. Furthermore, the direct causative association between hyperglycemia and the chronic complications of diabetes remained somewhat in question until the publication of the Diabetes Control and Complication Trial (DCCT), in 1993. This landmark study clearly demonstrated that intensive management of type 1 diabetes, resulting in an average 2% reduction in glycosylated hemoglobin (HbA$_{1c}$), yielded a 50–75% reduction in chronic complications over a mean 6-year follow-up. Although this study was performed in adults with type 1 diabetes, there was every expectation that results were relevant to microvascular complications in those with type 2 diabetes as well.

Reports from the Wisconsin Epidemiologic Study of Diabetic Retinopathy (WESDR) also showed a strong relation between HbA$_{1c}$ levels and complications in those with type 2 diabetes. Subsequently, a prospective study of insulin therapy in type 2 diabetes in Japan supported the conclusions of the DCCT with almost identical results from a very similar design. Finally, the recently reported results of the United Kingdom Prospective Diabetes Study (UKPDS) demonstrated the ability of oral agent or insulin therapy to safely reduce the progression of hyperglycemia and reduce complications.

There can now be no doubt that reducing blood glucose levels in patients with type 2 diabetes is advantageous. The general goal of therapy is to reduce the average glucose to a level near normal without causing excessive hypoglycemia. Although diet modification and exercise are important and indicated as the first interventions in this disease, they produce very limited long-term success in maintaining the desired level of glucose control. Consequently, pharmacological agents are necessary. Because insulin therapy has not been well accepted by patients or clinicians in the routine treatment of type 2 diabetes, the emphasis in treating this disease rests on effective use of oral agents.

As discussed elsewhere, the pathogenesis of type 2 diabetes is complex and our understanding of this process in individual patients continues to evolve. However, the three abnormalities that are typically seen include insulin resistance in muscle, increased endogenous glucose production (primarily from the liver), and beta-cell dysfunction. The increased hepatic glucose production (HGP) can also be considered a form of insulin resistance because insulin is a primary regulator of this process. This defect is largely responsible for fasting hyperglycemia in patients with type 2 diabetes. The beta-cell defect is evident first as loss of first-phase insulin release and, ultimately, as an overall reduction of insulin response to an oral glucose load. This defect initially contributes to postprandial hyperglycemia, and is progressive over time.

Blood glucose levels are ultimately determined by food intake, insulin supply, endogenous glucose production (HGP), and insulin-mediated glucose uptake into tissues, primarily the muscle. Accordingly, the development of pharmacological agents for treating type 2 diabetes has targeted these areas. Alternatively, one may divide available agents into two categories: those augmenting the supply of insulin, and those enhancing the effect of available insulin. Sulfonylureas and repaglinide enhance endogenous insulin secretion. All other oral agents contribute to improved effectiveness of endogenous or exogenous insulin. Metformin reduces primarily hepatic glucose production, although it may also have some limited benefit in increasing insulin sensitivity in the muscle. Troglitazone has its primary effect by improving insulin-mediated glucose uptake into muscle. The fifth oral agent, acarbose, delays the absorption of glucose from the small intestine, thereby reducing the requirement for immediate insulin secretion following a meal. Because weight loss medications reduce caloric intake and also improve insulin sensitivity through weight loss, they could also be considered in the category of agents improving insulin effectiveness. However, the few agents available in this treatment area have not been studied extensively in patients with diabetes, and no approved indications exist for their use in such patients. Therefore, the scope of this discussion will be restricted to those agents specifically approved for treatment of type 2 diabetes.

II. PRINCIPLES GUIDING TREATMENT WITH ORAL AGENTS

In simplest terms, the goal of any therapy for diabetes is avoidance of chronic complications. Because the relation between the mean glucose level and the occurrence of microvascular complications is essentially linear, the ultimate goal is the lowest glucose average that avoids problematic hypoglycemia. Although data are not as well-developed, improved blood glucose control also is likely to have beneficial effects on macrovascular disease. This benefit is proportionally less than that seen for microvascular complications and may eventually be shown to vary according to type of agent used.

In general, the occurrence of hypoglycemia in patients with type 2 diabetes is less frequent than that seen in treating type 1 diabetes. Factors such as other side effects, cost, age, physical disabilities, cardiac disease or other comorbidities, lifestyle, and patient compliance with monitoring will also affect the final glucose goals determined by the patient and provider. In numeric terms, the most often cited "ideal" goals of therapy include a fasting glucose level (FGL) less than 120 mg/dL and an HbA_{1c} of 7% (or 1% above the upper normal). "Acceptable" levels, as defined by the American Diabetes Association (ADA) and others are 140 mg/dL and 8% for the fasting glucose and HbA_{1c}, respectively. The 8% level is often quoted as the recommended "change point" for therapy, representing the level of control at which a change in therapeutic approach is necessary. However, initial therapy with oral agents is probably indicated at lower levels, such as HbA_{1c} of 7% or an FGL higher than 126 mg/dL, after an initial trial of lifestyle interventions emphasizing improved diet and exercise.

The potential benefit of identifying and treating patients with impaired glucose tolerance (IGT) to reduce the occurrence of macrovascular complications and delay progression to overt diabetes is intriguing. The Diabetes Prevention Program (DPP) is studying this issue, comparing lifestyle changes and metformin treatment with observation alone. Although troglitazone was removed from this trial owing to a patient death associated with hepatotoxicity, another study is forthcoming to investigate the use of this promising class of drugs in impaired glucose tolerance. At this time, pharmacological treatment of IGT is not considered standard care. Should these studies demonstrate a distinct advantage for early treatment, it is likely that pharmacological agents that improve insulin sensitivity and avoid hypoglycemia will also be implemented at lower glucose levels in those already carrying the diagnosis of diabetes.

Nearly all individuals are candidates for oral therapy of type 2 diabetes. In cases of severe liver disease or end-stage renal disease, insulin may be the preferred therapy until the underlying illness is resolved. Oral agents are contraindicated during pregnancy owing to lack of safety data. Similarly, the expanding group of children or adolescents with a diagnosis of type 2 diabetes has not been adequately studied for efficacy and safety of the various agents approved for treating adults. It is becoming common to treat these individuals using oral medications with which we have the most experience; namely, sulfonylureas or metformin.

Another problem of growing interest is the appropriate diagnosis and treatment of normal-weight hyperglycemic adults who may not have typical type 2 diabetes. Some of these individuals may have latent autoimmune diabetes of adults (LADA). Preliminary reports indicate that early treatment with insulin may help preserve beta-cell function in such cases. It has also been suggested that treatment with insulin secretagogues, such as sulfonylureas, may promote the autoimmune process by enhancing antigen presentation on the surface of cells. At this point the differential diagnosis of this group of patients relies mainly on clinical criteria that appear to be about 90% reliable. Experience with antibodies, such as antiglutamic acid decarboxylase (anti-GAD) and islet cell antibodies (ICAs), may lead to improved identification and treatment of these patients.

Finally, the degree of hyperglycemia at diagnosis may also create some uncertainty in initial therapy of type 2 diabetes. In some situations, such as delayed diagnosis or intercurrent physiological stress, patients may present with severe, symptomatic hyperglycemia. This is likely because of glucotoxicity (the reversible adverse effect of hyperglycemia on insulin sensitivity and insulin secretion), or the elevation of counterregulatory hormones (resulting in increased HGP and increased insulin resistance). Although at least one recent report has indicated sulfonylureas can effectively treat patients presenting with symptomatic glucose levels higher than 400 mg/dL, the general consensus has been to treat such patients initially with insulin. Not infrequently, however, these patients are unnecessarily left on the insulin therapy regimen indefinitely when oral agents are likely to be effective after a period of stabilization.

III. REVIEW OF ORAL AGENTS APPROVED FOR INITIAL THERAPY

A. Sulfonylureas

Sulfonylureas represent the oldest class of oral agents. The U.S. Food and Drug Administration (FDA) in 1957 first approved tolbutamide. By the mid-1960s there were four agents approved in the United States. Six different sulfonylureas are now available in the United States, two of which are also available in modified dosage forms (micronized glyburide and extended-release glipizide).

Sulfonylureas bind to the ATP-dependent potassium channel on the beta-cell, augmenting the effect of glucose to depolarize the cell membrane. This depolarization opens calcium channels, resulting in insulin secretion. Most sulfonylureas bind to a 140-kDa protein at the potassium channel. Glimepiride binds to a 65-kDa protein at the same site. There is no clear difference in effects attributed to these differences in binding. Although extrapancreatic effects have been attributed to sulfonylurea treatment, these apparent improvements in insulin sensitivity are likely the indirect effect of reduced glucotoxicity, rather than a direct effect of the agents.

Most sulfonylureas are metabolized in the liver and excreted through the kidney. Thus, this group of agents in usually contraindicated in progressive renal failure. Glipizide may have an advantage in renal insufficiency because it metabolites are inactive. Glimepiride also provides an advantage in this setting because its only active metabolite can be cleared by the liver. Because they are metabolized in the liver, sulfonylureas are also to be avoided in patients with significant liver dysfunction. Sulfonylureas are all highly bound to plasma proteins, but only the older first-generation agents are ionically bound, resulting in propensity for drug interactions. Competition for protein binding may be a problem during concurrent use of common drugs, including nonsteroidal anti-inflammatory agents, warfarin (Coumadin), salicylates, and β-adrenergic blockers. The reduced drug interactions characteristic of nonionically bound second-generation agents may also relate to their higher potency. However, greater potency does not render second-generation agents more effective, as all sulfonylureas are essentially equally effective in reducing hyperglycemia.

Most studies have demonstrated a 1.5–2.0% reduction in HbA_{1c} in sulfonylurea-treated patients on initial therapy. Approximately 20–30% of patients will experience inadequate response. This constitutes the group with "primary failure." Of the 70% with good initial results, 5–10%/year will go on to "secondary failure." Dose–response studies consistently show that most of the glucose-lowering potential is seen at 25–50% of the recommended maximum dose for all sulfonylureas. Few patients experience significant improvement when doses are increased beyond the 50% level. Food has some limited effect on absorption of sulfonylureas. Other than the extended-release form of glipizide, these agents are optimally taken 30 min before meals.

Sulfonylureas are the least expensive group of oral agents. Although most are available generically, even the branded once-daily forms, Glucotrol XL (extended-release glipizide) and Amaryl (glimepiride), are very reasonably priced, far less than other classes of oral agents. The primary side effect of sulfonylureas is hypoglycemia. This acute complication of therapy is most pronounced on initial therapy and can be a particular problem in elderly patients. Therefore, initiation of therapy requires small doses with frequent monitoring of blood glucose values in thin or elderly patients and in those with mild hyperglycemia. Because of the increased risk of hypoglycemia, patients must be cautioned about skipping or delaying meals or consuming alcohol. Although there was an association between increased hypoglycemic events and duration of action for earlier long-acting agents, glimepiride and Glucotrol XL have not shown this propensity.

The specter of cardiovascular toxicity has followed sulfonylurea therapy since the UGDP, despite several subsequent studies with contradictory findings. That benefit exceeds any cardiovascular risk can no longer be questioned based on the findings of the UKPDS during which sulfonylureas clearly reduced chronic complications without increasing cardiovascular events after 10 years of therapy. In fact, there was a statistically insignificant reduction in myocardial infarction in this relatively large group of sulfonylurea-treated patients. Nevertheless, one cannot exclude the possibility that a negative effect of sulfonylureas on vascular reactivity is overshadowed by the beneficial effects of glucose lowering. Given preliminary findings of different responses in such models as the diazoxide-induced forearm vasodilation, it has been proposed that glimepiride has potential cardiovascular advantages over glyburide and possibly other sulfonylureas. These are unsubstantiated claims at this point and probably play no role in agent selection.

Sulfonylureas are contraindicated in patients with sulfa allergies. Their use is associated with weight gain when patients experience significant improvement in blood glucose control. Other rare adverse effects include rashes, nausea, indigestion, and occasional abnormalities of liver enzymes. Chlorpropamide alone precipitates flush reactions with alcohol and can cause hyponatremia. Fewer than 2% of treated patients discontinue sulfonylurea therapy because of adverse events.

B. Meglitinides

Repaglinide is the first drug in a new class of insulin secretagogues representing a group of benzoic acid derivatives referred to as meglitinides. Repaglinide (Prandin) was newly approved in 1998, indicated for initial therapy and combination therapy with metformin. This agent has greatest affinity for binding to a site on the ATP-sensitive potassium channel receptor of the beta cell, separate from the site occupied with high affinity by sulfonylureas. Similarly, it stimulates glucose-mediated insulin secretion. However, it reportedly differs from sulfonylureas in its lack of inhibition of proinsulin biosynthesis and its lack of effect on insulin exocytosis.

Its greatest distinction comes from its pharmacokinetics. It is completely and rapidly absorbed. It has a rapid onset of action and a short half-life (1 h). Consequently, repaglinide has its dominant effect on postprandial glucose and a lesser effect on fasting blood glucose. An inherent advantage comes from the temporal relation of dosing and action with meal consumption. The drug is intended to be taken from 0 to 30 min before meals. If a meal is missed, repaglinide is not taken. Doses begin at 0.5 mg with each meal for those with HbA_{1c} levels lower than 8.0%. There is a dose-dependent response. Initial doses of 1–2 mg before meals are recommended for those with higher blood glucose levels. Maximum recommended doses are 4 mg before meals.

The liver is the single site of repaglinide metabolism and the primary site of excretion of its inactive metabolites. Thus, it should be used cautiously in the setting of significant liver dysfunction. Although it may be safe for treatment of those with renal failure, caution is advised until specific safety studies are available for these patients. No drug interactions have been noted with such common drugs as warfarin, digoxin, or cimetidine. However, repaglinide is metabolized by the cytochrome P-450 3A4 enzyme system and it may be affected by drugs that affect this system. Accordingly, metabolism is inhibited by ketoconazole and erthromycin and may be increased by agents inducing the enzyme system.

Available studies demonstrate effectiveness equivalent to that of sulfonylureas with HbA_{1c} reductions of 1.7–2.1%, compared with placebo groups. In head-to-head comparisons with various sulfonylureas, repaglinide showed equal efficacy relative to glyburide, gliclazide, and glipizide. Initial response rates are apparently similar to those of sulfonylureas. Secondary failure rates will not be available until the agent has a longer history, but they are also likely to be similar to rates seen with sulfonylureas.

The most common adverse effect experienced with repaglinide therapy is hypoglycemia, which occurs with a frequency comparable with that of sulfonylureas in routine controlled trials. In studies looking at the effect of missed meals, less hypoglycemia occurs when repaglinide is administered only when meals are consumed. Potential advantages in reduction of nocturnal or exercise-related hypoglycemia with repaglinide therapy have not been adequately studied. Weight gain on repaglinide therapy is probably no different from that seen with sulfonylureas. Other adverse effects appear to be rare. Because the drug is not sulfa-based, it should be safe for patients with a sulfa allergy. Cardiovascular toxicity has not been evident, but this has not been carefully evaluated in any large, long-term study.

C. Biguanides

Biguanides have been used in Europe since the 1950s. Phenformin was approved by the FDA in 1959 for treatment of type 2 diabetes. However, it was withdrawn from the market in the 1970s owing to its association with lactic acidosis. The other biguanide agent, metformin, continued to be available in several European countries for many years before its approval in the United States in 1995.

Metformin's mechanism of action remains somewhat unclear, despite 40 years of clinical use. Recent studies would suggest the primary benefit relates to reduction in hepatic glucose production, with a lesser and possibly indirect effect on insulin-mediated glucose uptake in muscle tissue. There may be a mild, poorly defined effect on glucose absorption as well. Insulin secretion is often reduced with metformin therapy as glucose levels decline. Therefore, hypoglycemia does not occur as a consequence of treatment with metformin alone. Metformin is cleared unmodified through the kidney and is contraindicated in renal insufficiency (serum creatinine > 1.3 in females or 1.4 in males). Minor, questionably significant drug interactions have been reported with furosemide and nifedipine. Cimetidine increases metformin levels and other cationic drugs, such as digoxin or triamterene, may also compete with metformin for renal tubular secretion.

Direct comparative studies have shown metformin's efficacy in monotherapy to be equivalent to that seen with sulfonylureas, both in terms of glucose reduction and frequency of adequate initial response. Likewise, despite its different mechanism of action, patients with secondary failure to sulfonylureas seldom respond well to substitution therapy with metformin. Recently, the UKPDS reported very good results with metformin in the long-term reduction of microvascular and macrovascular complications of type 2 diabetes in obese patients. On the surface, these benefits appeared to exceed those seen with sulfonylureas or insulin. However, in statistical comparison, improved outcomes were only significant when compared with the control group and not when compared with the patients treated with other agents. In addition to the avoidance of hypoglycemia during monotherapy, a second significant advantage to metformin therapy is the avoidance of weight gain. Some individuals will lose weight, a phenomenon seen even in nonobese patients. Finally, metformin also has a favorable effect on lipids, with mild reductions in low-density lipoprotein (LDL) and triglycerides.

The dose—response studies for metformin demonstrate benefit at doses as low as 500 mg/day, with progressive response to doses up to 2000 mg/day. Doses beyond 2000 mg/day, although safe and approved, render little additional benefit for most patients. Because of adverse gastrointestinal effects, doses are usually initiated at 500 mg once or twice daily, with increases as tolerated to 1000 mg twice daily with meals, if needed to accomplish blood glucose targets.

Lactic acidosis is a rare, but catastrophic, complication of metformin therapy. Its occurrence is much lower than phenformin-induced lactic acidosis. Most reported cases of lactic acidosis have occurred in patients having risk factors. For this reason, metformin is contraindicated in patients having renal insufficiency, congestive heart failure requiring pharmacological therapy, alcohol abuse, hepatic dysfunction, severe pulmonary disease, peripheral vascular disease, and acute illnesses potentially associated with hypotension and hypoperfusion. Patients receiving an intravenous radiographic dye load or having surgery should discontinue the metformin before the procedure and resume therapy only when a normal creatinine level is ascertained 48 h later. Lactic acid levels are not considered useful in monitoring for potential lactic acidosis in asymptomatic patients.

The most common metformin-induced adverse effects center on the gastrointestinal tract. Up to 30% of patients will experience nausea, abdominal bloating, abdominal cramping, or diarrhea. These symptoms are reduced somewhat by administration with food. Gastrointestinal symptoms are usually self-limited, but 5–10% of patients are unable to continue the drug long-term.

D. α-Glucosidase Inhibitors

Acarbose (Precose) and miglitol (Glyset) are the two α-glucosidase inhibitors presently marketed in the United States. This group of agents competitively inhibits α-glucosidase enzymes in the small intestine, including glucoamylase, sucrase, maltase, and isomaltase. Consequently, acarbose delays polysaccharide and disaccharide hydrolysis to absorbable monosaccharide (e.g., glucose) causing glucose absorption to occur over a greater portion of the bowel. The resultant glucose absorption curve is blunted, better allowing available insulin to dispose of the postprandial circulating glucose. These agents are minimally absorbed, but the absorbed drug is excreted through the kidneys. Therefore, use in severe renal insufficiency is not recommended. Drug interactions have not been a problem. To avoid side effects, miglitol and acarbose should be started at low doses and slowly increased over 6–8 weeks.

This group of agents appears to be modestly effective in treating diabetes. Postprandial glucose elevations are significantly reduced, but there is minimal effect on fasting glucose levels. Typically, studies have shown HbA_{1c} reductions of 0.5–0.9%. The degree of benefit correlates with relative carbohydrate content of the diet. Those persons eating diets with high carbohydrate content (e.g., >50% of daily calories) are likely to see the greatest reductions in HbA_{1c}.

The primary adverse effects associated with acarbose or miglitol therapy stem from the delivery of carbohydrates to the colon where a fermentation process produces gas. As many as 70% of patients will report flatulence. Abdominal pain and diarrhea are other frequent symptoms. Consequently, patient acceptance has been poor in the United States. If the drugs are started at low doses and slowly increased, side effects are usually tolerable. This group of agents should be avoided in patients with previously recognized symptomatic bowel disease. Despite the significant gastrointestinal side effects, patients do not tend to lose weight on this therapy. Liver enzyme elevations have been reported with very high doses of acarbose, but are rare.

These two agents will not result in hypoglycemia with monotherapy. However, when used in combination with other hypoglycemic medications, such as sulfonylureas, hypoglycemia can occur. In this case, patients should use glucose for treatment because complex carbohydrates will not be absorbed promptly.

E. Peroxisomal Proliferator-Activated Receptor-γ Activators

Peroxisomal proliferator-activated receptors (PPAR) are members of the steroid–thyroid superfamily of nuclear receptors that have been recognized only in the past decade. Once activated by ligand binding, PPARs form a heterodimer with retinoid X receptor (RXR) that then binds to DNA in the 5'-flanking region, resulting in transcriptional modulation. Among the three subtypes of PPARs, PPAR-γ influences carbohydrate and lipid metabolism. PPAR-γ is most abundant in adipose tissue, but is also found in skeletal muscle, liver, intestine, kidney, vascular smooth muscle, heart, and macrophages.

Thiazolidinediones were first identified in the early 1980s as agents that could affect glucose metabolism. It was a decade later that drugs from this class were found to be ligands for PPAR-γ. Troglitazone (Rezulin) is the first thiazolidinedione marketed in the United States. Rosiglitazone and pioglitazone were approved in 1999. Thiazolidinediones exert their effects through the PPAR-γ receptor. These agents, also referred to as "glitazones," reduce blood glucose by improving insulin-mediated glucose utilization, primarily in skeletal muscle tissue. Many consider these agents to be the best examples of true "insulin sensitizers." PPAR-γ activators may improve insulin sensitivity directly through their transcriptional effects in the muscle cells. However, alternative indirect effects are possible through reductions in free fatty acid (FFA) or tumor necrosis factor-α (TNF-α) production in adipose tissue where PPAR-γ receptors are most abundant. FFAs and TNF-α decrease insulin sensitivity in muscle tissue. Eventually, continued study of PPAR-γ–mediated responses could help us understand much more about insulin resistance.

Glitazones are rapidly absorbed following ingestion. Troglitazone absorption is enhanced in the presence of food; therefore, this agent is to be administered with a meal. The other glitazones can be taken at any time. Glitazones are metabolized through the liver. Rosiglitazone may have fewer drug interactions because it is metabolized through the CYP2C8 isoenzyme of the cytochrome P450 enzyme system, a route shared by relatively few drugs. Troglitazone is metabolized via CYP3A4, an enzyme system shared by multiple medications. It may induce this isoenzyme. Consequently, troglitazone has been shown to reduce estradiol and norethindrone levels by 30% when given in combination with oral contraceptives containing these two agents. Pioglitazone is metabolized via CYP2C8 and CYP3A4. Complete data on drug interactions is lacking though rosiglitazone has been more thoroughly evaluated. The dose of the glitazones need not be adjusted for renal insufficiency.

Troglitazone is no longer indicated for monotherapy due to its liver toxicity. Rosiglitazone and pioglitazone are indicated for monotherapy as well as combination therapy. In combinations, troglitazone can be started at 200 mg with maximum doses up to 600 mg daily. The initial dose of rosiglitazone is 4 mg daily with maximum doses of 4 mg bid. Four mg twice daily appears more effective than 8 mg daily. Pioglitazone can be started at 15 or 30 mg daily. Maximum dose is 45 mg daily.

As monotherapy, pioglitazone and rosiglitazone approach metformin and sulfonylureas in effectiveness. However, patient selection may influence the response rates. The best responses will likely occur in those with considerable endogenous insulin secretion but with significant insulin resistance, including obese patients. This group of drugs seems particularly effective in combination therapy.

All three agents produce modest increases in high density lipoprotein (HDL) as well as increases in LDL. Preliminary information suggests pioglitazone may cause the least elevation of LDL and rosiglitazone may cause the greatest elevation (up to 19%). However, lipoprotein B is not elevated and LDL increases are apparently due to increases in large, "fluffy" LDL, not the more atherogenic small, dense LDL. Triglyceride levels are reduced by troglitazone and somewhat by pioglitazone. Rosiglitazone seems to have no effect on triglycerides. Variations in lipid metabolism must be further evaluated.

Glitazones are generally well-tolerated. Plasma volume is increased, raising some concerns about use in congestive heart failure. New York Heart Association class III or IV heart failure is a relative contraindication for their use. Hemodilution results in mild decreases in hemoglobin but anemia seldom occurs. About 5% of patients experience peripheral edema, a figure that may be higher in combination with insulin. In clinical trials about 2% of patients on troglitazone were noted to have elevations of liver enzymes that were reversible after drug discontinuation. However, rare severe hepatic reactions have occurred resulting in death or liver transplant. This reaction is unpredictable. Troglitazone should not be started if transaminase levels are elevated 1.5 times the upper limit of normal. Furthermore, ALT levels should be checked every month for first year, than every 3 months. Rosiglitazone and pioglitazone clinical trials did not demonstrate any increased rate of liver enzyme abnormalities compared to placebo. No hepatic deaths have been reported with these two agents. However, more experience is required to exclude rare serious events. Accordingly, ALT levels are to be checked every two months for the first year and periodically thereafter.

IV. SELECTING THE INITIAL THERAPEUTIC AGENT

Each of the agents discussed in the foregoing is approved for initial treatment of type 2 diabetes with the exception of troglitazone. No one agent has been designated the "best" initial therapy for all patients. The characteristics noted in Table 1 will help guide the process of drug selection for individual patients.

Generally, for patients having fasting glucose values ranging from 126 to 150, it is best to select an agent that would avoid hypoglycemia. Metformin is an appropriate choice, particularly for the obese patient. In patients with relatively good blood glucose levels, sulfonylureas are more likely to precipitate hypoglycemia. This is a common problem when patients exercise or delay or skip meals. Patients for whom postprandial hyperglycemia is the dominant problem may be most effectively and safely treated with acarbose or possibly repaglinide at each meal. The usefulness of glitazones for monotherapy is limited by cost when other

Table 1 Therapy of Type 2 Diabetes Characteristics of Oral Agents

	Sulfonylurea	Repaglinide	Acarbose Miglitol	Metformin	Glitazones
Insulin levels	↑	↑	↔	↓	↓
Hypoglycemic potential	+ +	+ +	−	−	−
Convenience of flexibility	+ + +	+ + +	+	+ +	+ + + +
Weight	↑	↑	↔	↔↓	↔↑
Cost	+	+ + +	+ +	+ +	+ + + +
Monotherapy effect	+ + +	+ + +	+	+ + +	+ +
Side effects (1 + = least)	+	+	+ + +	+ +	+
	Hypoglycemia, hypersensitivity	Hypoglycemia	Flatulence, diarrhea	Diarrhea, nausea, anorexia	Edema
Safety profile (3 + = safest)	+ +	+ +	+ + +	+	+
				Lactic acidosis	Hepatoxicity (troglitazone)
Impact of renal status	+ +	−	+	+ + + +	−
Effect on triglycerides	↔	↔	↔	↓	↔↓

agents are perfectly acceptable. Nevertheless, rosiglitazone and pioglitazone can be very effective as monotherapy for obese patients who are likely to be highly insulin-resistant.

For patients with fasting blood glucose levels over 150 mg/dL, sulfonyl-ureas, metformin, or repaglinide, all are good first-line agents with significant and equal efficacy. Repaglinide is somewhat more costly and should be reserved for situations in which its flexible dosing with meals and short duration of action after the evening meal would provide an advantage over sulfonylureas. Metformin theoretically carries a distinct advantage in these patients, who are often obese and insulin-resistant. However, it is more costly and less well tolerated than sulfonylureas. Furthermore, no long-term prospective trials have demonstrated improved outcomes with metformin.

V. COMBINED THERAPY WITH ORAL AGENTS

There is ample evidence that any initially successful oral therapy tends to fail over time. In the UKPDS, when a second agent was added only when patients experienced symptomatic hyperglycemia or a fasting glucose level higher than 270 mg/dL, about 60% of the patients required a second agent by 6 years after randomization, whether the initial therapy was sulfonylureas or metformin. Secondary failure rates for newer agents are less well defined, but are likely to be similar. Despite the differing mechanisms of action, studies looking at "substitution therapy" (e.g., substitution of metformin for sulfonylureas[SU] after SU failure) have found no significant benefit to this strategy.

However, adding a second agent with a different mechanism has proved beneficial for all combinations studied to date. The relative responses of combined oral therapy are seen in Table 2. These data must be viewed cautiously, however,

Table 2 Approximate Relative Effects of Oral Agents Reduction in HbA$_{1C}$ [a]

	Sulfonylurea or Repaglinide	Acarbose Miglitol	Metformin	Glitazones
Single agent	1.5–2.0%	0.5–1.0%	1.5–2.0%	0.7–2.0%
Add to SU	—	0.5–1.0%	1.9%	1.3–2.6%
Add to metformin	—	0.5–1.0%	—	0.8–1.2%
Add to insulin	1.0%	0.4–0.7%	1.7–2.0% (+ insulin ↓)	1.0–1.4% (+ insulin ↓↓)

[a] These comparisons are limited by differences in the populations, initial level of glucose control (HbA$_{1c}$), duration of study, and other factors.

because the benefits of various combinations have not been measured in head-to-head studies employing the same patient group under the same study conditions.

It appears that combinations of an insulin secretagogue (e.g., sulfonylureas) and an agent enhancing the effect of insulin (e.g., metformin or glitazones) yield the greatest drop in blood glucose levels. Addition of acarbose or miglitol to sulfonylureas or metformin has a modest supplementary benefit (0.5–0.9% reduction in HbA_{1c}). Attesting to differing primary sites of action, the combination of metformin and a glitazone resulted in more than a 1.0% reduction in HbA_{1c} relative to use of either agent alone in obese patients with type 2 diabetes. At this point, use of insulin secretagogues plus metformin or a glitazone is becoming commonplace. Although some clinicians have begun to use combinations of a sulfonylurea, metformin, and a glitazone, this "triple" combination is neither approved nor supported by any prospective studies. A preliminary report indicates benefit from adding the third oral agent, but this strategy requires careful consideration of cost relative to the cost of initiating insulin after failure of two oral agents. Much remains to be learned about the relative benefits of various combinations.

The tactic of combined oral therapy has emerged from the need to regain glucose control after monotherapy failure. However, this tactic may also be useful in combining lower doses of two agents, thereby avoiding the adverse effects caused by treatment with maximal doses of a single agent.

VI. COMBINED USE OF INSULIN PLUS ORAL AGENTS

Most secondary drug failures in the treatment of type 2 diabetes relate to a progressive beta-cell defect. Accordingly, most patients with type 2 diabetes will eventually require insulin. The combination of sulfonylureas plus insulin has been used for over 15 years. Metaanalysis of this practice suggests modest reduction in HbA_{1c} and a slight reduction in insulin dose. The addition of evening insulin to daytime sulfonylurea therapy is quite reasonable as a transition approach because the evening insulin effectively reduces nocturnal hepatic glucose production with a simple and safe insulin regimen. However, using sulfonylureas with twice-daily insulin has very limited usefulness because it simply replaces part of the exogenous insulin requirement with endogenous insulin.

The more common use of oral agents with insulin involves insulin-sensitizing agents, such as glitazones or metformin. Studies evaluating the benefits of combining either of these agents with insulin have demonstrated significant reductions in HbA_{1c} as well as reductions in insulin requirements. There is a question of when metformin or a glitazone should be added. Simply increasing insulin doses will always improve glucose control, but resultant doses can be very large. Although the total daily insulin dose triggering the addition of an oral agent is quite arbitrary, using a limit of 70 U/day with inadequate glucose control (e.g.,

HbA_{1c} more than 8.0%) is common and reasonable. In many cases, insulin is added to previous oral therapy. We are still gaining experience with this transition, but it is likely that adding bedtime intermediate insulin may still be a preferred first step. Eventually, the requirement for two or more doses of insulin daily in addition to oral agents should lead to discontinuation of the oral agents until severe insulin resistance and poor control is again demonstrated. At this time the insulin-sensitizing agents may be added back.

VII. CONCLUSIONS

By mechanisms of action, four classes of oral agents are available for treating type 2 diabetes. Because diabetes is a progressive disease affecting both insulin supply and insulin function, combinations of oral agents are appropriate when initial therapy fails. Selection of agents is guided by a variety of therapeutic and pharmacokinetic characteristics. A logical progression of therapy is demonstrated in Fig. 1. Ultimately, a variety of approaches may attain good control without unacceptable adverse effects.

Goal HbA1C ≤ 7.0%   **Therapy Change Point = 8.0%**

Progress to pharmacologic therapy if FBG > 126mg/dl or HbA1C ≥ 7.0%
After HbA1C < 7.5% at any step, progress to next step when HbA1C rises ≥ 8.0%

◆ Step 1: *One month trial of diet and exercise* if FBG < 300 mg/dl without severe
       symptoms. Monitor q 2 weeks. Initiate education.
◆ Step 2: *Obese with normal renal function → metformin* if tolerated
       Nonobese → sulfonylurea or metformin
      • *Repaglinide* acceptable alternative for SU but more expensive
      • *Acarbose* or *miglitol* are options
      • *Rosiglitazone or pioglitazone* are options but quite expensive and lower
         response rate
◆ Step 3: *Sulfonylurea or repaglinide* **plus** *metformin*
       Or
       Sulfonylurea or repaglinide **plus** *troglitazone*
       Metformin **plus** *glitazone* (primarily in obese highly insulin resistant)
◆ Step 4: *Oral agent(s) plus evening insulin*
       Or
       Possible triple oral agent therapy (not well-substantiated)
◆ Step 5: *Multiple dose insulin therapy*
◆ Step 6: *Insulin plus Metformin or Glitazone*

Fig. 1 Suggested step therapy for type 2 diabetes.

BIBLIOGRAPHY

Baster B, IB Hirsch. The effect of improved glycemic control on complications in type 2 diabetes. Arch Intern Med 158:134–140, 1998.

Chiasson J-L, RG Josse, JA Hunt, C Palmason, NW Rodger, SA Ross, EA Ryen, MH Tan, MS Wolevert. The efficacy of acarbose in the treatment of patients with non–insulin-dependent diabetes mellitus. Ann Intern Med 121:928–935, 1994.

Dagogo-Jack S, JV Santiago. Pathophysiology of type 2 diabetes and modes of action of therapeutic interventions. Arch Intern Med 157:1802–1817, 1997.

Davidson MB, AL Peters. An overview of metformin in the treatment of type 2 diabetes mellitus. Am J Med 102:99–109, 1997.

DeFronzo RA, AM Goodman, the Multicenter Metformin Study Group. Efficacy of metformin in patients with non–insulin-dependent diabetes mellitus. N Engl J Med 333: 541–549, 1995.

Eastman PC, JC Javitt, WH Herman. Model of complications of non–insulin dependent diabetes mellitus. II Analysis of the health benefits and cost-effectiveness of treating NIDDM with the goal of normoglycemia. Diabetes Care 20:735–744, 1997.

Feinglos MN, MA Bethel. Treatment of type 2 diabetes mellitus. Med Clin North Am 82:757–790, 1998.

Garber AJ, TG Duncan, AM Goodman, DJ Mills, JL Rohlf. Efficacy of metformin in type 2 diabetes; results of a double-blind, placebo-controlled trial. Am J Med 103: 491–497, 1997.

Goldberg RB, D Einhorn, CP Lucas, MS Rendell, P Damsbo, W Huang, P Strange, RG Brodows. A randomized placebo-controlled trial of repaglinide in the treatment of type 2 diabetes. Diabetes Care 21:1897–1903, 1998.

Horton ES, F Whitehouse, MN Ghazzi, TC Venable, The Troglitazone Study Group, RW Whitcomb. Troglitazone in combination with sulfonylurea restores glycemic control in patients with type 2 diabetes. Diabetes Care 21:1462–1469, 1998.

Inzucchi SE, DG Maggs, GR Spollett, SL Page, FS Rife, V Walton, GI Shulman. Efficacy and metabolic effect of metformin and troglitazone in type II diabetes mellitus. N Engl J Med 338:867–872, 1998.

Johnson JL, SL Wolf, UM Kabadi. Efficacy of insulin and sulfonylurea combination therapy in type II diabetes: a meta-analysis of randomized, placebo-controlled studies. Arch Intern Med 156:259–264, 1996.

Johnson MD, LK Campbell, RK Campbell. Troglitazone: review and assessment of its role in the treatment of patients with impaired glucose tolerance and diabetes mellitus. Ann Pharmacother 32:337–348, 1998.

Lebovitz HE. alpha-Glucosidase inhibitors. Endocrinol Metab Clin North Am 26:539–551, 1997.

Maggs DG, TA Buchanan, CF Burant, G Cline, B Gumbiner, WA Hsueh, S Inzucchi, D Kelley, J Nolan, JM Olefsky, KS Polonsky, D Silver, TR Valiquett, GI Shulman. Metabolic effect of troglitazone monotherapy in type 2 diabetes mellitus: a randomized, double-blind, placebo-controlled trial. Ann Intern Med 128:176–185, 1998.

Riddle MC. Tactics for type II diabetes. Endocrinol Metab Clin North Am 26:659–677, 1997.

Rosenstock J, A Brown, J Fischer, A Jain, T Littlejohn, D Nadeau, A Sussman, T Taylor, A Krol, J Magner. Efficacy and safety of acarbose in metformin-treated patients with type 2 diabetes. Diabetes Care 21:2050–2055, 1998.

Schwartz S, P Raskin, Fonseca, JF Graveline. Effect of troglitazone in insulin-treated patients with type II diabetes mellitus. N Engl J Med 338:861–866, 1998.

Speigelman BM. PPAR-γ: adipogenic regulator and thiazolidinedione receptor. Diabetes 47:507–514, 1998.

Testa NA, DC Simonsen. Health economic benefits and quality of life during improved glycemic control in patients with type 2 diabetes mellitus. JAMA 280:1490–1496, 1998.

UK Prospective Diabetes Study Group. Intensive blood-glucose control with sulphonylureas or insulin compared with conventional treatment and risk of complications in patients with type 2 diabetes (UKPDS 33). Lancet 352:837–853, 1998.

UK Prospective Diabetes Study Group. Effect of intensive blood glucose control with metformin on complications in overweight patients with type 2 diabetes (UKPDS 34). Lancet 352:854–865, 1998.

Zimmerman BR. Sulfonylureas. Endocrinol Metab Clin North Am 26:511–537, 1997.

18
Insulin Therapy

Frank P. Kennedy
Mayo Clinic, Rochester, Minnesota

I. INTRODUCTION

Before the discovery of insulin by Banting and Best in the early 1920s, a patient who was diagnosed with type 1 diabetes had a few weeks to months to live. Following insulin's availability, microvascular and macrovascular complications have replaced diabetic ketoacidosis as the cause of death. All patients with type 1 diabetes require insulin, and about 35% of those with type 2 diabetes eventually use insulin.

Insulin was initially delivered, using glass syringes, by an intramuscular injection that was painful and often led to abscesses. Insulin syringes now have very fine needles, and injections are subcutaneous and mostly painless. Newer methods of insulin delivery also have been developed, including insulin pen systems that are widely used in many parts of the world, and aerosol injectors. Insulins themselves have improved markedly over time, both in purity and in the types of preparations, resulting in preparations with short to very long durations of action through altered subcutaneous absorption.

Arguably the greatest advance in the treatment of diabetes since the discovery of insulin has been the use of home blood glucose monitoring (HBGM), which replaced the inconvenient and inaccurate method of urine glucose testing. For the first time, HBGM allowed patients to truly manage their diabetes by adjusting insulin dosages to their calorie consumption, activity, and habits.

Insulin programs have also changed away from single or few doses of a long-acting insulin to smaller, more frequent (and more physiological) doses of insulin. This ability to change doses to compensate for hyperglycemia or hypoglycemia, meals, exercise, and illness has led to the development of intensive insulin therapy (IIT) programs that attempt to mimic normal insulin secretion in response to meals and other physiological events using subcutaneous insulin.

In 1993, the Diabetes Control and Complications Trial (DCCT) documented for first time that near-normal glycemic control reduces microvascular complications in type 1 diabetes. This relation between glycemic control, as measured by frequent HBGM or glycosylated hemoglobin (HbA_{1c}) levels, and microvascular complications has been confirmed by other studies for both type 1 and type 2 diabetes mellitus. Thus, today, our goal for most patients is to identify the insulin regimen that best allows them to safely achieve near normoglycemia.

Unfortunately, patients and many physicians view insulin therapy as a treatment of last resort. Patients commonly associate insulin as the "cause" of complications, and not the means to prevent them. Too often, those who take insulin have been poorly educated in its use, and end up fulfilling their initial fears of the negative consequences that come with starting a therapeutic insulin regimen. As physicians, it is our duty to become familiar in the use of insulin protocols that are best able to achieve optimal glycemic control. This includes educating patients in self-management of their diabetes in a proficient and proper manner. Multidisciplinary programs that educate patients in insulin administration, dose adjustment, treatment of hypoglycemia, and the relation between insulin dosage and their diet and physical activity should be part of every patient's care.

II. INSULIN PHARMACOLOGY

Insulin is an 86-amino acid, approximately 6000 molecular weight protein, that is synthesized in the beta cells of the islet of Langerhans. Between meals, insulin is released in a relatively constant amount (*basal secretion*) of about 1 U/h. When meals are consumed, insulin secretion and levels rise to five to ten times the basal rate within 30–60 min and then, returns to the basal rate over 2–3 h. The bioavailability of subcutaneously injected insulin is 55–77%. It is either excreted unchanged by the kidney, or metabolized by the liver or kidney. Once absorbed, the normal half-life is 0.8–1.5 h. Renal dysfunction has complex effects on insulin sensitivity, secretion, clearance, and renal glucose production. However, with uremia, a fairly substantial reduction in insulin requirements is generally found because of the markedly lowered insulin clearance. Insulin does not cross the placenta and is the drug of choice for the treatment of diabetes during pregnancy. There are no data on insulin crossing into breast milk.

Table 1 shows the average temporal profiles of the available insulin preparations. Several species are available—pigs (porcine), cows (bovine), human, or analogue. Porcine and bovine insulins differ from human insulin by one and three amino acids, respectively. Human insulin became available in 1982 through two biosynthetic processes, one that converted pork insulin to human, the other that

Table 1 Pharmacokinetics of Subcutaneous Insulin Preparations

Insulin	Onset of action	Peak of action	Duration of action
Lispro	5–15 min	1–2 h	3–5 h
Regular	30–60 min	2–4 h	6–8 h
NPH	1–3 h	5–7 h	13–18 h
Lente	1–3 h	4–8 h	13–20 h
Ultralente	2–4 h	8–14 h	18–30 h

used recombinant DNA technology. Human insulin is generally considered the insulin of choice. In reality, for most patients its advantages over animal insulins are minor to nonexistent, given the high purity of all commercially available insulins, so that patients who are doing well on animal insulin do not need to change, although their availability is diminishing and their cost now exceeds human insulin. Nor are there disadvantages of human insulin, and early concerns that it causes more frequent episodes of hypoglycemia have abated. However, human insulin is more rapidly absorbed than porcine insulin, probably owing to it being more hydrophilic, and there are a few patients who benefit from a change. On the other hand, there are a few patients who require porcine insulin owing to poorly defined problems with human insulin (see insulin allergy section).

There are many brands of insulin (Table 2). It is important that patients be consistent in the brand or manufacturer they use, because a change may somewhat

Table 2 Brand Names of Insulin[a]

Rapid-acting
    Human: Humulin R; Novolin R; Novolin R Penfill; Velosulin Human
    Modified human: Humalog
    Pork: Iletin II regular
Intermediate-acting
    Human: Humulin L; Humulin N; Novolin L; Novolin N; Novolin N Penfill
    Pork: Iletin II Lente; Iletin II NPH
    Beef/Pork: Iletin Lente; Iletin NPH
Long-acting
    Human: Humulin U
Mixtures
    Human: Humulin 50/50; Humulin 70/30; Novolin 70/30; Novolin 70/30 Penfill;
        Novolin 70/30 Prefilled

[a] Insulins are manufactured by Lilly and Novo Nordisk Corporations in the United States.

alter the dosage or its kinetic profile. Cost ranges from \$17 to \$25 per 10-mL vial, depending on the type. Humalog is the most expensive (Red Book, 1997). Insulin bottles are generally stable at room temperature for up to 6–8 weeks. However, it is recommended to use new bottles at least every month. Extremes in temperature should be avoided. Freezing causes more damage to insulin than temperatures up to 100°F (37.8°C). If the appearance of the insulin changes (for example, discoloration or solid particles appear), then the insulin vial should be discarded. It is also recommended not to leave bottles of insulin in direct sunlight. When patients cannot draw up their own insulin, prefilled syringes can be kept in the refrigerator for up to 3 weeks.

Only regular insulin should be used intravenously. Insulin in a parenteral solution is stable at room temperature or refrigerated temperatures (4°C) for 24 h. All intravenous lines should be flushed before infusion to prevent variable delivery because of adsorption to the tubing—it is recommended to wait 30 min after the initial flush, and flush again before initiating the infusion.

There is at least a 25% intraindividual variation, and possibly as much as a 50% variation in insulin absorption after subcutaneous injection. In general, human insulin has a slightly faster and shorter duration of action than animal insulins. Longer-acting insulins have a more variable absorptive pattern than shorter-acting insulins. This is one of the reasons that a dose of NPH or Lente insulin before the evening meal may last all night in one person, yet result in fasting hyperglycemia in another. The insulin analogue lispro appears to have the most consistency of absorption.

III. INSULIN PREPARATIONS

Insulin preparations are typically divided into three groups based on their speed of subcutaneous absorption (thus, time of onset and duration of action). The short-acting insulins are regular and lispro. Both types are clear in solution. *Regular insulin* or *cystalline zinc* (CZI) was the first type of insulin used for diabetes treatment. It is used today as a preprandial insulin that peaks 2–4 h after subcutaneous injection and has a duration of action that averages 6–8 h. The delay in absorption is due to the tendency of insulin to form hexamers in the presence of the zinc in standard buffers which slows absorption because only monomeric or dimeric forms of insulin can be absorbed. *Lispro insulin* is the first synthetically altered insulin (analogue) that consists of reversal of the proline residue at B28 and the lysine residue at B29. This change prevents lispro from being able to self-aggregate, keeping it as monomers in the subcutaneous space, which allows faster absorption. Lispro was released in 1996, and has become the ideal mealtime insulin, for it acts rapidly to reduce postprandial blood glucose concentrations, and then abates rapidly so that the frequency of postmeal hypoglycemia is less than with regular insulin. However, with meals that are low in carbohydrate, but high in fat, early postprandial hypoglycemia is not uncommon when this type of insulin is used immediately preceding the meal. An important difference between lispro and regular insulin is that lispro is given at the beginning of the meal, whereas regular insulin is typically injected 30 min before. Because of unknown teratogenicity and lack of long-term safety profile data, lispro insulin is not recommended during pregnancy or in women of childbearing potential. Lispro insulin has 50% more affinity for insulin-like growth factor I (IGF-1) receptors than human insulin, but this is just 10% of IGF-1's affinity, and no increase in cell growth has been demonstrated with lispro insulin.

The intermediate-acting insulins include *NPH* (neutral protamine Hagedorn or isophane) insulin and *Lente* insulin. These insulins are in a suspension as insulin crystals and thus appear cloudy in a vial. Lente has a slightly more prolonged duration of action then NPH, although that effect is clinically not generally useful. The human types of NPH and Lente are absorbed faster than the animal forms. However, there is a fair degree of variation in preparation of these insulins (lot-to-lot variation), making this difference of little clinical significance. Lente contains excess zinc as the basis for the crystallization that causes the slowed absorption and prolonged duration of action. This same effect can alter the profile of rapid-acting insulins that are mixed with Lente in the same syringe, and is more pronounced when the mixture remains in the syringe for more than a few minutes. Even when lispro insulin is mixed with Lente insulin, it is recommended it be injected within 5 min of drawing up this mixture. NPH contains protamine, which binds to the insulin and lowers its solubility. NPH mixtures appear less susceptible to alter the kinetics of short-acting insulins than does Lente.

There are two long-acting insulins, *Ultralente,* and *protamine zinc suspension* (PZI). PZI is rarely used today. Ultralente is often referred to as a ''basal insulin,'' although considerable confusion exists over its true kinetics. Most physicians were schooled when beef Ultralente was on the market, which had a very broad, almost nonexistent peak, and lasted on average 30 hs. Only human Ultralente is available now, which has a definite peak effect at 8–10 h and a duration of action closer to 18 h. It is sometimes used as a once-daily insulin, either at supper mixed with a short-acting insulin, or alone at bedtime. Intensive therapy programs often give Ultralente twice a day to minimize the broad rise and fall of the insulin effect with a single dose of this insulin, trying to mimic basal insulin secretion. Because of its long half-life, steady state is not reached for 3–4 days after a change in the dose.

There are several *insulin analogues* in clinical trials. Several short-acting insulin analogues besides lispro have been developed, including B28 Asp and B10 Asp. The latter has caused tumor growth in rats, which may be secondary to its high affinity for IGF-1 receptors, raising concerns about this insulin analogue's long-term safety. HOE-901 from Hoechst Roussel Pharmaceuticals is far along in development and may become be the first "true" basal insulin (long-acting analogue) owing to its nearly flat (no peak) absorption. It is a B31–B32 di-Arg-human insulin with substitution of asparagine by glycine at A21, with markedly decreased solubility at physiological pH (precipitates subcutaneously), thereby delaying its absorption. Although not currently available, it is in phase III clinical trials and is anticipated to be marketed in the year 2000. Another technique to prolong insulin absorption is to substitute cobalt for zinc because the cobalt–insulin hexamer dissolves more slowly than with zinc alone. Novo Nordisk is conducting studies on this type of insulin.

Proinsulin, which has 10% of the biological activity of native insulin, was initially reported to have a more potent effect in reducing hepatic glucose production than peripheral glucose disposal. Clinical studies noted an increased number of myocardial infarctions, resulting in discontinuation of investigating this drug. It may be possible to develop an insulin analogue with specific hepatic or peripheral effects by focused point mutations of the insulin molecule. This area of analogue development appears promising for the future.

IV. FACTORS THAT INFLUENCE SUBCUTANEOUS INSULIN ABSORPTION

A. Basic Insulin Injection Guidelines

Many factors can affect the absorption, and thus the bioavailability of subcutaneously injected insulin (Table 3). The correct technique, which ideally is taught by a certified diabetes nurse educator, is important for reproducible and accurate

Table 3 Factors Affecting Subcutaneous Insulin Absorption and Bioavailability

Type of insulin and insulin species
Insulin concentration
Insulin dose
Insulin mixing
Site of injection
Depth of injection
Local heat or massage
Exercise
Injection timing
Alteration in hepatic and renal function
Insulin antibodies or receptor defects
Unexplained daily variation

insulin administration. All insulins should be kept at room temperature. Before drawing up insulins that are in suspension (cloudy), the vial should be rolled gently between the hands to ensure a uniform suspension. The insulin vial is then turned upside down, and an equal amount of air is injected into the vial before withdrawing the proper amount of insulin. After drawing up the insulin, it is important to clear the syringe of any air bubbles. When mixing insulins, the regular or lispro (clear) insulin is drawn into the syringe first (to avoid contamination) followed by the longer-acting insulin, and quickly injected. When injecting, the tip of the needle should be pushed perpendicular into pinched up skin to ensure the insulin is injected into the subcutaneous fat. It is no longer advised to pull back on the plunger before injection, but simply inject once the needle has been inserted completely and the pressure of the "pinch" has been slightly released. In addition, the use of alcohol to cleanse the skin before injection is probably not necessary (and no longer recommended) because several studies have found no benefit of this practice. The insulin injection site should never be massaged.

B. Insulin Concentration

Less concentrated insulins such as U-40 (40 U/mL) are more rapidly absorbed than more concentrated insulins, such as U-100. This is partly due to a lower ratio of hexameric to monomeric forms with lower concentrations of insulin. U-100 insulin is the standard concentration in the United States. Patients should be cautioned when traveling abroad that U-40, U-80, and U-100 insulins are in common use outside the United States. Furthermore, physicians who take care of foreign patients must be familiar with the same principle. There is no inherent advantage to a certain concentration of insulin except to realize that the proper syringe must be used to ensure correct dosage delivery (i.e., U-100 syringe for U-100 insulin, and so on). For example, visitors to the United States who mistakenly use a U-40 syringe with U-100 insulin obtained in this country could develop dangerous hypoglycemia.

C. Insulin Dose or Volume

The higher the dose of insulin, and thus the larger the injected volume, the greater is the absorptive time of the insulin and the later the insulin peak. Larger doses also increase the variability of absorption. Unlike all other insulins, lispro's absorption appears unaffected by the given dose.

D. Mixing Insulins

The type of insulins mixed can affect the bioavailability of the mixture. Both Lente and Ultralente slow the absorption of regular insulin (owing to the excessive zinc found in Lente and Ultralente preparations), whereas NPH insulin has much less of this effect. Lispro insulin also appears to be delayed somewhat when mixed with Lente, but not NPH insulin. No such effect on lispro insulin has been clearly documented when mixing with Ultralente. The effect is minimized by injecting the mixed insulin as soon as it has been drawn up (within 3 min ideally). NPH insulin can generally be safely mixed with regular, and prefilled syringes stored in a refrigerator for up to 21 days for later use. Phosphate-buffered insulins, such as NPH, PZI, Velosulin, precipitate with zinc-containing insulins if mixed together. Lastly, the excess protamine in PZI insulin binds regular insulin, causing erratic absorption.

E. Site of Injection

Absorption is quickest in the abdomen, followed by the arms, then the buttocks, and thighs. These site differences are important, as random site injection may lead to variable blood glucose control. It is typical to recommend injection at one site, usually the abdomen, with rotation of the site in this same area to avoid local fat hypertrophy. In addition, the absorption of insulin from any one site is inversely related to the thickness of subcutaneous fat. Lispro insulin is less affected by the site of injection. Some physicians have suggested using site differences in their insulin programs: injecting the thigh or buttock before bedtime, which in theory, would slow the absorption and thus prolong its effect (all night, one hopes), whereas injecting into the abdomen would be ideal for preprandial insulin needs. However, we generally recommend that restricting all insulins to the abdomen and rotating within this area results in better, and more consistent, insulin and glucose profiles.

F. Depth of Injection

Depth of injection affects insulin absorption. Very shallow injections (intradermal) are not only painful, but are not well absorbed, whereas a deep intramuscular injection causes more rapid insulin absorption than in the subcutaneous fat. Repetitive intramuscular injections can cause formation of scar tissue.

G. Local Heat or Massage

Anything that increases subcutaneous blood flow will enhance insulin absorption. This includes exercise, saunas, or hot baths (which increase skin temperature) and local massage. These effects are more pronounced with regular insulin and least with lispro insulin. Inversely, smoking decreases subcutaneous blood flow and thus insulin absorption.

H. Exercise

Exercise increases insulin absorption by increasing blood flow, with this effect more pronounced with larger than with smaller doses of insulin. Thus, injecting into an extremity, which is then exercised, can significantly change absorption of the insulin. It is best to avoid injecting extremities for this reason and restrict injections to the abdomen, especially if physical activity is planned. Exercise also augments insulin sensitivity and thus may precipitate hypoglycemia in several different ways.

I. Injection Timing

All insulins have specific times to peak insulin levels. This is most critical in intensive insulin therapy programs in which either regular or lispro insulin is typically used before a meal, with the intention of matching the rise and fall in insulin effect and glucose level as closely as possible. Regular insulin usually requires a 20- to 30-min–lag time before the meal to match the peak insulin and glucose levels after consumption of a meal. Lispro, on the other hand, is given at the beginning of the meal owing to its faster absorption. Long-acting (Ul-tralente) and intermediate-acting insulin (NPH and Lente) is usually taken once (supper or bedtime) or twice a day (also at breakfast). If taken mixed with regular insulin, then the 20- to 30-min–lag time before meals is required. If taken alone or mixed with Lispro, they are taken at the meal time or prebed (not later than 11 PM).

V. INSULIN DELIVERY

Syringes are the mainstay of insulin delivery in the 1990s and in the foreseeable future. Today's syringes are a far cry from the glass syringes of the not so distant past that had long, painful needles that required resharpening and sterilization. Many kinds of syringes are widely available, with varying capacities (30–100 U), needle thicknesses (as small as 30-gauge needles), and needle length. For most patients, injections are nearly painless. Syringes are disposable and, under appropriate conditions and with education, are usually, reusable. Subcutaneous abscesses are a rare complication. Bruising and bleeding typically occur because of poor technique or reusing the syringe too many times.

Insulin pens (mechanical syringes) are also available, having been heavily used worldwide for more than 10 years, and they have been widely available in the United States for the last 2 years. There are generally two types of insulin pens: (a) prefilled pens that are disposed of once the insulin supply is exhausted and (b) pens with replaceable cartridges. Cartridges contain 150 U (1.5 mL) or

300 U (3.0 mL) of insulin. These devices allow convenience and easy portability; they are carried without refrigeration or special handling; thus, they are ideal for the noontime injections of rapid-acting insulin that are required for intensive insulin regimens. Precise dosing is another benefit, especially for patients who are unable to assess for air bubbles when filling a typical syringe or to easily visualize the lines on the syringe for accurate dosing: The insulin dose is dialed into the device by 1- or 2-U increments, and the plunger depressed after the needle is injected. Pens use disposable needles that are contained in plastic "caps" that make for easy disposal. The major disadvantage is the inability to mix insulins. Thus, two injections are needed for a mixed dose of NPH and regular or lispro unless one uses a premixed 70/30 or 50/50 cartridge. However, the intensive insulin regimen that is traditionally used with the pens avoids that problem by giving single insulin types four times daily (regular insulin premeals and NPH at bedtime).

There are air-jet insulin injectors that are more expensive and bulkier than insulin pens, and use high pressure air to inject a fine stream of insulin subcutaneously. Because the resultant subcutaneous depot of insulin is delivered over a larger surface area than from a syringe, the insulin is absorbed more rapidly. Although such devices seem to enhance absorption, there appears to be no evidence for improved intraindividual variability of absorption. Studies have found little advantage to such devices. Although purported to be needleless and painless, if used incorrectly the device can cause trauma to the skin. An American Diabetes Association (ADA) position paper recently advised against the use of high-pressure jet injectors for routine use.

Although oral insulin would be ideal, insulin is a protein and thus is destroyed by the gastrointestinal tract before it can reach the blood stream. There has been some work on an "insulin capsule," or liposomal insulin, which traverses the intestinal mucosa, allowing release of insulin into the blood. The most promising use of oral insulin may now be in the prevention of type 1 diabetes in identified high-risk individuals through a type of immunomodulation that is under investigation in an ongoing multicenter National Institutes of Health (NIH)-sponsored trial called the Diabetes Prevention Trial (DPT).

Insulin patches are being tested as a noninvasive means of delivering insulin. Hundreds of microscopic short needles (microneedles) arranged on a 2.5-cm–(1-in.)–square patch may be able to deliver insulin painlessly through the skin. Clinical trials are in progress. Other methods that have been tried to enhance insulin absorption through the skin have included electroporation (electrical charges alter the permeability) and ultrasound (induces air pockets in the stratum corneum).

Intranasal insulin has been of interest for several years. This avenue of delivery requires surfactants, such as bile acid salts (sodium glycocholate), that allow insulin to cross the nasal mucosa. Despite initial exciting studies that suggested this route of administration offered a means to deliver insulin quickly (peak concentration in less than 20 min), U-200–U-500 concentrations are required because of low bioavailability (5–10%). In addition, minor changes in the nasal mucosa by any type of inflammation results in large changes in insulin bioavailability and thus unstable blood glucose control. In addition, safety issues have been raised about the current surfactants. It is doubtful this will become a practical alternative route of insulin absorption in the near future.

On the other hand, intrapulmonary or aerosolized insulin delivery does not require surfactants, and its bioavailability through the alveoli is somewhat better (up to 50%). Insulin delivered in this manner peaks in 15–60 min. As with asthma inhalers, technique is crucial for adequate and reproducible dosing. Initial clinical trials have recently been reported, and appear promising as a means to deliver preprandial insulin.

External and surgically implanted programmable insulin pumps are available. The latter are still considered investigational. When used appropriately, they can obtain glycemic control that is similar to multiple, daily insulin injections. In the past, pumps used regular or Velosulin (phosphate-buffered regular insulin) insulin. Today, lispro is the insulin of choice in external pumps.

VI. INSULIN PROGRAMS

All patients with type 1 diabetes need insulin therapy owing to the autoimmune destruction of beta cells and the resultant loss of virtually all insulin production. Type 2 diabetes, especially in its early stage, is characterized more by both insulin resistance and a relative insulin deficiency. Therapy usually begins with diet, weight loss, and exercise, and if hyperglycemia persists oral agents are added. Insulin is typically added only if inadequate glycemic control persists. The recent United Kingdom Prospective Diabetes Study (UKPDS) clearly showed that many patients with type 2 diabetes will eventually need insulin.

Typically, patients who present with marked unexplained weight loss (even if obese) or with symptoms of marked polyuria and polydipsia, with or without ketonuria, require insulin therapy (sometimes temporarily), irrespective of the type of diabetes, as these symptoms are very suggestive of marked insulinopenia. Most pregnant patients with diabetes also require insulin therapy because oral hypoglycemic agents are contraindicated during pregnancy.

Insulin needs vary depending on the degree of obesity and physical activity of the patient. Dietary practices also are an important modulatory factor. In type 2 diabetes, patients with mild hyperglycemia typically require less insulin than those with marked hyperglycemia, reflecting the state of endogenous insulin secretion. Nonobese type 1 diabetes patients typically require 0.4–0.6 U/kg per day. However, patients in whom the diagnosis is new are usually started on a regimen of 0.2–0.4 U/kg, as they may go through a temporary phase of requiring small amounts of insulin, or even no insulin ("honeymoon phase"). Some authors advocate that some exogenous insulin should be maintained at this time to possibly reduce beta-cell destruction. Following the end of the honeymoon phase (usually less than 6 months), absolute insulinopenia occurs with onset of the normally expected daily insulin requirements. Furthermore, the fluctuating glycemia that characterizes type 1 diabetes becomes manifest; hence, multishot insulin programs that attempt to mimic normal insulin release by providing a basal dose of an intermediate- or long-acting insulin and premeal boluses of a short-acting insulin are advisable.

Type 2 diabetes usually requires much more insulin than type 1 diabetes, reflecting the frequent presence of obesity and insulin resistance. A bedtime dose of NPH insulin, with or without morning use of an oral agent, achieves excellent blood glucose control in many patients, especially those who exhibit their greatest hyperglycemia in the morning before breakfast.

Despite these comments, insulin programs are not disease-specific. Many patients with type 1 diabetes use conventional insulin regimens and, conversely, some patients with type 2 diabetes require intensive insulin programs. Choices reflect the patient's preferences and abilities for self-care; safety; lifestyle issues, such as jobs or hobbies that require flexibility in the insulin delivery; and the blood glucose goals that are set for each individual patient. Often it is best to begin with a simple insulin regimen, especially in type 2 diabetes, and modify it according to the blood glucose and HbA_{1c} values. The more common insulin programs are reviewed in Fig. 1.

A. Single or Twice-Daily Intermediate Insulin

When the goal of therapy is limited to abating symptoms of hyperglycemia, restoring a positive nutritional state, and improving overall sense of well-being, then a conventional insulin program suffices. Conventional insulin therapy is considered a once- or twice-daily regimen of insulin. It is simple to use, but does not mimic normal physiological insulin secretion. Thus, a general rule of thumb is that once- or twice-daily intermediate insulin is most appropriate for patients in whom achieving optimal glycemic control is not of paramount importance. However, in some type 2 patients with diabetes especially those who are obese, endogenous insulin secretion may be adequate to allow this type of insulin program to achieve excellent glycemic control. On the other hand, in established type 1 diabetes or any diabetic patient who lacks adequate endogenous insulin production (a common example is nonobese, elderly patients), glycemic control is typically poor, with large glucose variations throughout the day and a tendency for midafternoon and nocturnal hypoglycemia when the insulins are given prebreakfast and presupper.

Even in type 2 diabetes, twice-daily insulin regimens give a more stable serum insulin concentration, and thus glycemia, over once-daily regimens. Early-morning hypoglycemia can occur when the NPH or Lente is given before supper, often necessitating its use before bedtime. This effect is less pronounced in the elderly, who have a prolonged action of insulin because of the aging-associated reduction in renal function (and thus insulin clearance). Initially, patients typically monitor their blood glucose before breakfast and supper on a daily basis, then three to four times a week once goals are achieved. In addition, bedtime insulin and morning sulfonylurea (alternatively metformin alone or with a sulfonylurea) may conveniently control blood glucose, especially in patients with predominant fasting hyperglycemia on oral agents alone. Such patients typically still have considerable endogenous postprandial insulin secretion.

B. Split-Mix Insulin

This involves the use of NPH or Lente mixed with regular insulin or lispro, given before breakfast and supper. With increasing frequency, the second injection is split so that the regular insulin or lispro is injected before supper, and the NPH or Lente before bedtime. This is done because, in many patients (in particular the nonelderly), the intermediate-acting insulin effect wanes before breakfast when given at the evening meal. When first being started, this type of program requires HBGM (before each meal, bedtime, and weekly middle-of-the-night) and education in insulin dose adjustment based on the values. Once in place, patients measure their blood sugar four times a day, three or more times a week. The usual goals of HBGM are a fasting 80–120 mg/dL, 100–140 mg/dL before meals and at bedtime. Insulin regimens such as this are initiated with two-thirds of the total daily insulin dose given before breakfast, traditionally with two-thirds as intermediate-acting insulin and the remainder as rapid-acting insulin. The afternoon injection(s) is given as half of the remaining insulin as rapid-acting and the other half intermediate-acting (both one-sixth of the daily insulin dosage). Patients then adjust these doses according to the HBGM values, when appropriate, both on a daily basis with preset algorithms and over several days when insulin dosages prove incorrect. Patients need to be counseled in the importance of how changes in the timing of diet, or exercise affect their insulin program. They need to consume their meals at regularly scheduled times as well as being fairly consistent in caloric content, because taking the intermediate-acting insulin at breakfast to cover the lunchtime glycemic response minimizes flexibility and spontaneity in lifestyle.

This regimen is based on the premise that the combined injection of rapid-acting (regular or lispro) and intermediate-acting insulins (NPH or Lente) before breakfast and the evening meal results in four peaks of insulin action (see Fig. 1). In reality, the practice of drawing up two insulins in the same syringe tends to result more in a single, broad peak. Several factors contribute to this effect, including the time between the mixing of the insulins and their injection, the relative proportions of the two insulins, and the amount or volume injected. This is most evident with zinc-containing preparations (Lente and Ultralente), with a

- Single dose
  An injection of intermediate-acting insulin taken each morning.

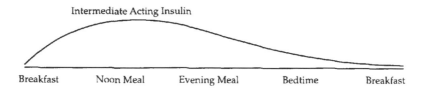

- Mixed dose
  An injection of both short-acting and intermediate-acting insulins mixed in one syringe taken each morning.

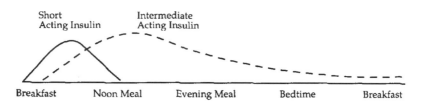

- Premixed single dose
  An injection of premixed insulin taken each morning.

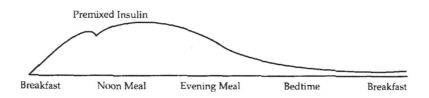

- Split dose
  Two injections of intermediate-acting insulin taken each day. These injections are usually taken before breakfast and before the evening meal or before breakfast and at bedtime.

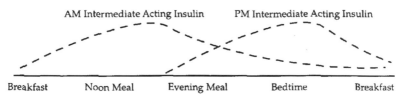

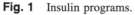

Fig. 1 Insulin programs.

- Split-mixed dose
  Two injections of short-acting and intermediate-acting insulins mixed in one syringe taken each day. These injections are usually taken before breakfast and before the evening meal.

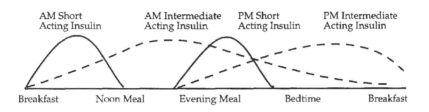

AM Short Acting Insulin   AM Intermediate Acting Insulin   PM Short Acting Insulin   PM Intermediate Acting Insulin

Breakfast   Noon Meal   Evening Meal   Bedtime   Breakfast

- Split-premixed dose
  Two injections of premixed insulin taken each day. These injections are usually taken before breakfast and before the evening meal or before breakfast and at bedtime.

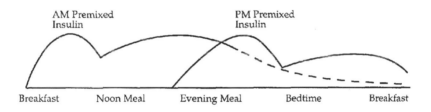

AM Premixed Insulin   PM Premixed Insulin

Breakfast   Noon Meal   Evening Meal   Bedtime   Breakfast

- Multiple daily injections
  Three or four injections taken each day. Short-acting insulin is used before all meals. Either intermediate-acting or long-acting insulin is taken with the evening meal short-acting insulin or as a separate injection at bedtime.

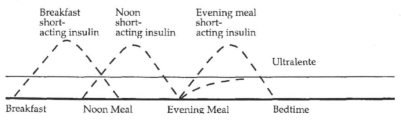

Breakfast short-acting insulin   Noon short-acting insulin   Evening meal short-acting insulin   Ultralente

Breakfast   Noon Meal   Evening Meal   Bedtime

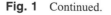

Fig. 1 Continued.

delay in the rapid-acting insulin effect occurring as soon as 2 min after mixing, and maximal after 5 min. It is much less a problem with NPH, thus a strong reason to use this type of insulin in mixed programs.

C. Premixed Insulin

Commercially available premixed insulins are a mixture of NPH and regular insulin. In the United States, 70:30 (70% NPH, 30% regular) and 50:50 admixtures are currently available, with several additional combinations available outside the United States. Although convenient, they present a lack of flexibility in the ability to alter the ratio of the intermediate to regular insulin to compensate for variances in daily routine. Thus, they are most appropriate for persons with regimented lifestyles (institutional living), or when individuals are not capable of mixing their own insulins because of poor dexterity or eyesight, an inability to follow instructions safely, or excessive age. Besides these special cases, premixed insulin offers few advantages otherwise, and the author limits their use to patients who cannot totally care for their diabetes by themselves.

D. Intensive Insulin Therapy

Also termed *multiple daily insulin* (MDI) or *basal-bolus therapy,* the goals of this therapy are to integrate food intake and lifestyle activities with the insulin doses. A commonly used approach is to inject Ultralente insulin at breakfast and supper (less commonly NPH) and either regular or lispro insulin before each meal to provide the basal need (background insulin required to maintain blood glucose control between meals and during the night) and to cover the meals (bolus). Some give Ultralente as a single dose before the evening meal. Experts vary somewhat as to three or five injections daily based on the level of concern over the mixing effect of Ultralente on the rapid-acting insulin. My own practice uses three injections for convenience (combined Ultralente and rapid-acting insulin at breakfast and supper). Lispro or regular insulin pens are both available, and are particularly convenient for the lunchtime injection at work, school, or elsewhere. When starting this regimen, the Ultralente dose is usually one-half of the total daily insulin dose (equally split between breakfast and supper although some recommend 60% prebreakfast and 40% presupper), but the actual doses vary among patients based on their level of insulin sensitivity and physical activity versus food intake (i.e., late teenage or young adult males sometimes require very large amounts of rapid-acting insulin to cover their high-caloric intake, and proportionately much smaller amounts of longer-acting insulin because of their extreme activity). The rapid-acting insulin given before meals is typically adjusted according to home blood glucose values by an algorithm (Table 4). Traditional starting doses are 40% of the rapid-acting insulin prebreakfast and 30% before lunch and supper; these amounts are adjusted based on the patient's dietary prac-

Table 4 Sample Algorithm for Premeal Insulin Supplements[a]

Premeal blood glucose	Insulin supplement (regular or lispro)
< 60	−2
60–79	−1
80–120	0
121–160	+1
161–200	+2
201–240	+3
> 240	+4

[a] Supplementation is an addition or substraction to the usual premeal dose of regular or lispro insulin in an intensive therapy program. This is not to be confused with sliding scales, which are commonly used by many patients and physicians to temporarily correct high blood glucose levels caused by illness, surgery, dietary indiscretions, or for no apparent reason. The regular use of sliding scales is discouraged.

tices. Generally, this kind of regimen is well accepted by patients, with the major positive being the mealtime and exercise flexibility in terms of being able to adjust insulin dosing accordingly. The major negative is that about 20% of persons experience middle-of-the-night hypoglycemia because of the "peak" effect of Ultralente that occurs 8–10 h after injection. If that occurs, the second Ultralente injection can be given at bedtime so that the patient now takes four injections (Ultralente/short-acting prebreakfast, rapid-acting prelunch, rapid-acting presupper, and Ultralente bedtime).

A second intensive insulin program is more frequently used outside the United States, reflecting the use of insulin pens that deliver a single type of insulin per injection. Regular insulin is given premeals and NPH at bedtime, thus four injections. The principle is identical with the foregoing Ultralente program, to deliver insulin in a basal-bolus program. The use of regular insulin is absolute, as its longer action over lispro is needed to preserve glucose control between meals (the prolonged effect of regular provides the basal insulin need between meals). The major positives of this regimen are the ability to use insulin pens at each injection, which for many patients provides convenience, ensures accurate dosing, and avoids having to mix. For those patients who develop nighttime hypoglycemia with Ultralente, switching to this regimen can reduce or eliminate the problem. The negatives are having to use regular insulin instead of lispro so that patients must still inject 30 min before their meal. Also, some patients do not like insulin pens, especially those who have had diabetes for many years and have a schedule and habits with which they are comfortable. Those patients can use this regimen with syringes, but it defeats the purpose, as they will inject four times daily as opposed to three times with the Ultralente regimen. When starting this regimen, the NPH dose is usually 30% of the total, and the regular insulin is divided generally in similar amounts per meal, unless unusual dietary practices suggest some other balance. Doses are then adjusted based on HBGM.

A major benefit of these insulin programs is that they allow a more liberal diet and flexible schedule for meals and activity because insulin is being taken at the time of each meal. An insulin pump or continuous subcutaneous insulin infusion (CSII) follows the same principle of basal and bolus dosing of insulin, and is described more fully in Chap. 19.

Intensive therapy programs typically use predetermined "algorithms" to supplement the bolus insulin (see Table 4) based on target blood glucose levels, food intake, exercise, or illness. This should not be confused with "sliding-scale insulin," which is an after-the-fact addition of short-acting insulin on the background of no, or inadequate insulin for that patient's usual needs. Algorithms are supplements to, or from, the patients usual insulin dose, and are intended to compensate for unusual factors that have influenced their insulin need at that particular time. The same concept is true for adjusting the dose to be taken for a planned variation in usual food intake or exercise. When used successfully, algorithms promote smooth glycemic controls, as opposed to sliding scales, which promote fluctuating glycemic control. The use of algorithms requires HBGM before each meal and at bedtime as a minimum expectation. Therefore patients need to be highly motivated and willing to take an active role in their own care. Moreover, despite the flexibility that these insulin programs allow patients for changing dietary and exercise habits, experience has shown that patients who are consistent in their timing and quantity of meals and exercise generally are most able to attain and maintain optimal glycemic control. The cost of intensive insulin therapy on average is about three times ($5000/year) that of nonintensive treatment programs. An intensive therapy program is best initiated in an environment that is familiar with using and teaching these programs, typically with a multidisciplinary team of an endocrinologist, certified diabetes nurse educator, dietitian, psychologist, and exercise physiologist. Important messages that should be given to patients considering moving to an intensive insulin program are that intensive programs bring flexibility, not rigidity, and use of mealtime insulin algorithms helps compensate for the lifestyle variations that characterize modern life, thereby promoting day-to-day glycemic control. For the latter, an alternative form of algorithm is based on ketone monitoring as a part of sick-day guidelines. (Table 5).

Goals for IIT must be individualized to the needs of each patient. A target HbA$_{1c}$ level of less than 7% (normal 4–6%) is generally recommended for most patients. However, IIT is sometimes chosen to lower the risk of severe nocturnal hypoglycemia or hypoglycemic events accompanying gastroparesis in which this overall level of control is not possible. Similarly, for those female patients desiring pregnancy, the target glycemic control is lower (HbA$_{1c}$ < 6%) before conception

Table 5 Insulin Supplements[a] for Ketones

If the urine ketone results reads	Take the following units of regular or lispro and recheck HBGM in 4 h
Trace or small	1–2 U (10%)
Moderate	2–3 U (20%)
Large	3–4 U (30% of usual short-acting premeal dose)

[a] An additional supplement of regular or lispro insulin may be needed when blood glucose levels are high and ketones are present in the urine. Urine should be measured for ketones whenever the blood glucose levels are higher than 300 mg/dL. Supplements should not be given at bedtime unless properly educated in doing this.

and during pregnancy to optimally lower the risk of maternal and fetal complications.

Contraindications to an intensive insulin therapy program include severe hypoglycemic unawareness, current substance abuse, severe psychopathology, a lifestyle not conducive to program compliance, cognitive impairment, and an unwillingness to do the necessary dietary, activity, HBGM, and insulin injection components of the program to make this a successful treatment option.

VII. ADVERSE EVENTS FROM INSULIN THERAPY

A. Hypoglycemia

The most frequent complication of insulin therapy, as well as oral agents, is hypoglycemia. Often patients think hypoglycemia is a unique problem of insulin. However, it occurs with at least an equal frequency with oral agents. Hypoglycemia is not a benign event. Studies have suggested up to 4–7% of deaths in patients with type 1 diabetes are due to hypoglycemia caused by such occurrencies as car accidents. Typically, hypoglycemia is mild and self-treated, with no lasting adverse effect. Yet, intensive insulin therapy increases the chance of severe hypoglycemia (defined as needing assistance) some threefold. The lower the HbA$_{1c}$ level, the higher the risk. Patients most at risk are those with "hypoglycemic unawareness," in whom there is impairment in counterregulatory hormone release to hypoglycemia. Some authors have advocated that a history of severe hypoglycemia is a relative contraindication for IIT, whereas others advocate the use of the more physiological IIT-type insulin regimens to lower the risk of hypoglycemia in susceptible persons. Patients taking insulin of whatever type and program need to be counseled about the risk of hypoglycemia (especially with IIT insulin programs) and the use of glucagon kits at home and work.

The symptoms of hypoglycemia are manifest initially by adrenergic symptoms (diaphoresis, tachycardia, tremor), and later by neuroglycopenic symptoms (change in behavior, confusion, seizures, coma). Nocturnal hypoglycemia can present as nightmares, night sweats, or morning headaches. When the patient is fully conscious, taking 15 g of a carbohydrate orally will typically correct the blood glucose level (Table 6). Patients should always carry carbohydrate, and identification. If unconscious, 1 mg of glucagon should be injected intramuscularly by a knowledgeable family member or friend.

Patients often fear hypoglycemia to the point of preventing them from fully attempting optimal glycemic control. Nocturnal hypoglycemia worries patients the most, and is unique to no one type of insulin program. Patients with bedtime glucose levels below 108 mg/dL (6.0 mM) are 80% more likely to have hypoglycemic reaction. In the DCCT, 43% of all severe reactions occurred at night. This risk seems to be reduced when lispro insulin is used in place of regular insulin at supper, and NPH or Ultralente is given at bedtime instead of before the evening meal. The most important tool to protect against severe hypoglycemia is to educate the patient in how to avoid and treat reactions. This includes educating the family in the use of glucagon for severe hypoglycemia, and making patients aware that increasing age, alcohol, physical activity, poor nutrition, and renal insufficiency, all increase the risk of severe hypoglycemia. Also, several medications affect insulin's hypoglycemic effect (Table 7).

Hypoglycemic unawareness is a common condition that stems from a lack of the normal glucagon and epinephrine response to hypoglycemia. Adrenergic symptoms that usually come from the epinephrine response are therefore, lost, so that patients are not warned of early hypoglycemia. Also, physiologically, the

Table 6   Treatment of Hypoglycemia[a]

Carbohydrates are used to increase the blood glucose level. Each of the following contains about 15 g of carbohydrate:

6 Lifesavers or other hard candy
2 teaspoons honey or syrup
2 sugar packets or 1 tablespoon of sugar
$\frac{1}{2}$ cup (4 ounces) regular soda
$\frac{1}{2}$ cup of fruit juice
3 glucose tablets (B-D brand)
9 jelly beans
3 graham crackers
1 fruit or starch exchange

[a] After 15 min, if symptoms still present, repeat the treatment.

Table 7 Drug Interactions with Insulin

Decrease hypoglycemic effect of insulin
    Corticosteroids
    Oral contraceptives
    Dextrothyroxine
    Diltiazem
    Dobutamine
    Epinephrine
    Niacin
    Smoking
    Thiazide diuretics
Increase hypoglycemic effects of insulin
    Alcohol
    α-Adrenergic blockers
    Anabolic steroids
    Nonselective β-adrenergic blockers
    Clofibrate
    Fenfluramine
    Guanethidine
    MAO inhibitors
    Pentamidine
    Salicylate
    Sulfinpyrazone
    Tetracycline

liver does not receive the normal signals to increased hepatic glucose output. Severe hypoglycemia presenting with neurological impairment and a blood glucose level of less than 40 mg/dL is the usual end result. This most typically occurs in patients who have had diabetes of long duration, and it is not necessarily associated with other complications, including autonomic neuropathy. Current research suggests recurrent or chronic hypoglycemia itself may cause this condition in some affected persons. The major treatment is avoidance of hypoglycemia, and education in insulin dose adjustment and hypoglycemia prevention and treatment.

The goal of insulin therapy is not just achieving optimal glycemic control based on some predetermined HbA_{1c} level, but it is also minimizing hypoglycemic episodes. At every patient visit, an assessment of hypoglycemic episodes should occur, including reviewing the patient's record book and discussing possible strategies to avoid future episodes, such as appropriate insulin timing, proper HBGM, a bedtime snack, and periodic 3-AM blood glucose checks.

B. Worsening Retinopathy

Several clinical studies have shown worsening of underlying retinopathy during
the first year after introduction of improved glycemic control. The risk appears
to correlate with the degree of poor control (degree of HbA_{1c} elevation) at the
time of initiating better control, and the decrease in HbA_{1c} level during the first
year. It occurs in both types 1 and 2 diabetes, and leads to serious proliferative
retinopathy, including blindness in a few patients. The basis is likely multifactorial, and includes retinal ischemia and elevated IGF-1 levels following the improved glycemic control. It is suggested that individuals with retinopathy when
beginning an intensive insulin program be evaluated by an ophthalmologist before
starting the program, and frequently thereafter.

C. Weight Gain

Weight gain is not unique to insulin therapy; it occurs with most of the oral
agents used in the treatment of type 2 diabetes. Regardless, weight gain is well
known to occur with insulin, especially intensive programs. In the DCCT (type
1 diabetes), the intensive insulin therapy group gained 5.1 kg versus 2.4 kg with
conventional therapy; the amount correlated with the initial and decremental
HbA_{1c} levels. In the UKPDS (type 2 diabetes), patients treated with insulin gained
more weight (10.4 kg) than those treated with sulfonylurea (3.7 kg) or metformin
(no weight change). The cause is likely multifactorial: treatment of increased
frequency of hypoglycemia, reversal of glycosuria, and a sodium retention effect
of insulin. Patients need to be counseled about possible weight gain, and the
recommended caloric intake lowered if their weight starts to increase. Physicians
need to appreciate that weight gain can be a crucial factor that prevents a patient's
willingness to comply with the prescribed program.

D. Insulin Allergy

With the advent of human insulin, there has been a marked decline in allergic
responses, such that they are a generally uncommon complaint to the physican.
Local or cutaneous reactions are the most common type, accounting for over
75% of allergic reactions. This includes pruritus, erythema, and induration at the
injection site. Such reactions typically last no more than 2–3 weeks after starting
insulin. Systemic allergic reactions present with generalized urticaria, angioneu-
rotic edema, or anaphylaxis, and are mediated by IgE antibodies. Thankfully,
they are rare today because of the high purity of modern commercially available
insulins. When a local or systemic allergy to insulin does develop within the first
month of treatment, it is often a patient who has resumed insulin therapy, or in
patients with a history of other drug sensitivities.

Local reactions, from animal insulins, that last more than 2–3 weeks are treated with antihistamines and switching to human insulin. If a reaction occurs with human insulin, switching to another brand of human insulin may help (may be a contaminant unique to that insulin brand).

E. Lipodystrophy and Lipoatrophy

Atrophy or hypertrophy of subcutaneous tissue can occur at insulin injections sites. This was common with the "impure" animal insulins of the past, but is relatively rare today with the use of human insulin. Areas of hypertrophy are less sensitive to pain and may be overused by the patient. They can be a source of erratic absorption of insulin, and they need to be identified and the patient counseled against injecting there. When hypertrophy develops, rotation of the injection sites away from the area of hypertrophy usually leads to its disappearance over time. Atrophy is more common during the first year of insulin use and is seen most frequently in women and children. It is believed secondary to an immune reaction, but is not associated with other allergic findings, and sometimes occurs at noninjection sites of subcutaneous tissue. It typically improves with purified or synthetic insulin injected into and around the affected area.

BIBLIOGRAPHY

Barmeth AH, Owens DR. Insulin analogues. Lancet 1997; 349:47–51.

Berger M, Cuppers HJ, Hegner H, et al. Absorption kinetics and biologic effects of subcutaneously injected insulin preparations. Diabetes Care 1982; 5:77–91.

Bolli GB. Counterregulatory mechanisms to insulin-induced hypoglycemia in humans: reference to the problem of intensive treatment of IDDM. J Pediatr Endocrinol Metab 1998; 11(suppl 1):103–115.

Burge MR, Schade DS. Insulins. Endocrinol Metab Clin North Am 1997; 26:575–598.

Diabetes Control and Complications Trial Research Group. Effect of intensive therapy on residual beta-cell function in patients with type 1 diabetes in the Diabetes Control and Complications Trial. A randomized, controlled trial. Ann Intern Med 1998; 128:517.

Edelman SV. Importance of glucose control. Med Clin North Am 1998; 82:665–687.

Fineberg SE. Insulin allergy and resistance. In: Lebovitz HE, ed. Therapy for Diabetes Mellitus and Related Disorders. 2nd ed. Alexandria, VA: American Diabetes Association, 1994.

Gnanalingham MG, Newland P, Smith CP. Accuracy and reproducibility of low dose insulin administration using pen-injectors and syringes. Arch Dis Child 1998; 79: 59–62.

Hirsh IB. Intensive treatment of type 1 diabetes. Med Clin North Am 1998; 82:689–719.

Joseph SE, Korzon-Burakowsk A, Woodworth JR, Evans M, Hopkins D, James JM, Amiel SA. The action profile of lispro is not blunted by mixing in the syringe with NPH insulin. Diabetes Care 1998; 21:2098–2012.

Kappel C, Dills DG. Type 2 diabetes. Update on therapy. Compr Ther 1998; 24:319–326.

Koivisto VA, Felig P. Alterations in insulin absorption and in blood glucose control associated with varying insulin injection sites in diabetic patients. Ann Intern Med 1980; 92:59–61.

Koivisto VA. The human insulin analogue insulin lispro. Ann Med 1998; 30:260–266.

Lee WL, Zinman B. From insulin to insulin analogs: progress in the treatment of type 1 diabetes. Diabetes Rev 1998; 6:73–88.

Saudek CD. Novel forms of insulin delivery. Endocrinol Metab Clin North Am 1997; 26: 599–610.

Trachtenburg DE. Ten errors to avoid in managing type 2 diabetes. Getting back to the basics. Postgrad Med 1998; 104:35–39,43.

UK Prospective Diabetes Study (UKPDS) Group. Intensive blood-glucose control with sulphonylureas or insulin compared with conventional treatment and risk of complications in patients with type 2 diabetes (UKPDS 33). Lancet 1998; 352:837–853.

Yki-Jarvinen H, Kauppila M, Kujansuu E, et al. Comparison of insulin regimens in patients with non-insulin dependent diabetes mellitus. N Engl J Med 1992; 327:1426–1433.

19

Insulin Pump Therapy: A Practical Tool for Treating Persons with Type 1 and Insulin-Requiring Type 2 Diabetes

Steven V. Edelman
University of California, San Diego, and VA Medical Center, San Diego, California

I. INTRODUCTION

Insulin pump therapy (continuous subcutaneous insulin infusion; CCII) is not for everyone. However, many persons with type 1 and type 2 diabetes could improve their glucose control with an insulin pump, while enjoying a much more flexible lifestyle. Many physicians are ignorant about insulin pumps and, as a result, they never think to offer them to their patients. Other caregivers are reluctant to prescribe insulin pumps because they do not want to create more work and "hassles" for themselves.

The truth of the matter is that the proper use of insulin pumps allows less work and fewer hassles for the caregiver in the long term. There are over 18,000 persons with type 1 and type 2 diabetes in the United States who are using insulin pumps. This number has grown quite dramatically since the results of the Diabetes Control and Complications Trial (DCCT) were reported in 1993. There have been many publications documenting the benefits of insulin pump therapy since it was popularized in the early 1980s (Table 1).

From a patient's point of view insulin pump therapy has proved to be beneficial in many aspects, including a much more flexible lifestyle while simultaneously enjoying improved glucose control. Insulin pump therapy permits increased flexibility in meal timing and amounts, increased flexibility in the time

Table 1   Proven Benefits of Insulin Pump Therapy

Improving glycemic control; thus preventing and delaying the complications of diabetes
Controlling the dawn phenomenon; early AM resistance to insulin contributing to fasting
  hyperglycemia
Reducing the incidence of extreme hyperglycemia and hypoglycemia
Improving growth and development in poorly controlled adolescents with type 1 diabetes
Improving insulin resistance and glucose toxicity in patients with type 2 diabetes in poor
  control

and intensity of exercise, improved glucose control while traveling across time
zones or with variable working schedules, and quality of life in terms of self-
reliance and control (Table 2).

Because pumps use only regular insulin, there is no peaking of injected
intermediate-and long-acting insulins, which do not provide a constant basal rate
owing to variable absorption and pharmacokinetics. Variable insulin absorption
and pharmacokinetics are probably responsible for up to 50–60% of the day-to-
day fluctuation in blood glucose values in patients using insulin therapy. Insulin
pump therapy permits more regular insulin absorption and pharmacokinetic profile, resulting in reproducibility in insulin availability and reduced fluctuations
in glycemic control. In addition, persons who are extremely insulin-sensitive
(total daily dose less than 20 U/day), find pump therapy very beneficial and
convenient because they can deliver insulin in very low doses with precision that
is not possible with normal injection methods.

II. INSULIN PUMP THERAPY IN INSULIN-REQUIRING PATIENTS WITH TYPE 2 DIABETES

Insulin pump therapy has been traditionally used mainly in persons with type 1
diabetes. However, insulin pump therapy is extremely valuable in patients with

Table 2   Advantages of Insulin Pump Therapy for the Patient

Flexible lifestyle
Flexibility in meal timing and amounts
Fewer and less severe hypoglycemic reactions
Avoidance of unconsciousness in individuals with hypoglycemic unawareness
Increased flexibility in exercise intensity and times
Improved control while traveling
Improved control with a variable work schedule
Quality of life in terms of self-reliance and control

insulin-requiring type 2 diabetes who have not achieved glycemic control with subcutaneous injections, or in those who are seeking a more flexible lifestyle. All of the benefits that are enjoyed by patients with type 1 diabetes, also apply to persons with type 2 diabetes. Many experts believe that because of the more physiological delivery of insulin, glucose control is achieved with less insulin than was needed with the subcutaneous insulin regimen. This may be due to a reduction in glucose toxicity and improvement of insulin resistance and beta-cell secretory function as a result of improved glycemic control with pump therapy. Weight gain is less of an issue because the patient is generally using less insulin than he or she was before insulin pump therapy. In addition, with the reduction of hypoglycemic events, there is less overeating to compensate for excessive insulin. Lastly, there is no doubt that there is less strain placed on the pancreatic beta cells of these patients with type 2 diabetes, and this definitely helps with overall glycemic control, because a functioning beta-cell can also autoregulate against hyper- and hypoglycemia, as seen in nondiabetic individuals.

Many older patients with the diagnosis of ''insulin-requiring type 2 diabetes'' have true late-onset type 1 diabetes. It has been documented in the literature when large groups of patients with insulin-requiring type 2 diabetes mellitus were tested for anti-glutamic acid decarboxylase (GAD) antibodies, with an approximate 5–8% positivity rate. These individuals are thinner at the time of diagnosis and generally do not respond well to oral agents and require insulin, although they do not present in severe diabetic ketoacidosis. In general, if a patient with insulin requiring type 2 diabetes cannot achieve glycemic control with an intensive insulin injection regimen, then insulin pump therapy should be considered.

III. IS YOUR PATIENT A CANDIDATE FOR AN INSULIN PUMP?

In general, any patient taking insulin with poor glycemic control, or who is requesting a more flexible lifestyle, should be considered for insulin pump therapy. Obviously, the patient must be reliable, be able to perform frequent home glucose monitoring, and have a fundamental understanding of diabetes and the importance of good control. The patient does not have to be a rocket scientist, and there is no real age limit, as patients who are between the ages of 8 and 80 can do well on pump therapy. It is also important that the patient can effectively understand, operate, and maintain the insulin pump and related catheter care. In summary, a good candidate for an insulin pump is someone who is interested in his or her diabetes and is reliable and compliant. If a patient comes to you requesting an insulin pump, he or she is probably a good candidate based on that fact alone.

One of the techniques I use to determine if a patient is a good candidate for an insulin pump, is that I put the individual on an intensive insulin regimen first. I usually prescribe human Ultra Lente with Humalog at breakfast and dinner, with an extra injection of Humalog at lunch and at other times for incidental hyperglycemia. This regimen requires at least four-times-a-day home glucose monitoring and prepares that person for an easy conversion to an insulin pump if indicated. If the patient can perform this regimen and perform frequent home glucose monitoring reliably, then he or she will do well with insulin pump therapy.

IV. DISADVANTAGES OF INSULIN PUMP THERAPY

In older text books, hypoglycemic unawareness is listed as a contraindication to insulin pump therapy because any therapeutic regimen that improves glycemic control, increases the chances for hypoglycemia. Insulin pump therapy reduces wide fluctuations in blood glucose values, including severe hypoglycemia. It is important to set the patient's goals at a higher range to avoid severe hypoglycemia. For example, the goals of glycemic control for an individual with hypoglycemic unawareness should be between the ranges of 120 and 180 mg/dL instead of the usual 70–160 mg/dL range in individuals without hypoglycemic unawareness.

In individuals who have frequent staphylococcal skin infections, insulin pump therapy may be problematic. In my experience, patients with poor glycemic control commonly develop frequent skin infections; and having a catheter or needle in the subcutaneous tissue over a long time period increases the chance of having an infection. However, with good glycemic control, many patients with a history of having frequent skin infections no longer have this problem.

Another potential disadvantage of pump therapy is the risk of sudden extreme hyperglycemia or diabetic ketoacidosis. This is especially true if the patient is using Humalog or lispro in the pump. Because only regular or fast-acting insulin is used, and if there is a prolonged interruption of insulin delivery, one can quickly develop extreme hyperglycemia and ketoacidosis. This is easily counteracted by always carrying an extra bottle of regular or Humalog insulin, as well as being knowledgeable about sick-day rules.

Financial concerns are always an issue, as the cost of insulin pump therapy with the accompanying supplies may be prohibitive if your patient does not have good insurance coverage. The pump itself costs 3000–4000 dollars and the supplies, which include insulin infusion lines, syringes, tape, and batteries, can run an additional 40–50 dollars a month. Most insurance companies will reimburse at least 80% with appropriately applied pressure by you and your patient. Representatives from the two insulin pump companies also have special staff to help you deal with the usual bureaucratic process.

Many patients who travel frequently will have hassles at the airport when they go through the airport security station. Sometimes, but not always, the insulin pump sets off the metal detector alarm, and your patient will have to explain that he or she is on an insulin pump. Lastly, some-individuals become tired of having

Table 3 Disadvantages of Insulin Pump Therapy

Risk of sudden extreme hyperglycemia and diabetic ketoacidosis
Skin infections and abscesses
Financial concerns
Hassles at the airport
Always having a bodily attachment

something ''connected to the body'' all of the time. When this occurs, I recommend a pump vacation, during which the patients goes back to multiple daily injections for a few days to weeks. The disadvantages of insulin pump therapy are listed in Table 3.

There are also many misconceptions about insulin pump therapy that you and your patients need to know (Table 4). Home glucose monitoring is still as important as ever with insulin pump therapy. When insulin pump therapy is initiated, more glucose monitoring is required, although later on, when the patient is well adjusted, the frequency of home glucose monitoring will be dependent on the variability of the patients day-to-day activities. Many patients think that insulin pump therapy will allow them to eat anything they want at anytime. It is important to realize that although meal times and amounts can be quite flexible with insulin pump therapy, the patient must maintain some degree of dietary discretion to maintain or improve glycemic control. In addition, unwanted weight gain occurs in some individuals who begin to overliberalize their diets, despite good glycemic control. Insulin pump therapy is not contraindicated for persons with hypoglycemic unawareness, and insulin pumps are not only for individuals with type 1 diabetes.

A great way to help your patient decide if he or she would be an insulin pump candidate is to talk to persons with personal experience. Have your patient check with the local American Diabetes Association or Juvenile Diabetes Foundation in your area to find a support group for persons who use insulin pumps. It is the individuals in these groups who will tell your patient the nitty-gritty of living

Table 4 Misconceptions About Insulin Pump Therapy

Home glucose monitoring is still needed as much
Insulin pumps for ''pigging out''
Contraindicated for persons with hypoglycemic unawareness
Insulin pump therapy is for type 1 diabetes only

with a pump on a day-to-day basis. In addition, both insulin pump companies have information that they will send to your patient, including video tapes and manuals. There are two insulin pump companies with excellent products (MiniMed Technologies; 1-800-933-3322, and Disetronic Medical Systems; 1-800-280-7801).

V. WHAT IS AN INSULIN PUMP AND HOW DOES IT WORK?

The pancreas of a nondiabetic individual secretes small amounts of insulin 24 h a day (basal rate), even if no food is ingested. Insulin is needed for normal metabolic function and the prevention of diabetic ketoacidosis. The pancreas also normally secretes larger amounts of insulin (bolus rates) when a person ingests a meal to prevent postprandial hyperglycemia. The insulin pump was designed to mimic, as closely as possible, a normal-functioning pancreas with basal and

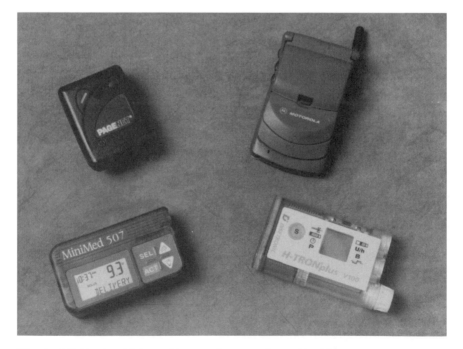

Fig. 1 MiniMed and Disetronic pumps in comparison with a beeper and a small cellular phone.

bolus rates that can be adjusted for individual needs based on prior experience and home glucose-monitoring results.

Insulin pumps are now about the same size as a deck of cards, a beeper, or a small cellular phone (Fig. 1). They weigh approximately 115 g (4 oz) and can be put in a pocket, on a belt, in a specially designed bra, inside a sock or panty hose, and many other ingenious areas that patients have discovered. You can make an analogy between an insulin pump and an automatic, computerized and mechanical insulin syringe that delivers insulin in a more physiological fashion. Insulin pumps have a lever that mechanically pushes down a plunger of a large insulin syringe (3.0 mL or 300 U of insulin) automatically 24 h a day (basal rate), and on demand before meals (bolus rate). The insulin then travels through a long infusion tube from the insulin syringe, that is housed in the insulin pump, to the subcutaneous tissue through an implanted-bent needle or a soft, flexible catheter. The infusion lines now have a quick-release mechanism and can be temporarily disconnected from the insertion site (Fig. 2). These quick-release

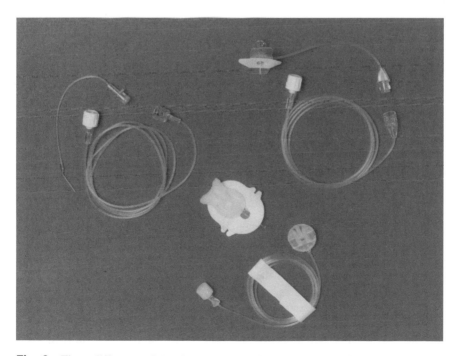

Fig. 2 Three different quick-release catheters for insulin pump therapy: bent needle (upper left), soft-set (upper right), and tender (bottom). Both catheter infusion lines are introduced with a needle that is removed after the catheter has been placed in the subcutaneous tissue.

catheters make showering, swimming, dressing, and other activities much more convenient.

Only regular or fast-acting insulin is used in the insulin pumps. The basal rate of the insulin pump replaces the intermediate- and longer-acting insulins, such as NPH, Lente or Ultra Lente. The boluses given before each meal are basically the same as with normal insulin injections of regular Humalog. Unfortunately, current insulin pumps do not have glucose sensors, although this technology is being advanced at a very rapid pace and may be available in the near future. Most pump wearers insert the catheter or bent needle in the abdominal area, although the upper outer quadrant of the buttocks, upper thighs and triceps fat pad of the arms can also be used (Fig. 3). It is recommended that the syringe and the infusion set be filled and changed every 3 days. However, many patients use their infusion sets much longer (up to 6 days) before changing. Prolonged use of the infusion set at a single site increases the likelihood of irritation or superficial abscess formation that may require antibiotic therapy or incision and drainage in the office setting. This scenario is very infrequent, and most irritated sites improve on their own without the need for antibiotics or other interventions. Insulin pumps have disposable batteries that last approximately 8 weeks. Both types of insulin pumps have built in alarms to prevent inadvertent insulin delivery or to warn the patient if the insulin pump is empty or if the infusion set becomes clogged or dysfunctional.

VI. INITIATING INSULIN PUMP THERAPY

In the ideal setting, successful initiation of insulin pump therapy should be orchestrated by an educated and motivated health care team, including a physician, diabetes educator, registered dietitian, and a pump counselor with access to an inpatient ward. However, outpatient initiation of insulin pump therapy is a more realistic setting for integrating pump routines into an individual's lifestyle and is a necessity because of third-party reimbursement plans. Before initiating insulin pump therapy, it is important to review several topics with the patient (Table 5). Both insulin companies have very knowledgeable professionals who are available to help educate your patients on these important topics before, during, and after initiation of insulin pump therapy.

Initiating insulin pump therapy as an outpatient is feasible and requires frequent contact with the patient for only 2–3 days. After the patient has been educated on the workings of the insulin pump and infusion lines, bolus and basal rates are determined and set. The patient is encouraged to follow his or her routine daily schedule with frequent home glucose monitoring. Blood glucose values should be obtained before and 1–2 h after each meal, at bedtime, and at 3 AM. These values will help you adjust the premeal bolus rates as well as the continuous

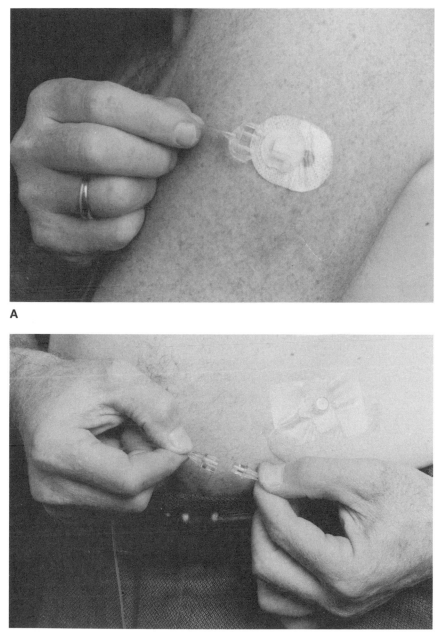

A

B

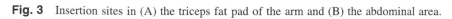

Fig. 3   Insertion sites in (A) the triceps fat pad of the arm and (B) the abdominal area.

Table 5   Topics to Review Before Initiating Insulin Pump Therapy

Target goals for glucose control
Prevention of diabetic ketoacidosis
Prevention of hypoglycemia
Insulin pump and infusion set operation (catheter care)
Guidelines for basal rate and bolus adjustments
Sick-day rules
Trouble-shooting for unexplained hyperglycemia

basal rates during a 24-h period and assess if the patient needs any secondary basal rates to counteract the dawn phenomenon, for example.

The initial bolus and basal rates can be based on the patient's prior insulin regimen or on the 24-h insulin requirements. I put most of my patients on an intensive insulin regimen using human Ultra Lente prebreakfast and predinner, with Humalog or regular insulin before each meal. In this manner I simply take the total Ultra Lente dose and divide it by 24 h to calculate the basal rate. If the patient had very good glucose control on the prior intensive insulin regimen with Ultra Lente and regular, I reduce the basal rate by 20% because many individuals need less insulin when initiating pump therapy. For the premeal boluses, I recommend the same Humalog or regular insulin doses.

The basal rate can also be calculated by taking 50% of the total combined insulin requirements of the patient and dividing it by 24 h. Once again I usually reduce this rate by 20% if the patient's glucose control was fairly good before initiating insulin pump therapy. For example, if a patient's total daily combined insulin dose is 50 U and the degree of control is quite poor, I would simply calculate the basal insulin dose as 25 U divided by 24 h equaling approximately 1.0 U/h.

Calculation of the basal rate can also be estimated or confirmed based on the patient's body weight. A conservative starting dose for the basal rate can be calculated, by using 0.22 U/kg body weight per day. For example, if a patient weighs 80 kg, then the basal rate should be 0.7 U/h (80 kg × 0.22 units ÷ by 24 h). If there is discrepancy in the estimated basal rate using these different techniques, the lower rate should be chosen for initiation of insulin pump therapy. It is also important to discontinue the patient's intermediate- or long-acting insulin at least 12–24 h before initiating pump therapy.   .

VII.   VERIFYING THE BASAL AND BOLUS RATES

To verify the overnight basal rate, the patient should try to avoid eating food after dinner and test the glucose value 2 h after dinner, at bedtime, 3 AM, and first thing in the morning. These values are very important to determine if the patient needs an increased basal rate in the early morning hours to counteract the dawn phenomenon (AM resistance to insulin caused by circulating growth hormone levels). In my experience, many patients will experience a rise in blood glucose values between 3 and 7 in the morning, requiring a 0.1 to 0.4-U/h increase during that time period. Occasionally a patient may experience a decrease in basal insulin requirements between the hours of 12 midnight and 3 AM. The majority of pump users will achieve excellent glycemic control with three or fewer basal rates per day.

Evaluating the daytime and evening basal rates can be determined by having the patient fast from the morning until dinnertime. If this is inconvenient, then I would suggest having the patient eat a very early breakfast, to skip lunch and monitor the blood sugars every 2–3 h up until dinner time. An adequate basal rate will allow ideal glucose control (between 70 and 110 mg/dL) while in the fasting state during the normal daily activities.

VIII. DETERMINING BOLUS RATES

The premeal bolus rates of insulin have usually been predetermined, before beginning insulin pump therapy, based on the patient's insulin regimen. The total daily dose of regular or Humalog insulin should be approximately 50% of the total daily insulin requirements. Some patients like to use the old dietary exchange system and others count carbohydrates and base their premeal regular dose on the total grams of carbohydrates. Many patients have been diabetic for several years and have a very good sense of how much insulin they need for any particular meal, based on years of prior experience. In general, the premeal insulin dose should be based on prior experience, the premeal glucose value, and any anticipated exercise after the ingestion of the meal.

When suggesting supplemental regular or Humalog insulin to counteract an elevated blood sugar level, one can use "1500" rule. The 1500 rule or sensitivity factor gives an estimation of how much the patient's blood sugar concentration will drop when given 1 U of regular or Humalog insulin. One simply takes the patient's total daily insulin requirements and divides that number into 1500. For example, if a patient uses 50 U of insulin per day, 1 U of Humalog or regular insulin will lower the blood sugar value by approximately 30 mg/dL (1500 divided by 50). This particular patient would take an additional 1 U extra of regular or Humalog insulin for every 30 mg/dL above the goal glucose value (i.e., 120 mg/dL).

Once the patient initiates pump therapy he or she should make contact with the caregiver at least once every 24-h period to go over the glucose values and to have answered any questions or concerns that have arisen. The glucose values could be easily forwarded to the caregiver by facsimile or e-mail before telephoning. In most patients after 2–3 days the bolus and basal rates are fairly close to the ultimate final values, and the patient can be seen in approximately 2–4 weeks.

IX. SPECIAL PRECAUTIONS AND EVERYDAY MANAGEMENT

One of the most important precautions for patients using insulin pump therapy is unexplained severe hyperglycemia and sick-day rules. Because there is no intermediate or long-acting insulin in the patient's circulation, a disruption in regular or Humalog insulin delivery can result in a fairly rapid rise in glucose concentration and subsequent development of diabetic ketoacidosis. The patient should be well trained in trouble-shooting and should always have a bottle of Humalog or regular insulin with a syringe or insulin pen. In general, I highly suggest using Humalog in the insulin pump, although it is not FDA approved at the current time. The benefits of Humalog or lispro insulin are an improved postprandial glucose value and a decreased incidence and severity of delayed hypoglycemia (i.e., 3–5 h after a meal), especially during exercise. The disadvantages of Humalog insulin for pump therapy are that if there is an unexpected discontinuation of insulin delivery (catheter dislodged, blockage, or an empty reservoir) the patient will experience a more rapid rise in the glucose value. In addition, temporary pump discontinuation for showers, exercise, and such, can be for only a very short time, no longer than 45–60 min.

I do not recommend initiating insulin pump therapy during pregnancy because a novice pump user would be at more risk for diabetic ketoacidosis than someone who is knowledgeable, comfortable, and had several months to years of experience with insulin pump therapy.

The new quick-release catheters are excellent for showering, bathing, and dressing, although if this type of catheter is not available, the pump can simply be put into a zip-lock bag and held in one hand or placed on a nearby shelf or soap dish during showering or bathing. Placement of the insulin pump during sleeping and sexual intimacy is usually not a problem, with occasional entanglement in body parts. Many patients use the quick-release catheters to free themselves from the insulin pump during sexual intimacy or short periods of intensive exercise.

Traveling with an insulin pump is very convenient, especially when crossing many time zones and having erratic meal amounts, types, and times. The only hassle is going through the airport security with fairly ignorant personnel. Many times the insulin pump will not trigger the airport security alarm, and I would suggest taking all pens, coins, beepers, and any other metal off before going through the security. This will help your patients avoid a hand search or a delayed passage through security.

Many patients enjoy a ''pump'' vacation from insulin pump therapy when they are enjoying a water sport weekend or just want to be totally free of any mechanically device connected to their body for a few days or weeks. In this case, I recommend that the patients go back to their previous intensive insulin regimen consisting of an intermediate- or long-acting insulin twice a day with regular or Humalog insulin before each meal.

X. CASE PRESENTATION

A 28-year-old man with a 15-year history of type 1 diabetes mellitus requests an insulin pump-because of difficulty controlling his diabetes. For the past 4 years, the patient has been on a multiple injection regimen consisting of human Ultra Lente insulin twice a day (8 U before breakfast and 12-U before dinner) and a regular insulin algorithm preprandially (approximately 5–10 U of regular insulin before each meal). He experiences extreme fluctuations in his daily blood glucose measurements, ranging between 40 and 400 mg/dL, despite testing his blood glucose levels four to eight times a day. Over the past 12 months, he has had two severe hypoglycemic reactions that occurred in the late afternoon and required assistance. The patient follows a fairly regular diet and exercise program, even though he is a traveling salesman and cannot always eat and exercise at the same times each day. He is not prone to bacterial skin infections and is very motivated to reduce the extreme highs and lows in his blood glucose levels as well as his gycosolated hemoglobin value (most recent value of 8.5%, normal 4–6%).

A. Case Discussion

Insulin pump therapy has several advantages that would help this particular patient, including (a) a significant reduction in the extreme high and low blood glucose values; (b) a reduction in the glycosylated hemoglobin value; (c) flexibility in lifestyle for time and quantity of meal and exercise scheduling; and (d) effective control of glucose values during the early morning hours (dawn phenomenon). This patient has one of the most important qualities of a pump candidate, which are reliability and compliance with treatment regimens and home glucose monitoring. He is knowledgeable on sick-day rules and knows how to adjust his dose of regular insulin, depending on his premeal blood sugar value. Because he does have the propensity for hypoglycemia unawareness, insulin pump therapy can be especially beneficial. The glycemic goal in patients such as this one with a history of hypoglycemia unawareness should be kept at a slightly higher and safer range to avoid unconscious reactions. The level should not be too high so that microvascular and macrovascular complications can be prevented or delayed. His glucose values should be kept in the mid−100- to 200-mg/dL range instead of the 70- to 160-mg/dL range that should be targeted in patients without hypoglycemic unawareness.

The hourly basal rate can be calculated by taking 50% of the total daily insulin requirements and dividing by 24 h. In this patient, the basal rate would be initiated at 0.7 U/h (20 Ultra Lente plus 20 regular) divided by 24 h. His initial preprandial bolus rates will be the same as they were on the multiple injection regimen which were based on his pre- and postprandial home glucose-monitoring results. Once this patient is comfortable using insulin pump therapy, I would convert him over to using the fast-acting insulin analogue lispro or Humalog.

XI. SUMMARY

Insulin pump therapy is a practical tool for treating patients with type 1 and insulin-requiring type 2 diabetes who have not achieved adequate glycemic control on conventional insulin injection regimens or are seeking an improved quality of life. Insulin pump therapy allows improved glycemic control, thereby preventing and delaying the complications of diabetes, in addition to reducing the incidence of extreme hyperglycemia and hypoglycemia. Insulin pump therapy can improve growth and development in poorly controlled adolescents with type 1 diabetes and reduce glucose toxicity, thus reducing insulin resistance and improving beta-cell function in persons with type 2 diabetes. From a patient's point of view insulin pump therapy has proved to be beneficial in many aspects, including a much more flexible lifestyle, while simultaneously enjoying improved glucose control. Insulin pump therapy permits increased flexibility in meal timing and amounts, increased flexibility in the time and intensity of exercise, and is invaluable for people traveling across time zones or with variable work schedules.

An appropriate insulin pump candidate should be someone who is interested in his or her diabetes and is reliable and compliant. Patients need to continue performing home glucose monitoring and be cautious about overliberalizing their diet. Initiating insulin pump therapy as an outpatient is easily achieved, especially if the patient has already been put on a multiple daily injection regimen. In general, 50% of the total daily insulin requirements are translated into a 24-h basal rate and the other 50% used as premeal boluses. Many patients need a secondary basal rate to cover the dawn phenomenon, and overall adjustment and acceptance of the insulin pump occurs quite quickly. Once a patient is instructed to adjust his or her diabetes on a day-to-day basis using home glucose monitoring, the work for the caregiver becomes quite minimal. More physicians and other caregivers need to become knowledgeable about insulin pump therapy so that they can at least offer them to potential candidates.

BIBLIOGRAPHY

Fredrickson L, ed. The Insulin Pump Therapy Book; Insights From the Experts. MiniMed Technologies, 1995.
Pickup JC, ed. Brittle Diabetes. Boston: Blackwell Scientific, 1985.
Walsh PA, Roberts R. Pumping Insulin; the Art of Using an Insulin Pump. MiniMed Technologies, 1989.
Walsh PA, Roberts R. Pumping Insulin: Everything in a Book for Successful Use of an Insulin Pump. 2nd ed. Torrey Pines Press, 1994, ii.

20
Pancreas Transplantation

Elizabeth R. Seaquist and David E. R. Sutherland
University of Minnesota, Minneapolis, Minnesota

I. INTRODUCTION

Pancreas transplantation has been used as therapy for type 1 diabetes mellitus for the last 20 or more years. It is the only therapy that successfully renders such patients insulin-independent and normoglycemic. However, successful transplantation requires subjects to be maintained on long-term immunosuppression, which increases their risk for infection and malignancy. Whether patients ultimately live longer and with less morbidity using life-long immunosuppression following pancreas transplantation than when using traditional insulin therapy is uncertain. Consequently, it is difficult for the practitioner to determine which patients would benefit most from pancreas transplantation. In this chapter, we will review the technique of pancreas and islet transplantation, discuss the risks and benefits of the procedure, and develop a list of indications and contraindications for this surgical therapy. At the end, clinicians will have a better understanding of the role pancreas transplantation plays in the treatment of their patients with type 1 diabetes.

II. TECHNIQUE OF PANCREAS AND ISLET TRANSPLANTATION

The goal of pancreas and islet transplantation is to provide a full complement of insulin-secreting pancreatic beta cells to a recipient with type 1 diabetes. This seemingly simple task is complicated by the complex structural and physiological relations present in the pancreas. The beta cells are the predominant cell type found in pancreatic islets, and they represent about 1% of the total pancreatic mass. The remaining 99% of the pancreas is composed of exocrine tissue that secretes digestive enzymes into the small intestine. Islets are composed of beta cells and three other types of endocrine cells: the glucagon-secreting alpha cell, the somatostatin-secreting delta cell, and the pancreatic polypeptide-secreting pp cell. To accomplish the goal of replacing the beta cells in a patient with type 1 diabetes, transplantation of isolated beta cells, isolated islets, or unmanipulated pancreatic tissue could be considered. The techniques necessary to isolate beta cells from the other islet cells have not yet been sufficiently well developed to render beta cells suitable for human transplantation. Isolation of functional islets from the exocrine tissue has been successfully performed for more than a decade, but survival of transplanted islets has been difficult to achieve. Consequently, insertion of unmanipulated pancreatic tissue has been and remains the transplant procedure of choice for patients with type 1 diabetes.

Most pancreas transplants involve the placement of an entire cadaveric pancreas into the abdomen of a recipient, although in some cases hemipancreas grafts have been used. In the vast majority of cases, a cadaver donor is used, but a very few centers will also consider using living donors. The most successful surgical approach has been to place the graft into the pelvis, anastamose the vasculature with the iliac artery and vein, and divert the exocrine secretions into either the urinary bladder or the native intestine (Fig. 1). Bladder drainage readily allows on-going noninvasive monitoring for graft rejection because the amount of amylase measured in the urine is high in patients with functioning pancreas grafts. If the quantity of amylase drops in the urine, graft rejection can be confirmed by biopsy before aggressively treating the patient before the endocrine tissue fails. Complications of diverting the exocrine effluent into the urinary bladder include excessive loss of bicarbonate and fluid into the urine and hemorrhage cystitis. If these complications cannot be overcome with medical therapy, a second operation in which the exocrine secretions are diverted into the intestines can be performed.

Much interest has been focused at the transplantation of isolated islets over the years. Most recently, the preferred route of administration has been as an intravenous injection into the umbilical vein. Islets then travel to the liver where they take up residence in the portal regions. Despite the simplicity of such an operation, islet transplantation has generally not been a successful procedure. The precise reason for its lack of success is uncertain, but may involve recurrence of autoimmune disease in the transplanted islets, drug toxicity, or immunological factors involved in the placement of the islets into the liver.

III. IMMUNOSUPPRESSION

All recipients of allografts require life-long immunosuppression to prevent graft rejection. Pancreas transplant recipients generally receive the same types of regi-

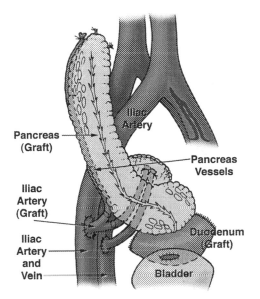

Fig. 1 Transplantation of a pancreas allograft: The donor organ is placed into the pelvis with exocrine effluent diverted into the bladder. Vascular anastomoses are established with the iliac artery and vein.

mens as other solid-organ recipients, with an effort over time to decrease the amount of prednisone prescribed or replace it with a newer agent. All immunosuppressive drugs carry the risk of increasing susceptibility to infections, particularly those that are viral and fungal in origin, and of malignancy. The drugs most commonly used and their individual side effects are listed in Table 1.

IV. SURGICAL COMPLICATIONS AND SURVIVAL RATES

Pancreas transplantation is associated with various surgical complications, including graft thrombosis, infection, graft pancreatitis, bleeding, and anastomotic leaks. In a retrospective evaluation of 445 consecutive transplants performed at our center, 35% of recipients experienced a significant surgical complication (1). The risk of developing a surgical complication in the first 3 months after transplantation was greater in those subjects undergoing simultaneous pancreas–kidney transplants (SPK) than in those who underwent a pancreas transplant alone (PTA) or after a kidney transplant (PAK) (2). Fortunately, the rate of graft failure from

Table 1 Immunosuppressive Drugs Used in Pancreas Transplantation

Drug name	Commercial name	Side effects[a]
Prednisone	Deltasone	Weight gain, osteoporosis, diabetes
Azathioprine	Imuran	Pancytopenia, nausea and vomiting
Cyclosporine	Neoral	Nephrotoxicity
Tacrolimus (FK 506)	Prograf	Nephrotoxicity, neurotoxicity (headache, tremor, motor dysfunction), hypertension
Mycophenolate mofetil	Cellcept	Diarrhea, neutropenia, fetal malformations

[a] All immunosuppressive drugs increase the risk of serious infections and lymphoproliferative disorders.

technical reasons in the United States is dropping over time in all patients (Table 2).

For those transplantation procedures that are technically successful, the greatest risk for subsequent loss of function is immunological. As immunosuppressive drugs have improved over the years, the rates of rejection have decreased (Fig. 2). The risk of immunological loss is greater in PTA cases than in the others.

With improved surgical techniques and better immunosuppression, the rates of overall graft survival have improved over the years (Fig. 3). For those patients who received transplants between 1994 and 1997, 73% remained insulin-independent at the end of the first year. Overall patient survival rates have also continued to improve. One-year patient survival rates for those receiving transplants in the

Table 2 Technical Failure Rates During the First Year After Transplant and Total Number of Operations Performed by Era in the United States

Type[a]	1990–1991		1992–1993		1994–1996	
	%	n	%	n	%	n
SPK	13	869	10	1077	8	1995
PAK	31	75	21	84	13	179
PTA	25	48	18	72	11	90

[a] SPK, simultaneous pancreas–kidney transplant; PAK, pancreas transplant after kidney transplant; PTA, pancreas transplant alone.
Source: Ref. 4.

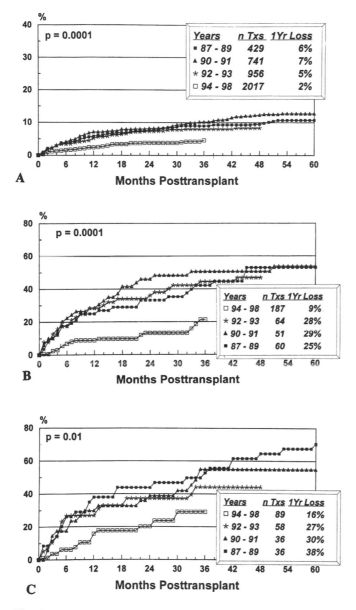

Fig. 2 Rates of immunological pancreas graft loss by era for all U.S. cadaver-drained pancreas transplants from 10/1/87 to 6/1/98: (A) simultaneous pancreas and kidney transplants; (B) pancreas transplant after kidney transplant; (C) pancreas transplant alone.

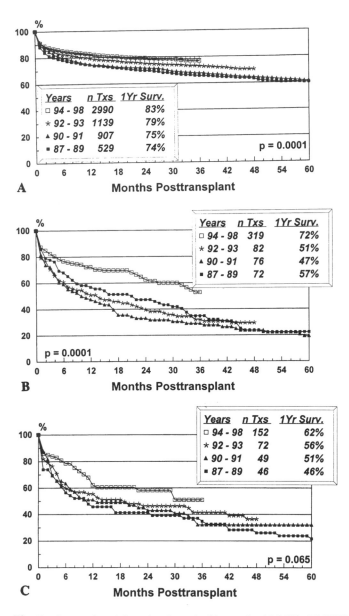

Fig. 3 Rates of graft functional survival by era for 10/1/87–6/1/98 U.S. cadaver pancreas transplants: (A) simultaneous pancreas and kidney transplant; (B) pancreas transplant after kidney; (C) pancreas transplant alone.

United States between 1994 and 1997 was 94% for those who received a pancreas and kidney transplant simultaneously, 95% for those who received a pancreas after a kidney transplant, and 93% for those who received a pancreas transplant alone (3).

Currently, many patients who require a kidney transplant for diabetic nephropathy are considered candidates for a simultaneous pancreas transplant. One concern about placing a pancreas graft in such patients is the influence such a procedure may have on graft and patient survival following kidney transplantation. Data from the United Network for Organ Sharing (UNOS) Registry from 1987–1996 demonstrate that the 1- and 3-year kidney graft survival rates were 90 and 68%, respectively, for patients with type 1 diabetes (4). In those patients who simultaneously received a pancreas and kidney grafts between 1987 and 1997, the kidney survival rates were 86 and 79%, respectively. However, in a nonrandomized and retrospective evaluation of the effect of pancreas transplantation on patient survival following kidney transplant, Manske and colleagues found that the 3-year patient survival rate is lower (68 vs. 90%) in patients who received simultaneous transplants than in those patients given a kidney alone (5). Unfortunately, not all of these patients received their transplants at the same center or were exposed to the same postsurgical care, suggesting that variables other than simultaneous pancreas transplant may have an influence on survival following a kidney transplant. In a separate study, Rosen and colleagues observed that patients receiving simultaneous kidney–pancreas grafts experience more frequent rejection episodes, more cytomegalovirus (CMV) infections, and more wound infections, and that these complications result in more hospitalizations than are seen in patients receiving a kidney alone (6). These investigations raise the question of whether simultaneous pancreas–kidney transplantation should be routinely recommended in patients with type 1 diabetes and diabetic nephropathy. Until a randomized trial is performed, perhaps only those patients without serious comorbidities should be considered for simultaneous transplantation.

V. METABOLIC CONSEQUENCES OF PANCREAS TRANSPLANTATION

Patients undergo pancreas transplantation to acquire insulin independence and avoid the long-term complications of diabetes mellitus. Insulin independence with normoglycemia occurs in more than 70% of pancreas transplant recipients at 1 year, and long-term follow-up demonstrates continued metabolic success in most subjects up to 5 years after transplantation (Fig. 4; 7). Following successful pancreas transplantation, patients with systemic venous drainage of their grafts uni-

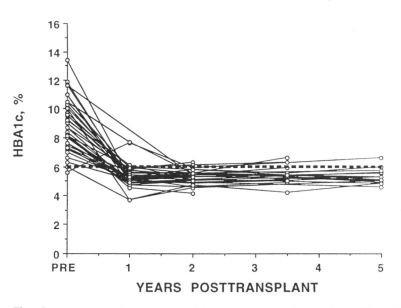

Fig. 4 Long-term glycemic control in pancreas transplant patients: Hemoglobin A_{1c} (HBA_{1c}) levels were measured on at least two occasions posttransplantation for as long as 5 years in 38 transplant recipients. The dashed horizontal line represents the upper limit of normal. (From Ref. 7.)

formly have basal hyperinsulinemia and increased insulin secretory response to intravenously administered glucose and arginine (8). Interestingly, the insulin secretory reserve capacity in recipients of a successful pancreas transplant is diminished, perhaps as a result of the immunosuppressive drugs used to prevent rejection (9). Despite this observation, some patients are at risk for the development of spontaneous hypoglycemia following pancreas transplantation, particularly after meals. In at least a few episodes, spontaneous hypoglycemia has led to serious sequelae in those patients with such problems after receiving transplants. Why some patients develop spontaneous hypoglycemia is uncertain.

Following pancreas transplantation, patients with type 1 diabetes mellitus once again regain their ability to secrete glucagon in response to hypoglycemia, although the secretory response is less exuberant than that seen in normal volunteers. With the return of hypoglycemia-induced glucagon secretion comes a return of hypoglycemia-induced endogenous glucose production. Observations such as these have made pancreas transplantation a particularly attractive option for patients with severe hypoglycemic unawareness.

VI. THE EFFECTS OF PANCREAS TRANSPLANTATION ON THE COMPLICATIONS OF DIABETES

Because the Diabetes Complications and Control Trial (DCCT) so clearly demonstrated that improving glycemic control prevents or forestalls the development of the microvascular complications of diabetes in patients with the type 1 form of the disease, more patients and physicians have considered the possibility of treating type 1 diabetes with pancreas transplantation. As noted previously, successful pancreas transplantation produces long-standing normoglycemia without the use of parenterally administered insulin or carefully monitored food plans. Consequently, one would expect that pancreas transplantation would decrease the risk of developing diabetic complications. Unfortunately, proving that successful pancreas transplantation prevents or reverses diabetic complications has been difficult, perhaps in large part because patients have received transplants late in the course of their disease, long after the first signs of diabetic complications have appeared.

In 1988, Ramsay and colleagues published the first report documenting the effect of successful pancreas transplantation on diabetic retinopathy in a small group of patients with type 1 diabetes and established retinopathy (10). After 2 years of successful graft function, no differences were noted in the rates at which retinopathy progressed in the eyes of successful pancreas transplant recipients as compared with the recipients of grafts that failed. Reports from other centers (4,11), but not all (12), replicated these findings and have led to the general agreement that, at least for those patients with established retinopathy, pancreatic transplantation is without obvious benefit on the progression of this complication (Table 3).

Table 3 Effect of Successful Pancreas Transplant on the Secondary Complications of Diabetes

Secondary complication	Effect of successful graft	Refs.
Retinopathy	No benefit	10
Peripheral neuropathy		
Clinical examination	No long-term benefit	13
Nerve conduction velocities	Beneficial	13
Autonomic neuropathy	Beneficial	13
Diabetic nephropathy	Beneficial effect noted after 10 years	17
Lipids	May worsen	19
Macrovascular disease	May increase risk	18
Quality of life	Very beneficial	20

Successful pancreas transplantation may provide more benefit to patients with established diabetic neuropathy. Most studies have demonstrated that patients may experience some symptomatic improvement within months of receiving a successful transplant, and small but significant changes in nerve conduction velocities have been consistently noted over time in patients with functioning grafts (13,14). Scores derived from a comprehensive clinical examination do not show much improvement in most patients over time, but the inevitable deterioration seen in similarly affected patients who did not undergo successful pancreatic transplantation appears to be halted. Consequently, it appears that pancreatic transplantation can halt the progression of peripheral neuropathy in patients with type 1 diabetes (see Table 3).

The effects of pancreatic transplantation on autonomic neuropathy also appears to be positive. In patients with established autonomic neuropathy, a successful pancreas transplant significantly slowed the rate at which cardiorespiratory reflex function declines during the first year. A successful graft in a patient with established autonomic neuropathy also provides a survival advantage because more of these patients were alive after 60 months of follow-up than were neuropathic patients who did not receive a successful graft. Unfortunately, the mortality rate of patients with autonomic neuropathy following an unsuccessful pancreatic transplantation was very high, suggesting that patients with autonomic neuropathy may experience substantial risk at the time of transplantation, but if the graft is successful, they have a greater chance of survival (see Table 3; 15).

Recent reports on the effect of pancreatic transplantation on diabetic nephropathy suggest that the procedure may ultimately reverse the nephropathic lesions associated with a strong likelihood of progression to end-stage renal disease. In 1989, Bilous and colleagues reported their observations of a group of successful pancreas transplant recipients who underwent their transplant some years after they had received a successful kidney transplant for diabetic nephropathy. When the biopsies from these transplanted kidneys were compared with the renal biopsies from matched kidney transplant controls with type 1 diabetes who had not undergone a pancreas transplant, the pancreas transplant recipients displayed less severe diabetic changes at the end of a mean of 2 years of follow-up (16). More recently, Fioretto and colleagues reported that the glomerular lesions associated with diabetic nephropathy in the native kidneys of patients with type 1 diabetes who underwent a successful pancreas transplant alone began to normalize after 10 years (17). Taken together, these observations suggest that the normoglycemia imposed by a successful pancreas transplant can probably prevent the progression of diabetic nephropathy and may even reverse this complication in patients with early-stage renal disease (see Table 3).

The macrovascular complications of diabetes appear to be increased in patients with type 1 diabetes who have received a successful pancreas transplant. Morissey and colleagues reported the results of a nonrandomized, retrospective controlled study in 1997 in which they found that despite the presence of fewer cardiovascular risk factors before undergoing pancreas transplant, recipients of a successful pancreas and kidney transplant experienced more complications attributed to peripheral vascular disease in the 4 years after surgery than did a similar group of patients with type 1 diabetes who received a kidney transplant alone (18). Some investigators have suggested this may be due to the hyperinsulinemia that invariably results from the systemic venous drainage of the pancreas graft. Interestingly, Bagdade and colleagues recently found that the recipients of successful pancreas transplants have the same proatherogenic level of cholesterol ester transfer as patients with type 1 diabetes, suggesting that the euglycemia imposed by the transplant may not necessarily lower the atherosclerotic risk for these patients (see Table 3; 19).

VII. EFFECT OF PANCREAS TRANSPLANTATION ON THE QUALITY OF LIFE

Many patients seek a pancreas transplant in an effort to improve their quality of life. They report that the daily demands of insulin therapy and consistent nutritional intake, with the attendant risk of hypoglycemia and long-term complications of diabetes, have a profoundly negative influence on their quality of life and that undergoing a pancreas transplant would be worth the risk of avoiding these ongoing concerns. Over the last decade, several groups have rigorously addressed the question of whether pancreatic transplantation alters the quality of life of patients with type 1 diabetes. Without exception, these studies demonstrate that those recipients of successful pancreas grafts rate their quality of life to be much higher after the transplant than before. Of interest, even the majority of patients who suffered from surgical complications and subsequently lost their graft in the first few months after transplantation report a desire to undergo a repeat pancreas transplant (20). Although these studies have all been performed in a select group of patients who actively sought a pancreas transplant, they are very consistent in demonstrating that pancreatic transplantation increases the quality of life for patients with type 1 diabetes (see Table 3).

VIII. INDICATIONS AND CONTRAINDICATIONS

Pancreatic transplantation offers patients with type 1 diabetes an alternative therapy to lifelong insulin administration. Indeed, the glycemic control provided by a successful pancreas transplant is probably superior to that provided by insulin therapy, and as patients with normoglycemia will have a reduced risk of diabetes complications, some assert that pancreatic transplantation is appropriate for all patients with type 1 diabetes who wish to avoid the long-term risks of persistently elevated blood glucose concentrations. Unfortunately, predicting which patients are at risk for developing complications, even in the face of the excellent level of glucose control that can be achieved by intensive insulin therapy, is not possible in the early stages of the disease, and the relative risks of long-term insulin therapy versus long-term immunosuppression have not been determined. In the absence of a controlled trial in which patients without complications are randomized to receive a pancreas transplant or intensive insulin therapy, clinicians and their patients are left to make their own decisions about who meets the conditions necessary to undergo a pancreas transplant.

Most clinicians have come to believe that pancreatic transplantation should be considered in all patients with type 1 diabetes who require a kidney transplant. Such patients will already be subjected to the risks of long-term immunosuppression to maintain their renal graft, and the anesthesia risk of a longer operation is felt to be low. However, data from nonrandomized studies suggest patients who receive a simultaneous pancreas–kidney transplant may have greater morbidity and mortality than patients who receive a kidney transplant alone. These data are very compelling, but arise from studies in which a substantial patient selection bias occurred. Consequently, at the University of Minnesota we continue to recommend that patients with diabetic nephropathy consider undergoing a simultaneous kidney–pancreas transplant whenever possible.

Some clinicians recommend that patients with severe hypoglycemic unawareness be offered pancreas transplant as an alternative therapy to insulin. Although successful pancreatic transplantation will usually avoid the recurrent problems with severe hypoglycemia experienced by such patients, merely stepping back from the intensity of insulin therapy is usually as successful in relieving their hypoglycemic symptoms.

Patients with debilitating complications from diabetes are often referred for pancreatic transplantation in the hope that the complications will be reversed by the surgery. Unfortunately, successful transplantation cannot reverse diabetic retinopathy, has limited benefit on symptomatic peripheral neuropathy, and may not alter the course of macrovascular complications. Patients with autonomic neuropathy may experience relief of their symptoms and may be appropriately referred for a pancreas transplant, but if it is unsuccessful, these patients appear to have greater mortality than patients who never underwent the operation. Recent data suggest that pancreatic transplantation may have a positive effect on the morphological lesions associated with diabetic nephropathy, but the magnitude of these changes are small; and their functional effect is unknown.

Despite all of the foregoing limitations, the effect of successful pancreas transplantation on the quality of life experienced by a patient has been well demonstrated. For this reason, we believe that pancreas transplantation can be considered as an alternative therapy for patients with type 1 diabetes at any stage of their disease. In deciding whether a pancreas transplant is the appropriate therapy for a patient, the clinician must work with the patient and their family members to ensure that they understand all the risks and benefits associated with the operation for the individual patient. For many patients, the risk of long-term immunosuppression outweighs any benefits of a successful pancreas transplant, but for some, the risk may be considered to be minor compared with ongoing insulin injections. Ascertaining the quality of another's life is difficult, at best, and if a well-informed patient with type 1 diabetes selects the risks of pancreas transplantation over the risks of insulin therapy, we believe their choice should be supported.

Contraindications for pancreas transplantation include the existence of other conditions that make long-term survival unlikely, such as advanced malignancy or end-stage human immunodeficiency virus (HIV) infection, or substantially increased surgical risk, such as uncorrectable coronary artery disease. For patients with severe hypoglycemic unawareness, failure to work closely with a physician and health care team skilled in the management of diabetes is a relative contraindication because appropriate diabetes management usually decreases if not removes the morbidity associated with this condition.

IX. MANAGEMENT AFTER TRANSPLANTATION

After a successful pancreatic transplantation, management focuses on appropriately adjusting the immunosuppressive drug regimen, monitoring for the toxicity and expected consequences of these drugs, and preparing to diagnose and treat risk factors that increase the likelihood of developing progressive diabetic complications. The immunosuppressive drug regimen used will be reduced in dose over time and may eventually require the administration of fewer drugs. To appropriately adjust drug doses, patients must be carefully monitored for evidence of graft rejection. For patients with diversion of their pancreatic exocrine effluent into the urinary bladder, this is easily accomplished by measuring the amount of amylase in the urine. For patients with enteric drainage, early signs of rejection, such as an increase in serum lipase, can be missed, and patients may display elevated blood sugar levels as their first sign of rejection. Suspected rejection episodes are confirmed by biopsy of the graft and aggressively treated with high-dose immunosuppression regimens.

The drugs used to suppress rejection are known to increase the risk of infection and malignancy, and management after transplant requires careful monitoring for these events. Viral infections, particularly with CMV, are common after a pancreas transplant, and most centers routinely use antiviral drugs as prophyalaxis in the early postoperative period. Transplant patients receiving immunosuppressive therapy who present with fever or other signs of infection need aggressive and comprehensive evaluation and treatment to prevent serious complications. Over time, patients on a immunosuppression regimen are at risk to develop many malignancies, particularly lymphoma and basal cell carcinoma. Careful evaluation of signs or symptoms of malignancy will allow early identification and treatment of these conditions.

After a successful pancreas transplant, patients remain at risk for the consequences of their diabetic complications. Retinopathy is unaffected by transplant and patients with advanced disease at the time of surgery will require ongoing ophthalmological care. Patients with existing diabetic nephropathy who do not undergo a kidney transplant at the time of their pancreas surgery may experience a rapid drug-induced worsening of their renal function and must be carefully monitored. Although some improvement in peripheral neuropathy can be expected after a successful transplant, patients still remain at risk for serious foot injury and must be instructed to continue to care for their feet. Macrovascular disease remains a big problem after transplant and may even increase. Consequently, attention to cardiovascular risk factors, such as lipids, smoking, and blood pressure, remain important parts of the long-term management of patients after successful pancreas transplantation.

REFERENCES

1. R Gruessner, D Sutherland, E Troppmann, N Hakim, D Dunn, A Gruessner. The surgical risk of pancreas transplantation in the cyclosporine era: an overview. J Am Coll Surg 185:128–144, 1997.

2. C Troppmann, A Gruessner, D Dunn, D Sutherland, R Gruessner. Surgical complications requiring early relaparotomy after pancreas transplantation. Ann Surg 227: 255–268, 1998.

3. A Gruessner, D Sutherland. Pancreas transplants for United States (US) and non-US cases as reported to the International Pancreas Transplant Registry (IPTR) and to the United Network for Organ Sharing (UNOS). In: CA, Terasaki, ed. Clinical Transplants. Los Angeles, CA: UCLA Tissue Typing Laboratory, 1997:45–59.

4. M Cecka, PI Teraski, eds. Clinical Transplants—1996. Los Angeles: UCLA Tissue Typing Laboratory, 1997.

5. C Manske, Y Wang, W Thomas. Mortality of cadaveric kidney transplantation versus combined kidney–pancreas transplantation in diabetic patients. Lancet 346: 1658–1662, 1995.

6. C Rosen, P Frohnert, J Velosa, D Engen, S Sterioff. Morbidity of pancreas transplantation during cadaveric renal transplantation. Transplantation 51:123–127, 1991.

7. R Robertson, D Sutherland, D Kendall, A Teuscher, R Gruessner, A Gruessner. Metabolic complications of long-term successful pancreas transplant in type I diabetes. J Invest Med 44:549–555, 1996.

8. P Diem, M Abid, J Redmon, E Sutherland, R Robertson. Systemic venous drainage of pancreas allografts as independent cause of hyperinsulinemia in type I diabetic recipients. Diabetes 39:534–540, 1990.
9. A Teuscher, E Seaquist, R Robertson. Diminished insulin secretory reserve in diabetic pancreas transplant and nondiabetic kidney transplant recipients. Diabetes 43: 593–598, 1994.
10. R Ramsay, F Goetz, D Sutherland, S Mauer, L Robison, H Cantrill, W Knobloch, J Najarian. Progression of diabetic retinopathy after pancreas transplantation for insulin-dependent diabetes mellitus. N Engl J Med 318:208–214, 1988.
11. A Scheider, E Meyer-Schwickerath, J Nusser, W Land, R Landgraf. Diabetic retinopathy and pancreas transplantation: a 3-year follow-up. Diabetologia 34(suppl 1): S95–S99.
12. A Konigsrainer, K Miller, W Steurer, G Kieselbach, C Aichberger, D Ofner, R Margreiter. Does pancreas transplantation influence the course of diabetic retinopathy? Diabetologia 34(suppl 1):S86–S88, 1991.
13. X Navarro, D Sutherland, W Kennedy. Long-term effects of pancreatic transplantation on diabetic neuropathy. Ann Neurol 42:727–736, 1997.
14. S Martinenghi, G Comi, G Galardi, G Di Carlo, V Di Carlo, G Pozza, A Secchi. Amelioration of nerve conduction velocity following simultaneous kidney/pancreas transplantation is due to the glycaemic control provided by the pancreas. Diabetologia 40:1110–1112, 1997.
15. X Navarro, W Kennedy, D Sutherland. Autonomic neuropathy and survival in diabetes mellitus: effects of pancreas transplantation. Diabetologia 34(suppl 1): S108–S112, 1991.
16. R Bilous, S Mauer, D Sutherland, J Najarian, F Goetz, MW Steffes. The effects of pancreas transplantation on the glomerular structure of renal allografts in patients with insulin-dependent diabetes. N Engl J Med 321:80–85, 1989.
17. P Fioretto, MW Steffes, DER Sutherland, FC Goetz, M Mauer. Reversal of lesions of diabetic nephropathy after pancreas transplantation. N Engl J Med 339:115–117, 1998.
18. P Morrissey, D Shaffer, A Monaco, P Conway, P Madras. Peripheral vascular disease after kidney–pancreas transplantation in diabetic patients with end-stage renal disease. Arch Surg 132:358–362, 1997.
19. J Bagdade, A Teuscher, M Ritter, R Eckel, R Robertson. Alterations in cholesteryl ester transfer, lipoprotein lipase, and lipoprotein composition after combined pancreas–kidney transplantation. Diabetes 47:113–118, 1998.
20. C Zehrer, C Gross. Quality of life of pancreas transplant recipients. Diabetologia 34:S145–S149, 1991.

21

Benefits of Intensive Diabetes Management

Bernard Zinman
University of Toronto, Mount Sinai Hospital, and The University Health Network, Toronto, Ontario, Canada

I. INTRODUCTION

Type 1 diabetes is characterized by autoimmune destruction of the beta cells of the pancreas, with resulting insulin deficiency. Despite 77 years of research and clinical experience since the discovery of insulin at the University of Toronto in the summer of 1921, our ability to achieve physiological insulin replacement and thus glycemic normalization remains illusive. Indeed, the inadequacies of contemporary diabetes management is exemplified by the fact that diabetes is the leading cause of blindness in adults, accounts for 30% of all causes of end-stage renal disease, is the most common cause of nontraumatic amputation of the lower extremity, and is a major risk factor for cardiovascular, cerebrovascular, and peripheral vascular disease. The debate on the importance of glucose control in the development of the microvascular complications of diabetes has been definitively answered with the publication of the Diabetes Control and Complications Trial (DCCT) results in 1993. The DCCT was a multicenter, randomized, prospective trial sponsored by the National Institutes of Health involving 1441 patients with type 1 diabetes in Canada and the United States. The study took its lead from several smaller European studies and addressed whether the complications of diabetes could be prevented with intensive diabetes management in individuals who had short-duration diabetes (1–5 years) and no complications at randomization (primary prevention) as well as patients with type 1 diabetes who had longer-duration diabetes (1–15 years) and early complications. The DCCT was stopped 1 year early because the magnitude of the beneficial effect of intensive diabetes

Table 1 The Diabetes Control and Complications Trial: Result Summary

Improved control of blood glucose reduces the risk of clinically meaningful
Retinopathy 76% (p < 0.002)
Nephropathy 54% (p < 0.04)
Neuropathy 60% (p < 0.002)

Source: Modified from DCCT, 1993.

management was so great that the study question had been definitively answered. As illustrated in Table 1, the implementation of intensive diabetes management dramatically reduces retinopathy, nephropathy, and neuropathy.

Another way of describing the benefits of intensive diabetes management is to evaluate the effect of this therapy on providing additional complication-free years of life. This is a useful way of illustrating the clinical influence of intensive diabetes management, and for some patients it is a great motivator. Examples of this kind of analysis in the context of specific complications and life expectancy are illustrated in Table 2.

II. HbA$_{1c}$ AND THE COMPLICATIONS OF DIABETES

The development and clinical utilization of glycosylated hemoglobin (HbA$_{1c}$) as an objective marker of glucose control has had a significant influence on both research and the clinical management of diabetes. From the DCCT it is clear that a curvilinear relation between HbA$_{1c}$ and the risk of developing complications exists for both intensive and conventionally treated patients (Fig. 1). The good

Table 2 Intensive Therapy Results in Additional Complication-Free Years

Complication	No. years
Peripheral retinopathy	4.7
Blindness	7.7
End-stage renal disease	5.8
Neuropathy	10.9
Lower extremity amputation	5.6
Additional years of life	5.1

Source: Modified from DCCT, 1996.

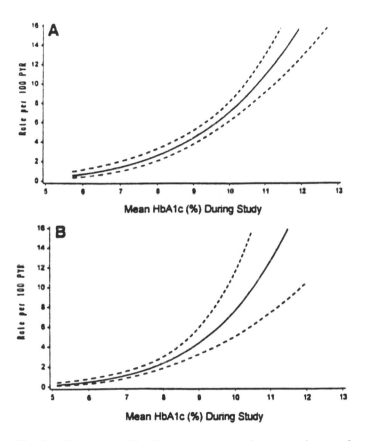

Fig. 1 The absolute risk of sustained retinopathy progression as a function of the mean HbA$_{1c}$: (A) conventional treatment group; (B) intensive treatment group. (From DCCT, 1995.)

Table 3   The Effect of Changing HbA$_{1c}$

Retinopathy	A 10% reduction in HbA$_{1c}$ (e.g., 9–8.1) equals a 45% lower risk of retinopathy progression
Hypoglycemia	A 10% reduction in HbA$_{1c}$ equals a 18% increase in the risk of hypoglycemia

Source: Modified from DCCT, 1995.

news about this relation is that any reduction in HbA$_{1c}$ is associated with an improvement in outcome. The not so good news is that to eliminate complications entirely HbA$_{1c}$ levels have to approach normal values. The relation between HbA$_{1c}$ and complications is a useful concept to use in encouraging patients to strive for better control. This is illustrated in quantitative terms in Table 3.

Unfortunately, the improvement in complication outcome associated with a drop in HbA$_{1c}$ is also associated with an increase in the risk of severe hypoglycemia. Indeed, in any particular patient a balance has to be achieved in which HbA$_{1c}$ is brought to the lowest possible level without excessive hypoglycemia. This will vary from patient-to-patient and, indeed, frequently determines the premeal and bedtime glycemic targets for that particular patient.

III.   IMPLEMENTING INTENSIVE DIABETES MANAGEMENT

One of the most important success factors in the context of achieving the goals of intensive diabetes management is appropriate patient selection. For this form of therapy to be effective the patient must assume day-to-day responsibility for adjusting the diabetes treatment regimen. To accomplish this successfully, he or she must be educated in all components of the treatment regimen and be empowered to make appropriate changes in response to daily living. The patient becomes the most important component of the diabetes health care team, which also includes the physician, the nurse educator, and the dietitian as core members. In addition, the diabetes health care team will employ other specialists in the context of the long-term complications of diabetes (ophthalmologist, nephrologist, and neurologist) and, not infrequently, an individual who focuses on psychosocial support.

To evaluate whether the patient is prepared to perform the self-care behaviors necessary for intensive diabetes management, we frequently ask individuals to do capillary self-monitoring of blood glucose valves four times a day for a period of at least 2 weeks and keep food and exercise records for a couple of days. Having established that a patient is a suitable candidate for intensive diabetes

Table 4 Curriculum Outline for Intensive
Diabetes Management

What is intensive therapy?
Getting started
Pattern management
Carbohydrate counting
Scales and supplements

management, we then proceed with a series of patient-centered workshops to provide the individual with the necessary skills to implement intensive diabetes management safely and effectively. These sessions usually involve four to six patients and consist of a combination of didactic material and patient problem solving. The educational programs are outlined in Table 4.

There are several key elements to the successful implementation of an intensive diabetes therapy program. Clearly, self-monitoring of blood glucose level is fundamental to the success of this program. If the patient is not willing to do at least four blood glucose self-monitoring measurements a day, they are unlikely to achieve any benefit from an intensive insulin therapy regimen. In addition, there are other key elements that appear to predict the successful outcome of intensive therapy. These are highlighted in Table 5.

In the context of the insulin treatment regimen, it is important that patients understand the concept of basal insulin requirements and meal insulin requirements. The use of insulin pumps for continuous subcutaneous insulin infusion (CSII) provides the most flexible means of replacing basal and meal insulin requirements. When used with a short-acting insulin analogue such as lispro (Humalog) CSII results in improved glycemic control and a reduction in hypoglycemia. Although insulin pump therapy has clear advantages in the context of

Table 5 Key Success Factors for Intensive Diabetes Management

Self-monitoring of blood glucose 4–6 times per day
A basal and meal insulin treatment regimen (multiple daily injections or continuous subcutaneous insulin infusion)
Individualized blood glucose targets
Self-adjustment of insulin dose based on premeal glucose level, amount of carbohydrate eaten, and planned postprandial exercise
Regular contact between health care team and patient
Family and psychological support

Table 6 Improved Glycemic Control in Type 2
Diabetes: Japanese Study

Improved control reduced the risk of:
Retinopathy by 65% (p = 0.007)
Severe retinopathy by 40%
Overall risk of nephropathy by 70% (p = 0.005)

Source: Modified from Ohkubo et al., 1995.

flexibility, in meal timing, and insulin dose adjustment, its utilization is limited by the cost of the pump and supplies, as well as the occasional adverse reaction to the subcutaneous infusion site. The newer pumps have appropriate safety alarms are easy to program, and are small enough to be worn innocuously. Currently, there are approximately 40,000–50,000 individuals with type 1 diabetes in the United States who are using insulin pumps to manage their diabetes. For those individuals who opt for multiple daily injections, it is our practice to start with a regimen of short-acting insulin before meals and NPH at bedtime. The pharmacokinetics of the newer short-acting insulin analogues (e.g., lispro) make them a more superior meal-time insulin than regular insulin. They can be administered immediately before the meal and provide improved postprandial glycemic control in both type 1 and type 2 diabetes. It is estimated that approximately 25% of individuals will not achieve satisfactory basal insulin replacement with a single injection of NPH insulin at bedtime, particularly if they are using short-acting insulin for meals. Under these circumstances, we add a second injection of NPH in the morning, and this generally provides adequate glycemic control. Long-acting insulin analogues are currently being developed to provide improved basal insulin replacement.

IV. WHAT DOES ALL THIS MEAN FOR TYPE 2 DIABETES?

Although it is clearly established that intensive diabetes management dramatically reduces the microvascular complications of type 1 diabetes, the same level of evidence is not yet available for type 2 diabetes. A randomized prospective trial entitled "The United Kingdom Prospective Diabetes Study" (UKPDS) will shortly report on the benefits of improved glycemic control in type 2 diabetes and will examine both micro- and macrovascular endpoints. The current evidence strongly supports a beneficial effect of improving glucose control in reducing retinopathy, neuropathy, and nephropathy in type 2 diabetes. A small prospective, randomized control trial with a design similar to the DCCT was completed in Japan and published in 1995. This study demonstrated that in lean type 2 Japanese patients the implementation of intensive therapy had effects essentially similar to that observed in the DCCT (Table 6). Whether glycemic control will have a similar positive effect on macrovascular disease endpoints (e.g., cardiovascular disease, stroke, and peripheral vascular disease) remains to be determined.

To summarize, the implementation of intensive diabetes management has major beneficial effects in both type 1 and type 2 diabetes. Improvement in microvascular disease outcome, empowerment of the patient, and increased flexibility in the context of daily living are associated with intensive diabetes management in many patients. Unfortunately, intensive therapy also results in two major adverse outcomes. The rate of severe hypoglycemia can increase significantly, and weight gain can be a consequence of improved control. Both of these adverse outcomes can be managed effectively. To avoid severe hypoglycemia, increased monitoring and an adjustment in the glycemic targets may be required. The problem of weight gain can be modified by reducing caloric intake by approximately 500 calories at the initiation of intensive therapy.

Given the current evidence the DCCT recommendation that intensive diabetes therapy with the goal of achieving near-normal glycemia should be implemented as early as possible in as many patients with type 1 diabetes as is safely possible, is well founded. Similar statements are likely to be appropriate for type 2 diabetes. Ultimately, the development of superior insulin treatment and glucose-monitoring techniques will make this goal easier to achieve.

BIBLIOGRAPHY

Diabetes Control and Complications Trial (DCCT) Research Group. The effect of intensive treatment of diabetes on the development and progression of long-term complications in insulin-dependent diabetes mellitus. N Engl J Med 1993a; 329:977–986.

DCCT Research Group. Lifetime benefits and costs of intensive therapy as practiced in the Diabetes Control and Complications Trial. JAMA 1996; 276:1409–1415.

DCCT Trial Research Group. Diabetes 1995; 44:968.

Egger M, et al. Risk of adverse effects of intensified treatment in insulin-dependent diabetes mellitus: a meta-analysis. Diabetic Med 1997; 14:919–928.

Holleman F, Hoekstra JBL. Insulin lispro. N Engl J Med 1997; 337:176–183.

Ohkubo Y, et al. Intensive insulin therapy prevents the progression of diabetic microvascular complications in Japanese patients with non–insulin-dependent diabetes mellitus: a randomized prospective 6-year study. Diabetes Res Clin Pract 1995; 28: 103–117.

Zinman B. The physiologic replacement of insulin. N Engl J Med 1989; 321:363–370.

Zinman B. Insulin regimens and strategies for IDDM. Diabetes Care 1993; 16(suppl 3): S24–S28.

Zinman B, et al. Insulin lispro in CSII—results of a double-blind crossover study. Diabetes 1997; 46:440–443.

22
Diabetic Eye Disease

Craig M. Greven
Wake Forest University School of Medicine, Winston-Salem, North Carolina

I. INTRODUCTION

Diabetic eye disease is a major public health concern. Retinopathy associated with diabetes mellitus is the leading cause of new cases of legal blindness (visual acuity of 20/200 or less) in the United States in persons between the ages of 20 and 74. Diabetic retinopathy is also a leading cause of blindness in England, Wales, Scotland, the Netherlands, and other developed countries. Over the past 30 years, growth in our knowledge of the epidemiology and pathogenesis and advances in technology have greatly enhanced our ability to treat diabetic eye disease. Studies have determined that the ocular complications of diabetes can be minimized by maintaining strict control of blood sugar levels. The efficacy of treatment modalities, such as laser photocoagulation, in minimizing diabetic blindness has also been proved. In this chapter, we will discuss how the advances in our understanding of diabetic eye disease have positively influenced our ability to minimize the devastating complication of diabetes-induced blindness.

II. DEMOGRAPHICS AND EPIDEMIOLOGY

Much of our information on the incidence, prevalence, and progression rates of diabetic retinopathy comes from data obtained from the Wisconsin Epidemiologic Study of Diabetic Retinopathy (WESDR)(1–6). This population-based study, commenced in 1979, consisted of a probability sample of over 10,000 patients with diabetes receiving care in an 11-county region of Southern Wisconsin. Patients were divided into three groups: (a) onset of diabetes younger than age 30, taking insulin; (b) onset at age 30 or older, taking insulin; and (c) onset of diabetes mellitus at age 30 or older, not taking insulin. These patients were followed prospectively for the progression and severity of diabetic retinopathy at 4 and 10 years. Retinopathy was assessed by an elaborate system of grading of fundus photographs by trained observers unaware of the patients' systemic health. The WESDR has shown that the factor most associated with increased prevalence and severity of diabetic retinopathy is longer duration of disease (1). When diabetes was diagnosed at an age younger than 30, 17% had evidence of some retinopathy within 5 years, and 98% had some retinopathy by 15 years. Similarly, in patients with diagnosis of diabetes who were 30 or older, 29% had retinopathy at 4 years, and 78% had retinopathy at 15 years (2). The increased prevalence of diabetic retinopathy in the older-onset diabetics compared with younger-onset diabetics at 5 years is probably related to difficulty in accurately determining the onset of diabetes in the older patients. In many of these patients the diagnosis is not made immediately; they may have had elevated blood sugar levels and subclinical diabetes for years before the time of diagnosis.

The rates of development of proliferative diabetic retinopathy in the younger-onset diabetics was 1.2% at 5 years, 56% at 15 years, and 67% at 35 years (1). In the older-onset diabetics, 2% had proliferative diabetic retinopathy at 5 years, and 15% at 15 years (2). The 10-year incidence of macular edema in the WESDR was 20.1% in the younger-onset group, 25% in the older-onset group taking insulin, and 14% in the older-onset group not taking insulin (3).

The 10-year incidence of legal blindness was approximately 2% for the young-onset diabetics, 4% for the older-onset diabetics taking insulin, and 5% for the older-onset diabetics not taking insulin.

A. Race

Most studies have found that the prevalence of retinopathy is equal among the different racial populations. However, occasionally retinopathy incidence and prevalence rates have been documented to be significantly higher in certain ethnic groups. For example, Pima Indians in Arizona have significantly higher rates of proliferative retinopathy than reported in the WESDR.

B. Age

The effect of increasing age on progression of diabetic retinopathy is variable. Prepubescent children rarely have detectable retinopathy. In the WESDR, children younger than 10 had the lowest incidence of retinopathy or progression to proliferative retinopathy at 10 years. Patients 10–29 had the highest rate of progression (6). In older-onset diabetics, there was an inverse relation between age and retinopathy progression, with onset between 30 and 60 showing a much greater progression of retinopathy than in patients older than 60 at the time of diagnosis.

C. Sex

The male sex has been associated with a statistically significant greater risk of developing diabetic macular edema than females (7). Male sex has also been related to increased severity of retinopathy. The WESDR preliminary report suggested that males with a diagnosis of diabetes when younger than 30 years of age had more severe retinopathy than females. However, in the 10-year study report of the WESDR, there was no significant difference in retinopathy incidence or progression to proliferative diabetic retinopathy in the three study groups described previously, based on sex (6).

D. External Factors

1. Cigarette Smoking

The role of cigarette smoking as relates to development and progression of diabetic retinopathy is somewhat controversial. It has been hypothesized that smoking-induced platelet aggregation, vasoconstriction, and the increased affinity of carboxyhemoglobin for oxygen decrease the available oxygen at the tissue level in cigarette smokers (8). Cross-sectional and longitudinal studies have suggested conflicting results for diabetic retinopathy progression and smoking. The WESDR reported at 10 years that neither smoking status nor pack-years smoked showed a significant association with the incidence and progression of diabetic retinopathy (9).

2. Alcohol

Results pertaining to alcohol intake and diabetic retinopathy are also somewhat controversial. Whereas the WESDR reported that alcohol consumption in moderation did not affect the occurrence of diabetic retinopathy (10), Young and associates found that higher alcohol intake (more than 10 pints of beer per week or equivalents) was associated with increased levels of exudation and proliferative diabetic retinopathy (11).

3. Physical Activity

Increased physical activity decreases mortality rates and large vessel complications in patients with insulin-dependent diabetes. Physical activity and its effect on diabetic retinopathy was evaluated by the WESDR, and in 1995, they reported a beneficial association between physical activity and progression of retinopathy or development of diabetic retinopathy (12). Additionally, no detrimental affect of strenuous physical activity, such as weight lifting, was detected.

E. Systemic Factors

1. Control of Blood Glucose Levels

The relation between blood glucose control and the development of diabetic eye disease and retinopathy was controversial in the 1960s and 1970s. In 1976, the American Diabetes Association (ADA) supported ''the concept that the microvascular complications of diabetes are decreased by reduction of blood glucose concentration (13). More recent studies have shown a positive correlation between diabetic retinopathy incidence and progression with elevated glycosylated hemoglobin (HbA$_{1c}$) levels (14,15).

The Diabetes Control and Complication Trial (DCCT) was a multicenter randomized clinical trial designed to determine whether intensive treatment reduced the development or progression of diabetic retinopathy. The details of the study are presented elsewhere in this book. To summarize the results, intensive treatment (three injections of insulin per day or the insulin pump) was compared with conventional treatment (one or two daily injections) in assessing the progression of diabetic retinopathy. The DCCT concluded that there was a substantial beneficial effect of intensive treatment in slowing progression of retinopathy, that this benefit increased with time, and was present in patients with no retinopathy to moderate nonproliferative diabetic retinopathy (16,17). Intensive treatment did not eliminate retinopathy or prevent its occurrence. Finally, the study showed that a beneficial effect of intensive treatment was not seen until after 3 years of intensive treatment.

Intensive treatment did reduce the risk of retinopathy developing or progressing to clinically significant degrees by 33–75%. Intensive therapy had its greatest effect when initiated early in the course of diabetes mellitus. The reduction of risk in the study is translatable into decreased need for laser photocoagulation and saved vision, and should be the cornerstone of any strategy aimed at limiting diabetic visual loss.

2. Blood Pressure

Acute and chronic hypertension causes narrowing of arterioles and vascular rigidity. Elevated blood pressure is a significant risk factor for mortality in diabetics. Numerous studies have assessed the relation between systemic hypertension and the presence of diabetic retinopathy. Elevated systolic blood pressure has been associated with an increased incidence of diabetic retinopathy (18), and diastolic hypertension has been associated with an increased risk of progression of diabetic retinopathy.

3. Renal Disease

The association of the comorbidities of diabetic eye disease and diabetic kidney disease are well-documented. Elevated serum creatinine and uremia have been associated with visually significant diabetic retinopathy.

The presence of microalbuminemia in all age groups of diabetics has been associated with an increased risk of diabetic retinopathy, and the development of proliferative diabetic retinopathy in younger-onset patients (19). These relations remained after controlling for hyperglycemia, blood pressure elevation, and other confounding variables. Additionally, in younger- and older-onset diabetics with gross proteinuria, the relative risk of developing proliferative diabetic retinopathy was 2.32 and 2.02, respectively, when compared with patients without gross proteinuria (20).

4. Pregnancy

It is hypothesized that the hypercoagulable state that occurs during pregnancy can exacerbate the hypercoagulable state that occurs in diabetics, and accelerate the progression of retinopathy. Studies have shown that pregnant diabetic patients have a higher incidence of retinopathy than a group of age-matched, duration of disease-matched, and blood glucose control-matched diabetic patients (21,22).

Deterioration of retinopathy may occur during pregnancy, particularly in patients with more advanced diabetic retinopathy at the onset of pregnancy. A positive correlation between severity of retinopathy and renal disease of pregnancy, preeclampsia, and perinatal deaths has been suggested. Because of these findings, the American Academy of Ophthalmology recommends that diabetics who become pregnant be evaluated at the time of diagnosis of pregnancy and subsequently during each trimester.

III. DIABETIC RETINOPATHY: SYMPTOMS

Patients with ocular complaints typically present with one of three symptoms: (a) blurred vision, (b) pain, or (c) redness. Persons with diabetes often are completely asymptomatic with 20/20 visual acuity despite having severe vision-threatening retinopathy. However, diabetics may complain of fluctuating vision, blurred vision, or floaters.

Diabetic retinopathy does not cause abnormalities in the external examination of the eye. Additionally, pain is not a symptom of diabetic retinopathy.

IV. DIABETIC RETINOPATHY: CLINICAL FEATURES

The classification of diabetic retinopathy has evolved as our understanding of diabetic eye disease has increased. Previously, diabetic retinopathy had been divided into background, preproliferative, and proliferative retinopathy. More recently, retinopathy has been graded as nonproliferative (mild, moderate, severe, and very severe) and proliferative diabetic retinopathy. The progression from mild, to moderate, to severe, nonproliferative diabetic retinopathy indicates progressive ischemia and an increased risk for the development of proliferative diabetic retinopathy and blindness.

Some of the clinical findings in nonproliferative retinopathy include microaneurysms, dot-and-blot hemorrhages, flame hemorrhages, exudates, cotton-wool spots, and venous beading. Proliferative diabetic retinopathy indicates that abnormal new blood vessels (neovascularization) are present either on the optic disc (NVD; neovascularization of the disc) or anywhere else in the retina (NVE; neovascularization elsewhere).

A. Nonproliferative Diabetic Retinopathy Features

1. Microaneurysms

Microaneurysms appear clinically as red or gray dots in the neurosensory retina. They are derived from retinal capillaries and are often located near occluded capillaries, suggesting an association with ischemia. These are typically the initial ophthalmoscopic sign of diabetic retinopathy. Their size ranges from 10 to 100 μm. Microaneurysms have incompetent tight junctions, and they are the source of transudation of lipoprotein moieties into the substance of the retina, leading to macular edema.

2. Intraretinal Hemorrhages

Intraretinal hemorrhages occur secondary to breakdown of capillaries, microaneurysms, and small venules. They are named according to their ophthalmoscopic appearance (Fig. 1). Flame-shaped or splinter hemorrhages occur in the superficial layer of the retina, the nerve fiber layer. In dot-and-blot hemorrhages, the accumulation of blood is in the outer plexiform layer. It is often impossible to clinically distinguish microaneurysms from small dot hemorrhages. Typically, hemorrhages resolve in 2–6 months, depending on their size.

Multiple hemorrhages in all quadrants of the retina are a sign of severe nonproliferative diabetic retinopathy and are associated with ischemia and an increased risk of the development of proliferative diabetic retinopathy (Fig. 2).

3. Hard Exudates

Lipid and protein molecules that leak from diabetic microangiopathy into the extracellular retina are hard exudates. These lesions appear refractile, are yellowish in color, and range in size from 30 μm to over a millimeter. Clinically, hard

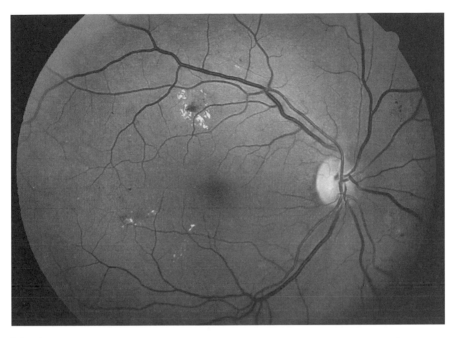

Fig. 1 Right eye: Mild nonproliferative diabetic retinopathy with exudates, microaneurysms, and dot-and-blot hemorrhages.

exudates are almost always accompanied by macular edema or retinal thickening. The deposition and resorption of hard exudates is an ongoing process. Resolution of exudate is thought to be mediated by macrophages. When massive amounts of exudate are present in the retina, one should consider the concomitant presence of an altered lipid state, such as hypertriglyceridemia.

4. Cotton-Wool Spots

Cotton-wool spots are nerve fiber layer infarctions caused by obstructions of terminal retinal arterioles. They signify ongoing retinal ischemia. Clinically, they appear as soft cotton-like patches, measuring 300 μm to 1 mm in size.

5. Venous Beading and Loops

Chronic ischemic of the retina leads to changes in the large-caliber retinal veins. Initially, venous dilation may occur, but with progressive ischemia, irregularities in the caliber of the vein, with focal constrictions and venous loops are present.

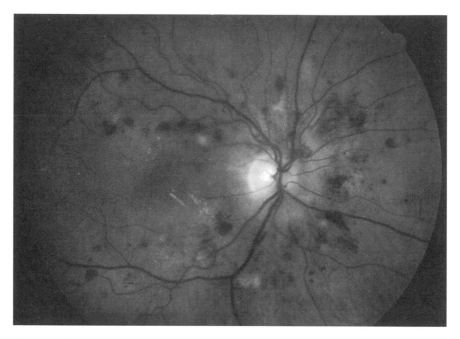

Fig. 2 Right eye: Severe nonproliferative diabetic retinopathy with multiple dot-and-blot hemorrhages and cotton-wool spots.

Venous beading indicates the presence of severe nonproliferative diabetic retinopathy.

6. Intraretinal Microvascular Anomalies

Dilated telangiectatic capillaries that shunt blood from arterioles to veins are termed intraretinal microvascular anomalies (IRMAs). They also represent progressive capillary closure and ischemia of the adjacent retina. IRMA is sometimes difficult to differentiate from early neovascularization of the retina.

B. Clinical Signs in Proliferative Diabetic Retinopathy

1. Neovascularization

Neovascularization is a term used to describe the proliferation of abnormal fibrovascular tissue on the surface of the optic disc and retina. With severe retinal ischemia, it is hypothesized that a vasoproliferative factor released from an ischemic retina causes diabetics to develop neovascularization of the optic disc

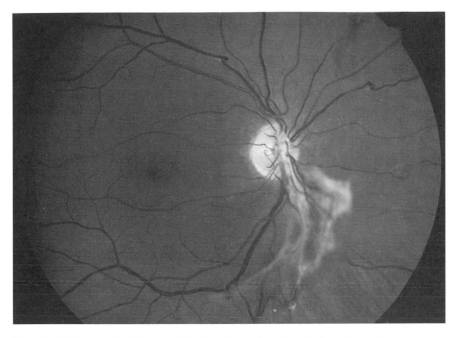

Fig. 3 Right eye: Proliferative diabetic retinopathy with gliotic and vascular neovascularization of the disc.

(NVD), the retina (NVE), and the iris (NVI). Early stage neovascularization of the disc appears as fine, vascular tufts growing on the optic disc vasculature. With progression, these vessels grow into the vitreous. Along with the vascular component, there is typically a glial component present (Fig. 3).

Neovascularization elsewhere in the fundus (NVE; Fig. 4) arises from veins and capillaries of the retina and grows into the vitreous cavity. These vessels progress in a random manner without directionality.

Complications occurring from neovascularization of the disc and retina are related to their interaction with the overlying vitreous. The abnormal blood vessels growing off the surface of the retina or optic nerve penetrate the vitreous cavity. The vitreous can respond by causing traction on these incompetent, weak vessels, leading to vitreous hemorrhage or traction retinal detachment.

a. Vitreous Hemorrhage

Blood within the vitreous cavity caused by traction on neovascularization can be minimal or can completely fill the vitreous cavity. The patient may perceive a mild vitreous hemorrhage as a few floaters, whereas a severe hemorrhage can

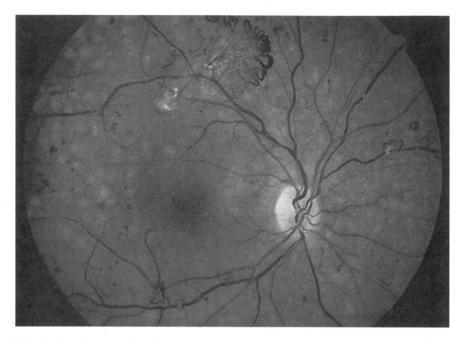

Fig. 4 Proliferative diabetic retinopathy with neovascularization elsewhere along the superotemporal arcade vessel. Note laser photocoagulation scars.

cause blindness. Some hemorrhages can resolve spontaneously, whereas more severe hemorrhages may require evacuation of the blood by vitreous surgery.

b. Traction Retinal Detachment

Extensive neovascularization of the disc and retina may have multiple areas of adherence to the vitreous. Progressive contraction of the vitreous jelly can lead to elevation of the neurosensory retina, termed a traction retinal detachment. If the macula is involved in this traction, it may be a blinding condition. Traction retinal detachments involving the macula require vitreous surgery to restore visual function (Fig. 5).

c. Diabetic Macular Edema

Diabetic macular edema is the accumulation of extracellular lipid, fluid, and protein in the macular region of the retina (Fig. 6). It occurs secondary to transudation of these materials across the damaged diabetic microvasculature. It is a leading cause of morbidity in the diabetic eye. It does not cause total blindness as do vitreous hemorrhage and traction retinal detachment, but causes loss of

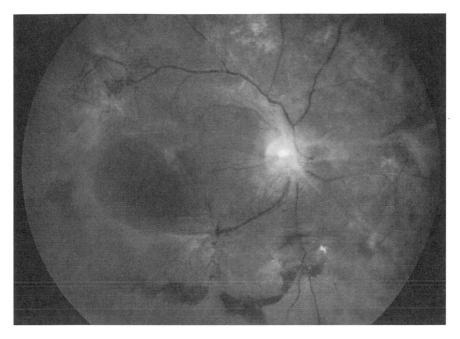

Fig. 5 Right eye: Proliferative diabetic retinopathy with traction retinal detachment and vitreous hemorrhage.

central vision and difficulty with reading and performing every day tasks such as driving. In advanced cases, vision can drop below the level of legal blindness.

d. Neovascularization of the Iris

In eyes with advanced ischemia, neovascularization may proliferate on the surface of the iris and into the trabecular meshwork. Although it can occur in eyes having no retinal or optic disc neovascularization, NVI usually occurs after the development of NVD or NVE. Untreated, this anterior segment neovascularization leads to severe, intractably elevated intraocular pressures and neovascular glaucoma, with the development of a blind painful eye.

V. MANAGEMENT OF EYE DISEASE

The cornerstone of the management of diabetic eye disease is appropriate management of blood glucose levels and the associated factors affecting retinopathy, such as blood pressure, serum lipids, and renal status. This is true not only in

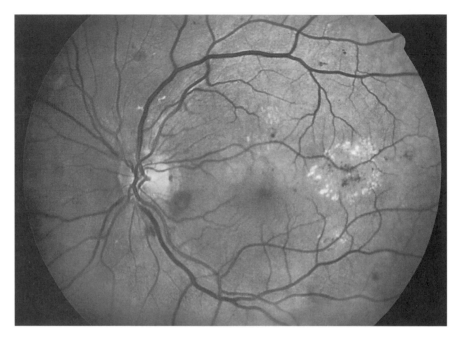

Fig. 6   Left eye: Diabetic macular edema with exudates encroaching on foveal region.

patients who have not yet developed significant retinopathy, but also in those who have advanced retinal diseases requiring local therapy. Two key studies have affected the way ophthalmologists manage diabetic retinopathy: the Diabetic Retinopathy Study (DRS) and the Early Treatment Diabetic Retinopathy Study (ETDRS). Both were randomized, controlled clinical trials sponsored by the National Eye Institute. They continue to serve as the gold standards in the management of diabetic retinopathy.

A.   Diabetic Retinopathy Study

The Diabetic Retinopathy Study (DRS) was designed to see if panretinal laser photocoagulation could prevent severe visual loss in eyes with high-risk proliferative diabetic retinopathy. *Severe visual loss* was defined as a visual acuity of 05/200 or worse; loss of vision to this level is severe enough that the patient could not ambulate in unfamiliar surroundings without assistance, and is usually caused by vitreous hemorrhage or traction retinal detachment. Patients with neovascularization of the disc greater than one-half disc area, or smaller amounts of neovascularization of the disc or neovascularization elsewhere associated with vitreous hemorrhage were randomized to either observation or panretinal laser photocoagulation.

Panretinal laser is an outpatient surgical procedure designed to destroy ischemic retina outside of the macular region. It is usually done in one to three sessions, with topical anesthetic, where approximately 1500–2000 spots of laser are placed in the retinal midzone and periphery. Panretinal laser photocoagulation (PRP) is felt to cause regression of retinopathy by several potential speculative mechanisms, including (a) destroying ischemic peripheral retina and thereby decreasing the production of vasoproliferative factors; (b) improving oxygenation of the retina from the choroid; and (c) allowing release of a vasoinhibitory factors causing regression of these vessels.

The DRS reported that 26% of control eyes had severe visual loss at 3 years, compared with only 10% in the laser-treated eyes (23–25). These results were highly statistically significant that PRP was beneficial in preventing severe visual loss in patients with high-risk proliferative diabetic retinopathy.

Many patients with proliferative diabetic retinopathy are asymptomatic with 20/20 visual acuity. These patients are hesitant to undergo any laser photocoagulation, as they do not perceive a visually significant threat present within their eyes. However, the data supplied to the clinician by this important study confirms the need for panretinal laser photocoagulation to prevent progressive loss of vision in this advanced form of diabetic retinopathy.

Complications of panretinal laser photocoagulation include an occasional mild decrease in central visual acuity. Additionally, because the laser spots are placed outside the macular region in the midzone and peripheral retina (Fig. 7). Patients may complain of decreased night vision and decreased peripheral vision.

B. The Early Treatment Diabetic Retinopathy Study

The ETDRS was also a National Eye Institute-funded study that sought to answer three main questions: (a) What effect does aspirin have on progression or regression of diabetic retinopathy? (b) Is focal laser photocoagulation effective in preventing visual loss in patients with clinically significant diabetic macular edema? (c) Would earlier panretinal laser photocoagulation be effective in decreasing the amount of visual loss in patients with advanced diabetic retinopathy?

Aspirin is a potent platelet inhibitor and its efficacy in preventing heart attacks and strokes has been demonstrated. Consequently, millions of Americans take aspirin daily. Patients with diabetic retinopathy and intraocular hemorrhage are often reluctant to take aspirin because of their concern about hemorrhagic complications. In the ETDRS, 3711 patients with mild nonproliferative to early proliferative diabetic retinopathy were randomly assigned to aspirin or placebo. The ETDRS concluded that aspirin was not effective in preventing the develop-

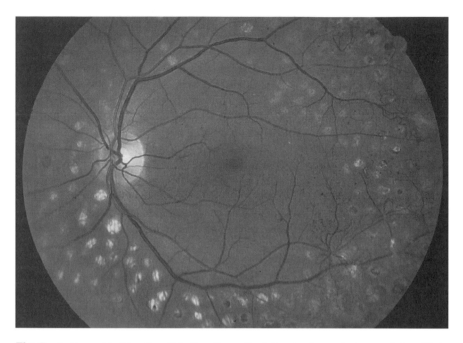

Fig. 7   Left eye: Proliferative diabetic retinopathy following laser photocoagulation. Note the lack of laser in the macular region. Visual acuity is 20/20.

ment of high-risk retinopathy, did not reduce the risk of visual loss, and did not increase the risk of vitreous hemorrhage (26,27). Because no statistically significant beneficial or harmful effects were seen, the study concluded that there are no ocular contraindications to aspirin in patients with diabetes.

Diabetic macular edema has already been described as thickening in the central retina related to diabetic microangiopathy. It is a major cause of ocular morbidity, and occurs in juvenile- and adult-onset diabetics.

Patients with visually threatening clinically significant macular edema, defined as thickening or exudate within 500 μm of the center of the fovea or an optic disc-sized area of thickening within 1.5 mm of the foveal center were randomized to focal laser photocoagulation or observation (28). The Early Treatment Diabetic Retinopathy Study determined that focal laser treatment to areas of leaky microangiopathy and nonperfused retina in the macular region was statistically effective in preventing visual loss in these diabetic eyes.

Focal laser photocoagulation is an outpatient procedure done in a single session (29). The patient is then followed for resolution of the macular edema. As only the involved abnormal retinal vasculature is treated, development of retinopathy in other areas can occur, necessitating additional focal photocoagulation treatments.

The ETDRS also suggested that eyes with both diabetic macular edema and proliferative diabetic retinopathy should have focal laser done before performing panretinal laser photocoagulation because macular edema can worsen in patients treated with panretinal treatment (28).

We learned from the Diabetic Retinopathy Study that panretinal laser can prevent severe visual loss in patients with high-risk retinopathy. The ETDRS questioned whether earlier treatment of diabetic retinopathy might decrease visual loss even more. In this arm of the study, patients with severe nonproliferative retinopathy were treated with panretinal laser and compared with an observation group. The ETDRS found that, with few exceptions, there was no significant beneficial effect of earlier panretinal laser, and suggested that deferral until high-risk characteristics developed was an appropriate management option (29).

C. Vitrectomy

Vitreous hemorrhage and traction retinal detachment are blinding events from diabetic retinopathy. Pars plana vitrectomy is a microsurgical procedure designed to remove blood from the vitreous cavity and repair traction retinal detachments by removing scar tissue from the surface of the retina and vitreous cavity. Vitrectomy is performed in the operating room under local or general anaesthesia. Typically, three 20-gauge incisions are made in the par plana region of the eye. An infusion cannula keeps the globe pressurized with physiological saline solution while a fiber optic light pipe provides illumination for the vitrectomy instrument to clear hemorrhage through a process of simultaneous suction and cutting. Microsurgical instrumentation allows intraocular scissors, membrane forceps, and laser photocoagulators into the vitreous to facilitate a good anatomical and visual outcome.

D. Other Ocular Conditions

Retinopathy is the number 1 cause of ocular morbidity and loss of vision in the diabetic patient. However, other ocular condition can occur in diabetics, leading to substantial visual loss.

1. Cataract

Cataract refers to opacification of the crystalline lens. It is typically an age-related phenomenon. In general, the risk of developing cataracts is greater in diabetics than in age-matched nondiabetic controls. Results of cataract extraction in diabetics without retinopathy are excellent, but there is an increased risk in patients with active retinopathy for the development of significant macular edema and proliferative retinopathy following surgery (30,31).

2. Glaucoma

Glaucoma is an optic neuropathy associated with elevated intraocular pressure. In association with the vascular complications of diabetes, it is felt that the optic nerve in diabetics may be more susceptible to elevated intraocular pressure than a nondiabetic patient.

Neovascular glaucoma develops in severely ischemic eyes. In this condition neovascularization of the iris (NVI) blocks outflow through the trabecular meshwork, causing severe intraocular pressure elevations and pain. It is managed by ablating ischemic retina with laser, but is often the terminal event in a blind diabetic eye.

3. Cranial Nerve Palsies

Ischemic mononeuropathies of cranial nerves III, IV, and VI lead to extraocular muscle paresis and subsequent double vision and motility disorders. Diabetes is a common cause of isolated cranial nerve mononeuropathies. They are often accompanied by pain. Typically there is resolution of the muscle paresis within 3 months. In third-nerve problems associated with diabetes, the pupillary fibers are spared and the pupil is normal. If the pupil is involved, one should suspect an intracranial aneurysm or other space-occupying lesion.

VI. CONCLUSION

The ocular complications of diabetes mellitus are related to ischemia. Control of blood sugar levels and medical management should be the cornerstone of any strategy designed to limit these ocular complications. In patients who develop retinopathy, laser photocoagulation may prevent visual loss. A close relation between the patient, the primary care physician, the endocrinologist, and the ophthalmologist with routine scheduled ophthalmic evaluations (Table 1) will enhance the likelihood of preventing diabetic blindness.

Table 1 American Academy of Ophthalmology Recommendations for Retinal Evaluation in Patients with Diabetes

	Initial evaluation	Minimum evaluation
Age younger than 30 at diagnosis	Within 5 years of diagnosis	Yearly
Age older than 30	At time of diagnosis	Yearly
Pregnancy	First trimester	Each trimester

REFERENCES

1. Klein R, Klein BEK, Moss SE, Davis MD, DeMets DL. The Wisconsin Epidemiologic Study of Diabetic Retinopathy. II Prevalence and risk of diabetic retinopathy when age at diagnosis is less than 30 years. Arch Ophthalmol 1984; 102:520–526.
2. Klein R, Klein BEK, Moss SE, Davis MD, DeMets DL. The Wisconsin Epidemiologic Study of Diabetic Retinopathy. III Prevalence and risk of diabetic retinopathy when age at diagnosis is 30 or more years. Arch Ophthalmol 1984; 102:527–532.
3. Klein R, Klein BEK, Moss SE, Cruickshanks KJ. The Wisconsin Epidemiologic Study of Diabetic Retinopathy XV. The long-term incidence of macular edema. Ophthalmology 1995; 102:7–16.
4. Klein R, Klein BEK, Moss SE, Davis MD, DeMets DL. The Wisconsin Epidemiologic Study of Diabetic Retinopathy. IX Four-year incidence and progression of diabetic retinopathy when age at diagnosis is less than 30 years. Arch Ophthalmol 1989; 107:237–243.
5. Klein R, Klein BEK, Moss SE, Davis MD, DeMets DL. The Wisconsin Epidemiologic Study of Diabetic Retinopathy. IX Four-year incidence and progression of diabetic retinopathy when age at diagnosis is 30 years or more. Arch Ophthalmol 1989; 107:244–249.
6. Klein R, Klein BEK, Moss SE, Cruickshanks KJ. The Wisconsin Epidemiologic Study of Diabetic Retinopathy. XIV Ten-year incidence and progression of diabetic retinopathy. Arch Ophthalmol 1994; 112:1217–1228.
7. Vitale S, Maguire MG, Murphy RP, et al. Clinically significant macular edema in type I diabetes. Incidence and risk factors. Ophthalmology 1995; 102:1170 1176.
8. Morgado, PB, Chen CH, Patel V, Herbert L, Kohner EM. The acute effect of smoking on retinal blood flow in subjects with and without diabetes. Ophthalmology 1994; 101:1220–1226.
9. Moss SE, Klein R, Klein BEK. Cigarette smoking and ten-year progression of diabetic retinopathy. Ophthalmology 1996; 103:1438–1442.
10. Moss SE, Klein R, Klein BEK. The association of alcohol consumption with the incidence and progression of diabetic retinopathy. Ophthalmology 1994; 101: 1962–1968.
11. Young RJ, McColloch DK, Prescott RJ, et al. Alcohol: another risk factor for diabetic retinopathy? Br Med J 1984; 288:1035–1037.
12. Cruickshanks KJ, Moss SE, Klein R, Klein BEK. Physical activity and the risk of progression of retinopathy or the development of proliferative retinopathy. Ophthalmology 1995; 102:1177–1182.
13. Cahill GF, Etzwiler LD, Frankel N. Editorial: "control" in diabetes. N Engl J Med 1976; 294:1004–1005.
14. Klein R, Palta M, Allen C, Shen G, Han DP, D'Alessio DJ. Incidence of retinopathy and associated risk factors from time of diagnosis of insulin-dependent diabetes. Arch Ophthalmol 1997; 115:351–356.
15. Goldstein DE, Blinder KJ, Ide CH, et al. Glycemic control and development of retinopathy in youth-onset insulin-dependent diabetes mellitus. Ophthalmology 1993; 100:1125–1132.

16. Diabetes Control and Complications Trial Research Group. Progression of retinopathy with intensive versus conventional treatment in the Diabetes Control and Complications Trial. Ophthalmology 1995; 102:647–661.

17. The Diabetes Control and Complications Trial Research Group. The effect of intensive diabetes treatment on the progression of diabetic retinopathy in insulin-dependent diabetes mellitus. Arch Ophthalmol 1995; 113:36–51.

18. Klein BEK, Klein R, Moss SE, Palta M. A cohort study of the relationship of diabetic retinopathy to blood pressure. Arch Ophthalmol 1995; 113:601–606.

19. Cruickshanks KJ, Ritter LL, Klein R, Moss SE. The association of microalbuminuria with diabetic retinopathy. The Wisconsin Epidemiologic Study of Diabetic Retinopathy. Ophthalmology 1993; 100:862–867.

20. Klein R, Moss SE, Klein BEK. Is gross proteinuria a risk factor for the incidence of proliferative diabetic retinopathy? Ophthalmology 1993; 100:1140–1146.

21. Moloney JBM, Drury MI. The effect of pregnancy on the natural course of diabetic retinopathy. Am J. Ophthalmol 1982; 93:745–756.

22. Axer-Siegel R, Hod M, Fink-Cohen S, et al. Diabetic retinopathy during pregnancy. Ophthalmology 1990; 103:1815–1819.

23. The Diabetic Retinopathy Study Research Group. Preliminary report on effects of photocoagulation therapy. Am J Ophthalmol 1976; 383–396.

24. The Diabetic Retinopathy Study Research Group. Photocoagulation treatment of Proliferative diabetic retinopathy: the second report of Diabetic Retinopathy Study findings. Ophthalmology 1978; 85:82–106.

25. The Diabetic Retinopathy Study Research Group. Photocoagulation treatment of proliferative diabetic retinopathy. 1981; 88:583–600.

26. Early Treatment Diabetic Retinopathy Study Research Group. Effects of aspirin on vitreous/preretinal hemorrhage in patients with diabetes mellitus. ETDRS Report No. 8. Ophthalmology 1991; 98:757–765.

27. Chew EY, Klein ML, Murphy RP, Remaley NA, Ferris FL. Effects of aspirin on vitreous/preretinal hemorrhage in patients with diabetes mellitus. ETDRS Report No. 20. Arch Ophthalmol 1995; 113:52–55.

28. Early Treatment Diabetic Retinopathy Study Research Group. Early photocoagulation for diabetic retinopathy. ETDRS Report No. 9. Ophthalmology 1991; 98:766–785.

29. Early Treatment Diabetic Retinopathy Study Research Group. Treatment techniques and clinical guidelines for photocoagulation of diabetic macular edema. ETDRS Report No. 2. Ophthalmology 1987; 94:761–744.

30. Jaffe GJ, Burton TC. Progression of nonproliferative diabetic retinopathy following cataract extraction. Arch Ophthalmol 1988; 106:745–749.

31. Benson WE, Brown GC, Tasman W, McNamara JA, Vander JF. Extracapsular cataract extraction with placement of a posterior chamber lens in patients with diabetic retinopathy. Ophthalmology 1993; 100:700–738.

23
Cardiac Disease in Diabetes Mellitus

Debasish Chaudhuri and William E. Hopkins
University of Vermont College of Medicine, Burlington, Vermont

I. INTRODUCTION

Diabetes mellitus is one of the leading public health problems worldwide and has a profound adverse effect on the cardiovascular system. Since the discovery of insulin therapy, death caused by diabetes mellitus (DM) has diminished considerably as a result of reduction in mortality and morbidity from diabetic ketoacidosis and infections. This has led to coronary artery disease (CAD) assuming a disproportionately larger responsibility for the morbidity and mortality experienced by diabetic patients. Diabetic patients suffer not only from an excess of CAD; they are also afflicted by diabetic cardiomyopathy and autonomic neuropathy. The diffuse involvement and aggressive progression of CAD in diabetics clearly separates them from the nondiabetic population and establishes diabetics as a high-risk group.

II. EPIDEMIOLOGY

A. Acute Myocardial Infarction and Cardiovascular Mortality

Epidemiological data derived from various studies, notably the Framingham Heart Study (13), has clearly established the alarmingly high rate of cardiac disease in patients with diabetes and the overall poor prognosis in this group of patients. The cardiovascular mortality rate is more than doubled in men and more than quadrupled in women who have diabetes, compared with their nondiabetic counterparts. The relative risk of myocardial infarction is 50% greater in diabetic men and 150% greater in diabetic women. Similarly, diabetic men succumb to sudden death 50% more often and diabetic women 300% more often than age-matched counterparts. Acute myocardial infarction (AMI) is said to account for approximately 30% of all deaths in diabetic patients. In fact, atherosclerosis and its sequelae have been estimated to account for 80% of all deaths and 75% of all hospital admissions in the diabetic population. Among those with type 1 DM the cumulative mortality from CAD is 35% by the age of 55, far higher than the 4–8% in patients without DM. In type 2 DM, coronary artery disease is the most common cause of death.

B. Prevalence and Extent of CAD

Data collected by using various diagnostic methods show an overall prevalence of CAD as high as 55% in the adult diabetic population, compared with 2–4% in the general population. Not only is the prevalence high, CAD is significantly more extensive in patients with DM. At coronary angiography or during autopsy, patients with DM have significantly more multivessel disease and less single-vessel disease than nondiabetics. The incidence of significant left main coronary artery disease in patients with DM is twice that in nondiabetic patients (13 vs. 6%). Interestingly, in a large autopsy study, 91% of patients with adult-onset diabetes and no known CAD had severe narrowing of at least one major epicardial artery, and 83% had severe two- or three-vessel involvement. In a group of adults of similar age without overt diabetes only 33% had severe single-vessel disease, and 17% had severe two- or three-vessel disease. In another autopsy study in patients with juvenile-onset DM, at least half of the overall length of the epicardial coronary arteries were narrowed by 50% or more, compared with less than 1% of the overall length being affected in nondiabetics.

III. PATHOLOGY

Although the major brunt of diabetes falls on the coronary arterial system, other structures are also significantly affected, for example, the myocardium and the autonomic nervous system supplying the heart. This is discussed in more detail in the subsequent sections.

A. Atherosclerotic Coronary Artery Disease

1. Acute Coronary Syndromes and Plaque Rupture

Factors responsible for the development and progression of atherosclerosis and subsequent clinical events are not fully understood. It is widely believed that in the major epicardial arteries the process is initiated by endothelial injury that leads to accumulation of extracellular matrix and lipid and proliferation of smooth-muscle cells in the arterial wall. Microthrombosis in the lumen may potentiate smooth-muscle cell proliferation by exposure of vascular wall constituents to mitogens associated with these thrombi. This process may constitute one of the key steps in initiation and proliferation of the plaque. Unstable plaques may proceed to rupture at their weakest point, which usually is toward the arterial lumen. This leads to platelet aggregation and thrombus formation and, if sufficiently occlusive, can cause an acute coronary syndrome—unstable angina or myocardial infarction. In contrast, if the endogenous fibrinolytic system (e.g., endogenous tissue plasminogen activator, t-PA) lyses the macrothrombus enough to prevent a clinical event, the episode of plaque rupture will be silent. However, this process of plaque rupture, thrombus formation, and spontaneous lysis leads to further progression of the atherosclerotic lesion. Highly fibrous or calcified plaques are more stable than lipid-rich plaques. With this as a background let us examine why DM causes diffuse and aggressive CAD.

2. Endothelial Dysfunction in DM

In recent years the seminal role played by the vascular endothelium in prevention of atherosclerosis and intraluminal thrombosis has become apparent. It appears that endothelial dysfunction antedates the development of macrovascular and microvascular complications of DM by a considerable time. Increased endothelial permeability, impaired endothelium-dependent relaxation, and increased expression of adhesion molecules, with increased monocyte adhesion, all have been described in DM. The normal endothelium also prevents platelet adhesion and activation of the coagulation cascade. Endothelial inhibition of platelet adhesion is also attenuated in patients with DM.

3. The Procoagulant Milieu in DM

Intraluminal thrombosis plays a key role in initiation and progression of the atherosclerotic plaque and is responsible for the acute coronary syndromes. The development and persistence of intraluminal thrombosis is a function of the local thrombotic activity, platelet aggregation, and the fibrinolytic system. Thrombotic activity is a dynamic equilibrium between prothrombotic and antithrombotic factors, whereas fibrinolytic activity is a dynamic equilibrium between plasminogen activators, primarily t-PA, and the primary physiological inhibitor of plasminogen activation, plasminogen activator inhibitor type-1 (PAI-1).

Platelet aggregation plays a key role in the development of intraluminal thrombus, and heightened platelet adhesiveness and aggregability increases the risks of an acute coronary event. Several studies have shown platelet hyperaggregability in DM. Also, there is a higher proportion of activated platelets in the circulation of diabetics, even in the absence of an ongoing acute coronary syndrome. Increased levels of coagulation factor VII and of fibrinogen have been demonstrated in patients with DM and appear to decrease with tight glycemic control. Fibrinogen has an independent correlation with increased risk of CAD.

There is also evidence of an attenuated fibrinolytic system in patients with DM. Expression of the surface molecules thrombomodulin and t-PA—naturally occurring anticoagulant and fibrinolytic proteins—is reduced, resulting in the shift of balance tilted in favor of procoagulants. This is reflected by enhanced tissue factor-mediated procoagulant activity and increased PAI-1 expression on the surface of endothelial cells. Increased circulating PAI-1 levels have been associated with hyperinsulinemia and with insulin resistance and are consistently found in hyperinsulinemic type 2 DM.

4. Lipoprotein Abnormalities in DM

Abnormalities in lipoprotein metabolism may contribute significantly to the increased cardiovascular risk in DM. The nature of lipoprotein alteration is complex and is dependent on multiple variables (e.g., type of diabetes, level of control, presence of nephropathy, and others). In poorly controlled type 1 DM, a rise in triglycerides, a moderate rise in low-density lipoprotein (LDL) cholesterol and a low high-density lipoprotein (HDL) cholesterol are the predominant abnormalities. Interestingly, good glycemic control in type 1 DM can normalize the lipoprotein abnormality unless the patient has established nephropathy, when normalization of a lipoprotein abnormality is considerably difficult.

In type 2 DM the principal lipoprotein abnormality appears to be elevated triglycerides, often in association with a low HDL cholesterol level and a normal to mildly elevated LDL cholesterol level. The triglyceride abnormality appears secondary to the overproduction and reduced clearance of large triglyceride-rich VLDL. Whether high triglycerides are an independent risk factor for CAD continues to be debated. In contrast with type 1 DM the lipoprotein abnormality in type 2 DM is much more related to the insulin-resistant state than the glycemic control. Interestingly, even though LDL cholesterol levels may be normal with even modest glycemic control in both types of DM, increased LDL glycosylation owing to raised blood glucose levels makes it more susceptible to oxidation, which is thought to be a key step in atheroma formation. In type 2 DM there is also a predominance of small, dense LDL believed to be associated with the insulin-resistant state and which appears to be atherogenic, as these forms are more susceptible to oxidation.

5. Glycemic Control and Diabetic Nephropathy

The issue of glycemic control and its effect on the initiation and progression of atherosclerosis continues to be unclear. This is most apparent in type 2 DM for which the degree of hyperglycemia and the duration that it has been present, does not appear to have a consistent association with the development of CAD and other macrovascular complications. Also unclear is the relative contribution of the insulin-resistant state itself and of hyperinsulinemia that is present before failure of the beta cells ensues. There is, however, substantial evidence implicating each of these variables in the pathogenesis and progression of atherosclerosis. In a recent trial intensive glycemic control in diabetic patients after a myocardial infarction was associated with a 52% reduction in 1-year mortality and demonstrates that glycemic control may be important even with established disease (7). More light will be shed on this issue by a number of ongoing trials looking at the benefits and risks of intensive glycemic control with emphasis on cardiovascular complications.

In type 1 DM, the duration of hyperglycemia seems to have a more consistent relation to CAD. Irrespective of the age of onset of type 1 DM, CAD is rare before the age of 30 years, but the risk increases exponentially after the age of 40 years. The Stockholm Diabetes Intervention Study demonstrated that tight glycemic control retards the development of atherosclerosis in type 1 DM patients. The excess of insulin required to achieve good control is usually not significantly higher than that for modest control and appears unlikely to accelerate the risk of cardiovascular disease.

An issue of great concern is the alarming rise in cardiovascular risk in patients with diabetic nephropathy. Once persistent proteinuria develops, the cardiovascular mortality risk increases from 4.2 times without proteinuria to about 37 times, compared with the nondiabetic population. The risk of developing CAD is 15 times higher in diabetics with nephropathy compared with diabetics without nephropathy. It seems that nephropathy unfavorably alters the lipoprotein profile, increases the hypercoagulable state, and may herald the onset of hypertension.

B. Diabetic Cardiomyopathy

A large body of evidence in experimental animals and in human autopsy studies confirms the presence of a unique cardiomyopathy in diabetes that is not related to epicardial coronary artery disease or to hypertension. Clinically, the earliest impairment is diastolic performance. Although systolic function is initially normal, in the later stages it too can be affected. Cardiac hypertrophy can be present owing to diabetic cardiomyopathy even in the absence of hypertension, although the presence of the latter accentuates both the hypertrophy and the degree of diastolic dysfunction. Diabetic cardiomyopathy may be one of the reasons for the four- to fivefold increase in congestive heart failure seen in DM patients, excluding prior CAD or rheumatic heart disease. The risk of developing diabetic cardiomyopathy is increased even when other factors such as hypertension, age, CAD, weight, and abnormal lipids are corrected for. The exact cause and pathogenesis of diabetic cardiomyopathy is unknown. Deranged myocardial calcium handling, abnormal collagen deposition by advanced glycosylation end products, and abnormal glucose metabolism, all have been implicated. Tissue characterization with sophisticated cardiac ultrasound suggests increased fibrosis, even in diabetics with normal left ventricular diastolic and systolic function.

C. Cardiac Autonomic Dysfunction

Numerous noninvasive, invasive, and autopsy studies have shown that the autonomic nervous system, including that of the heart, is affected by DM. It appears that demonstrable cardiac autonomic dysfunction may be present earlier in the course of DM than somatic autonomic involvement. Both the sympathetic and parasympathetic nervous system are involved and, in fact, can lead to total cardiac denervation. It has been suggested that the parasympathetic system is involved initially, leading to relatively increased sympathetic activity, as evidenced by resting tachycardia. Lack of parasympathetic tone may cause or exaggerate inappropriate coronary vasoconstriction. Sympathetic involvement usually occurs within 5 years of parasympathetic involvement, the principal clinical manifestation being postural hypotension.

Sudden cardiac death is the most ominous complication of cardiac autonomic dysfunction and is thought to be due to malignant ventricular tachyarrhythmias precipitated by heightened sympathetic tone or prolonged QT interval (owing to repolarization abnormality) or both, especially in patients with impaired left ventricular function.

The other major clinical sequela of cardiac autonomic dysfunction is impaired perception of cardiac pain during ischemia or infarction, leading to late or misdiagnosis of CAD, an issue discussed in more detail in a later section. The rate of painless ST segment depression on stress testing is twice as common in the diabetic than in the nondiabetic population, and diabetics perceive ischemia later in the course of the event than nondiabetics do.

In a review of diabetic autonomic neuropathy, Ewing and Clarke (9) outlined five tests that can be used to test parasympathetic and sympathetic function.

1. Heart rate response to the Valsalva maneuver: ratio of the longest R–R interval after Valsalva to the shortest R–R interval during Valsalva of 1.10 or less. The normal ratio is 1.2, or higher.
2. Heart rate variation during deep breathing: lack of beat-to-beat heart rate variability on ECG recording of 10 beats per minute, or fewer. The normal variation is 15 beats, or more.
3. Immediate heart rate response to standing: ratio of the 30th beat to the 15th beat, after standing, of 1.0 or less. The normal ratio is 1.04, or more.

4. Blood pressure response to standing: fall in systolic blood pressure of 30 mmHg or more after standing. The normal fall in systolic blood pressure is 10 mmHg, or less.
5. Blood pressure response to sustained handgrip: rise in diastolic blood pressure of 10 mmHg, or less. The normal increase is 16 mmHg, or more.

In their review, Ewing and Clarke (9) outline the optimal ways to perform these tests. The first three test parasympathetic function and the last two test sympathetic function. Patients have normal autonomic function if all five tests are normal. They have early parasympathetic damage if one of the first three tests are abnormal and definite parasympathetic damage if two or more of the first three tests are abnormal. Combined parasympathetic and sympathetic damage if present if at least one of the two tests for sympathetic function is abnormal in addition to abnormal parasympathetic function.

IV. CLINICAL FEATURES OF CAD IN DIABETIC PATIENTS: SYMPTOMS OF ISCHEMIA OR INFARCTION

There is no doubt that diabetics with cardiac autonomic neuropathy have altered and delayed perception of ischemia and can present with quite atypical symptoms leading to a delay in the correct diagnosis or a misdiagnosis of CAD, thereby leading to suboptimal therapy. Moreover, diabetic patients may underestimate the gravity of the symptoms and delay seeking medical help. Studies have shown a much higher incidence of inappropriate triaging of diabetic patients with atypical symptoms as well as significantly delayed presentation of diabetic patients for medical treatment, which may play a role in the higher incidence of cardiogenic shock and peri-infarction morbidity and mortality seen in diabetics.

Autopsy studies show a much higher incidence of myocardial scar, suggestive of past infarctions, in diabetics with no prior cardiac history than in nondiabetic individuals. Some controversy exists over the true incidence of silent myocardial infarction in diabetics, with some investigators suggesting that this phenomenon may be more of a myth than reality. As was shown in the Framingham Study about 25% of the infarctions went unrecognized. However, half of these patients had atypical symptoms not recognized as cardiac ischemia, thus it appears that only 12% of patients had truly silent infarctions. Most studies do show a higher trend of silent infarction in diabetic patients, but lack the statistical power for conclusive proof. However, there appears to be little doubt that a high index of suspicion is warranted in diabetics presenting with atypical symptoms, such as confusion, nausea, vomiting, or shortness of breath. An ECG at presentation may be very helpful in such situations, particularly if there is a previous

ECG for comparison. A baseline ECG should be obtained and available in all diabetic patients.

V. DIAGNOSIS OF CAD IN DIABETIC PATIENTS

A. Stress Testing

Although the prevalence of CAD is higher in the diabetic population, routine stress testing in asymptomatic diabetics with no known disease has not previously been recommended. Given the high prevalence of CAD in diabetics the American Diabetes Association (ADA) and American College of Cardiology (ACC) held a consensus development conference (6) in February 1998 and recommended stress testing in diabetic patients with any of the following:

1. Typical or atypical cardiac symptoms
2. Resting ECG suggestive of ischemia or infarction
3. Peripheral or carotid occlusive arterial disease
4. Sedentary lifestyle, age 35 years or older, and plans to begin a vigorous exercise program
5. Two or more of the following five risk factors:
    Total cholesterol 240 mg/dL or higher, LDL cholesterol 160 mg/dL or
        higher; or HDL cholesterol less than 35 mg/dL
    Blood pressure higher than 140/90 mmHg
    Smoker
    Family history of premature CAD
    Positive micro- or macroalbuminuria test

There are now various diagnostic stress test modalities that can be confusing to individuals who do not perform these tests on a regular basis. Simply put, these tests use either exercise or pharmacological forms of stress. In addition, a stress test can be a nonimaging (ECG only) or imaging test (nuclear or echocardiography). The following is a brief account of these tests, including their advantages and disadvantages.

1. Exercise Stress Test (ECG)

Although this is the most frequently requested test for diagnosis of CAD, it has the lowest sensitivity and specificity compared with the imaging tests (approximately 70% for each). It requires the patient to exercise to at least 85% of maximal predicted heart rate (MPHR), below which the rate of a false-negative result is increased. Also, it requires the ECG to be normal at baseline, as superadded ST-T wave changes on preexisting abnormalities are not specific markers of CAD. Women tend to have more false-positive results for unclear reasons. Unfortunately, the presence of ST-T wave changes at baseline is increased in diabetics owing to the presence of hypertension, cardiomyopathy, conduction abnormalities, and other unknown reasons. Also the presence of impaired and delayed ability to perceive ischemic cardiac pain can lead to confusion. Even so, a nonimaging ECG stress test can be used as a diagnostic test in diabetics with atypical symptoms and a normal ECG, and to assess prognosis and functional capacity of patients with known CAD and following uncomplicated myocardial infarction.

2. Pharmacological Stress Tests

Such tests are extremely valuable for patients who cannot reliably exercise on a treadmill or bicycle. There are two categories of pharmaceuticals used as stressor agents, sympathetomimetic agents, and coronary vasodilators. Of the sympathetomimetic agents available, dobutamine is the most commonly used. It increases the ionotropic state of the heart, the heart rate, and at times blood pressure, all of which increase myocardial oxygen consumption. Peak heart rates of 85% are usually attainable (sometimes needing supplemental atropine administration). When used for the diagnosis of CAD, dobutamine stress echocardiography entails a stepwise increasing dose of dobutamine ($10–40$ μg/kg per minute) and multiple tomographic echo images of the heart at baseline, low-dose, middose, and peak dobutamine infusion. Ischemia is diagnosed based on a new regional wall motion abnormality. Dobutamine can also be used as a stressor in conjunction with nuclear myocardial perfusion imaging (see following discussion). Antianginal medications should optimally be withdrawn before the test, particularly β-adrenergic blockers that inhibit the chronotropic and inotropic effects of dobutamine.

The coronary artery vasodilators commonly used are dipyridamole and adenosine. They induce maximum coronary vasodilation and are used most often in conjunction with nuclear perfusion imaging. Dipyridamole blocks the facilitated transport of adenosine into the cell, thereby raising extracellular levels of adenosine which, in turn, causes coronary vasodilation by binding with the adenosine A_2 receptors in the cell membrane. Ischemia is diagnosed if the regional hyperemic response is attenuated by the presence of a coronary arterial stenosis. This results in a "perfusion defect" on the nuclear image that is not present at rest. Both the vasodilators can worsen bronchospasm in patients with hyperactive airway disease. Caffeinated beverages should be avoided for at least 24 h, and theophylline-containing medications need to be discontinued at least 48 h before these agents can be used as stressors. This is because methylxanthines competitively bind to the adenosine receptors and inhibit vasodilation.

3. Stress Echocardiography

Stress echocardiography can employ either exercise or a pharmacological agent (see foregoing) as a stressor. Whichever mode of stress is used, the two most important factors for a successful test is the quality of images and the expertise of the interpreter. When these are met, the sensitivity and specificity of this test is equal to that of myocardial perfusion imaging. The sensitivity and specificity will be reduced in patients with marginal or poor quality images, which is common in obese individuals or individuals with chronic obstructive lung disease. Stress echocardiography provides information about dynamic valvular function and is less expensive than perfusion imaging.

4. Stress Perfusion Myocardial Imaging

This is still the most widely used stress-imaging technique, with a sensitivity of 85–90% and a specificity of 75–85%. In the current era, the two most common imaging agents are thallium and technetium-labeled sestamibi (Cardiolite). Single-photon emission computed tomographic (SPECT) imaging has improved overall image quality and thus, the ability to differentiate myocardium supplied by the left anterior descending, circumflex, and right coronary arteries. Although obesity causes attenuation of the nuclear signal, the image quality is not as adversely affected as echocardiographic images. Because baseline ECG abnormalities and obesity are common in diabetics, nuclear perfusion myocardial imaging is commonly used in these individuals. As it does not rely on the development of ischemia, a diagnostic test can still be performed if the patient is taking antianginal medications.

5. Recommendations

Although stress testing is not officially recommended for all asymptomatic individuals with diabetes, we recommend a low clinical threshold for such individuals and agree with the recommendations of the ADA and ACC consensus document (6) outlined earlier. Rigorous history taking should be employed to determine if patients experience any signs consistent with ischemic heart disease. Chest pain may be absent although many patients with ischemia experience dyspnea. A standard exercise stress test should be used for patients who can exercise and have a normal baseline ECG. Patients who cannot exercise adequately should undergo pharmacological stress testing. Baseline ECG abnormalities or pharmacological stress requires an imaging stress study. The choice of stress echo or nuclear perfusion imaging should depend on local expertise and availability. Coronary angiography should be used in patients with obvious ischemic symptoms.

B. Preoperative Cardiac Risk Evaluation for Noncardiac Surgery

This is a clinically important issue given the prevalence of CAD in diabetics. Although the general principles of risk assessment and treatment are similar for diabetics and nondiabetics, the very presence of DM places the patient in an intermediate-risk category for a perioperative cardiac event. As with nondiabetics, preoperative cardiac symptoms and the nature of surgery are key factors. Patients with DM who have the aforenoted indications for a diagnostic stress test should undergo stress evaluation before elective noncardiac surgery. Those low-risk patients without the aforenoted indications for stress testing should undergo preoperative stress evaluation before moderate to high-risk surgical procedures, such as major vascular, intrathoracic, or intraperitoneal surgery. Diabetic patients with a high probability of CAD should undergo coronary angiography before elective surgery. Detailed discussion of the preoperative cardiovascular evaluation of patients before noncardiac surgery is available in the 1996 American College of Cardiology (ACC)/American Heart Association (AHA) Task Force Report (2).

VI. TREATMENT OF CAD IN DM

A. Acute Myocardial Infarction

About 7–27% of patients presenting with an acute myocardial infarction are diabetic. Several studies both in the prethrombolytic and thrombolytic era have clearly demonstrated that the in-hospital mortality is 1.5–2 times higher in diabetic patients compared with their nondiabetic counterparts. In particular, diabetic women have twice the mortality rate of diabetic men and four times that of nondiabetic men.

In the era before coronary care units, in-hospital mortality of diabetic patients presenting with an acute myocardial infarction was 40–60%. With the introduction of coronary care units, the mortality rate dropped to 27–36% compared with 17–19% in nondiabetics. The introduction of early thrombolytic therapy saw a further reduction in mortality in diabetics to 10–17% in those treated with thrombolytics within the first 6 h as compared with 6–7.5% in nondiabetics so treated. Given the higher mortality risk in diabetics with infarction the relative benefit of early thrombolysis is accentuated in diabetics. It is estimated that early thrombolysis results in 15 lives saved per 1000 in nondiabetics compared to 37 lives saved per 1000 myocardial infarctions in diabetic patients. In spite of this, diabetes remains an independent predictor of a fatal outcome at 1 month and also confers a worse prognosis at 1 year, with a 1-year mortality of approximately 14.5% compared with 9.1% in nondiabetics.

In early thrombolytic trials, there was some suggestion that diabetics may be more resistant to the effects of thrombolysis because of the impaired fibrinolytic state discussed earlier. More recently, the Global Utilization of Streptokinase and Tissue Plasminogen Activator for Occluded Coronary Arteries (GUSTO-I; 10) trial showed similar early angiographic patency rates of the infarct-related artery in diabetics and nondiabetics. However diabetics also had a higher reocclusion rate. Fortunately, the important side effects of thrombolytics are similar in diabetics, for there does not seem to be any significant difference in the rates of hemorrhagic complications or of cerebrovascular accidents caused by thrombolytics. Of particular note is that retinal or preretinal hemorrhage is extremely rare, even when thrombolytics were given to patients with known diabetic retinopathy. Percutaneous coronary artery interventions can be used as primary therapy in diabetics with an acute myocardial infarction, to establish normal flow in the infarct-related artery in the face of continuing ischemia, or as a rescue to failed thrombolysis.

The increased mortality in diabetics following a myocardial infarction is predominantly because of an increased incidence of congestive heart failure (CHF), although reinfarction and recurrent ischemia may also be contributory. Many studies have shown a disproportionate increase in CHF and cardiogenic shock in diabetics compared with nondiabetics with a similar infarction size and similar loss of left ventricular systolic function. This has been attributed to less compensatory hyperkinesis in the noninfarcted walls that may be due to more extensive atherosclerotic epicardial coronary artery disease, previous unsuspected myocardial infarction, presence of diabetic cardiomyopathy, autonomic neuropathy, or secondary to abnormalities in the microcirculation. There is no evidence that diabetics sustain larger infarctions than their nondiabetic counterparts. Diastolic dysfunction owing to the presence of diabetic cardiomyopathy or hypertension or both should be suspected if there is overt heart failure in the face of a clinically small infarct and relatively preserved systolic function.

B. Secondary Prevention of Cardiac Events in DM

1. Aspirin

Aspirin is of benefit in the secondary prevention of unstable coronary syndromes and myocardial infarction both in nondiabetics and in diabetics. The exact dose of aspirin continues to remain unclear, as does the issue of whether diabetic patients with a significantly greater baseline level of platelet activation need a higher dose of aspirin to achieve the same level of platelet inhibition as their nondiabetic counterparts. In the Second International Study of Infarct Survival (ISIS-2; 12) diabetic patients receiving 160 mg of aspirin had no reduction in mortality. Although there has been a trend toward using lower doses of aspirin in patients with CAD, diabetics should receive 325 mg of aspirin per day.

2. β-Adrenergic Blockers

Despite their adverse metabolic effects β-adrenergic blockers are effective in reducing reinfarction and sudden death in diabetic patients, perhaps to a greater extent than in nondiabetic individuals. Early treatment in MI with β-blockers produced a 13% short-term mortality reduction in all patients, compared with 37% mortality reduction in diabetic patients. With longer follow-up, mortality was reduced by 33% in all patients and 48% in diabetic subjects. β-Blockers should be used in patients with preserved left ventricular function and in patients with dysfunctional left ventricles. Deterioration in glycemic control or blunted counterregulatory response to hypoglycemia is seldom a serious clinical issue.

3. Angiotensin-Converting Enzyme Inhibitors

The role of this group of drugs is well established in reducing morbidity and mortality in patients with left ventricular systolic dysfunction, especially when due to coronary artery disease (ischemic cardiomyopathy). They have also been effective in the secondary prevention of reinfarction in diabetic patients. They are particularly attractive in diabetic patients owing to their renal protective and antihypertensive effects.

C. Treatment of Lipid Abnormalities in DM

The specific lipid abnormalities that occur in DM have been described in the foregoing. Aggressive treatment of lipid disorders is recommended for all patients with DM (primary and secondary prevention). As in nondiabetic individuals, lipid levels may be affected by factors unrelated to glycemia or insulin resistance, such as renal disease, hypothyroidism, and familial lipoprotein disorders (e.g., familial hypercholesterolemia, familial combined hyperlipidemia, and familial hypertriglyceridemia). These genetic disorders should be suspected in patients with severe hypercholesterolemia or hypertriglyceridemia. Alcohol and estrogen use may also contribute to hypertriglyceridemia. *It is suggested that adult patients with diabetes receive a full fasting lipoprotein analysis annually.*

The American Diabetes Association has made recommendations for both medical nutrition therapy (MNT [dietary therapy]) and physical activity. Maximal MNT typically reduces LDL cholesterol 15–25 mg/dL. Thus, if the goal LDL reduction exceeds 25 mg/dL the physician may decide to institute drug therapy at the same time as behavioral therapy. In other patients, behavioral interventions may be evaluated at 1-month intervals. Consideration of drug therapy should not be delayed beyond 3–6 months.

There have been four major lipid-lowering trials published this decade. Each compared a hydroxymethylglutaryl coenzyme A (HMGCoA) reductase inhibitor or "statin" with placebo in patients with hypercholesterolemia. None of the clinical trials exclusively enrolled patients with DM. In fact, there were surprisingly few diabetics in the four trials. In both primary prevention trials (WOSCOPS, pravastatin; and AFCAPS/TexCAPS, lovastatin) the cardiovascular event rate was significantly decreased with lipid-lowering therapy. However, only

1% of patients in WOSCOPS and 3% of patients in AFCAPS/TexCAPS were diabetics. There was no significant reduction in cardiovascular events in the small number of patients with DM. In the Scandinavian Simvastatin Survival Study (4S) (15) trial, patients with moderate to severe hypercholesterolemia (total cholesterol 210–310 mg/dL) and angina or a previous MI (secondary prevention trial) were randomized to either simvastatin or placebo. Simvastatin significantly reduced the incidence of nonfatal MI, cardiovascular mortality, and total mortality. Of the 4444 patients enrolled in the 4S trial, 201 were diabetics. Despite the limited number of diabetic patients, simvastatin showed even greater efficacy in diabetic individuals than in the overall study group. The 6-year relative reduction in all cardiovascular events for the diabetic group taking simvastatin was 55%. In the Cholesterol and Recurrent Events (CARE) study, 4159 patients with mild to moderate hypercholesterolemia (total cholesterol < 240 mg/dL) and a previous myocardial infarction (secondary prevention trial) were randomized to either pravastatin or placebo (14). Pravastatin significantly reduced the combined endpoint of death and nonfatal myocardial infarction by 25% in diabetics (586 of 4159 patients enrolled) and 23% in nondiabetic patients.

The National Cholesterol Education Program (NCEP) recommends that the LDL cholesterol be reduced to less than 100 mg/dL in all patients with known CAD, to less than 130 mg/dL in patients without known CAD and two or more risk factors, and to less than 160 mg/dL in patients without known CAD and one or no risk factors. However, recent data revealed that over 5–7 years of follow-up, diabetics without known CAD have cardiovascular event rates equal to that of nondiabetics who have had a previous cardiovascular event (11). For that reason, we and many others feel that all diabetics should be treated aggressively, and the LDL should be less than 100 mg/dL.

1. Pharmacologic Therapy

The HMGCoA reductase inhibitors (statins) remain the first choice in reducing LDL cholesterol levels as multiple primary, and secondary prevention trials have proved their efficacy and safety (1). There are numerous drugs with a wide range of potencies to choose from in this group. Minimal reductions in LDL may be achievable with all the statins, whereas greater reductions in LDL levels will require the more potent agents atorvastatin and simvastatin. It is currently argued whether individual statins have other unique cardioprotective effects independent of reduction in lipid levels, or whether the magnitude of the LDL reduction is the sole consideration for efficacy. A detailed discussion of this controversy is beyond the scope of this chapter. The choice of the statin should depend on the magnitude of LDL reduction desired, the initial LDL levels, and the judgment of the prescribing physician. For patients who cannot tolerate a statin or who need a second agent a bile acid-binding resin should be used. Fibric acids, such as gemfibrozil, should be used primarily in diabetic patients with significant hypertriglyeridemia who are at risk of pancreatitis (see later discussion).

A low HDL cholesterol level is a powerful predictor of CAD in diabetics. However, raising HDL levels is difficult. Behavioral modifications, such as weight loss and especially exercise cause a modest increase in HDL levels, and smoking should be strongly discouraged. The combination of a statin with nicotinic acid is extremely effective in modifying diabetic dyslipidemia (with the largest increase in HDL cholesterol), unfortunately the combination can significantly worsen hyperglycemia. Thus, if used, low doses of nicotinic acid ($\leq$ 2 g of nicotinic acid per day), with frequent glucose monitoring is recommended. The use of combinations of a statin and gemfibrozil or nicotinic acid causes more hepatic toxicity and myositis.

In diabetics, a triglyceride level of 200–400 mg/dL may be commonly found; and the best initial therapy is improving glycemic control, weight loss, increased physical activity, and moderation of alcohol consumption. For this degree of triglyceride elevation, clinical judgment must be exercised whether to initiate drug therapy. For triglyceride levels higher than 1000 mg/dL, severe dietary fat reduction ($<$ 10% of calories) in addition to pharmacological therapy is necessary to reduce the risk of pancreatitis. Fibric acid derivatives are the drugs of first choice for triglyceride reduction with statins being modestly effective in high doses in hypertriglyceridemic patients who also have high LDL cholesterol. The morbity and mortality associated with pancreatitis should be stressed to all patients with significant hypertriglyceridemia.

D. Coronary Artery Interventions and Bypass Surgery

Because of the severity and prevalence of CAD, many patients with DM undergo revascularization procedures (i.e., percutaneous transluminal coronary angioplasty [PTCA] or coronary artery bypass surgery [CABG]). Typically 20–25% of patients referred for percutaneous coronary angioplasty are diabetics. The correct choice of the revascularization strategy, although obviously important can sometimes be difficult, as discussed in the following section.

1. Single-Vessel Disease

In the nondiabetic population, symptomatic single-vessel disease in most instances is treated with PTCA (if technically possible), especially if medical therapy has already failed. The same usually holds true for diabetic patients, especially as recent large studies have not shown any significant increase in in-hospital complications in diabetic patients and the procedural success rate is equivalent. However, the issue is complicated because with simple balloon angioplasty the restenosis and late vessel closure rate is almost twice that in the nondiabetic population (47–69 vs. 28–40%) as has been consistently reported in all major trials. DM has been described as an independent risk factor for restenosis after balloon angioplasty. Atherectomy (rotational or directional) is similarly plagued by this high restenosis rate in the diabetic population.

Restenosis after PTCA results from a combination of mechanical forces (immediate vessel recoil), proliferative changes (neointimal hyperplasia), and late changes in the vessel geometry (remodeling). Stenting greatly eliminates the early recoil and late constrictive remodeling. Whether neointimal hyperplasia (which is the main cause of in-stent restenosis) is more pronounced in diabetics than nondiabetics is not currently known. It does appear that the use of metallic stents has made a significant effect on the restenosis rates. Trials have consistently demonstrated a drop in the restenosis rate to at least the 25–30% range in diabetics compared with 15–20% in nondiabetics. Some studies have failed to demonstrate an increased restenosis rate in diabetics. The stent restenosis rate may be higher in diabetics receiving stents in saphanous vein grafts.

Patients with single-vessel disease presenting with angina usually have preserved ventricular function and, according to several trials, there is no significant survival benefit between CABG, PTCA, or medical therapy. Patients treated medically or with PTCA, however, are more prone to recurrent symptoms and require more hospitalizations. They are also likely to need more revascularization procedures. Following PTCA there is a statistically insignificant lowering of the incidence of acute myocardial infarction between 2 and 5 years. At the present time with improved expertise and technology, it appears that PTCA combined with stent deployment for the relief of angina, is an acceptable form of treatment in the diabetic population.

2. Multivessel Disease

When Andreas Gruentzig first introduced balloon angioplasty in 1977, focal, noncomplex single-vessel disease was considered suitable for PTCA to delay the requirement for CABG which was the accepted gold standard for revascularization. The 1980s saw an explosive growth of PTCA as an alternative revascularization strategy, as improved operator skills and technology resulted in percutaneous interventions on more complex lesions and on multivessel disease. This led to a head-to-head comparison between CABG and PTCA in patients with multivessel CAD. Between 1986 and 1991, six randomized, controlled trials (ERACI, RITA, CABRI, GABI, EAST, and BARI) enlisted an aggregate of 4310 patients with multivessel disease who were thought suitable for either PTCA or CABG (note: this excluded patients with more severe forms of disease who could be treated with surgery only). The results from these trials were remarkably concordant. CABG was associated with a slight (not statistically significant) survival advantage, less angina, and fewer revascularization procedures. PTCA led to a slight (not statistically significant) reduction in myocardial infarction over the subsequent 2–5 years.

How do these overall results compare with analysis of the diabetic subpopulation in these trials? The oft quoted BARI study (4,5) showed that at 5-year follow-up treated diabetic patients (insulin or oral hypoglycemic agents) had a significant survival advantage with CABG compared with PTCA (80.6 vs. 65.5%; p = 0.003). The survival curves began to separate as early as 6 months after randomization. Importantly, this advantage was seen only in those patients who received an internal mammary artery graft and not in patients who received all venous grafts. A more recently published trial by Weintraub et al. from Emory University, Atlanta showed that in the insulin-treated subgroup 5- and 10-year survival rates were 68 and 36% after PTCA and 75 and 47% after CABG, respectively (16). In both studies PTCA patients needed more repeat revascularization procedures.

Of importance is that these trials were all conducted in an era when stenting was not as commonly practiced as it is today. Given that stenting significantly reduces the rate of restenosis and late vessel closure, it is not known what effect it would have on the foregoing data.

Also to be considered is that diabetics fare much worse than their nondiabetic counterparts with bypass surgery. In the Emory experience the in-hospital mortality rate was 5% in the bypass group compared with 0.36% in the PTCA group. In BARI the in-hospital mortality rate was double (1.2 vs. 0.6%) for surgically treated patients with diabetes. Finally, the BARI study again demonstrated that surgically treated diabetic patients have a worse 5-year survival than do nondiabetics (80.6 vs. 91.4%). Repeat revascularization was higher and coronary event-free survival was less in diabetics than in nondiabetics. The incidence of sternal wound and other in-hospital infections and renal failure were higher in diabetics as well (see also Refs. 4,5,8).

The therapeutic modality to choose in the stent era may be a dilemma. At this time, the data we have may favor surgical intervention for multivessel disease in treated diabetic patients at least until we have randomized trial data of diabetic patients whose multivessel disease was uniformly treated with stenting. Also still unknown, is what effect newer therapeutic modes (e.g., oral platelet glycoprotein IIb/IIIa receptor blockers, and radiation therapy) is going to have on restenosis rates following percutaneous interventions. Also, it is unclear whether strict glycemic control in the peri- and postprocedural period after coronary angioplasty would reduce the restenosis rate. *What is clear, however, is that diabetic patients fare relatively poorly compared with nondiabetic patients after multivessel revascularization, independent of the treatment modality chosen.*

VII. FUTURE DIRECTIONS

There is no doubt that atherosclerotic complications are accelerated in diabetics with profound clinical and socioeconomic effects. The onus is on the medical community to concentrate research activities on the elucidation of the unique mechanisms that lead to accelerated atherosclerosis in diabetic and insulin-resistant patients. The pathogenesis and clinical significance of diabetic cardiomyopathy and autonomic neuropathy also needs to be further elucidated. Efforts to reduce restenosis rates in diabetes are of prime importance. Diabetics should now be treated aggressively with appropriate primary and secondary preventative measures, and available diagnostic studies should be employed as outlined in this chapter.

REFERENCES

1. American Diabetes Association. Management of dyslipidemia in adults with diabetes. Diabetes Care 1998; 21:179–182.
2. American College of Cardiology/American Heart Association Task Force Report. Guildlines for perioperative cardiovascular evaluation for noncardiac surgery. Report of the American College of Cardiology/American Heart Association Task Force on Practice Guildlines. Circulation 1996; 93:1278–1317.
3. Aronson D, Rayfield EJ. Diabetes. In: EJ Topol, ed. Textbook of Cardiovascular Medicine. Philadelphia: Lippincot–Raven, 1998, pp. 185–208.
4. BARI Investigators. Comparison of coronary bypass surgery with angioplasty in patients with multivessel disease. N Engl J Med 1996; 335:217–225.
5. BARI Investigators. Influence of diabetes on 5-year mortality and morbidity in a randomized trial comparing CABG and PTCA in patients with multivessel disease. The Bypass Angioplasty Revascularization Investigation (BARI). Circulation 1997; 96:1761–1769.
6. Consensus Development Conference on the Diagnosis of Coronary Heart Disease in People with Diabetes. Diabetes Care 1998; 21:1551–1559.
7. The DCCT Research Group. The effect of intensive diabetes management on macrovascular events and risk factors in the Diabetes Control and Complications Trial. Am J Cardiol 1995; 75:894–903.
8. Ellis SG, Narins CR. Problem of angioplasty in diabetics [editorial]. Circulation 1997; 96:1707–10.
9. Ewing DJ, Clarke BF. Diagnosis and management of diabetic autonomic neuropathy. Br Med J 1982; 285:916–918.
10. Gusto-I Angiographic Investigators. Angiographic findings and outcome in diabetic patients treated with thrombolytic therapy for acute myocardial infarction: the GUSTO-I experience. J Am Coll Cardiol 1996; 28:1661–1669.
11. Haffner SM, Lehto S, Ronnemaa T, Pyorala K, Laakso M. Mortality from coronary heart disease in subjects with type 2 diabetes and in nondiabetic subjects with and without prior myocardial infarction. N Engl J Med 1998; 339:229–34.

12. ISIS-2 Collaborative Group. Randomized trial of intravenous streptokinase, oral aspirin, both, or neither among 17187 of suspected acute myocardial infarction—ISIS-2. Lancet 1998; 2:349–360.

13. Kannel WB, McGee DL. Diabetes and glucose tolerance as risk factors for cardiovascular disease: the Framingham Study. Diabetes Care 1979; 2:120–126.

14. Sacks FM, Pfeffer MA, Moye LA, et al. The effect of pravastatin on coronary events after myocardial infarction in patients with average cholesterol levels. N Engl J Med 1996; 335:1001–1009.

15. Scandinavian Simvastatin Survival Study Group. Randomised trial of cholesterol lowering in 4444 patients with coronary heart disease: the Scandinavian Simvastatin Survival Study (4S). Lancet 1994; 344:1383–1389.

16. Weintraub WS, et al. Outcome of coronary bypass surgery versus coronary angioplasty in diabetic patients with multivessel coronary artery disease. J Am Coll Cardiol 1998; 31:10–19.

24

Gastrointestinal Complications of Diabetes Mellitus

Bernard Coulie and Michael Camilleri
Mayo Clinic and Mayo Foundation, Rochester, Minnesota

I. INTRODUCTION

Gastrointestinal symptoms are frequently encountered in patients with diabetes mellitus. Diabetic enteropathy may result in dysphagia, heartburn, nausea and vomiting, abdominal pain, constipation, diarrhea, and fecal incontinence (7). Although not generally considered important causes of morbidity in diabetic patients, these symptoms can be encountered in up to 75% of diabetic outpatients evaluated at a tertiary referral center. The prevalence of gastrointestinal symptoms among community diabetic patients is, however, lower. A recent questionnaire-based study in Olmsted County, Minnesota, showed that only constipation and use of laxatives were more prevalent in diabetics than in controls matched for age and gender (17). The high prevalence of functional gastrointestinal disorders, such as irritable bowel syndrome, constipation, and functional dyspepsia in Western civilizations confounds any estimates of the prevalence of diabetic enteropathy based on symptoms alone. Nonetheless, the nature of the symptoms suggests that many may result from motor and sensory abnormalities of the gastrointestinal tract, which reflects alterations in neural control, impaired intestinal absorption or secretion, and deranged pancreatic function (Fig. 1).

This chapter reviews the pathophysiology of gastrointestinal symptoms in patients with diabetes mellitus, and emphasizes current diagnostic and therapeutic approaches in their management.

II. ETIOLOGY AND PATHOPHYSIOLOGY

A. Motor Dysfunction

The pathogenesis of abnormal gastrointestinal motility in diabetes mellitus is incompletely understood and is likely multifactorial, including extrinsic denerva-

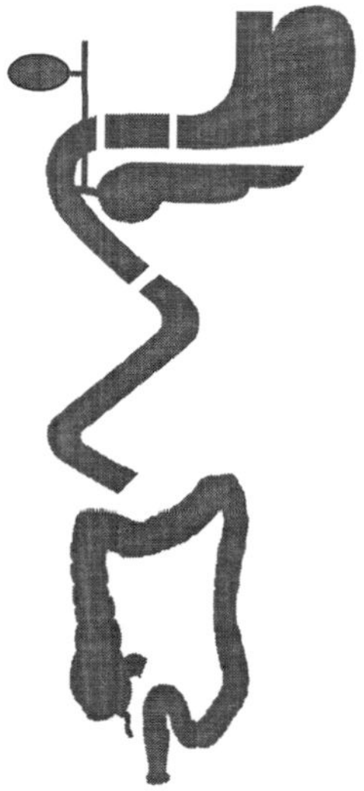

GI manifestations of diabetes	Associated disease	Clinical presentation
↓ gall bladder motility		gall stones
antral hypomotility, pylorospasm		gastric stasis, bezoars
↓ α_2-adrenergic tone in enterocytes	exocrine pancreatic insufficiency, celiac sprue, SB bacterial overgrowth, bile acid malabsorption	diarrhea, steatorrhea
SB dysmotility		gastric or SB stasis, rapid SB transit
colonic dysmotility		constipation, diarrhea
anorectal dysfunction, sensory neuropathy, sympathetic (IAS) or pudendal (EAS) neuropathy		diarrhea, incontinence

Fig. 1 Mechanisms of GI symptoms in patients with diabetes mellitus.

tion, enteric neuropathy, and hyperglycemia (1,9,12,14). These result in impaired gastric contractility or abnormal myoelectrical control (1). The syndrome is typically seen in patients with type I or insulin-dependent diabetes mellitus (IDDM). Peripheral neuropathy is present in the majority of patients with enteropathy, and other forms of autonomic neuropathy are common. Previous work has attributed these motility disorders to mainly vagal nerve dysfunction, although dysfunction of the sympathetic innervation has also been implicated and probably causes a reduced internal anal sphincter tone, resulting in nocturnal stool incontinence. Motor abnormalities of the small intestine observed in symptomatic diabetic patients are often indistinguishable from those seen in patients with other syndromes affecting postganglionic sympathetic function. The relative contributions of parasympathetic and sympathetic nerve damage to diabetic visceral neuropathy in the nonsphincteric regions of the digestive tract remains unclear. Vagal dysfunction is probably critical in gastric stasis, but it is unclear whether rapid small bowel transit and diarrhea result from vagal neuropathy or from loss of tonic inhibitory sympathetic input. Electrolyte imbalances caused by diabetic ketoacidosis (e.g., hypokalemia) and uremia may further aggravate impaired motor function in diabetic patients.

Apart from these disturbances in the extrinsic neural control of the gut, there is also some degree of histological damage and biochemical impairment in the enteric nervous system in patients with long-standing diabetes. In an early study, some nerves were reported to show swollen, irregular processes, vacuolation or fragmentation of the dendrites, and Schwann cells (5A). Myenteric plexus nerves appear morphologically normal in diabetic animal models, even in viscera that are clearly affected by diabetic autonomic neuropathy. Immunohistochemical studies of the enteric nervous system in rats with experimental diabetes have shown increased levels of the inhibitory neurotransmitter vasoactive intestinal polypeptide (VIP) and reduced concentrations of nitric oxide (NO), neuropeptide Y, serotonin, substance P, and calcitonin gene-related peptide (CGRP). These findings are relevant because they may explain alterations in visceral sensation and in the control of motor functions, such as the peristaltic reflex. Histopathological abnormalities observed in gut smooth muscle may be secondary to ischemia; primary smooth muscle failure seems unlikely, because diabetic intestinal muscle retains its tensile properties and affinities for several agonists in vitro and its sensitivity to cholinergic stimulation in vivo.

In recent years, it has been suggested that glycemic control alters several gastrointestinal functions (9), such as gastric emptying, gastric myoelectric activity, antroduodenal motor activity, gastric visceral sensation, and the colonic response to feeding. Alterations in glucose control may also alter glucose counterregulatory hormones, some of which directly affect gastrointestinal motility. These include glucagon, glucagon like peptide 1, amylin, epinephrine, somatostatin, growth hormone, and cortisol. The effects of autonomic nerve damage on release of these hormones from the pancreas, intestine, and liver could also contribute to the motor dysfunction.

Work from our laboratory suggests that autonomic dysfunction has a more significant role in the pathogenesis of gastric dysmotility than glucose homeostasis per se, for patients with non–insulin-dependent diabetes mellitus (NIDDM) without evidence of autonomic neuropathy have normal gastric emptying of solids despite elevated blood glucose and glycosylated hemoglobin (HbA$_{1c}$) levels (8). Similarly, a hyperglycemic clamp did not significantly alter the colonic motor response to feeding, when compared with euglycemia in health (16).

B. Abnormal Mucosal Fluid Absorption

In diabetic animal models, the enterocyte has impaired α_2-adrenergic tone (5). This led to therapeutic use of the α_2-adrenergic agonist clonidine (0.1–0.3 mg, b.i.d., as tolerated), in the treatment of diabetic diarrhea in humans. Disturbances of fluid transport and motor dysfunction probably coexist in these patients, and agents such as clonidine may correct both alterations of enteric function.

C. Abnormal Mucosal Sensation

Abnormal mucosal sensation is an important mechanism in patients with diabetes and constipation or incontinence (19). It results from pudendal nerve dysfunction.

There is also evidence that the absence of severe symptoms in patients with diabetic gastroparesis may reflect impairment of gastric afferent sensory function.

III. CLINICAL MANIFESTATIONS AND INVESTIGATION OF DIABETIC ENTEROPATHY

A. Dysphagia and Heartburn

1. Symptoms

Esophageal symptoms are frequent in diabetic patients. Abnormal esophageal pressure profiles in diabetic patients, particularly in the lower esophageal sphincter, and in amplitude, frequency, and shape of propagated esophageal contractions correlate with signs of peripheral or autonomic neuropathy, but do not always correlate with esophageal symptoms. Reflux symptoms may be aggravated by impaired gastric emptying. Rarely, recurrent vomiting may lead to Mallory-Weiss tears and bleeding.

2. Investigations

Specialized tests that assess esophageal motor function play a relatively minor role in clinical practice. Dysphagia and heartburn should prompt upper gastrointestinal endoscopy to exclude gastroesophageal reflux disease and other incidental mucosal diseases (e.g., candidiasis or neoplasms). Because of the high incidence of coronary atherosclerosis among diabetic patients, chest pain should not be attributed to disturbed motor function of the esophagus, and appropriate tests need to be undertaken to exclude coronary artery disease.

B. Nausea, Vomiting, and Dyspepsia

1. Symptoms and Signs

Nausea and vomiting, often accompanied by weight loss and early satiety, are common gastrointestinal symptoms among patients with diabetes. Episodes of nausea and vomiting may last days to months, or occur in cycles, and blood glucose concentrations may be poorly controlled. Frequent episodes of hypoglycemia are encountered when food delivery to the small bowel for absorption is not sufficient to match the hypoglycemic effect of exogenously administered insulin. Kassander termed the syndrome of impaired gastric emptying often associated with impaired glycemic control "diabetic gastroparesis" (12). It is frequently associated with retinopathy, nephropathy, peripheral neuropathy, and other forms of autonomic dysfunction, including abnormal pupillary responses, anhidrosis, gustatory sweating, orthostatic hypotension, impotence, retrograde ejaculation, and dysfunction of the urinary bladder. A succussion splash or large gastric residual after overnight fast may be documented clinically. Rarely, patients with gastroparesis present with retrosternal or epigastric pain, and cardiac, biliary, or pancreatic disease may be considered.

Dyspepsia refers to postprandial upper abdominal discomfort, early satiety, bloating, distension, as well as nausea and vomiting. There are some patients who have increased gastric sensitivity, whereas others lack an accommodation response to feeding. Food ingestion stimulates tension receptors in the nonaccommodating gastric wall, resulting in perception of bloating, early satiety, nausea, indigestion, or pain. Vagal neuropathy is likely cofactor preventing the gastric accommodation response.

2. Investigations

The algorithm shown in Fig. 2 should encompass exclusion of incidental conditions by endoscopy, even when gastroparesis is suspected: gastric outlet obstruction from chronic peptic ulcer disease (including tests for *Helicobacter pylori*) or neoplasms. Other factors can cause a deterioration of gastric emptying, including metabolic derangements (such as diabetic ketoacidosis or uremia) and medications commonly used in treating other problems in patients with diabetes mellitus

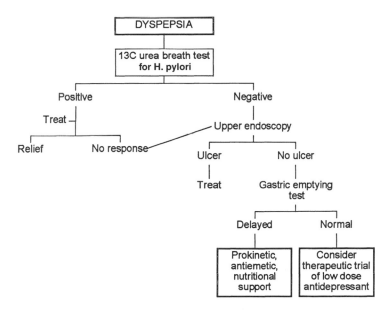

Fig. 2 Management of dyspepsia in patients with diabetes mellitus.

(e.g., anticholinergics, phenothiazines, antihypertensives, tricyclic antidepressants, serotonergic agents, dopaminergic drugs, opiates, and calcium channel blockers).

a. Measurement of Gastric Emptying

The positive diagnosis of diabetic gastroparesis requires demonstration of a delay in gastric emptying. Barium studies and scintigraphy using labeled liquid meals are of limited use, because the gastric emptying of liquids and semisolids (e.g., mashed potatoes) is often normal, even in the presence of moderately severe symptoms. Assessment of the emptying of solids is a more sensitive test. The choice of the radiolabeled marker is important, as the emptying of digestible and nondigestible solids of different sizes varies considerably. Each laboratory must standardize its method and develop normal data in healthy subjects.

At Mayo Clinic, we use ^{99m}Tc-labeled eggs that are cooked to a firm consistency to provide a solid medium, which is emptied linearly from the stomach when the solid component of the meal has been broken down to a particle size of less than 2 mm. This can be measured as part of a whole-gut transit test (Fig. 3). Larger indigestible particles are emptied with the antral component of the interdigestive migrating motor complex (MMC) and, hence, may reflect interdigestive motility and may not accurately assess postprandial function.

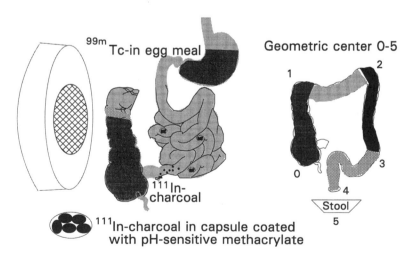

Fig. 3 Whole-gut scintigraphic transit test: an isotope-labeled egg meal serves to measure gastric and small-bowel transit; a delayed-release pH-sensitive capsule that dissolves in the ileum and contains a different isotope facilitates measurement of colonic transit.

A sequence of three scans is taken 2, 4, and 6 h after ingestion of a standard breakfast meal (4). The proportion of radioisotope emptied from the stomach at 2 (24–47%) and 4 h (> 50%) distinguishes normal function from gastroparesis, with a sensitivity of 90% and a specificity of 78%. This accuracy is comparable with that obtained from more detailed methods requiring repetitive scans and costly analyses, and this strategy has been replicated in a prospective study. Colonic filling at 6 h provides an estimate of orocecal transit rate.

With the recent introduction of stable isotope breath test technology, alternative methods have become available to noninvasively measure gastric emptying of solids. The stable, nonradioactive isotope ^{13}C, bound to a medium-chain triglyceride (octanoic acid) or a proteinaceous algae (*Spirulina*) substrate, can label the solid component of a test meal (Fig. 4). The ^{13}C-labeled substrate is absorbed in the duodenum, metabolized in the liver and excreted as breath $^{13}CO_2$. By collecting breath samples at specific time points after ingestion of the meal (e.g., 75, 90, and 180 min with ^{13}C-*Spirulina*), the $^{13}CO_2$ enrichment of breath can be measured by mass spectrometry, and gastric emptying parameters can be calculated accurately in healthy and in diabetic patients (10,13). Because data on the sensitivity and specificity of the breath test for detection of gastroparesis are currently lacking, further validation studies in diabetic gastroparesis are necessary. If an accuracy similar to the scintigraphic gastric emptying test is demon-

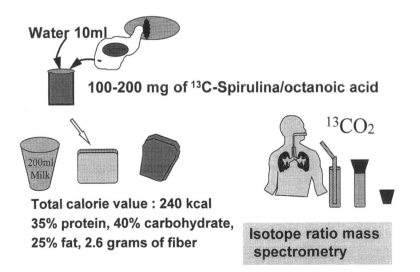

Fig. 4 Stable isotope breath test to measure gastric emptying of solids. A ^{13}C-substrate is incorporated in a meal and the rate of breath excretion of $^{13}CO_2$ is used to calculate gastric emptying rate.

strated, breath tests will be valid alternatives and provide considerable advantages because of the absence of any radiation exposure and the opportunity to measure gastric emptying in the diabetes clinic or doctor's office and embark on community-based studies in diabetes mellitus.

b. Measurement of Gastric Accommodation and Sensitivity

The tests available are cumbersome and incompletely validated for clinical practice and remain research tools. A therapeutic trial with a low dose of an anticholinergic antidepressant agent, such as amitryptiline, 10–25 mg, o.d. or b.i.d., is the most practical approach to reducing gastric symptoms such as pain and early satiety. This agent may relax the stomach and possibly reduce visceral afferent sensitivity.

C. Gastric Bezoar

Gastric bezoars form when fasting antral motor function is deficient. When bezoars are found endoscopically or on a barium x-ray films, they are a sign of antral hypomotility. Other motor dysfunctions contribute to gastric stasis in patients with diabetes mellitus, such as pylorospasm and small bowel dysmotility. The role of altered gastric accommodation in gastric stasis and bezoar formation is unclear. However, altered accommodation may contribute to dyspeptic symptoms, such as early satiety, bloating, and abdominal distention. Measurement of pressure profiles in the stomach and small bowel confirms the motor disturbance (1) and may provide important information before selecting patients for enteral feeding. Thus, patients with a selective abnormality of antral function may tolerate feeding delivered directly into the small bowel; on the other hand, those with a more generalized motility disorder may not tolerate enteral feeding.

D. Diarrhea

1. Symptoms

The frequency of diarrhea in patients with diabetes seen at university medical centers has been reported to vary from 8 to 22%. However, it is far less frequent when assessed by self-reported questionnaires (17). Several factors may result in diarrhea in patients with diabetes mellitus. Diarrhea caused by diabetes is typically chronic, can be severe, and occurs in patients with a long history of diabetes and insulin treatment. Diarrhea can occur at any time, but is often nocturnal, and may be associated with anal incontinence, indicating internal anal sphincter dysfunction. Bouts of diarrhea can be episodic with intermittent periods of normal bowel movements, or even constipation, making it sometimes difficult to differentiate this form of diarrhea from the much more common irritable bowel syndrome.

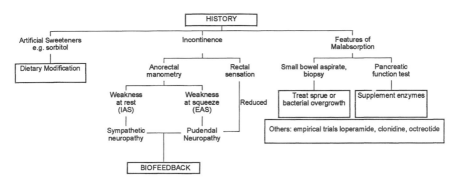

Fig. 5 Management algorithm for patients with diabetes mellitus and diarrhea.

2. Mechanisms

''Diabetic diarrhea'' is only one of the reported causes of chronic diarrhea in patients with diabetes, although its precise etiology is unclear and is often multifactorial. Thus, various mechanisms may result in chronic diarrhea in these patients and form the basis for the management strategy (Fig. 5). These mechanisms include the following:

1. Autonomic neuropathy secondary to diabetes may result in small-bowel dysmotility (abnormal pressure profiles have been documented during fasting and postprandially) or colonic dysmotility, but the literature on small-bowel transit shows conflicting results, that is, either delayed or accelerated transit.

2. Altered intestinal secretion results from impairment of water and electrolyte transport owing to reduced α_2-adrenergic tone in enterocytes.

3. Small bowel bacterial overgrowth is an infrequent finding among diabetic patients with chronic diarrhea (22). It results in bile salt deconjugation, fat malabsorption, and diarrhea.

4. Bile acid malabsorption also has been reported, but may be secondary to rapid ileal transit which may result from autonomic neuropathy. Colonic secretion may result from increased concentrations of deconjugated bile acids in the colon.

5. Anorectal dysfunction is a relatively common problem among patients with diabetes; fecal incontinence is experienced by approximately 20% of patients with long-standing diabetes mellitus in a tertiary referral population (19,21). The experience of diabetologists and community-based posted questionnaires (17) suggest these prevalence data cannot be extrapolated to the diabetic patients in general. Incontinent patients

with diabetes (21) demonstrate decreased anorectal sensation, and significantly reduced resting anal sphincter pressures (a function of the internal anal sphincter and sympathetic innervation), but usually normal squeeze pressure (a function of the external sphincter and parasympathetic innervation). Although rare in diabetes, external sphincter dysfunction, may be associated with dysfunction of the urinary bladder and indicate a pudendal neuropathy.

Diarrhea among diabetic patients may be secondary to associated disorders, the prevalence of which appears to be greater than in nondiabetic controls: (a) exocrine pancreatic dysfunction which may result from pancreatic atrophy, disruption of enteropancreatic reflexes, or elevated serum hormonal levels of glucagon, somatostatin, and pancreatic polypeptide, which reduce pancreatic enzyme secretion; (b) celiac sprue appears to be more common in patients with type I diabetes than in control subjects, and the common HLA haplotype HLA_1B_8 suggests an underlying genetic predisposition.

3. Investigations

A detailed dietary and medication history are key (see Fig. 5). For example, sorbitol-containing dietetic foods may cause an osmotic diarrhea, and laxatives or antacids may cause diarrhea. We also specifically search for features that suggest fecal incontinence or malabsorption (20). Patients with fecal incontinence frequently complain of "diarrhea," even though stool volume or consistency may be unaltered. The anorectal examination allows assessment of the resting and squeeze anal sphincter pressures; lack of sensation in the rectum and perianal skin may indicate the presence of a significant neuropathy (21). Absence of the cutaneous anal "wink" reflex indicates sacral root dysfunction. Evaluation of anorectal function should include anorectal manometry, and testing of rectal compliance and sensation to balloon distension. Other methods are available to confirm pudendal neuropathy or pelvic floor dysfunction, such as electromyography, or pudendal nerve conduction tests, but these, for the most part, are used as research tests. Anal endosonography is useful to identify defects in the anal sphincter or thinning of the perineal body that may coincide and are common in multiparous women. Defecating proctography evaluates rectal anatomy and may identify rectoceles or intussusception and the function of the pelvic floor during the process of defecation. Rectoceles are considered to be significant if they fill preferentially and fail to empty during attempted defecation.

The presence of anemia, macrocytosis, hypoalbuminemia, or excess stool fat suggest intestinal malabsorption, and specific tests are indicated to diagnose small-intestinal bacterial overgrowth, celiac disease, or pancreatic exocrine insufficiency. These are relatively infrequent causes of diarrhea in diabetes. Quantitation of stool fat over 48 or 72 h is the ideal way to assess steatorrhea, although a quantitative measurement (Sudan stain) is a good screening test. However, moderately increased fecal fat excretions ($\leq$ 14 g/day) may also result from altered small-bowel motor or secretory function. Hence, fecal fat outputs within the range of 7–14 g/day may not distinguish nutrient malabsorption from an intestinal motor or secretory disorder.

Bacterial overgrowth in the small intestine is usually diagnosed by quantitative culture of jejunal aspirates in preference to breath tests after an oral carbohydrate load (reviewed in Ref. 20), a count of more than 10^5 aerobes or more than 10^3 per mL anaerobes is diagnostic. Alternatively, one may use the breath excretion of H_2 or $^{14}CO_2$ after oral ingestion of simple substrates, such as glucose or D-[^{14}C]xylose that are metabolized by enteric bacteria. Anemia and low serum folate suggest celiac sprue and mandate a small bowel biopsy. Exocrine pancreatic insufficiency caused by diabetes can be identified by direct pancreatic function testing following intravenous cholecystokinin (CCK) stimulation. It is rarely severe enough to cause steatorrhea. The rare patient with bile acid malabsorption is typically treated with cholestyramine, which may be used as a therapeutic trial, or by slowing small bowel transit pharmacologically.

Intestinal motor dysfunction is best demonstrated by radioisotopic transit measurements. Abnormal small bowel pressure profiles require intubation and do not distinguish patients with slow transit or those with diarrhea and rapid transit. Estimation of breath hydrogen after ingestion of substrates, such as lactulose, is a suboptimal measure of orocecal transit. It can be difficult to interpret breath hydrogen tests if gastric emptying is abnormal or small bowel bacterial overgrowth is present. More accurate, noninvasive radioisotopic techniques are now available to simultaneously measure gastric emptying, and small-bowel and colonic transit of solid particles (see Fig. 3). Perfusion studies that may detect abnormalities in intestinal absorption or secretion are rarely, if ever, necessary. A clinical response to the α_2-adrenergic agonist clonidine may suggest impairment of intestinal absorption as a cause of diarrhea (6).

E. Constipation

1. Symptoms

Constipation is probably the most common gastrointestinal symptom among patients with diabetes. In an epidemiological study based on a mailed questionnaire, constipation or use of laxatives were the only symptoms more frequent in diabetes than in age- and gender-matched controls (17). Constipation is typically intermittent and may alternate with episodes of diarrhea; its pathophysiology remains unclear. Constipation may result from a disturbance of colonic transit or a disturb-

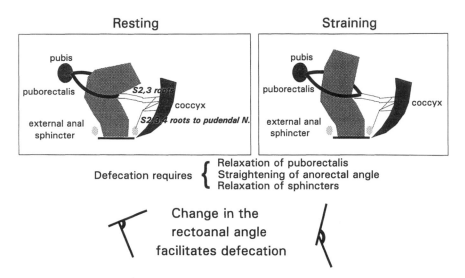

Fig. 6 Dynamics of defecation: defecation requires coordinated relaxation of the puborectalis (pelvic floor) and external anal sphincter, while increased abdominal pressure or colonic contractions propel stool through the straightened rectoanal angle.

ance in the process of defecation (Fig. 6). The colonic motor response to a meal (or gastrocolonic reflex) is impaired in patients with IDDM who have evidence of peripheral neuropathy and symptoms of severe constipation. However, colonic smooth-muscle contractile activity in response to cholinergic stimulation is normal (2). A pilot study suggested that community diabetes have a higher frequency of evacuation disorders or slow transit constipation than matched constipated controls (15). Larger studies are warranted to elucidate the role of regional colonic functions, the contribution of pelvic floor disorders, and impaired rectal sensation secondary to pudendal neuropathy, resulting in the absence of a normal peristaltic motor response during distention by stool.

A careful rectal examination during relaxation and straining is needed to exclude rectal mucosal lesions and to detect the presence of rectal prolapse, rectocele and excessive perineal descent, or failure of the puborectalis to relax.

2. Investigations

A stepwise, empiric approach is recommended (Fig. 7). First, patients should be encouraged to increase dietary intake of fiber to 20 or 30 g/day, and to add an osmotic laxative (e.g., milk of magnesia, sorbitol). High-fiber diets from nondigestible solid may aggravate symptoms of gastroparesis or even precipitate bezoar

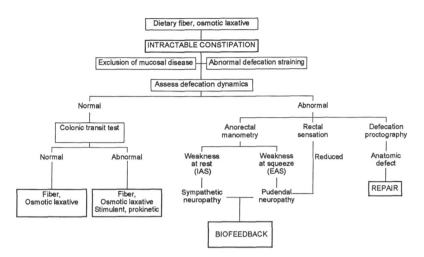

Fig. 7 Management algorithm for chronic constipation in patients with diabetes mellitus.

formation, and soluble forms of psyllium are likely to empty from the stomach more easily; however, their effectiveness in alleviating constipation in diabetic patients has not been formally studied. If constipation persists, proctosigmoidoscopy should be directed toward identification of a rectal or colonic mucosal lesion, such as cancer or a stricture caused by diverticulitis. If mucosa is normal, evaluation of anorectal and pelvic floor function is essential, as disorders of the defecation dynamics (see Fig. 6) may be present either from complications of diabetes, or from an unrelated problem. Outlet obstruction to defecation is an important cause of constipation in the general population. Clinically, these disorders present as an inability to initiate defecation, digitation to facilitate defecation, assumption of contorted postures during elimination of the fecal bolus, a sense of incomplete evacuation, or rectal discomfort, and the frequent and often ineffective use of laxatives or enemas. As for the investigation of incontinence, anorectal manometry, and anal ultrasound are essential. Neurophysiological evaluation of the pelvic floor muscles or pudendal nerve are needed in only a few patients. If pelvic function is normal, colonic transit time should be evaluated using noninvasive, reliable, and inexpensive tests, such as radiopaque markers or scintigraphy. Simultaneous measurement of gastric emptying and small-bowel transit also allows assessment for associated symptoms, such as nausea, vomiting, and bloating.

F. Chronic Abdominal Pain

Diabetic patients are susceptible to the usual causes of abdominal pain seen in the general population. However, there is an increased prevalence of gallstones, owing to altered gallbladder contractility, and of mesenteric ischemia owing to generalized atherosclerosis. Thoracolumbar radiculopathy may result in pain in a girdle-like distribution. Specific tests are indicated if the clinical features of pain suggest these disorders. A careful history is essential.

IV. TREATMENT OF DIABETIC ENTEROPATHY

General points in the management of diabetic enteropathy include optimal control of blood glucose levels, restoration of hydration, nutrition, and normal intestinal propulsion; and treatment of complications, such as bacterial overgrowth or intractable pain.

A. Esophageal Symptoms

There is no specific treatment for the esophageal symptoms experienced by diabetic patients. Reflux esophagitis requires use of conservative measures, antacids, or antisecretory agents and, if there is associated gastric stasis, a prokinetic agent (see following section).

B. Diabetic Gastroparesis

1. Medications

Patients with severe exacerbation of symptoms should be hospitalized and may require nasogastric suction. Intravenous fluids should be provided, and metabolic derangements (ketoacidosis, uremia, hypo- or hyperglycemia) corrected. Parenteral nutrition may become necessary in cases of malnutrition. Bezoars may be mechanically disrupted during endoscopy, followed by gastric decompression to drain residual nondigestible particles. Erythromycin at a dose of 3 mg/kg body weight intravenously every 8 h appears to be effective in clearing residue, as it induces dumping from the stomach. A week's treatment with oral erythromycin, 250 mg, t.i.d., is worthwhile once patients begin to tolerate oral intake of food. Because both liquids and homogenized solids are more readily emptied from the stomach than solids, liquid or blenderized food will be better tolerated. Frequent monitoring of blood glucose levels is essential during this phase. Rarely, it is necessary to bypass the stomach with a jejunal feeding tube if the motor dysfunction is limited to the stomach and there is no response to prokinetic therapy. This procedure should be preceded by a trial for a few days of nasoenteric feeding with infusion rates of at least 60 mL/h of iso-osmolar nutrient. Jejunal tubes are best placed by laparoscopy or minilaparotomy, rather than by percutaneous endoscopic gastrostomy tubes. Such tubes allow restoration of normal nutritional status, but they are not without adverse effects.

If the patient remains symptomatic, prokinetic agents may be considered as adjuncts. The results of subjective and objective efficacy in several medium- and long-term studies of prokinetic agents in patients with diabetic upper gut stasis have been reviewed in depth (3) and are summarized briefly. Metoclopramide is a peripheral cholinergic and antidopaminergic agent with central antiemetic activity. During brief administration, it initially enhances gastric emptying of liquids in patients with diabetic gastroparesis, but its symptomatic efficacy is probably related to its central antiemetic effects. However, its long-term use is restricted by a decline in efficacy and by a troubling incidence of central nervous system side effects.

Domperidone is a peripherally acting dopamine antagonist without cholinergic activity. Brief administration enhances gastric emptying of both solids and liquids. After prolonged administration, domperidone has no significant effect on gastric motor function, but may still improve symptoms of gastroparesis. Central nervous system side effects are less frequently observed with domperidone than with metoclopramide. Other adverse effects observed with both metoclopramide and domperidone are hyperprolactinemia and galactorrhea.

The substituted benzamide, cisapride, has a general stimulatory and prokinetic effect on the gastrointestinal tract. It acts by activation of a serotonin-4 receptor which results in enhanced release of acetylcholine from nerve endings within the myenteric plexus. Prolonged use of cisapride is not associated with undesirable hormonal and neurological side effects, and there is less tachyphylaxis during long-term treatment, compared with metoclopramide and domperidone. Briefly administered cisapride enhances gastric emptying in gastric stasis, and it has been effective in the treatment of diabetic gastroparesis when administered for 4 weeks. Its long-term efficacy has been demonstrated in open trials, although less convincingly in medium-term, controlled trials. Recently published case reports indicate that cisapride in high doses or combined with other medication that interact with cytochrome P-450 (e.g., macrolide antibiotics, phenothiazines, antifungal medication) potentially induces long QT syndrome, increasing the risk for ventricular tachycardia (''torsade de points'').

The macrolide antibiotic erythromycin is a potent gastroprokinetic, particularly in diabetic gastroparesis patients. It acts as an agonist at both neural and muscular motilin receptors, which are located throughout the mammalian gastrointestinal tract. Erythromycin was introduced into the clinical motility arena by Janssens et al. (11), who demonstrated that brief administration of this macrolide antibiotic accelerated gastric emptying of solids and increased antral contractions in patients with diabetes, some of whom also had evidence of gastric stasis. Despite its efficacy in the immediate management of symptomatic patients with gastroparesis, there is little evidence that it improves symptoms over the long term. Erythromycin loses much of its stimulatory effect beyond the first few weeks of treatment, possibly owing to down-regulation of motilin receptor expression.

Currently, intravenous erythromycin (3 mg/kg every 8 h by infusion) is a useful adjunct in the acute exacerbations of gastroparesis or clearance of gastric bezoars. In most patients, it is stopped after 5–7 days, as intolerance or tachyphylaxis develops. Macrolide prokinetics (e.g., EM574, ABT-229) without bacterial properties (''motilides'') are currently under investigation for various dysmotility states, including diabetic gastroparesis. EM574 dose-dependently accelerates gastric emptying of solids in healthy humans.

2. Gastric Pacing

Diabetic gastroparesis has been attributed to impaired myoelectrical activity in the antrum. Antral contractile activity and propulsion is regulated by underlying electrical slow-wave activity, that originates in the pacemaker region of the stomach (at the transition between fundus and corpus on the greater curvature) and which migrates aborally toward the pylorus. Hence, it has been postulated that gastric pacing could be able to correct and entrain gastric slow-wave activity, and thereby, improve gastric emptying. However, studies to this point have produced conflicting results. Recent data from McCallum and associates (18), in five patients with diabetic gastroparesis, showed that gastric pacing was able to improve symptoms of gastroparesis and to accelerate gastric emptying, thereby resulting in less fluctuation of blood glucose and better day-to-day control. Further placebo-controlled studies are warranted to assess the real value of this new, invasive, and expensive technique in the treatment of diabetic gastroparesis.

3. Surgery

Surgical intervention should be avoided in gastroparetic patients. A few anecdotal reports of antrectomy with vagotomy, gastrectomy, or pyloroplasty have demonstrated a poor clinical outcome. Decompression by percutaneous or operative gastrostomy may provide symptomatic relief and possibly assist in those selected for jejunal tube feeding. This can also be achieved by laparoscopic placement of jejunal tubes.

C. Diabetic Diarrhea

The initial management of the patient with diabetes and chronic diarrhea should be directed to the correction of water and electrolyte imbalance, rigorous control of the blood glucose levels, and restoration of nutrition, if necessary, with intravenous hyperalimentation. We have suggested a diagnostic algorithm for evaluation of these patients (see Fig. 5).

Treatment should be directed at the identified cause of diarrhea, rather than sequential empiric trials. For small-bowel bacterial overgrowth, antibiotics are administered on a rotational basis for 1 week out of 2–4 weeks to avoid bacterial resistance. These include doxycycline, 100 mg b.i.d.; metronidazole, 250 mg t.i.d.; co-trimoxazole, 800/160 mg b.i.d.; and ciprofloxacin, 500 mg b.i.d.. Other treatments include a gluten-free diet for celiac disease, pancreatic enzyme supplementation for exocrine insufficiency, and biofeedback techniques aimed at retraining rectal sensation for fecal incontinence. Bile acid malabsorption is usually treated with cholestyramine (up to 16 g/day) or by decreasing small-bowel transit with loperamide. For patients in whom the pathogenesis of diarrhea is unclear, antidiarrheal agents, such as loperamide and diphenoxylate, can reduce the number of stools, particularly if diarrhea is associated with rapid intestinal transit. Decreasing motility may actually promote stasis and potentially aggravate bacterial overgrowth; hence, exclusion of bacterial overgrowth is essential before embarking on an empirical, long-term therapy with antidiarrheals.

Clonidine, at doses of 0.1–0.6 mg, b.i.d. orally, reduces the number and volume of stools in a small number of patients with diabetic diarrhea. Clonidine may be associated with significant adverse effects, such as orthostatic hypotension or worsening of gastric emptying, which limit its use. Transdermal clonidine may control diarrhea without causing hypotension. Verapamil (40 mg b.i.d.) may also help control diarrhea, probably by delaying colonic transit.

The long-acting somatostatin analogue octreotide has been proposed as an alternative treatment of chronic diarrhea in patients with diabetes mellitus. Somatostatin inhibits stimulated water secretion in animals and humans, increases gut absorptive capacity, and suppresses gastrointestinal hormones that are potentially diarrheogenic. Octreotide retards small-bowel transit in health, and is administered as a subcutaneous injection of 50–75 μg twice a day. However, at higher doses, octreotide may inhibit pancreatic exocrine secretion, aggravate nutrient malabsorption, and induce gallstone formation. Octreotide LAR, a depot preparation administered once monthly, is now available and might provide long-term relief of diarrhea; however, formal studies are needed.

D. Constipation and Incontinence

Pelvic floor dysfunction, incontinence, and rectal sensory disturbances should first be treated with biofeedback. This approach requires patients to observe their own pelvic floor movements and external anal sphincter pressure recordings while straining or squeezing. Repeated training sessions are needed, at which patients are instructed how to normalize expulsion patterns. In the absence of pelvic floor dysfunction, management of constipation should include use of bulk or osmotic laxatives. If these measures fail to control symptoms, an enema program may be necessary.

In patients in whom colonic transit time is abnormally prolonged, stimulants of colonic motility such as bisacodyl, senna alkaloids, or glycerine suppositories that stimulate propulsive high-amplitude colonic contractions may be helpful. Novel, more colon-selective prokinetics (e.g., prucalopride and tegaserod) are being studied to assess their effect on symptoms and colonic transit in patients with slow-transit constipation, and they may also play a future role in treatment of constipation in diabetics.

V. SUMMARY AND A LOOK AT THE FUTURE

Thus, patients with enteropathies caused by diabetes mellitus present a spectrum of clinical manifestations with diverse pathophysiologies. A simple test that documents the mechanism contributing to these symptoms is helpful in the selection of therapy. These patients need a single physician who coordinates and prioritizes treatment of the protean manifestations and complications of diabetes mellitus. In particular, medications used to treat depression and hypertension have marked effects on gut motor function, and alternatives without such effects may correct the disturbance and relieve patient's symptoms.

Despite specific approaches to the treatment of diabetic enteropathy and the availability of prokinetic agents to treat motility disorders, management has been only partially successful. Reversal of the derangements that cause the abnormal gut functions would clearly be preferable, but no medical therapy is of proved benefit in restoring the underlying disorders of nerve function. Therefore, current therapy is based on restoration of euglycemia and symptomatic control. The prospect of complete euglycemic control with pancreas transplantation offers the chance of better control in the future. With improved immunosuppressive regimens and surgical techniques, graft survival rates are now similar to those of other organ transplants. Whether pancreatic transplantation reverses diabetic enteropathy is uncertain, because pancreatic transplantations have been performed for indications other than the management of diabetic enteropathy. Novel, effective therapies are needed to enhance and refine the empiric approaches discussed.

REFERENCES

1. Abell TL, Camilleri M, Hench VS, et al. Gastric electromechanical function and gastric emptying in diabetic gastroparesis. Eur J Gastroenterol Hepatol 3:163–167, 1991.
2. Battle WM, Snape WJ Jr, Alavi A, et al. Colonic dysfunction in diabetes mellitus. Gastroenterology 79:1217–1221, 1980.

3. Camilleri M. Appraisal of medium- and long-term treatment of gastroparesis and chronic intestinal dysmotility. Am J Gastroenterol 89:1769–1774, 1994.

4. Camilleri M, Zinsmeister AR, Greydanus MP, et al. Toward a less costly but accurate test of gastric emptying and small bowel transit. Dig Dis Sci 36:609–615, 1991.

5. Chang EB, Fedorak RN, Field M. Experimental diabetic diarrhea in rats. Intestinal mucosal denervation, hyposensitivity and treatment with clonidine. Gastroenterology 91:564–569, 1986.

5A. Duchen LW, Anjorin A, Watkins PJ, Mackay JD. Pathology of autonomic neuropathy in diabetes mellitus. Anals Internal Medicine 92:301–303, 1980.

6. Fedorak R, Field M, Chang E. Treatment of diabetic diarrhea with clonidine. Ann Intern Med 102:197–199, 1985.

7. Feldman M, Schiller ER. Disorders of gastrointestinal motility associated with diabetes mellitus. Ann Intern Med 98:378–84, 1983.

8. Frank JW, Camilleri M, Thomforde GM, et al. Postprandial hyperglycemia in type II diabetes mellitus: role of glucagon, gastric emptying, and glucose absorption. Gastroenterology 106:A500, 1994.

9. Fraser RJ, Horowitz M, Maddox AF, et al. Hyperglycemia slows gastric emptying in type I (insulin-dependent) diabetes mellitus. Diabetologia 32:151–159, 1989.

10. Ghoos YF, Maes BD, Geypens BJ, et al. Measurement of gastric emptying rate of solids by means of a carbon-labeled octanoic acid breath test. Gastroenterology 104: 1640–1647, 1993.

11. Janssens J, Peeters TL, Vantrappen G, et al. Improvement of gastric emptying in diabetic gastroparesis by erythromycin: preliminary studies. N Engl J Med 322: 1028–1031, 1990.

12. Kassander P. Asymptomatic gastric retention in diabetics (gastroparesis diabeticorum). Ann Intern Med 48:797–812, 1958.

13. Lee J-S, Camilleri M, Burton D, Zinsmeister AR, Klein PD. ^{13}C-Spirulina breath test for gastric emptying: validation vs. scintigraphy and a new accurate method for data analysis of a 3-hour test. Dig Dis Sci 43:1587, 1998.

14. Lincoln J, Bokor JT, Crowe R, et al. Myenteric plexus in streptozotocin-treated rats: neurochemical and histochemical evidence for diabetic neuropathy in the gut. Gastroenterology 86:654–661, 1984.

15. Maleki D, Camilleri M, Burton DD, Rath-Harvey DM, Oenning L, Pemberton JH, Low PA. A pilot study of the pathophysiology of constipation among community diabetics. Dig Dis Sci 43:2373–2378, 1998.

16. Maleki D, Camilleri M, Zinsmeister AR, Rizza RA. Effect of acute hyperglycemia on colorectal motor and sensory function in humans. Am J Physiol 273:G859–864, 1997.

17. Maleki D, Camilleri M, Zinsmeister AR, Van Dyke CT, Leibson C, Melton LJ III, Yawn B, Locke GR III. Prevalence of gastrointestinal symptoms in insulin-(IDDM) and noninsulin-dependent diabetes mellitus (NIDDM) in a U.S. community. Dig Dis Sci 41:1900, 1996.

18. McCallum RW, Chen JD, Lin Z, et al. Gastric pacing improves emptying and symptoms in patients with gastroparesis. Gastroenterology 114:456–461, 1998.

19. Schiller LR, Santa Ana CA, Schmulen AC, et al. Pathogenesis of fecal incontinence in diabetes mellitus. N Engl J Med 307:1666–1671, 1982.

20. Valdovinos MA, Camilleri M, Zimmerman BR. Chronic diarrhea in diabetes mellitus: mechanisms and an approach to diagnosis and treatment. Mayo Clin Proc 68: 691–702, 1993.

21. Wald A, Tunuguntla K. Anorectal sensorimotor dysfunction, fecal incontinence and diabetes mellitus. N Engl J Med 310:1282–1287, 1984.

22. Whalen GE, Soergel KH, Geenan JE. Diabetic diarrhea: a clinical and pathophysiological study. Gastroenterology 56:1021–1032, 1969.

25
Diabetic Kidney Disease

Virginia L. Hood
University of Vermont College of Medicine, Burlington, Vermont

> End-stage renal disease from diabetes can be prevented or delayed for many
> years with appropriate management.

I. EPIDEMIOLOGY

Diabetes is the leading cause of end-stage renal disease (ESRD) in the United
States and a risk factor for ESRD ascribed to other causes. Diabetes accounted
for 40% of new cases and 30% of those in the ESRD program in 1996. Twenty
to forty percent of persons with diabetes develop renal disease and have the
potential to progress to ESRD. Presently, at end stage, there are similar numbers
of men and women and similar numbers of those with type 1 and type 2 disease.
However, because the incidence of ESRD from type 2 is twice that of type 1,
type 2 will soon exceed type 1 as the major cause of diabetes-associated ESRD.
This is not unexpected, as type 2 accounts for 80–90% of all diabetes. Those at
risk are developing diabetes at younger ages and are living longer, thus increasing
the risk for macro- and microvascular complications.

II. PATHOGENESIS

A. Pathology

The histopathology of diabetic nephropathy is identical in type 1 and type 2
disease. Before nephropathy is manifested clinically, thickened glomerular basement membranes and an increase in the amount of mesangial matrix can be seen
in renal biopsy specimens. Persistence of the diabetic state over time is associated

with mesangial matrix expansion and, to a lesser degree, an increase in mesangial cellularity. Eventually, the nodular glomerulosclerosis described by Kimmelsteil and Wilson that typifies diabetic nephropathy appears. Tubulointerstitial abnormalities occur in concert with the glomerular pathology, starting with thickening of tubular basement membrane, then progressing to fibrosis, with mononuclear cell infiltrates and tubular atrophy. Initially, there is an increase in glomerular and tubular size. Increased overall kidney size has been reported in 20% of those investigated. Although with progressive sclerosis, kidney size may decrease, many kidneys remain of normal size even when end-stage disease is present.

B. Pathophysiology

Renal damage results from the interaction of metabolic, hemodynamic and genetic factors. Hyperglycemia causes glycosylation of proteins in membranes of small blood vessels and glomeruli. The resultant thick, leaky membranes allow increased passage of blood constituents (protein and lipid) into the mesangium. Mesangial reaction with proliferation of cells and expansion of the mesangial matrix results in glomerulosclerosis. The abnormal metabolic milieu in diabetes causes renal hemodynamic changes that result in high pressures and flow within the glomeruli (hyperfiltration) which exacerbate the processes leading to glomerulosclerosis. Systemic hypertension, which can result from renal damage in type 1 or be present before renal damage in type 2 also contributes to the pathology. Although as yet undetermined, it seems likely that genetic susceptibility operates through these processes (Fig. 1; Table 1).

1.   Metabolic Factors

The major pathogenic factor producing diabetic nephropathy is hyperglycemia. The first glycosylation step occurs when glucose reacts nonenzymatically with amine groups on macromolecules, including peptides, lipids, and DNA. This process is reversible with glucose control and may be modified by pharmacological agents, such as aminoguanidine, which are currently being investigated. With persistent hyperglycemia, the glycosylated products are converted to advanced glycosylation end products (AGE) that alter structural proteins and binding sites, and cause other abnormalities that result in disruption of enzyme, cytokine, and macrophage systems. These latter changes are not responsive to glucose control. Glycosylation is responsible for the thickening of the glomerular basement membrane and initial increase in the amount of mesangial matrix. Circulating glycosylated proteins, such as albumin, when deposited in the glomerulus can add to the damage. Hyperglycemia and the accompanying deranged metabolic milieu in diabetes contribute to renal hyperperfusion that also contributes to progression of nephropathy.

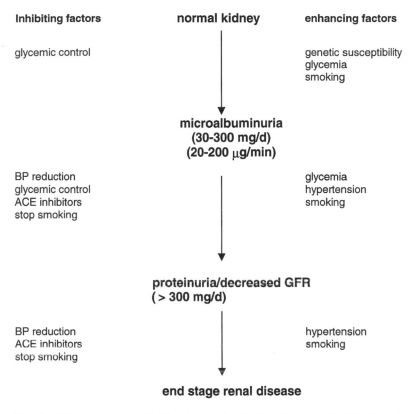

Fig. 1 Enhancing and inhibiting factors for the development of diabetic nephropathy. Diabetic nephropathy develops over 10–30 years in 20–40% of persons with type 1 or type 2 diabetes.

2. Renal Hemodynamic Factors

In the preclinical phase, an increase in glomerular filtration rate (GFR) is found in 25–50% of those patients with type 1 and a considerable proportion of those with type 2 diabetes. Numerous hormonal, dietary, growth, and vasoactive substances have been implicated as mediators of the increased renal plasma flow and glomerular capillary pressure that bring about this hyperfiltration state. This form of local hypertension can disrupt the normal filtration barrier, magnifying

Table 1   Risk Factors for the Development or Progression of Diabetic Nephropathy

---

Development
    Genetic: family history of renal disease, hypertension, cardiovascular disease
    Metabolic: hyperglycemia, duration of diabetes
    Hemodynamic: hypertension
    Other: smoking
Progression
    Metabolic: hyperglycemia
    Hemodynamic: hypertension
    Other: smoking, coincident renovascular disease, superimposed renal injury

---

the mesangial cell proliferation, the mesangial matrix expansion, and the basement membrane thickening that occur as the result of hyperglycemia.

3.   Systemic Hemodynamic Factors

Systemic hypertension is present in 50% of those with type 2 diabetes at presentation and may or may not predate proteinuria. In type 1, hypertension is rarely present before the onset of established clinical nephropathy (proteinuria and reduced GFR). However, a familial tendency for hypertension has been implicated as a significant risk factor for the development of nephropathy in those with type 1 disease. Systemic hypertension is an important mediator of progression of disease in both type 1 and type 2 conditions.

4.   Genetics

Genetic susceptibility to diabetic nephropathy is suggested by familial clustering, similar renal pathological changes over time in sibling pairs, the association of nephropathy with a family history of hypertension, and an as yet unconfirmed relation of nephropathy with the insertion deletion polymorphism of the angiotensin-converting enzyme inhibitor (ACEI) gene. Although the incidence of diabetic nephropathy is two to three times higher in African Americans and six times higher in Native or Hispanic Americans, there is considerable heterogeneity within these populations relative to the development of nephropathy.

5.   Smoking

Smoking is a strong predictor of renal risk in type 1, the presence of proteinuria in type 2, and a risk factor for progression of disease in both conditions. Stopping smoking has been associated with reduced risk of progression in type 1. Smoking is also a predictor of renal artery stenosis and atheroembolic renal disease, both conditions that occur commonly in those with type 2 diabetes and can contribute to renal dysfunction.

III. CLINICAL COURSE

A. Natural History

The first clinical sign of kidney involvement is excretion of a greater than normal quantity of protein (albumin) in the urine. The initially small, but excess amount of albumin excretion is known as *microalbuminuria* and is defined as 30–300 mg/day, or 20–200 μg/min, or an albumin/creatinine ratio of 30 μg/mg creatinine. Microalbuminuria appears 5–15 years after the onset of type 1 diabetes. It is followed in 5–10 years by the presence of dipstick-positive proteinuria ($>$ 300 mg/day or $>$ 300 mg/g creatinine). Proteinuria can vary in amount and may reach nephrotic range ($>$ 3.5 g/day or 3 g/g creatinine). Once proteinuria is persistent, there is an inevitable decline in renal function to ESRD over a period of 2–10 years (decreases in GFR of 5–14 mL/min per year), the shorter course being in those with nephrotic range proteinuria and uncontrolled hypertension. During this phase, systemic hypertension is frequently present and exacerbates the rate of decline in renal function. Those with type 2 diabetes often have proteinuria, high blood pressure and sometimes, impaired renal function at the time of presentation with diabetes. Factors influencing progression rates include persistent hyperglycemia, uncontrolled hypertension, and continuation of smoking.

B. Signs, Symptoms, and Clinical Presentation

For the purposes of investigation and treatment, diabetic nephropathy can be divided into three main stages although, as previously mentioned, the pathological processes are a continuum. The three stages are incipient nephropathy, characterized by normal renal function and microalbuminuria; overt nephropathy, characterized by proteinuria and eventually accompanied by impaired renal function and usually hypertension; and end-stage renal disease, characterized by the need for renal replacement therapy. Subsets of overt nephropathy that require special consideration are the nephrotic syndrome, type 4 renal tubular acidosis, renal insufficiency, and pre–end-stage renal disease.

Incipient nephropathy is asymptomatic and recognized only by screening for microalbuminuria. Screening should begin 5 years after onset of type 1 and at diagnosis in type 2 disease.

Overt nephropathy, characterized by proteinuria > 300 mg/day or > 300 mg/g creatinine is also usually asymptomatic and is recognized during routine physical examinations when proteinuria is noted on urinalysis and subsequently quantitated. Proteinuria may be accompanied by increased blood pressure or decreased renal function (elevated serum creatinine). Symptoms are only present when large quantities of proteinuria result in hypoalbuminemia and edema (nephrotic syndrome). Hematuria is present in up to 30% of persons with overt nephropathy and red blood cell casts are occasionally noted.

Nephrotic syndrome is characterized by proteinuria greater than 3.5 g/day or greater than 3g/g creatinine. If protein production does not equal protein excretion, hypoalbuminemia, hypercholesterolemia, lipiduria, and edema occur. Unlike the proteinuria that occurs in idiopathic nephrotic syndrome, diabetes-associated heavy proteinuria often persists even when glomerular filtration is markedly reduced.

Type 4 renal tubular acidosis (RTA), characterized by a metabolic acidosis with normal anion gap, elevated serum potassium, is usually associated with mildly impaired renal function (serum creatinine 1.5–3.0 mg/dL). Diabetes-associated type 4 RTA is due to a defect in the renin angiotensin aldosterone axis, known as hyporenin hypoaldosteronism. Hemodynamic or tubular solute delivery-mediated changes in juxtaglomerular apparatus function reducing renin output, or insulinopenia-mediated intracellular potassium alterations reducing aldosterone production, have been postulated as causes. The acidosis is usually mild (serum bicarbonate 15–23 mEq/L) and the hyperkalemia modest (serum potassium 5.0–7.0 mEq/L). Other causes of hyperkalemia should be sought and corrected wherever possible.

Renal insufficiency is characterized by GFR less than 30 mL/min (serum creatinine levels higher than 3 mg/dL). In this phase, anemia, resulting from reduced erythropoietin production, and disorders of calcium and phosphorus metabolism, resulting in hyperparathyroidism and metabolic bone disease, begin to appear.

Pre–end-stage renal disease is a loosely defined phase of overt nephropathy that occurs when GFR is reduced to 10–20 mL/min (serum creatinine 5–10 mg/dL), and symptoms and signs of uremia or volume excess have begun to be more apparent. Any or all of these symptoms or signs may occur at lesser degrees of renal dysfunction than found in those with nondiabetic renal disease. One prominent manifestation is symptomatic gastroparesis, which results from the interaction between diabetic neuropathy and uremia. Also a manifestation of autonomic neuropathy is orthostatic hypotension, which may become more symptomatic in this period and, frequently, interferes with the maintenance of optimal blood pressure control. Anemia is nearly always present and contributes to the fatigue, dyspnea, and cardiac dysfunction that develop as renal function declines.

IV. DIAGNOSIS

A. Diagnostic and Monitoring Tests

1. Renal Excretory Function

The GFR is best assessed in clinical situations by measurement of the serum creatinine concentration, because it is readily available, reliable, and its limitations are fewer than other measures. The major limitation of using creatinine in the clinical setting is that it underestimates true GFR in persons with reduced muscle mass; however, by using a formula such as the Cockcroft–Gault equation (Fig. 2), a truer estimate of GFR can be made. This is important when using GFR to assess medication dosage. One other limitation is conceptual. Because the relation between serum creatinine and GFR is exponential, a small change in serum creatinine indicates a large loss of renal function when serum creatinine is in the lower ranges, but not when it is high. A change in serum creatinine from 1 to 2 mg/dL represents a 50% loss of renal function, whereas a change from 9 to 10 mg/dL is only a 10% loss. A 24-h urine collection to measure creatinine clearance is rarely used to assess GFR because it is more prone to measurement error and no more precise than the Cockcroft–Gault formula. In clinical trials, GFR is estimated by lothalamate clearance, but this measurement is rarely useful in a clinical setting.

Serum creatinine should be measured at diagnosis in type 2, at 5 years after onset of diabetes in type 1, and then at least yearly in both conditions.

2. Proteinuria

Microalbuminuria refers to small, but abnormal amounts of albuminuria (> 30 mg/day; Fig. 3). Patients with microalbuminuria are likely to progress to proteinuria (> 300 mg/day). Proteinuria is also referred to as *macroalbuminuria,* clinical albuminuria, or persistent proteinuria. Estimates of the presence of microalbuminuria or proteinuria can be made by measuring the ratio of microalbumin to creatinine, or of protein to creatinine, on single urine samples. These measurements correlate well with 24-h or timed (4-h) urine collections for microalbumin or

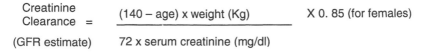

$$\text{Creatinine Clearance} = \frac{(140 - age) \times weight\ (Kg)}{72 \times serum\ creatinine\ (mg/dl)} \times 0.\,85\ \text{(for females)}$$

(GFR estimate)

Fig. 2 Estimate of glomerular filtration rate (GFR) using serum creatinine concentration. Not reliable in pregnancy, obesity, or if renal function is not stable. (From Cockcroft and Gault, Nephron 1976.)

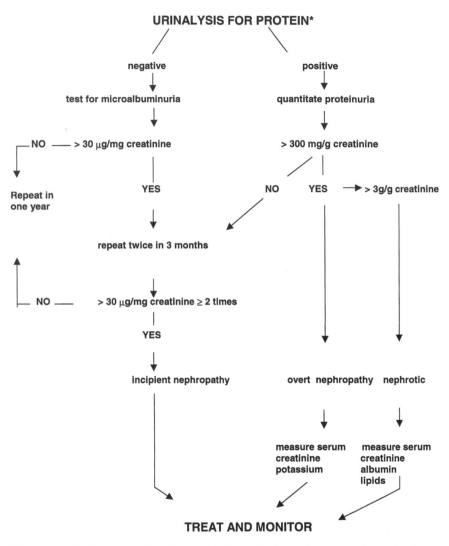

URINALYSIS FOR PROTEIN*

* Test when patient has no condition that may interfere with urinary albumin excretion such as fever, congestive heart failure, marked hyperglycemia, marked hypertension, or within hours of energetic exercise or following a large intake of protein. Test at diagnosis in Type 2, at 5 years after diagnosis in Type 1 and yearly thereafter in both.

Fig. 3 Suggested schemes for testing for proteinuria.

protein. Separate biochemical assays are required to detect microalbumin and protein. Compared with biochemical assays, dipstick methods are not as sensitive, hence they should not be used for screening; nor are they as specific, hence positive tests should be confirmed by more specific methods. In those with standard dipstick-negative urine, microalbuminuria should be quantitated at diagnosis for type 2, at 5 years after onset of disease in type 1, and yearly in both. A similar time line should be used to quantitate proteinuria for those patients with dipstick-positive urine.

Because there is day-to-day variability in urinary albumin excretion, neither diagnosis nor change in diagnostic category should be made unless elevated levels are detected in at least two of three urine samples over a 3 to 6-month period. Increases in urinary albumin excretion occur as the result of energetic exercise, fever, congestive heart failure, marked hyperglycemia, marked hypertension, and a large protein intake.

3. Urinalysis

Dipstick-positive or microscopic hematuria is present in up to 30% of those with diabetic nephropathy. Oval fat bodies may be seen in the urine of those with the nephrotic syndrome. With deterioration of renal function, waxy or granular casts are frequently seen with microscopy.

4. Renal Biopsy

A renal biopsy should be considered when there is a suggestion that a renal disorder other than diabetes is present (Table 2).

Table 2 Indications for Evaluating Other Causes of Renal Disease or Renal Artery Stenosis

---

Renal disease
    Proteinuria in persons with type 1 diabetes for fewer than 10 years or without diabetic retinopathy
    Decline in GFR of more than 15 mL/min per year
    Hematuria ± RBC casts without proteinuria
    Hematuria and proteinuria with evidence of systemic vasculitis
Renal artery stenosis
    Decline in GFR (increase in serum creatinine) following treatment with ACE inhibitors or angiotensin II receptor antagonists
    Asymmetrical kidney size
    Sudden worsening of blood pressure control or loss of renal function plus evidence of systemic atherosclerotic vascular disease, hyperlipidemia, or smoking

---

5. Radiological Studies

Radiological studies can be used to assess renal size and parenchyma or to investigate renovascular disease and urinary tract abnormalities. Intravascular radiocontrast agents should be used with caution in those patients with impaired renal function. Normal intravascular volume should be present before use of these agents in all persons. When indicated and available, carbon dioxide angiography is a useful alternative for investigation of renovascular or peripheral vascular disease.

B. Differential Diagnosis

Proteinuria and impaired renal function are manifestations of many forms of renal disease. When there is a sudden decrease in renal function, prerenal causes such as volume depletion or ''effective volume depletion'' (seen in heart failure, and states in which serum albumin is low), postrenal causes, such as obstruction to urinary outflow, and other glomerular or tubulointerstitial causes should be considered. Sudden worsening of blood pressure control may warrant investigation of renovascular disease. Other causes of nephrotic syndrome should be considered when it is present in persons without long-standing diabetes, without coincident diabetic retinopathy or in those whose clinical course is not suggestive of diabetic nephropathy. The presence of white blood cells (WBC) or WBC casts on urinalysis warrants investigation of urinary tract or renal infection. Hematuria, with or without red blood cell (RBC) casts in the absence of proteinuria, or found in a clinical setting not consistent with overt nephropathy, should trigger investigation of other urinary tract or renal disorders.

V. TREATMENT

Normalization of blood sugar concentrations and discontinuation of smoking reduce the risks of developing diabetic renal disease. Control of hypertension and proteinuria prevent or slow its progression. In several large clinical trials in this decade blood glucose control, blood pressure control, use of ACE inhibitors, and modest dietary modifications, have decreased the development of chronic renal disease by at least 50%. Treatment goals are outlined in Table 3.

Table 3 Treatment Goals

Blood pressure less than 130/85 mmHg
Normal blood glucose and blood lipids
No smoking
Stable or reduced microalbuminuria or proteinuria
No other injury to the kidneys

Because the critical outcomes of renal disease—death, the need for dialysis, or transplantation—appear 5–30 years after the appearance of clinical disease, studies of treatment effectiveness frequently use surrogate outcomes that predict the critical outcomes, with varying degrees of accuracy. Those that are generally accepted are the rate of decline in GFR, time to doubling of serum creatinine, and change in protein excretion.

A. Metabolic Control

Control of blood glucose levels reduces the development of incipient nephropathy and, to a smaller extent, the progression to overt nephropathy in both type 1 and type 2 disease. The Diabetes Control and Complication Trial (DCCT) achieved glycemic control that resulted in a glycosylated hemoglobin (HbA$_{1c}$) averaging 7% in the intensive treatment group, compared with 9% in standard treatment group. In the intensive treatment group the development of microalbuminuria (incipient nephropathy) was reduced over 6 years by 35%, and persistent protein-uria (overt nephropathy) was reduced by 56%. A historical but longer-term study from a district in Sweden—followed 197 persons who developed type 1 diabetes before the age of 15 between 1961 and 1980 to their death or to 1991. In this study, Bojestig and colleagues showed a remarkable reduction in the 15 year cumulative incidence of overt nephropathy from 30% in those whose disease was diagnosed between 1961 and 1965 to 5.8% in those whose disease was diagnosed between 1971–1975, and zero in those whose diagnosis was made between 1976 and 1980. In the later groups excellent glycemic control was obtained (HbA$_{1c}$, 6–7%). The development of proteinuria was highly correlated with HbA$_{1c}$. The U.K. Prospective Diabetes Study (UKPDS) examined the influence of blood sugar control in 3867 subjects with type 2 diabetes. Subjects in the intensive treatment group whose HbA$_{1c}$ averaged 7%, compared with 7.9% in the conventional treatment group, had a 30% relative risk reduction for the development of microalbuminuria over 9–12 years, and a 75% relative risk reduction in doubling of the serum creatinine over 12 years.

B. Blood Pressure Control

There is overwhelming evidence that blood pressure (BP) control reduces the progression of nephropathy in type 1 and type 2 disease, and that lowering blood pressure is the most important factor for slowing the rate of progression. Parving noted in 1983 that blood pressure control reduced proteinuria and slowed the rate of decline in GFR. Since then, hundreds of studies have confirmed these findings. A metanalysis of 100 studies found that each 10-mmHg decrease in BP was associated with 3.7 mL/min higher GFR (clinically significant better renal function) and less proteinuria. In a series of studies involving small numbers of partici-

Table 4 Treatment of Hypertension: Goal: BP < 130/85 mmHg

Lifestyle modifications
    Reduce dietary sodium
    Increase exercise
    Limit alcohol
    Weight loss (if indicated)
ACE inhibitors or angiotensin II receptor antagonists
Other antihypertensive agents as needed
    Diuretic (low-dose thiazide or loop)
    Calcium channel antagonists
    α_1-Adrenergic antagonists
    β-Adrenergic blockers
    Other

pants with type 1 and type 2 disease, the rate of deterioration in renal function was correlated with the level of the blood pressure achieved during long-term follow-up. The Modification of Diet in Renal Disease (MDRD) study, which included 840 persons with a variety of renal diseases, including type 2 diabetes, evaluated the effect of BP control in addition to that of reduced dietary protein. Those with proteinuria higher than 1 g/day who achieved BP of 130/80 mmHg had the slowest rate of progression. The UKPDS also demonstrated the value of tight BP control (average 144/82 mmHg) in preventing macrovascular and microvascular complications in type 2 diabetes. In this study equally favorable effects were seen with captopril (an ACE inhibitor) and atenolol (a β-adrenergic blocker).

There are several large ongoing trials in Europe and the United States to examine the optimum goal for BP control in persons with both diabetic and nondiabetic renal disease. The current recommended goal is less than 130/85 mmHg.

Specific treatment strategies are outlined in Chapter 34. However, a general approach is to use an ACE inhibitor, add a diuretic, then a vasodilator, such as a calcium channel antagonist or α_1-adrenergic antagonist or a β-adrenergic blocking agent to control heart rate. Many patients will require more than one agent and 30% of patients are likely to require three or more agents to adequately control BP (Table 4). Although debate continues over effects of specific antihypertensive agents on the course of renal disease, controlling blood pressure, by any means, is the most effective measure known for slowing progression to ESRD.

C. Angiotensin-Converting Enzyme Inhibitors

The ACE inhibitors have a beneficial effect on slowing the progression of diabetic nephropathy independently of BP control, and this has now been demonstrated in persons with type 1, with type 2, and in those with and without hypertension and with and without proteinuria. The major limiting factors are hyperkalemia and a reversible increase with serum creatinine; hence, these values should be carefully monitored when ACE inhibitors are used. The likelihood of the serum creatinine and or serum potassium increasing is greater as renal function deteriorates, and during intercurrent illnesses accompanied by volume depletion, effective volume depletion, or the use of nonsteroidal anti-inflammatory drugs (NSAIDs). There is no identified threshold at which ACE inhibitors are contraindicated.

In 1992, Björck and colleagues reported that, despite similar blood pressure control in two small groups of patients with type 1 diabetes, those treated with enalapril had less proteinuria and a slower decline in renal function than those taking metoprolol. They also noted that at every level of BP, the enalapril-treated group had less proteinuria than the metoprolol-treated group. The significance of these findings was reinforced by the larger study of Lewis and colleagues in 409 persons with type 1 diabetes and proteinuria greater than 500 mg/day and serum creatinine less than or equal to 2.5 mg/dL. Those receiving 25 mg of captopril three time daily had a 50% risk reduction for reaching ESRD or 48% risk reduction for having their serum creatinine double over 3 years, compared with those taking placebo and other antihypertensive agents. This effect was most pronounced in those whose serum creatinine valves were higher than 2 mg/dL. Although blood pressures were slightly lower in the captopril-treated group (MAP 96 ± 8 vs. 100 ± 8 mmHg), the beneficial effect of the ACE inhibitor was still present when the analysis was adjusted for mean arterial pressure (MAP). The effect was also seen in subjects without hypertension. Of the study participants 25% had blood pressures less than 140/90 mmHg. There are similar results with other ACE inhibitors and in persons with type 2 diabetes with normal blood pressure and microalbuminuria. A metanalysis of 100 studies of blood pressure control in type 1 and type 2 diabetes confirmed that ACE inhibitors had an independent beneficial effect on proteinuria and protective effect against worsening renal function. Every ACE inhibitor investigated appears to have a renoprotective effect in doses equivalent to captopril 25 mg t.i.d. or enalapril 10 mg q.d.

There is also evidence that in nondiabetic renal disease, in addition to the blood pressure-lowering action, ACE inhibitors reduce proteinuria and facilitate a reduction in the decline of renal function.

D. Other Antihypertensive Agents

Debate continues over whether other antihypertensive agents have protective effects on renal function in addition to the benefit of maintaining optimal blood pressure. Of the calcium channel antagonists (CCAs) only diltiazem and verapamil have reduced proteinuria in a manner similar to the ACE inhibitors. However, there is accumulating evidence that a variety of CCAs, with or without ACE inhibitors, attenuate or stabilize the progression of renal disease. Studies are underway to assess the effects of angiotensin II receptor antagonists for reducing proteinuria and slowing the progression of renal disease in both diabetic and nondiabetic renal disease. Despite the lack of information, it is currently common practice to substitute angiotensin II receptor antagonists for ACE inhibitors in those patients for whom cough prohibits ACE inhibitor use.

E. Diet

That the rate of progression of renal disease could be reduced by modification of the diet was first described by Walker and colleagues in a small group of patients with diabetic nephropathy. Other studies with few patients and short follow-up have shown a small benefit from moderate protein restriction. Overall, the magnitude of any additional benefit, over that achieved by other measures that slow progression of disease, has not been impressive. Interestingly, the composition of the diet consumed by Walker's subjects was very similar to that recommended by the American Diabetes Association (ADA) for all persons with diabetes. Because there is no guarantee that a protein intake of less than 0.8 g/kg per day over a long period will not result in malnutrition, lower protein intakes should be considered in only those patients with pre–end-stage renal disease (serum creatinine valves higher than 5 mg/dL) in whom their use for short periods can help control symptomatic uremia (Table 5).

F. Avoid Additional Injury to Kidney

Claude Bernard said that the function of the kidney is to protect the body's *mileur interieur*. However, the kidney needs protection from the exterior milieu from which radiocontrast agents; nephrotoxic chemicals and drugs; infection, inflammation, obstruction, ischemia, and volume depletion threaten its integrity and function. In persons with renal impairment, every attempt should be made to recognize and treat urinary tract infections, ensure adequate drainage of the urinary tract, and avoid or promptly correct volume depletion. In addition, potentially nephrotoxic agents or drugs, such as NSAIDs, radiocontrast agents, and aminoglycoside antibiotics, should be used with caution. In any person with nephropathy

Table 5 Diet

Protein	0.8–1 g/kg/day
Fat	30% of total calories
Fiber	40 g/day
Sodium	2 g/day (for hypertension)
Potassium	3 g/day (for hyperkalemia)

Table 6 Prevent Additional Injury to the Kidney

Ensure adequate drainage
Avoid or correct volume depletion
Treat infection
Use nephrotoxic agents or drugs with caution (NSAIDs, radiocontrast agents, aminoglycosides)
Use angiographic procedures with caution

and especially, those taking ACE inhibitors, renal function should be carefully monitored during intercurrent illnesses or during use of NSAIDs. The diabetic kidney appears to be particularly susceptible to toxicity from radiocontrast materials when there is impaired renal function. When using these substances, volume deletion should be avoided and a normal-volume state attained before their administration. When indicated and available, carbon dioxide angiography is a useful alternative for investigation of renovascular or peripheral vascular disease (Table 6).

G. Treatment Strategies

Individual patient management must be tailored to the stage of diabetic nephropathy and the coexisting co-morbid conditions. Strategies for a variety of clinical presentations are outlined in Table 7.

Table 7 Treatment Strategies

A. No Clinical Nephropathy (no proteinuria, normal BP): general measures
     Control blood glucose, blood lipids
     Optimize weight
     Encourage exercise
     Heart healthy diet
     Stop smoking
     Monitor microalbuminuria and serum creatinine each year
     Monitor blood pressure each visit
B. Incipient nephropathy (> 30 μg albumin per milligram creatinine in the urine) with normal BP
     General measures (see under A)
     If incipient nephropathy persists after 6 months of general measures use ACE inhibitors to stabilize or reduce albuminuria
     Monitor serum creatinine, potassium, urinary albumin/creatinine every 3–6 months until stable, then each year

(continued)

Table 7   (Continued)

C. Overt nephropathy (> 300 mg protein per gram creatinine in the urine) with normal
    BP and normal renal function
        General measures (see under A)
        ACE inhibitors to stabilize or reduce albuminuria
        Monitor serum creatinine, potassium, urinary albumin/creatinine every 3–6
            months until stable, then each year
D. Overt nephropathy with hypertension (BP > 130/85 mmHg)
        As for overt nephropathy (see under C)
        As for hypertension (see Table 4)
E. Overt nephropathy with renal insufficiency (serum creatinine > 3 mg/dL)
        General measure (see under A)
        Use ACE inhibitors with caution
        Monitor renal function during intercurrent illnesses that include volume changes
            or the use of nephrotoxic agents or medications
        Avoid excess protein in diet (0.8–1 g/kg/day)
        Avoid other injury to kidney
        Evaluate and manage anemia, calcium, and phosphorus metabolism
        Monitor serum creatinine, electrolytes, calcium, phosphorus, and hematocrit
            every 3–6 months
        Consider nephrology consultation
F. Overt nephropathy with nephrotic syndrome (> 3.5 g protein per gram creatinine in
    the urine)
        Control blood pressure
        ACE inhibitors to stabilize or reduce proteinuria
        2 g sodium, 1 g/kg/day protein diet
        If symptomatic use loop ± thiazide-like diuretics
        Control hyperlipidemia
        Monitor serum creatinine, potassium, albumin, urinary protein/creatinine at least
            every 3 months
        Nephrology consultation
G. Overt nephropathy with hyperkalemia (K > 5.5 mEq/L) or type 4 RTA
        General measures
        3-g potassium diet
        Avoid salt substitutes containing potassium chloride (KCl)
        Reduce dose or discontinue ACE inhibitors or angiotensin II receptor antagonists
        Avoid β-adrenergic blockers
        Control blood glucose
        If indicated use loop or thiazide-like diuretics
        Avoid potassium-sparing diuretics
        Nephrology consultation if serum potassium remains > 6.0 mEq/L

VI. RENAL REPLACEMENT THERAPY

A. Dialysis

Renal replacement therapy (RRT) for those with diabetes is usually instituted when there is less renal impairment than in those without diabetes because symptoms appear at an earlier stage from the interaction between the manifestations of uremia and diabetic neuropathy and vasculopathy. Frequently, despite an adequate GFR, it is impossible to maintain acceptable extracellular fluid (ECF) volume (the absence of pulmonary and severe peripheral edema) without unacceptable "levels of uremia," or vise versa. Hence, RRT is usually started when the GFR is 15–20 mL/min (serum creatinine 5–8 mg/dL), rather than less than 10 mL/min (serum creatinine > 10 mg/dL) as is most common in those without diabetes. Early institution of dialysis improves symptoms of gastroparesis, controls volume, and may enhance nutrition by improving dietary intake.

Age-adjusted 5-year survival for all patients on dialysis is 19–47% of that of the U.S. population as a whole. For patients with diabetes, survival on dialysis has improved by 14% over the 10 years from 1985 to 1995, although it remains significantly lower than in nondiabetic patients. Survival on dialysis is similar for type 1 and type 2 patients. As in all persons with ESRD, the major cause of death is cardiac disease (52%). Recognizing and revascularizing those with significant coronary artery lesions (including those without symptoms of cardiac ischemia) improves survival compared with medical treatment alone. There are currently no studies of the effects of atherosclerotic risk factor reduction, either before or during RRT, on cardiovascular morbidity or mortality. The macrovascular and microvascular complications of diabetes progress at at least the same, if not a greater rate during RRT than would be expected from the natural history of the disease. The adverse consequences of neuropathy, retinopathy, and peripheral vascular disease develop at an alarming rate. In addition, the creation and maintenance of natural or synthetic arteriovenous accesses are frequently problematic because of extensive vascular disease. One factor exacerbating dialysis-associated vascular pathology is the accumulation of advanced glycosylation end products that are produced in greater amounts in those with diabetes and are not cleared in those with renal failure. Although high-flux dialysis clears these substances the most efficiently of all the modes of dialysis, levels at best are three to six times higher normal.

There is little known about either the benefits of tight control of blood glucose levels or the standard by which to measure it in dialysis patients. The standard high-performance liquid chromatography (HPLC) method for determining HbA_{1c} provides altered values in dialysis patients because of carbamylation of hemoglobin. In addition diabetic dialysis patients have lower HbA_{1c} than expected for given levels of glucose, making it inaccurate to use the recommended guidelines for control.

B. Renal Transplantation

Renal transplantation is the optimal treatment for patients with diabetic nephropathy. However, successful transplantation depends on donor organs being available, rejection prevented or reversed, and the recipient surviving the surgery and the complications of immunosuppression. Patients with type 1 and type 2 disease have 5-year graft survival similar to those with transplants without diabetes, but higher mortality rates because of higher rates of infection and coronary artery disease in the peri- and posttransplant periods. Because pretransplant recognition and treatment of hemodynamically significant coronary artery lesions improves survival, pretransplant coronary angiography is indicated in those at greatest risk. This includes asymptomatic persons age 45 and older, with diabetes for more than 25 years, or with a smoking history, as well as persons with symptoms of coronary artery disease, an abnormal ECG or abnormal stress test.

Complications of renal transplantation include increased insulin requirements because of increased insulin clearance as the result of restored kidney function, increased insulin resistance from the effects of prednisone, weight gain, and treatment with cyclosporine or tacrolimus. Diabetic nephropathy can develop in the transplanted organ through the same processes that caused the native kidney disease. This can be prevented by a concomitant pancreas transplant (see Chap. 20) or minimized by tight control of blood glucose levels, as was shown in the DCCT trial. As in patients without diabetes, the transplanted kidney is also at risk for damage from cyclosporine and tacrolimus.

Diabetes can develop de novo following renal transplantation for the same reasons that control of blood glucose may worsen. Posttransplantation diabetes (PTD) occurs in up to 20% of those taking regimens containing cyclosporine and prednisone, and in up to 30% of those whose regimens include tacrolimus and prednisone. All three agents reduce insulin secretion and increase insulin resistance. Other risk factors include a family history of type 2 diabetes, increasing age, African American heritage, and high-dose steroid antirejection therapy. PTD appears 6–12 months after transplantation and is pathogenetically similar to type 2 diabetes. However it is reversible in 20–50% of patients despite continuing immunosuppression and, in nearly all, if immunosuppression is withdrawn. Posttransplant diabetes is associated with reduced patient and long-term graft survival.

VII. INDICATIONS FOR REFERRAL

Referral to a nephrologist can be helpful for assistance with diagnosis, treatment, and for discussion of the timing and nature of renal replacement therapy. Common indications are listed in Table 8.

Table 8 Indications for Referral

Diagnostic
  Nephrotic syndrome or urinary protein/creatinine > 3
  Suspicion of renovascular or other nondiabetic renal disease
  Serum potassium higher than 6.0 mEq/L
Treatment
  Blood pressure not at goal
  Serum creatinine > 3 mg/dL or doubling in less than 1 year
  Discussion about renal replacement therapies
Anytime for questions or concerns

BIBLIOGRAPHY

Björck S, Mulec H, Johnsen SA, Nordén G, Aurell M. Renal protective effect of enalapril in diabetic nephropathy. Br J Med 304:339–343, 1992.

Bojestig M, Arnqvist JH, Hermansson G, Karlberg BE, Ludvigsson J. Declining incidence of nephropathy in insulin-dependent diabetes mellitus. N Engl J Med 330:15–18, 1994.

Brancati FL, Whelton PK, Randall BL, Neaton JD, Stamler J, Klag MJ. Risk of end-stage renal disease in diabetes mellitus. A prospective cohort study of men screened for MRFIT. JAMA 278:2069–2074, 1997.

Cockcroft D, Gault M. Prediction of creatinine clearance from serum creatinine. Nephron 16:31–41, 1976.

Diabetes Control and Complications Trial Research Group. The effect of intensive treatment of diabetes on the development and progression of long-term complications in insulin-dependent diabetes mellitus. N Engl J Med 329:977–986, 1993.

Diabetic Nephropathy. In: RW Schrier, CW Gottschalk, eds. Diseases of the Kidney. 6th ed. Boston: Little Brown, 1997:2019–2062.

Epstein M. Calcium antagonists and renal disease. Kidney Int 1998; 54:1771–1784.

Kasiske BL, Kalil RNS, Ma JZ, Liao M, Keane WF. Effect of antihypertensive therapy on the kidney in patients with diabetes: a meta-regression analysis. Ann Intern Med 118:129–138, 1993.

Lewis EJ, Hunsicker LG, Bain RP, Rohde RD for the Collaborative Study Group. The effect of angiotensin-converting-enzyme inhibition on diabetic nephropathy. 329:1456–1462, 1993.

Orth SR, Ritz E, Schrier RW. The renal risks of smoking. Kidney Int 51:1669–1677, 1997.

Parving H-H, Smidt UM, Andersen AR, Svendsen PA. Early aggressive antihypertensive treatment reduces rate of decline in kidney function in diabetic nephropathy. Lancet I:1175–1178, 1983.

Pedrini MT, Levey AS, Lau J, Chalmers TC, Wang PH. The effect of dietary protein restriction on the progression of diabetic and nondiabetic renal diseases. A meta-analysis. Ann Intern Med 124:627–632, 1996.

Peterson JC, Adler S, Burkart JM, Greene T, Hebert LA, Hunsicker LG, King AJ, Klahr S, Massry SH, Seifter JL. Blood pressure control, proteinuria, and the progression of renal disease. The modification of diet in renal disease study. Ann Intern Med 123:754–762, 1995.

Ravid M, Lang R, Rachmani R, Lishner M. Long-term renoprotective effect of angiotensin-converting enzyme inhibition in non–insulin-dependent diabetes mellitus. Arch Intern Med 156:286–289, 1996.

U.K. Prospective Diabetes Study (UKPDS) Group. Intensive blood-glucose control with sulphonylureas or insulin compared with conventional treatment and risk of complications in patients with type 2 diabetes (UKPDS 33). Lancet 352:837–853, 1998.

U.K. Prospective Diabetes Study Group. Tight blood pressure control and risk of macrovascular and microvascular complications in type 2 diabetes: UKPDS 38. Br Med J 317:703–713, 1998.

U.S. Renal Data System, USRDS 1998 Annual Data Report. National Institutes of Health, National Institute of Diabetes and Digestive and Kidney Diseases. Bethesda, MD, April 1998.

Walker JD, Dodds RA, Murrells TJ, Bending JJ, Mattock MB, Keen H, Viberti GC. Restriction of dietary protein and progression of renal failure in diabetic nephropathy. Lancet II:1411–1414, 1989.

26

Erectile Dysfunction in Diabetes Mellitus

Kenneth J. Snow
Joslin Clinic, Boston, Massachusetts

André Guay
Lahey Clinic Northshore, Peabody, Massachusetts

I. INTRODUCTION

A. Definition

Sexual dysfunction can include difficulties with libido, penile erections, and ejaculations, with erectile difficulties constituting the vast majority of this group. Previously, the term impotence was used interchangeably for all aspects of sexual dysfunction, leading to confusion. In 1992, the National Institutes of Health (NIH) Consensus Conference recommended that the term *erectile dysfunction* (ED) be used to described problems relating to penile erections. This statement defined ED as the inability to achieve or maintain an erection long enough to permit satisfactory sexual intercourse. Decades before, Masters and Johnson gave a definition that may be preferable. It was the inability to achieve or maintain an erection long enough to complete intercourse in more than 25% of cases. This definition seems more clinically relevant, as it conveys the fact that men will occasionally fail and still be considered normal.

B. Prevalence

Because of cultural and religious taboos, the medical community has only recently discussed the extent of sexual problems. Kinsey's initial data in 1948 revealed an incidence of less than 3% in men younger than 45, but 25% by age 75. Further studies have increased this percentage, which most agree increases with age. The recent Massachusetts Male Aging Study that evaluated nearly 1300 males, found some degree of erectile difficulty in 52% of men age 40–70.

Before 1960, physicians at psychiatric clinics evaluated most men for sexual difficulties and, not surprisingly, the evaluation found a psychological cause in most men. This belief is being reversed as more comprehensive medical evaluations are carried out. The categories of etiological causes will vary depending on the medical specialty (or bias) of the physicians involved. The number of patients felt to have organic causes for their ED has increased to over 70% in recent years.

C. Specific Causes of ED

It is difficult to evaluate the specific causes because various investigators categorize by general topics, such as vascular and neurological, whereas others give more specific diagnoses. Most authors believe that vascular risk factors, such as diabetes, hypercholesterolemia, hypertension, and smoking, cause most cases of ED. Similar etiological factors were found by Kaiser in 1988, but she stressed the more important concept that many patients have multiple causes of ED, a concept mirrored by others.

II. NORMAL-AGING CHANGES

Some men seeking help for presumed ED may be having only normal-aging changes. Table 1 reviews these changes. As men age they lose the ability for spontaneous erections from fantasy or looking at suggestive pictures. More direct genital stimulation (foreplay) is needed. Problems arise when the partner refuses to participate. Also, as a man ages, sexual activity needs to be attempted in a

Table 1 Normal Aging Sexual Changes in Men

Decreased ability for spontaneous erection
More foreplay needed
Penile sensitivity decreased
    Decreased premature ejaculation
    Increased retarded ejaculation
Refractory period lengthens
Episodes of detumescence without orgasm
Loss of focus may cause loss of erection

quiet place with minimum distractions. A loss of focus invites detumescence as does attempting sexual activity when fatigued.

Penile sensation decreases with age, and this may be difficult to separate from diabetic neuropathy. There is less premature ejaculation with age, but the patient may also notice retarded ejaculation or anejaculation. This may lead to fatigue and detumescence without orgasm. The refractory period is the time from ejaculation to the next penile erection. This time element lengthens with age and may be 30 min at age 20 but 2 days at age 70.

III. NORMAL PENILE PHYSIOLOGY

To have normal penile erections, adequate blood flow and neural stimulation is necessary. This concept has special meaning to the diabetic patient who has microneurovascular changes at the medium- and small-vessel level. In the past, poor vascular response was understood to mean decreased vascular flow to the penis, and this does occur in the man with diabetes, as there is increased atherogenesis in his blood vessels. More importantly, however, is the intrapenile vascular supply, which we have began to appreciate only recently. Intrapenile blood supply is more dependent on neural impulses and chemical substances that affect intracavernosal smooth muscle and vascular tone.

A recent review by Hakim and Goldstein explains the current concepts involved, and these are summarized in Table 2. The penis has two elongated shafts, corpora cavernosa, which comprise multiple sacs surrounded by smooth muscle. The basal state is under adrenergic tone that keeps these muscles con-

Table 2 Mechanism of Local Control of Trabecular Smooth Muscle in the Corpora Cavernosa

Neural mechanisms
    Adrenergic (constrictor): detumescence
    Cholinergic (dilator): tumescence
    Nonadrenergic, noncholinergic (dilator): nitric oxide for tumescence
Chemical mechanisms
    Nitric oxide (dilator): endothelium-derived relaxing factor in human corpora cavernosum
    Prostaglandins (both constrictor and dilator)
    Endothelin (constrictor)
    VIP: enhancer for NO-mediated dilation
    Prostacyclin (dilator)
    Norepinephrine (constrictor)

tracted and the penis detumesced. This state may be aided by the endothelium-derived constrictor, endothelin. On sexual stimulation, cholinergic fibers from the brain release acetylcholine, which partially blocks the adrenergic fibers. The major substance formed from the stimulation of the nonadrenergic, noncholinergic nerve fibers is nitric oxide (NO). There are also neurotransmitters that may also be important relaxers of the corporal smooth muscle. A neural comediator that has a smaller, but still important, role is vasoactive intestinal peptide (VIP).

As the muscle relaxes, the corporal sacs dilate and fill with blood, increasing the intracavernosal pressure. The expanding sacs press the exiting veins against the elastic outer membrane, the tunica albuginea, and effectively decreases the efflux of blood, thereby, further increasing the intracavernosal pressure. Ejaculation causes a reversal of these effects, especially by contraction of the cavernosal smooth muscle, with resulting detumescence.

IV. DIABETES MELLITUS AND ED

A. Prevalence

In a 1987 review, Braunstein found that the incidence of erectile dysfunction in diabetic men varied from 27.5 to 75% in various studies. Other reviews varied from 30 to 60%. As the age of the study population increased, the prevalence was higher, with up to 95% of diabetic men older than 70 having some degree of dysfunction. In diabetic men younger than 30, 20% had ED, and a substantial number may suffer from infertility.

B. Pathophysiology of ED

Although some investigators have stated that ED does not correlate with the patient's age or the duration and severity of the diabetes, the majority do feel that the incidence of ED is definitely related to the age of the patient, duration of the diabetes, control of the blood sugar levels, and presence of diabetic complications. Lack of glycemic control and the presence of diabetic complications seems to increase the incidence of erectile problems. The incidence of ED is higher in diabetic men who have an elevated HbA_{1c}.

The main pathology related to diabetic ED involves vascular and neural changes, in the form of cavernosal artery insufficiency and autonomic neuropathy. Detailed analysis of patients may find vascular or neurological pathology in nearly 90%, and both factors in 40%. The sympathetic nervous system keeps the muscles of the corpora cavernosum contracted, which produces the basal state of detumescence. Men with diabetes have the same increased adrenergic tone as other men with ED. Furthermore autonomic dysfunction, not only of the adrenergic system, but also of the cholinergic nerves, is present. Impairment of the acetylcholine synthesis is no different in type 1 diabetes than in type 2 diabetes, but it is worsened with the duration of diabetes. Central autonomic dysfunction may aggravate the penile autonomic abnormalities.

Morphological studies reveal structural damage to the penile autonomic nerves. Alterations have been shown in smooth muscle and nerve tissue, and these changes are seen not only in patients with diabetes, but also in those with other diseases, such as hypertension and tobacco abuse. Other studies have shown more penile arterial fibrosis than damage to the penile nerve fibers. The vascular pathology may be compounded by other arterial risk factors, such as tobacco abuse and hypertension, both of which are common causes of ED, even in a general population of men.

Apart from structural alterations, there are changes in chemical mediators in penile tissue. The major chemical mediator of smooth-muscle relaxation in the corpora cavernosum is the nitric oxide (NO) that is produced by both the nonadrenergic, noncholinergic nerve fibers, as well as endothelial cells. Its activity is deficient in diabetic rabbits, as well as in diabetic men. The degree of reduction in the level of NO may not be as affected as the decrease in its pharmacological action, and the impairment of the endothelium-dependent vasodilation may be more important than any change in the smooth muscle itself. Diabetes may also affect other modulating transmitters. Not only NO, but also VIP immunoreactivity is decreased in diabetic nerves. Studies on rats with diabetes have demonstrated defects in the VIP receptor. Similar experimental studies on diabetic rats have suggested that the vasodilator prostacyclin may be decreased.

A further determinant in the pathophysiological mechanism may be hypogonadism, which is not uncommon in diabetes. Nitric oxide synthase activity was decreased in this situation and seemed to be related to androgen deficiency. Dihydrotestosterone may be the active hormone necessary for the production of nitric oxide-mediated erections.

The other endocrine glands are also implicated in the causation of erectile dysfunction. Up to one-third of men complaining of impotence have abnormalities of androgen, thyroid, or prolactin hormones. Spark had previously found defects in testosterone production in 35% of 105 impotent patients, and correction of the androgen deficiency corrected 33 of the 37 patients. In a recent study of 659 men, all 67 years of age, a low testosterone level correlated with elevated blood sugar levels. Many of these men had previously undiagnosed diabetes or glucose intolerance. Another study confirmed the relation between elevated blood sugar values and low levels of free testosterone and dihydroxyepiandrosterone (DHEA) sulfate levels, and these low androgen values were also inversely related to insulin concentrations.

The testosterone levels also appear to be lower when diabetes control is poor. A failure to show a difference in testosterone levels between men with diabetes and controls may have been due to the use of total testosterone values and a population that may have been biased toward psychological problems.

There are a variety of medications that can affect sexual function. Libido, erectile capacity, or ejaculatory mechanisms may be affected. Table 3 lists some of the more commonly used medications, especially in the diabetic male.

Because many men with diabetes have hypertension, these drugs need to be scrutinized. Many of the older medications, such as reserpine, guanethidine, and hydralazine had a high rate of sexual side effects. The next generation of

Table 3 Commonly Used Drugs That Affect Sexual Function

Central nervous system-acting drugs
    Antidepressants
    Antipsychotics
    Tranquilizers
    Anorexiants
Cardiovascular
    Digoxin
    Older antihypertensives (reserpine, guanethidine, hydralazine)
    β-Adrenergic blockers (especially propranolol, metoprolol, penbutolol, pindolol, timolol)
    Certain α-adrenergic blockers (clonidine, guanfacine, prazosin)
    α-Adrenergic and β-adrenergic blockers (labetalol)
    α-Methyldopa
    Thiazide diuretics
    Spironolactone
    Calcium channel blockers (fairly low risk)
Allergy-related
    Corticosteroids
    Theophylline
    Bronchodilators
Antifungals
    Fluconazole, ketoconazole, itraconazole
Recreational
    Marijuana
    Alcohol
Miscellaneous
    Metoclopramide, flutamide, clofibrate, gemfibrozil
Nonprescription
    Antihistamines (chlorpheniramine, diphenhydramine, chlotrimeton)
    Decongestants
    Cimetidine

drugs, mainly the β-adrenergic blockers and thiazide diuretics also produced definite problems. The earlier drugs, such as propranolol, caused more difficulties than the more recent ones, such as atenolol, which is less lipid-soluble. Even the local β-adrenergic blocker for glaucoma, timolol, may affect erections.

Many over-the-counter drugs, such as pseudoephedrine and certain antihistamines such as diphenhydramine and chlorpheniramine, have caused problems for years. One recent problem is the declassification of some medications that are now available without a prescription, such as cimetidine. Men with diabetes and gastroparesis might be given metaclopramide, which may elevate prolactin levels. Many central nervous system (CNS)-active drugs may inhibit sexual function by directly acting on the central neurological impulses or by production of prolactin.

Men with diabetes are not immune from having performance anxiety and relationship problems. Various studies have shown a predominantly psychogenic causation from less than 10% to over 33% of men with diabetes and ED. Other patients may have mixed organic–psychogenic causation.

V. DIAGNOSTIC EVALUATION

A. History

As part of the evaluation of ED, one should take a history and perform a physical examination, with emphasis placed on the sexual history and pertinent medical history (Table 4). The first question needs to center on exactly what is the problem, for many patients may complain of impotence, who have a primary problem of erectile dysfunction, decreased libido, or ejaculatory problems. When dealing with erectile dysfunction, the duration of the problem and its presentation—whether sudden or gradual, with or without progression—provides information to suggest a greater or smaller likelihood of organic disease. The presence of morning erections suggest a psychogenic component to the ED, although their absence does not dispute it because morning erections decrease in frequency as men age.

As poor control of blood sugar concentrations increases the likelihood of ED, one must ascertain the patient's glycemic control as well as the presence of diabetic complications. Concomitant medical illnesses should be identified, with particular attention paid to vascular disease and to medications used for the treatment of these problems.

B. Psychological

The initial interview with the diabetic male presenting with sexual difficulties should be undertaken, if possible, with the sexual partner present. If not, at the

Table 4 Evaluation of Men with Diabetes and Erectile Dysfunction

---

History (with partner)
    Control of blood sugar levels
    Complications of DM
    Other medical conditions
    Medications (prescription and nonprescription)
    Performance anxiety
    Relationship problems
    Health of partner
Physical examination
    Blood pressure
    Breast examination
    Cardiac examination
    Vascular examination
    Neurological examination
    Genital examination
Diagnostic tests
    HbA_{1c}, free testosterone
    Nocturnal penile tumescence and rigidity (for possible psychological etiology)

---

next visit, because relationship problems may be a primary or aggravating factor in the difficulty with sexual function.

Despite the presence of neuropathy in a high percentage of diabetic, impotent men there is still a significant percentage of psychological problems and relationship problems. Various psychometric tests have been used. The Florida Sexual History Questionnaire is a simplified test that can be used as a screening tool in the office. Investigators have shown its validity in discriminating primary organic from primary psychogenic disease.

C. Physical Examination

The physical examination should focus on evidence of normal virilization, a testicular examination, and any anatomical changes such as Peyronie's disease or hypospadias, as well as evidence of vascular or neurological deficits.

D. Testosterone Measurement

Apart from blood sugar-related determinations to assess the control of the diabetes, the minimum hormonal measurement that should be performed is a serum, free testosterone. It is now fairly well agreed that testosterone, especially free

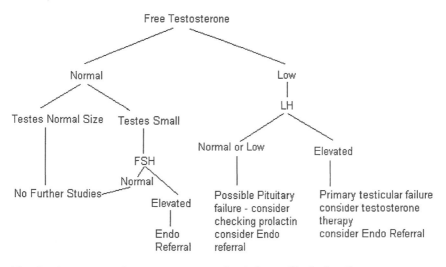

Fig. 1 Assessment of serum testosterone levels in erectile dysfunction.

testosterone—or bioavailable testosterone—decreases with age. The free testosterone declines with a drop of 1.2%/year beyond the age of 40, and sex hormone binding globulin rises with age, rendering the total testosterone measurement inaccurate, for it measures the amount bound to its carrier protein. When interpreting the level of free testosterone, the age of the patient should be taken into account, but many laboratories do not give age-related ranges for testosterone. When levels are questionably low, then a decision on an empiric therapeutic trial of testosterone should be considered.

If the free-testosterone level is normal and the physical examination is normal, then no further laboratory evaluation is needed. If testicular volume is decreased in the presence of a normal testosterone value, one must consider Sertoli cell dysfunction and check a follicule-stimulating hormone (FSH) level. If the free-testosterone level is low, then one must differentiate whether this situation is primary testicular failure or central hypogonadism. In primary testicular failure luteinizing hormone (LH) levels increase in response to the decreased level of testosterone. In central hypogonadism, LH levels are decreased which, in turn, causes a lowered testosterone level. Figure 1 presents one approach to the assessment of testosterone levels.

E. Nocturnal Penile Tumescence and Rigidity Monitoring

If the differentiation between organic and psychogenic erectile dysfunction is difficult to determine, measurement of nocturnal penile activity may be beneficial.

Early studies were performed in sleep laboratories while also studying polysomnography. They showed that men with diabetic impotence had more severe impairment of erectile parameters compared with most categories of nondiabetic, impotent men. Some studies questioned the validity of the results, as nondysfunctional, diabetic men showed abnormal studies compared with age-matched normal controls. This may be partly attributed to the technique of measuring rigidity in a sleep laboratory, or to the lack of rigidity measurements. We are also not absolutely sure how much departure from "normal" a man has to be before this translates into sexual difficulty.

In the last decade, a portable home monitor, RigiScan, was developed that could measure tumescence and rigidity while the patient slept in the privacy of his own home. It is much more convenient and cost-effective. Sleep disorders, especially sleep apnea and nocturnal myoclonus, may invalidate the results, and the patients should be screened with questions beforehand.

F. Vascular

Diabetic men have a high incidence of vascular disease. Patients with severe autonomic neuropathy have a more severe decrease in the intrapenile circulation. An earlier standard test was to measure the penile–brachial index, for which the systolic blood pressure of the cavernosal artery divided by the brachial artery pressure gave an index of penile blood flow. The predictive power of this test was less in men with diabetes than in patients with severe peripheral vascular disease. In fact, an abnormal penile–brachial index (< 0.75) correlated better with coronary artery disease than with erectile dysfunction.

Greater precision has been achieved by using duplex ultrasound to monitor cavernosal artery pressure after the intracavernosal injection of papaverine or prostaglandin-E_1. Caution must be used in interpreting these results as decreased blood flow (versus controls) is seen in diabetic men who have normal erectile function. The more risk factors that exist for arterial insufficiency, such as aortoiliac disease, history of tobacco abuse, and hypertension, the greater the chance that intrapenile blood flow is decreased. There is still no satisfactory substitute for a reliable history and examination of the femoral arteries for pulses and bruits.

G. Neurological

The patient's history and physical examination will generally disclose the presence of neuropathy. Unfortunately, diabetic neuropathy is still a diagnosis of exclusion, and other causes must be considered.

With various methods of measuring pudendal nerve function, impotent diabetic men have abnormal results. It should not be forgotten that decreased penile sensation, along with decreased conduction velocities, are normal-aging phenomenon in all men, not only in men with diabetes; where normal-aging neurological symptoms end and diabetic neuropathic symptoms begin may be difficult to determine.

VI. TREATMENT

A. Correct What Can Be Corrected

The first consideration in a diabetic man with erectile dysfunction is optimal control of his blood sugar level, with avoidance of hypoglycemia. If the patient is taking a drug that is well known to affect erectile function, consider changing the medication if possible to an agent less likely to be a problem. Even if the agent is not the entire cause for the ED, it may be contributing along with other factors.

B. Sex Therapy

A qualified sex therapist should be part of the health team. Not every psychologist has had the training and experience necessary to treat these disorders. In the past, the outcome using long-term psychotherapy was controversial, but brief therapy with behavioral methods seems to achieve better results. The sex therapist may have multiple roles. At times, performance anxiety needs to be addressed, and in other cases, relationship issues may be dominant. This may be true after years of erectile dysfunction during which avoidance of each other is a major stumbling block with the couple. Some couples have to be taught about the need for more foreplay with aging. At times, decreased libido problems may point to an underlying conflict that has to be evaluated.

C. Hormone Treatments

Thyroid disorders, whether overactive or underactive, should be treated with appropriate medications. Generally, borderline thyroid levels contribute very little to a sexual problem. Some patients with low libido and subclinical hypothyroidism may respond to thyroid replacement therapy. Corticosteroids should be withdrawn whenever possible when used to treat conditions other than adrenal insufficiency. Elevated prolactin levels may respond to withdrawing any offending medications. Pituitary tumors may need to be ruled out if prolactin levels are quite high. Hyperprolactinemia of any cause, may be treated with the dopamine agonists bromocriptine or pergolide.

Patients with primary gonadal failure need permanent testosterone replacement. Apart from helping with libido and erectile problems, testosterone deficiency may also cause lethargy, depression, anemia, muscle weakness, and osteoporosis. The choice is generally either long-acting testosterone esters by intramuscular injections, or with the newer testosterone patches. Not all men with low testosterone levels and ED will respond to testosterone replacement. The presence of vascular disease may partially predict a nonresponse. In essence, the more the medical risk factors for erectile dysfunction, the less likely is the response to testosterone replacement alone.

Because testosterone may aggravate a preexisting prostate cancer, a prostate-specific antigen (PSA) should be assessed before testosterone treatment. One can then check the PSA again after a few months of treatment, then yearly thereafter. Hemoglobin and hematocrit levels should also be checked regularly because of the risk of polycythemia, especially in smokers.

Men with diabetes often have secondary hypogonadism. These patients may also be treated with testosterone directly, but this may further suppress the central axis, which may have been suppressed from uncontrolled diabetes, multiple medications, alcohol excess, or stress. One can treat these patients by stimulating the central axis with clomiphene citrate. The response may be better in younger patients and, again, those with fewer medical risk factors.

VII. MEDICAL THERAPIES FOR ED

If controlling the blood sugar level, changing medications, or replacing deficient hormones is not sufficient to reestablish normal sexual function, one must consider other methods (Table 5).

Table 5 Frequently Used Therapies for Erectile Failure in the Man with Diabetes

Nonpharmacological therapy
    Penile constriction rings
    Vacuum tumescence devices
    Penile implants
Local pharmacological therapy
    Penile injections
    Intraurethral suppositories
Oral therapy
    Sildenafil
    Yohimbine

A. Nonpharmacological Therapy

1. Constriction Rings

Patients who have no trouble in producing an adequate erection with foreplay, but who lose it prematurely before ejaculation, are said to have early detumescence or venous leakage. They may not need medications or devices to produce an erection, but rather just something to prevent detumescence. Kits are available with rubber rings of various sizes that can be placed at the base of the penis after a suitable erection has been produced. These can be cumbersome and are relatively expensive. A newer, simplified adjustable latex ring called the Actis Venous Flow Controller is available (Vivus, Menlo Park, CA). It is simple, safe, and inexpensive. Early experience indicates better acceptance by the patient and partner.

2. Vacuum Tumescence Devices

Vacuum pumps are plastic cylinders that are placed over the penis. Air is evacuated, creating a negative pressure that draws blood into the penis. A ring is placed around the base of the inflated penis which will retain the erection. Various models have been developed over the past two to three decades. Satisfactory erections are obtained in about 75% of patients, whereas about 50% of patients have long-term satisfaction. It is safe, but quite mechanical. A certain percentage of partners may fail to accept this technique. Younger men and those patients who do not have a long-term relationship may find this technique cumbersome and embarrassing. Vacuum devices may be useful for diabetic men who have a significant vascular component and in whom other therapies have had no effect.

3. Penile Implants

The penile implant was one of the first modes of therapy for erectile dysfunction. With the development of newer therapies, the number of implants performed yearly has substantially decreased. There are two basic types. The semirigid rod and the inflatable rod. The latter has more hardware that is placed in the penis, scrotum, and suprapubic area, thus increasing the risk of mechanical failure or infection. The earlier models had a high rate of mechanical failure, but this has decreased significantly with engineering improvements. Satisfaction rates among diabetic men and their partners vary depending on the study. It should be stressed, however, that preoperative counseling should be given to the couple to dispel any unrealistic expectations. Although decreased, infections are still a concern in the diabetic population.

B. Local Pharmacological Therapy

1. Intracavernosal Injection Therapy

Intrapenile injection with vasoactive substances has been taught for the past 15 years. Initially, papaverine was used, but there was a high incidence of penile fibrosis, which was decreased when phentolamine was added. The addition of prostaglandin E_1 improved the results, with up to 90% of patients responding. However, studies have revealed a loss of nearly half of the patients to this treatment in the first year. Infection is uncommon, but is more prone to occur in the diabetic patient who uses this technique.

Recently, the use of prostaglandin E_1 (Caverject; Upjohn and Edex, Schwarz) alone has increased, as it is the only intrapenile chemical officially approved for use by the U.S. Food and Drug Administration (FDA). It does not appear to be as effective in diabetic erectile dysfunction as the papaverine–regitine mixture (52% effective vs. 79%), or as effective as other vasoactive mixtures. Acceptance of this therapy has been limited by the patient's willingness to perform intrapenile injections.

2. Intraurethral Therapy

Recently, prostaglandin E_1 has been formulated into an intraurethral suppository that is absorbed into the corpora spongiosum of the glans penis and migrates rapidly into the corpora cavernosa. Up to 60% of patients with diabetes attain adequate erections in our experience with this therapy. The response rate is not as dependable as for intrapenile injections, but there are fewer potential complications, such as penile scarring and priapism.

C. Oral Medication

1. Sildenafil

Sildenafil (Viagra; Pfizer, Inc.) is an oral agent released in early 1998. During stimulation, nitric oxide (NO) is released in the corpus cavernosum, which activates guanylate cyclase and results in increased levels of cyclic guanosine monophosphate (cGMP). This causes smooth-muscle relaxation in the corpus cavernosum, allowing blood to flow in. Sildenafil inhibits phosphodiesterase type 5 (PDE-5) which degrades cGMP. Thus, inhibition of PDE-5 by sildenafil causes an increase in cGMP, with subsequent increased vasodilation.

The drug is rapidly absorbed, with peak serum levels about 30–120 min after taking it. One should, therefore, instruct patients to take the medication about 1 h before attempting intercourse and that sexual stimulation (foreplay) is necessary.

The drug improves erections in up to 80% of patients, although is more likely to help patients with a psychological basis for their ED. Patients with complete or near complete loss of erectile function have a lower response rate. Most common side effects include headache, flushing, dyspepsia, and nasal congestion. The drug is contraindicated for patients taking nitrates.

Sildenafil has occasionally increased sensitivity to light and affected blue-green color discrimination. As yet, there are no studies evaluating the effect of this agent on retinal blood vessels in patients with diabetes. Because of its vasodilatory action, there is concern over its use in patients with retinopathy, especially those patients with proliferative disease.

The recommended starting dose is 50 mg, taken as needed, 30 min to 4 h before sexual activity. The dosage can be increased to 100 mg if needed or decreased to 25 mg if side effects occur. A patient should not take more than one dose each day.

2. Yohimbine

Yohimbine, an α_2-adrenergic blocker, is an extract of the yohimbe tree in Africa. Its usage predates the existence of the FDA, which was founded in 1938. Its efficacy is controversial. Studies have shown yohimbine to be more efficacious in psychological impotence, but its overall positive response may be as high as 30–40%. The starting dose is usually one 5.4-mg tablet three times a day. It may take 2 weeks to notice an effect, and if there is to be a response, it will generally occur in the first month. If there is a response, patients may need only one or two tablets about 1 h before desired sexual activity.

D. Approach to Therapy

There are multiple possibilities for the nonspecific treatment of ED. For patients with venous leakage, a venous flow controller might be the first choice if the patient will accept it, because it is inexpensive and has no side effects.

For those with a significant psychogenic component, counseling along with an oral agent, such as yohimbine or sildenafil, has a high likelihood of working. For the vast majority of diabetic patients who have a significant neurovascular component as the cause of their ED, one may start with sildenafil. If the drug is contraindicated or unsuccessful, second-line therapy could include either intraurethral therapy or a vacuum tumescence device, depending on patient desire.

E. Referral

After performing the initial evaluation, one may wish to begin therapy if the cause of the ED is clear and the physician is comfortable with the use of oral therapy for ED. If the cause is unclear, one should consider consultation at that time. Certainly, if a patient fails oral therapy, one should refer that patient for further treatment, unless the physician is quite comfortable with the various forms of therapy available.

BIBLIOGRAPHY

Braunstein GD. Impotence in diabetic men. Mt Sinai J Med 54:236–240, 1987.

Drugs that cause sexual dysfunction: an update. Med Lett 34:73–78, 1992.

Feldman HA, I Goldstein, DG Hatzichristou, RJ Krane, JB McKinley. Impotence and its medical and psychosocial correlates: results of the Massachusetts Male Aging Study. J Urol 151:54–61, 1994.

Geisser ME, FT Murray, MS Cohen, PJ Shea, RR Addeo. Use of Florida Sexual History Questionnaire to differentiate primary organic from primary psychogenic impotence. J Androl 14:298–303, 1993.

Guay AT. Treatment of erectile dysfunction in men with diabetes. Diabetes Spectr 11:101–111, 1998.

Hakim LS, I Goldstein. Diabetic sexual dysfunction. Endocrinol Metab Clin North Am 25:379–400, 1996.

Kaiser FE, SP Viosca, JE Morley, AD Mooradian, SS Davis, SG Korenman. Impotence and aging: clinical and hormonal factors. J Am Geriatr Soc 36:511–519, 1988.

Masters WH, VE Johnson. Human Sexual Inadequacy. Boston: Little Brown, 1970.

NIH Consensus Development Panel on Impotence. JAMA 270:83–90, 1993.

Spark RF, RA White, PB Connolly. Impotence is not always psychogenic: newer insights into hypothalamic–pituitary–gonadal dysfunction. JAMA 243:750–755, 1980.

27

Peripheral Vascular Disease in Diabetes

Gary W. Gibbons
Boston University Medical School, Boston Medical Center, Boston, Massachusetts

I. INTRODUCTION

Lower extremity peripheral vascular disease (PVD) is among the most important reasons for disabling pain, nonhealing ulcerations, and amputation in individuals with and without diabetes. The incidence of PVD in diabetic patients is at least ten times that of nondiabetics and increases with age and duration of diabetes. PVD results in decreased arterial perfusion to the lower extremity and foot. It contributes to pain, limb ulceration, impaired wound healing, and decreases the ability to fight infection by delaying or preventing the delivery of oxygen, nutrients, the components of a proper immune response, and antibiotics to the infected area. Pecoraro and colleagues noted that critical ischemia was associated with 62% of cases in whom there was nonhealing ulceration and was a causal factor in 46% of amputations. Unrecognized or untreated PVD increases the risk for amputation. The purpose of this chapter is to review the signs, symptoms, evaluation, and therapies for PVD to help the primary care physician in his day-to-day management of diabetic patients. The bottom line: ''modern revascularization procedures offer great hope to diabetic patients with limb-threatening ischemia and should be considered before any thought of amputation.''

II. HOST CONSIDERATION, RISK FACTORS, AND PREVENTION

Although PVD can singularly lead to amputation, it is the triad of neuropathy, vascular insufficiency, and an altered response to infection that collectively makes the diabetic uniquely susceptible to foot problems. In population-based studies, pulse deficits were found in approximately 10% of diabetic subjects and absent pulses in approximately 20–30%. Females with diabetes develop PVD at the same rate as males, and for all, there are increased morbidity and mortality, particularly if foot ulceration, infection, or gangrene occur. Although diabetes is an important risk factor for PVD, hypertension, smoking, hyperlipidemia, obesity, and family history are well-established risk factors and contribute additional risk for patients with diabetes. Prevention or delaying the onset of PVD must be a primary goal of practitioners, and this is best achieved by the elimination of risk factors, including cigarette smoking, good control of diabetes, control of hypertension and dyslipidemias, maintaining ideal weight, and routine and proper exercise.

It is important to note that diabetic patients can effectively live their lives with neuropathy, vascular insufficiency, and an altered response to infection. Patient and physician education and understanding correlate directly with the successful management of foot problems. Minor trauma continues to be the single most important contributor to ulceration, especially when associated with other pathophysiological, behavioral, and educational risk factors. The primary care physician must educate diabetic patients on the importance of proper hygiene, daily shoe and foot inspection, the wearing of appropriate shoes, and rotation of shoes at least twice each day to vary the stress and pressure points. The simple technique of testing for sensory neuropathy with a monofilament can be used to identify patients at risk for ulceration and, therefore, most in need of preventative intervention or referal to a specialist. This is especially true if there is associated deformity and diminished circulation. Periodic vascular examination, including noninvasive testing when appropriate, helps identify patients at risk who can be observed more carefully or be referred to a vascular specialist. We cannot underscore enough the importance of a multidisciplinary team approach that tailors individual diabetes management, control of other associated risk factors, periodic vascular examinations, proper foot care, and continued education.

The relation between the major arterial circulation and the adequacy of the cutaneous circulation of the lower extremity and foot requires understanding because adequate cutaneous perfusion depends not only on the underlying arterial circulation, but also may be significantly influenced by other factors, including skin integrity, pressure necrosis from repetitive mechanical pressure, tissue edema, uncontrolled infection, autonomic dysfunction, cardiac conditions, such as congestive heart failure and cardiomyopathy with low output, and medications, especially those with the side effect of vasoconstriction.

III. PATHOPHYSIOLOGY

Optimal management of diabetic, lower-extremity PVD requires an understanding of the specific pattern of its involvement. All diabetics do not have poor circulation. Although the pathology of atherosclerosis is similar in both diabetic and nondiabetic patients, several distinguishing features characterize diabetic lower extremity PVD. In the diabetic patient, there is a predisposition for macrovascular occlusive disease to involve primarily the tibial and peroneal arteries between the knee and the foot, as is evidenced by the finding that 40% of diabetic patients with gangrene have a palpable popliteal pulse. The dorsalis pedis artery and foot vessels, however, are usually spared. No occlusive microvascular disease of the diabetic foot exists that precludes revascularization. This misconception from the early 1950s has been refuted by many observers and was reviewed by LoGerfo and Kaufman in 1984 in the *New England Journal of Medicine.* Unfortunately, the misconception of an occlusive microvascular lesion affecting the diabetic foot fosters an attitude of hopelessness in many health care professionals and is responsible for inappropriate vascular care extended to many patients. Because there is sparing of the foot vessels, especially the dorsalis pedis artery, tissue perfusion in the ischemic diabetic foot can be restored with appropriate vascular reconstruction.

Although there is no microvascular occlusive disease, there is microvascular dysfunction that begins early in diabetic life with an increased microvascular pressure and flow that lead to endothelial injury with sclerosis (basement membrane thickening) and a limited capillary capacity, with loss of autoregulatory function, including the abolition of a vasoconstrictor response. This microvascular dysfunction is not an occlusive lesion and does not preclude revascularization; on the contrary, it supports an aggressive approach to restore circulation. Rather than reporting to the patient and family that the situation is hopeless, the practitioner or health care professional should be saying that when ischemia is complicating a diabetic foot problem, perfusion to the foot can be restored with appropriate modern revascularization techniques.

Diabetic lower-extremity PVD is also associated with a diminished ability for collateral circulation to develop, especially around the distal profunda femoris artery and the infragenicular arteries. This may explain why arterial occlusions or stenosis (especially multilevel disease) have more serious limb-threatening consequences for the diabetic than for the nondiabetic, not because of involvement of the foot arteries.

Diabetics also have a propensity for calcification involving the intimal plaque and media (medial calcinosis or Monkeberg's sclerosis). Although this is probably neuropathic in origin, it frequently involves diabetic arteries at all levels, but again often spares the foot vessel. Medial calcinosis can result in erroneous noninvasive test results, especially elevating segmental systolic pressures along the lower extremity and the ankle/brachial ratio. It also complicates surgical, laser, or balloon angioplasty treatment.

To summarize, all diabetic patients should undergo routine foot examination and periodic vascular examination. Diabetic patients can live with PVD until a traumatic event initiates an ulcer or fissure. If there is any question about the adequacy of the circulation, or there is a change in symptoms or examination results, noninvasive vascular evaluation is helpful to compliment the clinical impression. Elective vascular consultation to someone experienced with diabetic patients is appropriate, especially if any type of foot surgery or problem exists. These patients fall into the high-risk category for ulceration, so routine inspection and care of the feet, with prescription of appropriate footwear, is mandatory.

Vascular evaluation and consultation should be strongly recommended for patients whose ulcers are thought to have an ischemic component or fail to heal within a specific time period (assuming that appropriate treatment has been rendered), including incisions from local procedures that failed to heal and areas that recurrently breakdown. It must be remembered that there are a few diabetic patients who have significant enough ischemia that they do not heal, even in the presence of palpable foot pulses at rest because they have enough collateral circulation. This tenuous blood supply becomes insufficient with any increased demand.

IV. CLINICAL PRESENTATION

Health care professionals see diabetic patients every day who harbor major arterial occlusive disease yet are asymptomatic. The clinical presentation of patients with major artery occlusions or hemodynamically significant stenoses varies depending on their activity level and the adequacy of the collateral pathways. Establishing the diagnosis of ischemia in the diabetic is made more difficult by the presence of peripheral and autonomic neuropathy.

Claudication is usually the first symptom of significant PVD involving the lower extremity. It is the inability to walk a given distance (usually expressed in blocks) because of muscle pain or cramping secondary to inadequate arterial blood supply. Diabetics with neuropathy may describe claudication more as a numbness or a dead feeling or just as a need to stop at a given distance. The location of the muscle grouping involved in claudication helps distinguish proximal inflow (aortoiliac) occlusive disease from that of distal outflow (femoral–popliteal–tibial). The more proximal the muscles involved, the more proximal the occlusive disease. The occlusive disease is usually one level above the symptomatic muscle group. As an example, calf claudication (the most frequent type of claudication) usually signifies superficial femoral artery disease. Claudication is worsened by an incline or a faster pace and is almost always relieved by rest. Symptoms of aortoiliac occlusion may progress to those of the classic Leriche's, but impotence in the diabetic may also be secondary to autonomic neuropathy. Distinguishing claudication from symptoms of nerve root irritation caused by spinal stenosis, intervertebral disk herniation, or neuropathy itself can be quite challenging.

Intermittent claudication is not a precursor to limb loss, especially the early stages, and conservative management is recommended because only 10 to 15% of patients progress to more-threatening complications. Regression in diabetics is more common than in nondiabetics, especially in patients who continue to smoke or fail to correct other risk factors. Vascular consultation and more invasive intervention are indicated in patients with claudication, after walking usually less than one-half to one block, that interferes with the patients lifestyle or work. Again, it is important to remember that symptoms in the diabetic patient with severe diffuse arterial occlusive disease may be masked by neuropathy until some type of minor trauma results in ischemic ulceration.

Vascular consultation is recommended for patients presenting with limb-threatening indications, such as rest pain, tissue loss (ulceration or gangrene), or reconstructive foot surgery incisions that will not heal. Rest or night pain (a deep aching in the foot) is usually distinguishable from neuropathy, especially when combined with the clinical features of ischemia. Patients with rest pain often obtain some relief by getting up and walking or hanging their feet in a dependent position. Rest pain is a precursor of tissue ulceration or gangrene if not corrected. Ischemic ulceration, fissures, and dry gangrene demand vascular consultation and intervention, depending on the patients associated risk factors and well-being. Gangrene has other causes, such as infection and pressure. Any ulcer or incision from a local foot procedure that does not heal should be reevaluated for ischemia that may have been underappreciated earlier.

V. CLINICAL EVALUATION

Clinical evaluation, judgment, and experience remain the most important means for assessing vascular insufficiency in the diabetic lower extremity (Table 1). Routine examination of both feet is necessary with periodic vascular evaluation that seeks pallor or dependent rubor, loss of hair, atrophy of the skin, or cornification of the nails. Fissures or ulcerations should be evident, as should temperature demarcation. The palpation of pulses, although difficult at times, is most important, as are listening for bruits and palpation of thrills. Determination of the venous-filling time is more important than simple evaluation of capillary filling, which because of autonomic neuropathy, may remain normal, despite the presence of significant ischemia. It must be emphasized that it is inappropriate for any health care professional to press on the end of the toe, blanch the nail bed, and based on this conclude that there is good capillary filling and, therefore, adequate circulation.

Table 1   Signs and Symptoms of Peripheral Vascular Disease

Intermittent claudication
Feet cold to touch
Nocturnal and rest pain relieved with dependency
Absent pulses
Blanching on elevation
Delayed venous filling after elevation (> 25 s)
Dependent rubor
Atrophy of subcutaneous fatty tissue
Shiny appearance of skin
Loss of hair on foot and toes
Thickened nails, often with fungus infection
Gangrene or nonhealing ulcer of surgical procedure
Miscellaneous: blue toe syndrome, acute vascular occlusion

Because of neuropathy, clinical assessment may be difficult and should be complemented with noninvasive testing by whatever means the evaluator has in his or her laboratory (Table 2). We have not found any noninvasive tests for the diabetic patient that uniformly characterizes the degree of vascular insufficiency or predicts primary healing (with or without vascular reconstruction) or amputation level. We reported that because of medical calcinosis, the interpretive results of standard noninvasive tests, such as systolic blood pressure and the ankle/brachial ratio are often misleading and incorrect when applied to the diabetic lower extremity. Despite this, insurers and other health care agencies rely on ankle/brachial ratios in an inappropriate manner. In 1998 the primary practitioner or health care professional should recommend vascular consultation and probable arteriography if there is any question of ischemia complicating a diabetic foot problem.

Table 2   Noninvasive Vascular Tests

Doppler systolic pressure measurements
Doppler ankle pressure measurements and ankle/brachial index
Doppler waveform analysis
Pulse volume recordings
Toe pressures
Transcutaneous oxygen pressure
Duplex color flow scanning
Magnetic resonance (MR) angiography

VI. ARTERIOGRAPHY

Arteriography is still the most effective means for definitive evaluation of diabetic PVD. Precision arteriography is mandatory, however, because it most influences the surgeons decision for vascular reconstruction by whatever means. Because of the association of dye-related transient renal compromise in the diabetic, careful preparation, especially adequate hydration, is required, as is discontinuing any potential nephrotoxic drugs and the avoidance of elective major revascularization immediately following arteriography. Digital subtraction arteriography with proximal pressure measurements decreases the dye volume needed for performance of a complete study, including visualization of the foot arteries, which is mandatory. With current arteriographic techniques, more than 90% of diabetic patients with ischemic foot lesions have surgically correctable occlusive disease. Although magnetic resonance (MR) angiography and color flow duplex scanning hold promise for the future, especially in patients with renal compromise, arteriography is still the gold standard at present. In our experience, the use of ionic and nonionic contrast has not influenced the incidence of renal failure.

Many diabetic patients with PVD are deemed nonreconstructable because of an inadequate arteriogram. The practitioner or any health care professional should be involved with the actual interpretation of the arteriogram, demanding visualization of the foot vessels, which should be correlated with an audible doppler signal over the dorsalis pedis or distal posterior tibial arteries or branches. An inadequate arteriogram presents additional risk for the patient, especially if it must be repeated, because it is costly and can lead to an inappropriate revascularization procedure or complications. This obviously requires team work, but in our experience, the diabetic patient with threatened limb loss and only an audible dorsalis pedis doppler signal, still has a 50% chance of a successful revascularization procedure. More experienced vascular consultation by someone knowledgeable about diabetic PVD should always be an option when there is a question.

VII. PATIENT ASSESSMENT AND PREPARATION

Vascular intervention depends on the patients associated risk factors and well-being. Patients who have severe dementia or mental deterioration and do not ambulate are certainly not candidates for revascularization. Patients with extensive tissue destruction with possible limb salvage, even if circulation was restored, must be carefully evaluated for whether they would be better served with primary amputation. Age is no contraindication to an aggressive approach to limb salvage, including revascularization. It is important to assess carefully all of the risk factors and comorbid conditions that might affect patency and success. Current revascularization techniques allow a flexible approach with many procedures, both for inflow (aortoiliac) and outflow (infrainguinal) that can be tailored to individual patient requirements on the basis of preoperative assessment and preparation.

It is not surprising that coronary artery disease and left ventricular dysfunction are the leading causes of morbidity and mortality in all major revascularization procedures. Cardiac involvement may be asymptomatic because of sensory and autonomic neuropathy. An abnormal electrocardiogram or a history of significant coronary artery disease or left ventricular dysfunction (congestive heart failure) requires further preoperative evaluation. The presence and time interval of a previous myocardial infarction as well as left ventricular dysfunction affect perioperative mortality and morbidity. Echocardiography and nuclear stress testing are adjunctive tests that may lead to cardiac catheterization and coronary revascularization before elective major revascularization procedures. Renal function should be returned to baseline, and discontinuation of nephrotoxic agents should be attempted before revascularization if possible. Compromised pulmonary function must be evaluated and treated because it may influence the type of revascularization procedure and the anesthesia recommended. Medications are reviewed and adjusted. Use of medications affecting the clotting cascade should be discontinued in advance of planned revascularization procedures. Control of the blood sugar level is a prerequisite for revascularization procedures unless it is an emergency.

An absolute requirement before any revascularization is the control of all active infection. Infected wounds must be carefully probed, and all necrotic tissue must be debrided and dependently drained. Appropriate adjunctive intravenous antibiotics are administered throughout the revascularization period. Team work is needed so that there is preparation to move quickly to revascularization after adequate control of infection to prevent further ischemic necrosis.

VIII. PERIOPERATIVE MANAGEMENT

Anesthesia is tailored to the individual patients needs and the procedure that is to be performed. General endotrachial, spinal, and epidural anesthesia, all are equally effective, appropriate, and safe. To reduce or prevent cardiac morbidity, invasive cardiac monitoring utilizing a Swan Ganz catheter is continued until the patient has shown an ability to mobilize and eliminate third-space fluid. Nutritional replenishment and control of edema are also extremely important.

Although early postbypass ambulation is desired, it is delayed in patients with open, dependent ulcers and in patients who undergo reconstructive foot surgery or local toe or forefoot amputation. These patients should, however, have active and passive range of motion exercises. Early ambulation without weight-bearing on the affected side is encouraged by the use of walkers or crutches. Weight-bearing should be increased slowly and progressed to prevent the development of an acute Charcot foot, the incisional disruption of local foot procedures, or recurrence of a recently healed ulcer. Healing sandals with appropriate molded inserts and proper foot wear require expertise to prevent breakdown or recurrence.

IX. TREATMENT

The criteria for any revascularization (restoring circulation) are the right indications, the potential for rehabilitation, and an appropriate conduit. Claudication is rarely an indication for revascularization unless it is disabling by interfering with the patients work or lifestyle. Claudication is first treated by controlling risk factors including weight reduction, the cessation of smoking, control of lipid abnormalities and hypertension, good diabetic control, and an active and aggressive exercise program. Medications, such as pentoxifylline, vasodilators, or calcium channel blockers are relatively ineffective for most diabetic patients with PVD. Again, teamwork is needed because protective footwear and continuous inspection are important during exercise to protect high-risk areas that are neuropathic. Diabetics can live with significant PVD without incident until a traumatic event initiates an ulcer.

Ischemic rest pain and night pain are indications for some type of revascularization procedure as is tissue ulceration, gangrene, and the inability of a surgical procedure to heal because of ischemia. Again, if there is any question about ischemia, referral to a vascular surgeon knowledgeable about diabetic vascular disease and its treatment is recommended. Diabetic patients tolerate revascularization procedures extremely well, with morbidity and mortality results equal to those of the nondiabetic and no greater than amputation.

X. ENDOVASCULAR PROCEDURES

Endovascular procedures (balloon angioplasty, atherectomy, laser angioplasty) note a significant difference in success based on the location of the atherosclerotic disease, the length of the lesion being treated, local versus diffuse vascular involvement, and the composition of the plaque. There is diminishing success with more distal disease, longer length of lesions, more diffuse disease, and heavily calcified plaques, the typical disease presentation in diabetic patients. Our experience has shown that the best endovascular results are achieved with balloon angioplasty of short isolated iliac artery stenoses or occlusions. There is diminishing success as one progresses distally in the arterial tree, especially angioplasty involving the popliteal, tibial, or peroneal arteries. Angioplasty is adjunctive for patients presenting with inflow (aortoiliac) and outflow (femoral–popliteal–tibial) disease. One must correct the inflow first, and successful balloon angioplasty avoids a surgical procedure saving it for the more distal disease. The routine use of stents requires further clinical evaluation because they are costly, and long-term results of their placement in different locations is lacking.

Gene therapy holds promise for the future. Injecting short stretches of DNA containing the genetic code for vascular endothelial growth factor, a protein that simulates the growth of new blood vessels has been done, but more clinical studies are needed to prove its cost effectiveness before this therapy becomes routine. Gene therapy is also being studied to prevent blockage in bypass grafts after revascularization procedures. While we are all fascinated with space-age technology, new therapies should not be recommended or performed routinely until controlled clinical trials demonstrate their proper indications and cost effective results.

XI. REVASCULARIZATION PROCEDURES

The type of major revascularization procedure depends on the findings of the total arteriogram that visualizes the foot vessels, the patients condition, and the presence of comorbidities. All revascularization procedures can be tailored to individual patient needs.

A. Management of Aortoiliac Occlusive Disease (Inflow Procedures)

Although atherosclerotic PVD has a propensity for the more distal arteries of the lower leg, aortoiliac involvement (inflow disease) does occur, especially in diabetics with a history of smoking. Inflow must be restored before or concomitant with more distal infrainguinal (outflow disease) revascularization. Aortoiliac (inflow) procedures are performed similarly in diabetic and nondiabetic patients and usually require the use of synthetic grafts. Inflow procedures can be tailored to each patient's needs, depending on the location and extent of disease, associated risk factors, and the patients well-being.

B. Infrainguinal Outflow Procedures (Femoral/Popliteal/Tibial/Pedal)

Sophisticated and aggressive distal revascularization techniques have demonstrated excellent graft patency and limb salvage in the diabetic lower extremity. Autogenous vein (either saphenous or arm) is the conduit of choice, with synthetic grafts, such as polytetrafluorethylene, used only as a last resort. The distal revascularization should be tailored to the amount, size, and quality of vein available; the patients indications and associated risk factors; and the actual anatomical setup as determined by complete arteriography visualizing the foot vessels. This flexible approach also allows the decision to place the vein in the reversed or nonreversed (in situ or ex situ) position based on individual patient needs.

It is important to discuss the purpose of the bypass. Is it needed to cure claudication, or to restore foot perfusion to heal extensive tissue loss or a previously performed foot procedure? The simplest and most effective bypass would be one that bypasses a blockage or disease in the superficial femoral artery, with restoration of flow to the popliteal, tibial, and peroneal vessels, with continuity down into the foot. Unfortunately, this bypass is often impossible in the diabetic, so a flexible approach with discussion of all available options for each case is desirable preoperatively. For claudication or rest pain a more proximal infrainguinal bypass usually suffices. We do not advocate distal bypass grafting especially to the dorsalis pedis artery for relief of claudication or rest pain, especially when a more proximal bypass will adequately take care of the problem.

Restoration of pulsatile blood flow to the foot is important to heal extensive tissue loss, gangrene, or incisions from local forefoot procedures. Again, a flexible approach allows the use of an inflow source that is most distal, such as the popliteal artery, when arteriography shows there is patency all the way to that level. In general, it is most desirable that the larger part of the vein be placed to the more proximal larger artery and to use the smaller end of the vein for anastamosis to the distal artery, which at times can be 1 mm in diameter.

Once circulation to the foot is restored, more localized debridement, reconstructive foot surgery, or amputation or revision may be performed, or an area left open to heal.

All active infection must be controlled before any revascularization procedure, which includes debridement of all necrotic tissue and tissue and bone, and dependent drainage of pus. Most bypass grafts lie adjacent to the lymphatic channels, which can be involved with the infectious process. Once infection is controlled, one must be prepared to move immediately to arteriography and revascularization to prevent further ischemic tissue loss. Appropriate, effective adjunctive intravenous antibiotics are also essential during this revascularization period.

XII. RESULTS OF DISTAL BYPASS GRAFTING

We have learned that to achieve the most rapid and durable healing of an open foot ulcer one needs to restore a pulse to the foot by a distal revascularization to an artery, with direct continuity to the dorsalis pedis, posterior tibial, or plantar arteries themselves. Bypassing only to the more proximal popliteal or tibial–peroneal arteries may be inadequate for the diabetic patient with extensive tissue loss for the reasons mentioned previously. In summary, the best results of distal revascularization are achieved when the bypass is extended to the most proximal tibial outflow vessel in direct continuity with the pedal circulation, rather than bypassing to a blind popliteal segment or peroneal vessel. We prefer to do direct pedal artery grafting in situations where pulsatile flow is essential to promote the healing of ulcerations, minor amputations, or to facilitate reconstructive foot surgery.

Since 1995 the pedal artery bypass now constitutes about 25% of our revascularization procedures. Initial 3-year results of this procedure show an 87% graft patency and 92% limb salvage. At 5 years the primary and secondary patency rates are 68% and 81%, respectively. Limb salvage in this group exceeds 87% at 5 years. Regional as well as general anesthesia are equally safe, and routine perioperative invasive cardiac monitoring is mostly responsible for our operative mortality of only 1.8% and cardiac morbidity of 5.4%. These complication rates are comparable with those of diabetic patients undergoing major amputation alone and, again support an aggressive approach to limb salvage.

Diabetic patients are rarely candidates for distal balloon or laser angioplasty for limb salvage because of their vulnerability for diffuse, extensive, infrapopliteal disease and medial calcification, both of which limit the success of these procedures. These procedures rarely restore adequate tissue perfusion to the foot. Since 1984 our multidisciplinary team approach to the diabetic foot has demonstrated a significant reduction in every category of amputation at the Beth Israel Deaconess Medical Center and the Joslin Diabetes Center. From the patient's perspective this aggressive approach relieves their pain, heals their wounds, and allows them to better return to function and well-being. Working as a team, we have also been able to reduce our length of stay and cost of care. There are advantages to preserving as much of the foot as possible. By restoring foot perfusion, our podiatry colleagues have been able to perform direct foot-sparing surgery, such as local excision of ulcerations and infected bony prominences, osteotomys or athroplasties, which have often eliminated the need for toe or forefoot amputation. In conjunction with the plastic surgery, rotational or free flaps are occasionally required to achieve healing and return of function. Fitting and wearing shoes are easier when the foot remains intact. Obviously careful follow-up and protection are crucial.

XIII. THE CHALLENGE

Peripheral vascular disease is a known complication of diabetes. Lower extremity ulcers, especially those leading to amputation, represent a major concern for patients with diabetes and health care professionals who treat them, from both a quality of life and an economic standpoint. An aggressive approach to limb salvage is no more costly and carries no greater risk than the alternative of major amputation, which is the diabetics greatest fear. Although life expectancy for the diabetic with limb-threatening ischemia is reduced, other factors, such as quality of life and the ability to live and function independently, are important considerations. In this chapter I have reviewed peripheral vascular disease as it affects the diabetic patient and our team approach that has documented cost-effective, value-added care. It remains my belief that quality of care is the best way to reduce the cost of care.

BIBLIOGRAPHY

Caputo GM, Cavanaugh PR, Ulbrecht JS, Gibbons GW, Karchmer AW. Assessment and management of foot disease in patients with diabetes. N Engl J Med 1994; 33: 854–360.

Gibbons GW. Vascular evaluation and long-term results of distal bypass surgery in patients with diabetes. Clin Pod Med Surg 1995; 12:129–40.

Gibbons GW, Marcaccio E Jr, Freeman DV, Campbell DR, Miller A, LoGerfo FW. Improved quality of diabetic foot care 1984 vs 1990: reduced length of stay and costs, insufficient reimbursement. Arch Surg 1993; 128:576 581.

Gibbons GW, Burgess AM, Guadagnoli E, et al. Return to well-being and function after infrainguinal revascularization. J Vasc Surg 1995; 21:35–45.

Gibbons GW, Habershaw GM. The septic diabetic foot ''foot sparing surgery.'' In: Ernst CB, ed. Advances in Vascular Surgery. Chicago, IL: Mosby-Year Book, 1995; 211–226.

LoGerfo FW, Coffman JD. Vascular and microvascular disease of the foot in diabetes: implications for foot care. N Engl J Med 1984; 311:1615–1619.

Pecoraro RE, Reiber GE, Burgess EM. Pathways to diabetic limb amputation: basis for prevention. Diabetes Care 1990; 13:513–521.

Pomposelli FB, Jepson SJ, Gibbons GW, et al. A flexible approach to infrapopliteal vein grafts in patients with diabetes mellitus. Arch Surg 1991; 126:724–729.

28
Management of the Diabetic Foot

Geoffrey M. Habershaw
Beth Israel Deaconess Medical Center, Boston, Massachusetts

I. INTRODUCTION

Before World War II, the first foot operation experienced by the unfortunate diabetic patient was an above-the-knee amputation. Dr. Eliott Joslin began to realize that most of what he saw happening to the lower extremities of his diabetic patients was preventable. He uttered one of his more memorable statements by indicating that he believed that "Diabetic gangrene was not heaven-sent, but earth borne." As a response to this, he hired Dr. John Kelly in 1928, a podiatrist, to man the first "foot room", in the New England Deaconess Hospital. Dr. Kelly became the first podiatrist in the United States to be on the staff of a university-affiliated hospital. Dr. Joslin also teamed with Dr. Leland McKitterick, a distinguished general surgeon from the Massachusetts General Hospital, to help him with his diabetic patients. Dr. McKitterick was the first surgeon to employ the use of a "foot-sparing" amputation on patients with diabetes. This was the transmetatarsal amputation (TMA; Fig. 1), and it can be considered to be the first diabetic foot operation, reported by Dr. McKitterick in 1949. This procedure removed all the toes and the forefoot, but left enough of a weight-bearing surface that the patient could still use it to walk. Patients would sometimes spend as much as 8 weeks in bed, waiting for the foot to heal enough to be able to move about. The TMA saved thousands of feet that would otherwise have been lost, and remains a durable procedure to this day.

The TMA was the mainstay of diabetic foot salvage when Dr. Frank Wheelock joined the surgical staff in the early 1950s. He applied vascular surgical technique to the diabetic foot. This added further to the number of extremities that could be saved, and remained the mainstay of diabetic foot salvage throughout the 1950s, 1960s, and 1970s.

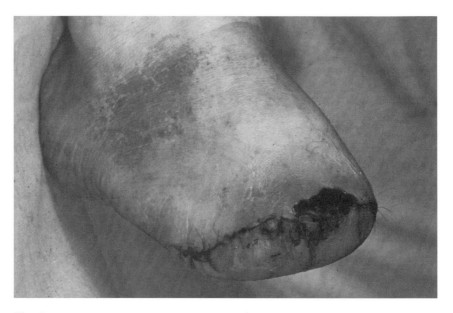

Fig. 1 Transmetatarsal amputation: Photograph taken February 12, 1947. This was one of the original patients with diabetes who had the "first diabetic foot operation." The surgeons would wait for the eschar to heal or not. Healing meant a walking foot could be maintained. Nonhealing meant below-knee amputation.

Dr. Frank LoGerfo joined the vascular surgical staff in the 1980s as Chief of Vascular Surgery, and had been performing infrapopleteal bypass since the mid-1970s with good success. This procedure remains as the diabetic foot operation to the present. The application of the femoral to the dorsalis pedis bypass graft, along with enhanced-imaging technique, better and safer antibiotics, better diabetic heart disease and kidney management, foot-sparing surgical techniques, and education, have lessened the primary amputation at the Beth Israel Deaconess Medical Center to 5%. This is down from 33% in the early 1970s.

Sixty to seventy percent of diabetic foot ulceration takes place because of neuropathy and 30–40% because of ischemia in combination with neuropathy. Most of these problems are preventable with an understanding of how neuropathy, ischemia, and mechanics interrelate to allow soft-tissue breakdown.

A. Diabetic Neuropathy

Peripheral neuropathy of diabetes will have three major effects on the lower extremity: sensory, motor, and autonomic. The major function of the sensory nerves on the lower extremity is to act as an alarm system for perception of injury. Immediate perception of injury is vital to healing. Injury caused by disruption of the skin is made worse with each successive step when pain perception is absent.

Pain or hyperesthesia, may be the first symptom of peripheral neuropathy. Painful peripheral neuropathy may even persist for years as the main manifestation. We do not see foot ulcers develop during this time owing to restricted activity and the development of habits by the patient that make the feet and legs more comfortable. Along with restricted activity, they will rotate shoes and socks several times a day. This will allow greater comfort because of lessened friction and changed pressure points. When painful neuropathy subsides, hypoesthesia or lessened sensation may begin, causing lessened sensory input from the lower extremities. This is when injury may occur without perception of pain. There is a "lack of limp" with injury.

Somatosensory dysfunction at the level of the joints and tendons will affect the ability to perceive where the foot is in space and time. This dysfunction of the Golgi tendon bodies and Pascinian corpuscles may lead to awkward, unsteady gait and additive microtrauma causing neuropathic injury such as Charcot fracture.

Motor nerve dysfunction will cause foot deformity and weakness. The intrinsic musculature of the hand allows fine motor control of the fingers to permit writing, buttoning, turning a key, and such. The intrinsic musculature of the foot helps hold the toes on the ground during the powerful contraction of the muscles in the legs. With intrinsic muscular dysfunction, the toes will contract causing hammertoes (Fig. 2). This will cause pressure points to develop on the tips and tops of the toes. There will also be greater pressure beneath the metatarsal heads at the ball of the foot. The relative cavus attitude of the foot will also cause greater pressure below the heel. This is the foot "at risk" with peripheral neuropathy of diabetes and should be identified early and protected by appropriate care and shoeing.

Proximal muscular weakness develops slowly in peripheral neuropathy of diabetes. The anterior leg will develop slow weakness and may first be noticed by the patient when tripping becomes more frequent, especially when fatigued. This can progress, in time, to a full-blown footdrop, without spasticity, as seen with central motor neuron deficit. It then becomes necessary to use bracing for the safe ambulation of the patient (Fig. 3).

Autonomic neuropathy will allow drying of the skin owing to sweat gland dysfunction which may lead to cracking. Thickening of the nails may occur, making it difficult for them to be cared for without professional help. Arteriovenous shunting and peripheral vasodilation may occur causing faulty temperature regulation and swelling of the extremities.

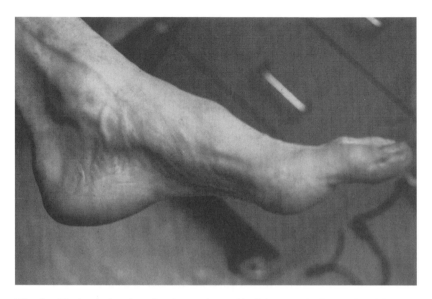

Fig. 2 The intrinsic minus foot in a patient with diabetes and advanced peripheral neuropathy: Pressure points are accentuated at the ball of the foot, heel, and hammertoes. It needs protection from friction with appropriate shoeing and orthotics.

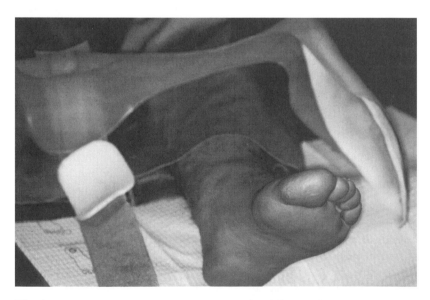

Fig. 3 Drop-foot brace in a patient with paresis of the anterior musculature of the leg. Uncontrolled foot drop will cause a high probability of falls and injury. Notice the soft foot pad in the brace to help prevent friction and blistering.

B. Soft Tissue Biomechanics

During walking the skin on the plantar surface of the foot remains fixed to the weight-bearing surface, while the musculoskeletal elements inside the foot move over it. The forces produced are from the combination of body weight (vertical force) and the motion of the bones (shear force) within the foot. Pronation and supination of the foot will permit a rotation of the metatarsal heads, causing shear of the skin. The skin may respond to these forces by thickening and causing callus formation (Fig. 4). The forces will be greater with greater deformity, such as bunions or hammertoes. The combination of structural deformity, excess dynamic forces, and neuropathy of diabetes is the most common cause of neuropathic ulceration.

Active disruption of the skin occurs with high stress, 700–1000 lb/in.^{2}. This might occur by stepping on a nail or piece of broken glass. It is not the most common cause of ulcers. Low stress, 2–3 lb/in.^{2} may disrupt the skin in a bedridden patient by decubitus ulcer formation, and will be more common in the neuropathic patient. It will not, however, cause plantar foot ulcers in the walking

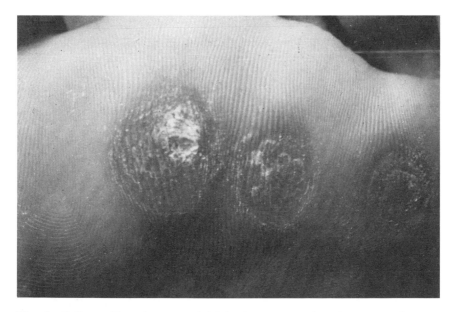

Fig. 4 Calluses: These become painful in the sensate patient. Insensate patients may not feel the pain, will not compensate their gait, and may blister below the callus. This may then become infected and develop into ulceration. Shoeing, orthotics, and regular care by the podiatrist will help avoid these complications.

neuropathic patient. Foot ulcers are caused by repetitive moderate stress, 40–60 lb/in.^{2}. These are the forces transmitted to the skin by the normal motion of the bones. The resultant callus formation fails to be painful, the patient does not limp, and ulcer formation may result.

C. How Ulcers Heal

An understanding of how ulcers develop is important to attempt their prevention, but once they occur, the earlier an aggressive treatment approach is begun, the more likely and sooner they will heal.

There are four essential elements that need to be addressed so that ulcers will heal:

1. There must be adequate arterial flow to the foot, preferably palpable pedal pulses. Wounds may still heal without pulsitile flow to the foot, but it will be delayed.
2. There must be absence of infection, infection is not to be confused with colonization of wounds. All superficial wounds are colonized by bacteria, but not all wounds are infected. Wounds that probe deeply into the foot—for example, to bone or deep spaces—should be considered infected even if there are no signs and symptoms. Because of immunosuppression, patients with diabetes may not mount an appropriate response to infection.
3. There must be adequate medical management of the patient. Cardiac disease, including coronary artery disease and congestive heart failure, will cause inadequate perfusion of the tissues, lessening blood flow needed to deliver infection-fighting cells, nutrients, and antibiotics. Consistently high blood sugar levels will delay healing by a blunted inflammatory response that stops production of collagen needed to close the wounds. Chronic renal failure will delay healing by persistent high concentrations of metabolic byproducts and fluid balance disturbances. Proper nutrition is also imperative for wound healing.
4. There must be pressure relief from the ulcerated site. Repetitive mechanical irritation of a wound will always lead to failure of healing.

D. Evaluation of Ulcers

When confronted with a foot ulcer, a decision must be made to treat the patient as an outpatient or as an inpatient. Mild ulcerations that are superficial can usually be managed as an outpatient. Deep ulcerations that probe into subcutaneous struc-

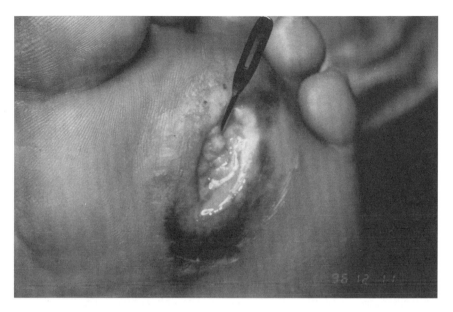

Fig. 5 Severe ulceration: This is a 6-in sterile, stainless steel probe that has fallen (not pushed) into a neuropathic ulcer. A wound that probes this deeply will need to be opened in the operating room, and cleared of all necrotic tissue and infection before delayed primary closure. Failure to be aggressive early will lead to abscess and possible limb loss.

tures are usually treated as inpatients along with incision and drainage type surgery (Fig. 5). Tables 1 and 2 highlight other factors.

II. OUTPATIENT MANAGEMENT OF ULCERATION

When it has been established that arterial flow is adequate, infection has been controlled, and medical issues are under control, then it is appropriate to turn

Table 1 Mild Ulcers (Outpatient Management)

Superficial	Weekly debridement
No osteomyelitis	Dressing changes q.d. or b.i.d.
Minimal to no cellulitis	Rest of the injured part
Palpable pedal pulses	Oral antibiotics initially
No systemic symptoms	
Reliable patient	
Good support system	

Table 2   Severe Ulcers (Inpatient Management)

Deep tissue involvement	Hospital admission
Osteomyelitis probable	Incision and drainage
Presence of cellulitis	Bed rest
Poor arterial flow	Deep culture and sensitivity
Systemic symptoms	Intravenous antibiotics
	Revascularization

attention to pressure relief of the ulceration. Ulcers should heal if the patient is compliant and all other factors are controlled. When healing does not progress, one must them reevaluate all other factors that could delay it; for example, vascular status, infection, medical condition, pressure-relieving techniques, nutrition, and compliance.

There is no substitute for non–weight-bearing, the most efficient pressure-relieving technique. This requires the use of crutches, walker, or wheelchair. Most of our neuropathic patients will use these devices only sporadically; therefore, it is necessary to have a substitute technique for pressure relief when the ulcerated foot touches the floor.

A.   The Felted Foam Dressing

The felted foam dressing is an accommodative pad designed to relieve 60–80% of vertical forces from the ulcerated site on the plantar surface of the foot when it hits the ground. The materials necessary to place this pad are as follows:

> Rubber cement
> 2-in. Fabco gauze
> Felted foam, 1/4 in.
> 2 × 2 gauze pad (sterile)

1. The pad is cut out to accommodate the ulcerated site (Fig. 6).
2. Rubber cement is painted on the felt surface of the pad and on the skin, both plantar and dorsal, not the ulcer itself (Fig. 7).
3. The pad is bonded to the skin and wrapped with Fabco in a recurrent fashion, so as not to circlage the forefoot and cut off circulation (Fig. 8).
4. A window is cut in the pad and a topical agent of choice may be used on the ulcer and covered with a 2 × 2 pad (Fig. 9).

The felted foam dressing is left on the foot for 1 week. It is kept dry during this time. A postoperative shoe (Fig. 10) may be used for additional protection

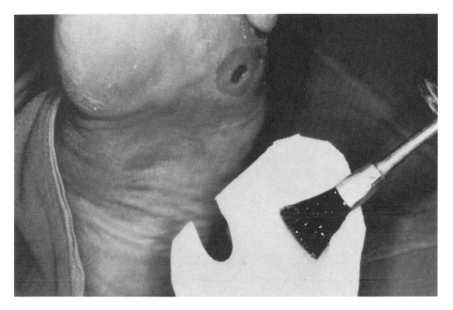

Fig. 6 The felted foam pad is cut out to accommodate the ulcer. The pad will extend into the arch, but not cover the heel. Rubber cement is placed on the felt side of the pad.

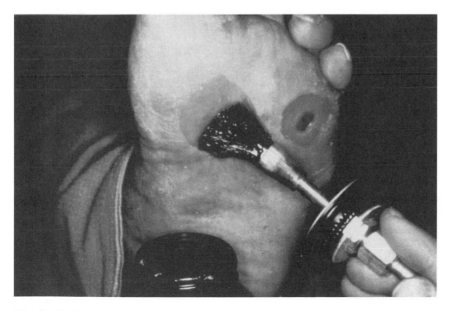

Fig. 7 Rubber cement is also placed on the foot, but not on the ulcer.

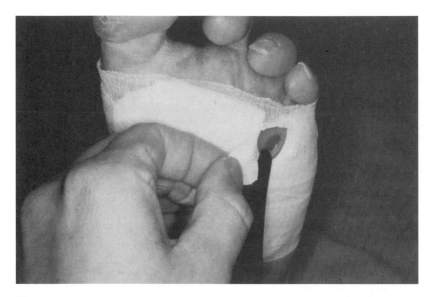

Fig. 8 The pad is placed on the skin where the rubber cement will bond it in place. The pad is then wrapped with Fabco and a window is cut in the pad so that a topical agent of choice can be placed on the ulcer.

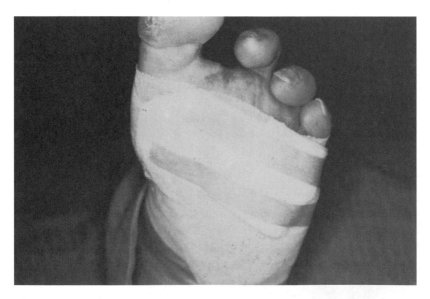

Fig. 9 The window is then covered with a 2 × 2 gauze pad. The patient is encouraged to stay off the foot as much as possible. The pad is kept dry. It should be replaced in 1–14 days.

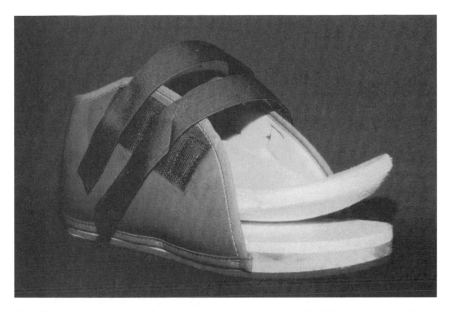

Fig. 10   Healing sandal: A postoperative shoe with a molded Plastazote insole is used by the patient with a felted foam dressing. A conventional shoe would be too tight with the pad in place.

when the foot hits the floor (Fig. 11). The 2 × 2 pad is changed once or twice a day. A sock is worn over the pad at all times except when the 2 × 2 is being changed. When the pad is removed in the office the following week, most of the rubber cement comes off with the pad. It should be removed slowly to prevent an unlikely skin tear. The foot can then be washed and a new pad applied. The ulcer should be measured or traced at each visit to document healing. The pad can continue to be used as long as healing is progressing. No ulcer should take more than 12 weeks to heal.

Total-contact casts are also an effective method for pressure relief. When appropriately applied, ulcers can be expected to heal without incident. It is a labor-intensive technique and should be applied only by the experienced professional (Fig. 12).

B.   Ulcer Debridement

Along with weekly ulcer debridement, the overall condition of the patient should be accessed during inspection. Questions such ''How are you feeling? Is the

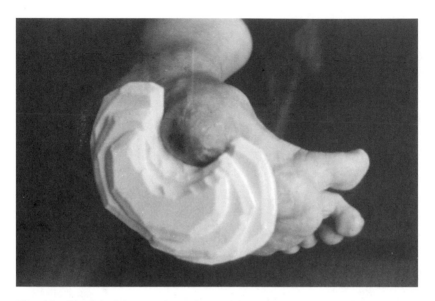

Fig. 11 The felted foam pad may be used for ulcers in any part of the foot. Here it is being used on an ulcer along the medial column of a Charcot foot. Notice how the felted foam may be layered to relieve additional pressure.

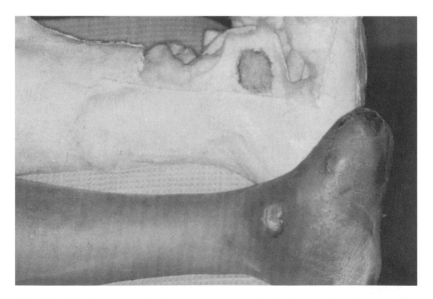

Fig. 12 This is a misapplied total contact cast. Notice the cast abrasion over the medial malleolus. Appropriately applied total contact casts can be very effective, but one must be careful in patients who have fluid balance problems that manifest in the lower extremity.

diabetes under control? Has there been fever or chills? Are you staying off your foot?'' are appropriate to ask. The ulcer should be examined to check for depth with a probe and signs of infection. Foot pulses should be checked at each visit. All excess tissue should be removed around the circumference of the ulcer, except vascularized dermis. A macerated rim around the ulcer means that the patient is not staying off the foot. A curved jaw tissue nipper, along with a sharp scalpel will work most efficiently for ulcer debridement (Fig. 13).

III. INPATIENT MANAGEMENT OF ULCERS

Such patients have been admitted because they will likely be brought to the operating room. An acutely ill patient with an abcess in the foot should be taken to the operating room as soon as possible to drain all sepsis. Dependent drainage should be achieved so that all fluids will run out of the foot with the patient at bed rest (Fig. 14). Synthetic drains (Penrose, Nu gauze, ingress–egress) should not be used. Long incisions that will promote drainage are best. All necrotic tissue should be removed, including infected bone. Deep specimens for cultures should be taken, preferably before the patient receives the first dose of intravenous antibiotics. These culture studies should include aerobic, anaerobic, and cultures for fungi and acid fast bacilli. The wounds are packed open with saline-soaked gauze. Circulatory status is monitored and absence of pedal pulses should prompt at least noninvasive vascular studies or arteriogram if vascular status is critical.

The wound is continually debrided on a daily basis on daily rounds. When necrosis becomes extensive, one should never hesitate to bring the patient back to the operating room for further extensive debridement.

Closure of the wound is dependent on eliminating all necrotic tissue, osteomyelitis and pathogens. The techniques of closure are the following:

1. Primary
2. Delayed primary
3. Secondary
4. Split-thickness skin graft
5. Local rotational Flap
6. Free flap

Primary closure of a wound can be performed when acute infection is not present, the patient is metabolically stable, and there is no abcess or deep necrotic tissue encountered at the time of surgery. The deep involved tissue is all removed, the wound is power irrigated, and closed with full-thickness sutures. No deep absorbable sutures are used.

Delayed primary closure is performed when there is necrotic tissue or abcess, and the wound is packed open at the time of surgery. The wound is debrided

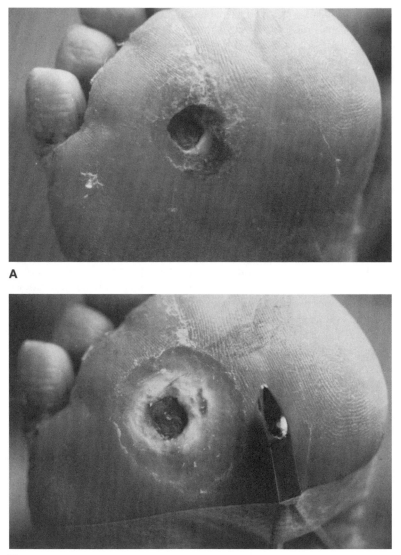

Fig. 13 (A) Mild neuropathic ulcer—predebridement: There is a thick layer of callus surrounding the ulceration. Debridement of this tissue will stimulate growth factors and enhance granulation tissue formation. (B) Mild neuropathic ulceration—postdebridement: The callus has been removed with a 4-in curved jaw tissue nipper. The ulcer does not probe deeply, which indicates it can be treated as an outpatient. The healthy granulation tissue indicates adequate circulation. The white, macerated rim around the ulcer will disappear when the pressure is off the foot.

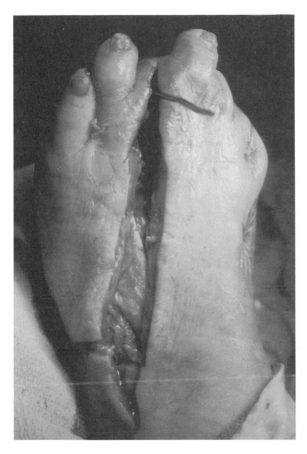

Fig. 14 Dependent drainage of infection: A plantar ulcer eroded through the foot to the dorsum, and an abscess developed along the extensor tendon sheath. Aggressive dependent incision and drainage will ensure drainage of infectious material into the dressings. This will also facilitate daily debridements.

daily, and when two successive cultures, 3 days apart are negative for pathogens, the wound is closed. This also is done with full-thickness sutures.

Closure by secondary intention is performed by allowing the wound to completely epithelialize on its own. It is usually not a large area and is not directly below a plantar pressure point, for example, below a metatarsal head.

A split-thickness skin graft is used when there is a large area to be closed and it would be unreasonable to allow it to heal by secondary intention. This will

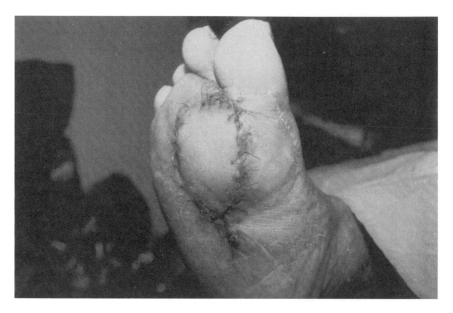

Fig. 15 Local rotational flap: This full-thickness flap with blood supply intact was advanced from proximal to distal, to cover a noninfected ulcerated site. It is imperative to maintain 6 weeks of non–weight-bearing after this, and to follow-up with appropriate shoes and orthotics.

usually be in areas where large portions of necrotic skin had to be removed in the process of draining infection.

Local rotational flaps are full-thickness pedicle flaps that maintain their own blood supply (Fig. 15). They are used mostly on the plantar surface of the midfoot to help close ulcers after removal of bony prominences, especially in the Charcot foot. It is usually necessary to place a split-thickness skin graft at the donor site.

The free flap is a full-thickness graft transplanted from another part of the body, with its arterial and venous supply brought with it. It is commonly used to close large defects where more resilient tissue is needed, such as the heel. It requires microvascular skills and is usually performed by plastic surgery.

Plantar wounds that have been primarily closed require at least 4 weeks of non–weight-bearing. Skin grafts and flaps should not be walked on for 8–10 weeks. Failure to comply with this may undo the surgery and require further hospitalization and additional surgery.

IV. THE CHARCOT FOOT

Charcot neuropathic arthropathy occurs in about 1:700 patients with diabetes mellitus. It will not develop without the presence of peripheral neuropathy, and it is not exclusive to the patient with diabetes mellitus. It can occur in any disease that damages the peripheral nerves or posterior column of the central nervous system. Diabetes is certainly the most common cause, with alcoholic-induced neuropathy second, and hereditary insensitivity to pain third. Other causes may be syringomyelia and tabes dorsalis.

A. Etiology of Charcot

Vascular dysfunction and somatosensory nerve dysfunction have been implicated in the development of the Charcot foot. Some investigators have also implicated the excessive nonenzymatic glycosylation of bone collagen. It is believed by us that there is a combination of these factors that allow it to occur.

B. Pathogenesis

The patient may remember an injury in about 40% of cases, but usually will just notice unilateral unexplained swelling of one foot that may or may not be painful. The swelling may be down by the morning, but will come back again during the day early in the course of the process. Later on the swelling will always be present and, indeed, may begin to become painful.

C. Physical Findings

The foot is warm and swollen, but will usually not show deformity in the early stages. When there is deformity, crepitus may be felt at the level of the midfoot. This is pathognomonic for active fracture. When deformity occurs, it is usually in the midfoot (Lisfranc's joint) at the tarsometatarsal junction; 60% of cases will occur at this level. The remaining 40% will occur at the metatarsophalangeal joints, talonavicular joint level, talocalcaneal joints, and the ankle joint. The more proximal the fracture (i.e., the closer to the ankle joint) the more severe the fracture in terms of treatment and rehabilitation.

D. Diagnosis of Charcot

A high index of suspicion is a must for the effective diagnosis of Charcot fracture. A unilaterally swollen foot in a neuropathic patient without foot ulceration should be considered to be Charcot fracture until proved otherwise. Infection and deep venous thrombosis need to be ruled out. Plain x-ray films will many times be negative early because Charcot fracture will begin as ligmentous injury with no overt evidence of bone disruption. Bone scintigraphy will be useful at this time owing to its sensitivity to accelerated bone metabolism. It is not necessary to obtain bone scans if fracture is seen on plain films. Unilateral Charcot is the most common presentation, but disease can be present. When it is diagnosed unilaterally, the contralateral foot will develop the fracture 30–40% of the time within a year.

E. Treatment

The mainstay of treatment continues to be non–weight-bearing. There is no better substitute for crutches, walker, or wheelchair. Casting may be done, but it should be a non–weight-bearing cast. Removable, bivalve casts will permit daily inspection of the skin and may work as well as closed casting, as long as weight-bearing is restricted. Patients who cannot be non–weight-bearing may be placed in ''off-the-shelf'' walking casts, which will give some protection and allow healing at a slower rate. Non–weight-bearing should be 3 months. This may be adjusted up or down depending on the clinical situation.

Signs of healing will be temperature reduction, resolution of swelling, and absence of crepitus on clinical examination. Serial x-ray films taken each month should show fracture healing with evidence of sclerotic bone changes. Active fracture will give way to coalescence as non–weight-bearing is continued. Crepitus must be gone before weight-bearing begins. Swelling and temperature increase may persist owing to the inevitable degenerative arthritis that will now develop. It may take a full year for all of the swelling to diminish.

Resolution of weight-bearing should be gradual and partial. Osteopenia will be an inevitable side effect of adjacent bony structures. Partial, gradual weight-bearing over 4–6 weeks is necessary to help avoid further injury (Fig. 16).

V. SHOEING THE NEUROPATHIC FOOT

The shoe that will not allow ulceration to develop in the neuropathic patient does not exist. Only restoration of protective sensation to the extremities would do that. Because there is no perfect shoe, they must be selected according to their ability to be ''least likely'' to cause soft-tissue breakdown. This requires cushioning, support, and enough room for digital and metatarsal deformity. This ''fallibility'' of shoes is overcome by insisting that our neuropathic patients rotate their shoes and socks every 3–4 h, and this is why:

1. It gives an insensate patient a brief moment to inspect the foot for undetected injury that may have occurred over the past few hours.

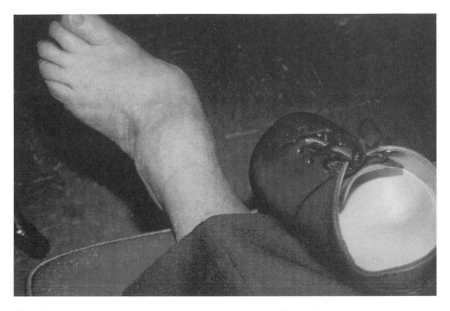

Fig. 16 Charcot foot with molded shoe: This foot will not fit into a store-bought shoe. Molded shoes are necessary with this degree of deformity. A molded Plastazote orthotic is necessary to provide total contact for the foot.

2. Pressure points are changed by rotating to another pair of shoes.
3. All shoes begin to lose cushioning and support after about 3 or 4 h of use, which allows friction to increase.

Rotating shoes and socks during the day is the single most powerful weapon the neuropathic patient has in preventing the development of new ulceration.

A. Over-the-Counter Shoes

The modern-day athletic–walking shoe qualifies as an effective shoe for the neuropathic patient (Fig. 17). It has a rounded toe box, soft upper, cushioned collar, cushioned midsole, laces to toe that allow for swelling, and a removable insole that can be replaced with an orthotic if necessary.

Shoes with extra depth and rounded in the toe box are especially useful for patients with digital deformity. Orthotics will also fit nicely because of the extra room (Fig. 18).

Molded shoes should be used when there is sufficient deformity that conventional shoes cannot be worn. They should be made with deep, rounded toe

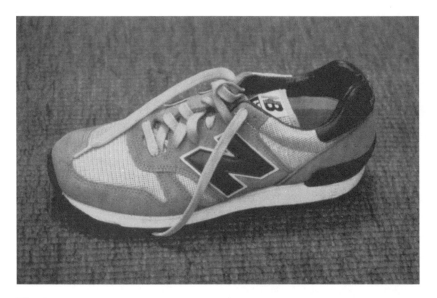

Fig. 17 Running and walking shoes provide cushioning and support for the neuropathic foot. It is still necessary to advise the neuropathic patients to rotate their shoes and socks every 3–4 hours.

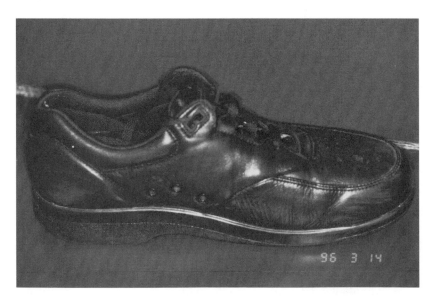

Fig. 18 The extra-depth shoe has a rounded deep toe box that will allow accommodation of hammertoes and prominent metatarsal heads. There is also enough room for a molded, soft orthotic.

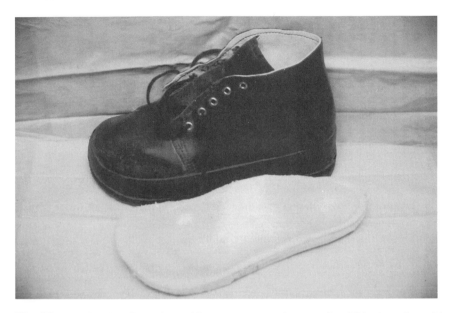

Fig. 19 Molded shoe for patient with a transmetatarsal amputation. This short shoe with molded orthotic will help prevent excessive pressure at the distal end of the foot.

boxes and a wide heel. They should be laced to the toe and have 1/2-in.–removable, full-length soft orthotics.

Patients with partial foot amputations may need special accommodation. Patients with transmetatarsal amputation need a shoe that will grip the ankle so it will not fall off during walking (Fig. 19). The patient with Charcot fracture may also need "chukka" shoe height to accommodate soft, thick orthotics and adapt to an altered gait because of the fracture.

A patient will often inquire about wearing dress shoes. They may be worn for short periods with very limited walking, as long as there has been no recent history of ulceration. I let my patients know that I consider them to be "sitting shoes."

B. Orthotics

Orthotics function to limit musculoskeletal motion and also to cushion vertical forces. The neuropathic foot does better with soft orthotics, rather than rigid ones. Heat-molded Plastazote in various densities is easily adapted to athletic, extra depth, and molded shoes. The orthotics may be covered with Spenco or PPT to help minimize shear.

Both shoes and orthotics should be kept in good repair. Worn out shoes and orthotics will cause increasing friction, leading to skin breakdown.

VI. ADVICE FOR PATIENTS: DOs AND DON'Ts

Patients should not

> Go barefoot at any time, even inside the house
> Wear tight or worn out shoes
> Use any sharp instruments on the feet to trim calluses
> Wear medicated corn pads
> Use any form of external heat, including heating pads and hot water bottles
> Soak feet in hot water
> Smoke or be near people who are smoking

Patients should

> Wash the feet and dry them well and use a mild soap
> Wear padded socks to help absorb friction
> Wear shoes that fit and ones that do not have to be broken in
> Change their shoes and socks twice a day
> Check their feet for any breaks in the skin and report it to their physician
> Keep their blood sugar level in good control
> Make sure to remind their primary doctor to check their feet at each visit
> Have primary doctor refer them to podiatrist if self-care becomes very difficult

29
Diabetic Neuropathy

Peter D. Donofrio
Wake Forest University School of Medicine, Winston-Salem, North Carolina

I. EPIDEMIOLOGY

It is estimated that 16 million people in the United States have diabetes. The frequency of neuropathy in this group depends on the method used to define neuropathy (i.e., symptoms, clinical signs, electrophysiology, nerve pathology, or a combination). Pirart reported from his large study of 4400 patients that the prevalence of polyneuropathy was 8% in diabetics at the time of diagnosis (1). This percentage rose to approximately 40% after 20 years and 50% at 25 years (1). Pirart defined *neuropathy* for his study as the loss of Achilles or knee reflexes or both and diminished vibration perception. Neuropathy occurs in the same frequency in type I and II diabetes. Little objective data are known about the effect of neuropathy on morbidity and mortality. Yet, anyone with experience caring for patients with diabetic neuropathy can attest to the severe morbidity that arises from their deficits of weakness, pain, paresthesias, imbalance, and autonomic dysfunction.

II. CLASSIFICATION OF DIABETIC NEUROPATHY

Because the neuropathy associated with diabetes can have many presentations, several classifications have been proposed. Some have been based on the major clinical presentation (e.g., paralytic, ataxia, neuralgia), whereas others have addressed the symmetry or asymmetry of the process, or have divided neuropathies into those that are symmetrical, focal, or multifocal. Given that no classification system is acceptable to everyone, the division of neuropathy developed by Dyck

Table 1 Classification of Diabetic Neuropathy

I.	Symmetrical distal polyneuropathy
II.	Symmetrical proximal neuropathy
III.	Asymmetrical proximal neuropathy
	A. Cranial
	B. Trunk radiculopathy or mononeuropathy
	C. Limb plexus or mononeuropathy
	D. Multiple mononeuropathy
	E. Entrapment neuropathy
	F. Ischemic nerve injury from acute arterial occlusion
IV.	Asymmetrical neuropathy and symmetrical distal polyneuropathy

Source: Ref. 2.

and colleagues best encompasses grouping by symmetry, anatomy, and distribution of symptoms and signs (Table 1) (2).

Symmetrical distal polyneuropathy is the most common presentation of diabetic neuropathy (3). It typically involves sensory more than motor fibers and manifests as numbness, paresthesia, and pain in the feet and lower legs. The symmetrical proximal neuropathies are rare and typically occur in association with a symmetrical distal polyneuropathy. The asymmetrical neuropathies are clustered together in Dyck's classification only for convenience. Several are acute or subacute in presentation and may share a common vascular pathogenesis. The fourth category is the detection of any of the first three neuropathic presentations in a patient with an underlying symmetrical distal polyneuropathy.

A. Symmetrical Distal Polyneuropathy

Epidemiological studies have shown a symmetrical distal polyneuropathy to be the most common neuropathy observed in diabetes (3). Its frequency increases with age, quadrupling in prevalence during the first 20 years of diabetes. Risk factors for developing symmetrical distal neuropathy include: duration of diabetes, increasing body weight, age, retinopathy, overt albuminuria, height, duration of hypertension, insulin use, and race or ethnicity (4).

Symptoms typically begin in the toes and soles of the feet. Common complaints include numbness, tingling, burning, achiness, pins-and-needles sensations (paresthesias), twisting, heaviness, and sharp, shooting pains. Patients may complain of a deadness in their feet or liken their feet to be immersed within blocks of ice. On examination, patients often have abnormalities that reflect large nerve fiber loss (vibration, position sense, and light-touch impairment) and small fiber involvement (pinprick and cold perception loss). Dysesthesias may be produced by light touch or pinprick applied to the affected limb. Ankle muscle stretch reflexes are commonly reduced or diminished. Foot ulcers, usually located on the plantar aspect of the toes or metatarsal heads, may arise in patients with insensate feet. Infrequently observed is a neuropathic arthropathy (Charcot joint) of the interphalangeal or metatarsophalangeal joints associated with sensory loss and recurrent trauma. Motor nerve loss is less common and severe and may not follow sensory involvement for months to years. Typically, the first motor functions lost are toe extension and flexion, later followed by weakness of ankle dorsiflexion and eversion. In most patients, diabetic symmetrical distal polyneuropathy obeys the length-dependent principle of distal greater than proximal. The process begins distally and as the disease advances progresses to proximal sites. Typically, when diabetic polyneuropathy advances to the level of the knee, patients begin to experience similar symptoms in the finger tips. Further worsening of the disease results in spread of the symptoms to areas above the knees and wrists. In severe disease, this length-dependent process may also affect the sensory and motor fibers innervating the chest and abdomen. Distal nerve loss in this area results in sensory abnormalities that resemble a shield as nerve fibers die back toward cell bodies in the dorsal root ganglion. Unless this sensory loss is interpreted within the framework of a diabetic polyneuropathy, the neurological findings may be misconstrued as reflecting a myelopathy, leading to an erroneous diagnosis and unnecessary testing. Weakness of abdominal muscles produces laxity of the abdominal wall, outpouching of the abdomen, and weakness in sitting up from the supine position.

In rare instances, a symmetrical distal polyneuropathy may present suddenly in a diabetic whose glucose control is poor but not out of control. Often this is associated with weight loss, anorexia, severe neuropathic pain, and tactile hyperesthesia (diabetic cachexia). Neuropathy may also suddenly develop after institution of insulin therapy, a condition sometimes referred to as ''insulin neuritis.''

Autonomic symptoms and signs commonly accompany sensory loss and can affect any organ that receives innervation from autonomic fibers. The reported prevalence of autonomic dysfunction varies widely in the literature, with some authors describing percentages as high as 80%. Cohen and colleagues reported a prevalence of autonomic neuropathy of 44.9% in their subjects in the ABCD Trial (4). Patients with dysfunction of thermoregulation describe excessive coldness or warmth in their feet. On clinical examination, the clinician may note hair loss, atrophic skin changes, anhydrosis or hyperhidrosis, and a red or white discoloration of the toes and feet. Dependent ankle and foot edema may be observed, a condition resulting from abnormal arteriovenous shunting and venous pooling of blood.

Cardiovascular autonomic dysfunction may be of two types: the commonly observed postural hypotension and the relatively asymptomatic resting tachycardia and fixed heart rate. Symptoms reported by patients with orthostatic hypotension include syncope, postural weakness, faintness, dizziness, vertigo, visual blurring, and syncope. Not infrequently, orthostasis becomes symptomatic or is unmasked when the patient is treated with a new medication, such as a diuretic, tricyclic antidepressant, or vasodilator. Symptoms may arise when the patient becomes dehydrated or unexpectantly develops congestive heart failure. Orthostatis is explained by the failure of reflex tachycardia and vasoconstriction to maintain cardiac output and arterial pressure when the patient assumes the upright position, and uncompensated venous pooling occurs in the legs.

Gastrointestinal function from the esophagus to the anus may be affected by diabetic autonomic neuropathy. In the esophagus, radiologic and manometry studies have shown abnormalities of primary peristalsis, tertiary contractions, and delayed transit. Fortunately, the clinical correlation with these abnormalities is poor and most patients are asymptomatic. Diabetic gastroparesis is one of the most recognized autonomic dysfunctions affecting the gut. This term refers to delaying gastric emptying, which may be asymptomatic or may manifest as anorexia or as abdominal fullness during or for prolonged periods after meals. Gastroparesis has been attributed to vagal nerve denervation of the gastric muscular wall. Diarrhea in a diabetic patient, particularly at night, may signify autonomic impairment of the small intestine and the prolonged intestinal transit and small intestinal bacterial overgrowth that produces these symptoms. Constipation is probably the most common gastrointestinal autonomic complaint of a diabetic with neuropathy. Not unexpectedly, autonomic dysfunction of the large colon produces atony and lost of the gastrocolic reflect after feeding.

Bladder abnormalities are common in men and woman with advanced diabetic neuropathy. Most commonly seen is the hypotonic, insensitive, distended bladder prone to overflow incontinence and urinary tract infections. Impotence is another frequent presentation of autonomic dysfunction in diabetes. A commonly quoted estimation of impotence is 75% of all diabetic men who are older than 50 years (5). Impotence is usually attributed to a combination of vascular abnormalities and autonomic dysfunction of the parasympathetic and sympathetic nerves. In most instances, impotence progresses from partial to complete over 2 years and remains irreversible. Given the pathogenesis of impotence in diabetes, hormonal therapy is ineffective. Retrograde ejaculation and impotence often coexist in the same patient.

Abnormalities of pupillary constriction to bright light and dilatation to darkness can be recorded in diabetics with autonomic dysfunction. Fortunately, this dysfunction rarely produces clinical complaints. Similarly, autonomic dysfunction of the respiratory system is asymptomatic.

B. Symmetrical Proximal Neuropathy

Symmetrical proximal neuropathy is the least common and poorest understood of the neuropathies discussed in this chapter. Symmetrical proximal neuropathy is typically observed in patients older than 50 years, who complain of poorly localized pain in the lower back and hip region. Usually within several days, they develop symmetrical or asymmetrical weakness of hip flexion, knee extension, and neighboring muscles subserving hip and knee movement. The patient may comment on unexplained weight loss during the period of pain and weakness. Sensory loss in the region of pain and weakness is either absent or unimpressive. Many patients with symmetrical proximal neuropathy have a superimposed distal symmetrical polyneuropathy. In most patients the condition is self-limited and improvement may coincide with the initiation of insulin therapy. Pain typically improves over several months, whereas strength may not return to normal for 1–2 years. The site of pathology in symmetrical proximal neuropathy is not well understood. The pathological process may involve the anterior horn cell, lumbosacral plexus, or multiple mononeuropathies. Symmetrical proximal neuropathy is thought to be slower in progression, less painful, and associated with less weight loss than the asymmetrical form.

C. Asymmetrical Proximal Neuropathy

1. Cranial Mononeuropathies

Four cranial mononeuropathies have been observed more commonly in diabetic patients than the general public. They include neuropathies of the third, fourth, and sixth nerves (diabetic ophthalmoplegia) and the seventh nerve. The most dramatic and impressive is the diabetic third nerve palsy. This condition typically presents suddenly in patients older than the age of 50, often beginning with a frontal headache or severe pain in or behind the eye. Within a few days there is profound ptosis and outward deviation of the ipsilateral eye. In most cases, the examiner finds sparing of the pupil and partial or complete weakness of eye elevation, downward movement, and adduction. Symptoms persist for several weeks, usually followed by complete recovery in 3–5 months. The abrupt presentation of diabetic ophthalmoplegia is frequently misinterpreted as a stroke or an aneurysm of the posterior communicating artery.

Diabetic sixth nerve palsies usually are unilateral and present with diplopia and weakness of eye abduction. Similar to oculomotor palsies, abducens palsies improve over weeks to months and recovery is full. Extremely rare is the trochlear or fourth nerve palsy. In this condition, patients complain of constant diplopia that is improved by tilting the head away from the affected eye (Bielschowsky's sign) and accentuated by tilting in the opposite direction.

Bell's palsy occurs much more commonly in diabetics than in a control population. One study from Japan reported that 77% of patients with Bell's palsy had abnormally high hemoglobin $A_{1C}(HgA_{1C})$ levels (6). Another study found a twofold higher risk for Bell's palsy in patients with diabetes (7). Surprisingly, the results of one study suggested that the prognosis for recovery was better in diabetics with Bell's palsy than in patients without systemic disease.

Truncal or thoracoabdominal neuropathy or radiculopathy is an uncommon condition, with a unique and characteristic presentation. Typically observed in patients older than 50, this condition presents with acute unilateral pain and dysesthesia in a thoracic or abdominal dermatomal pattern. The pain is often severe and has been described by a myriad of terms, ranging from aching and boring, to sharp, tearing, or jabbing. The pain may encompass a complete radicular pattern or may affect only portions of the posterior or anterior rami. The skin over the chest or abdomen may be extremely sensitive and may be irritated by contact with clothing. In over half of patients with thoracoabdominal radiculopathy, there will be loss of appetite and unexplained weight loss of 20–25 lb, raising a suspicion for a paraneoplastic or infiltrating process. Not uncommonly, patients undergo an exhaustive and costly evaluation for cardiac, intrathoracic, intra-abdominal, orthopedic, and psychiatric disorders before an association with diabetes and diabetic neuropathy is considered. This condition is often observed in the first few years of diabetes and in patients with mild disease. Examination discloses hypesthesia to pinprick in a dermatomal pattern and weakness of thoracic or abdominal muscles innervated by the affected root(s). A diagnostic evaluation, usually consisting of plain spine films, spinal magnetic resonance imaging (MRI), and screening blood tests, is usually unremarkable. An electromyogram (EMG) of thoracic, abdominal, and paraspinal muscles will yield denervation in a high percentage of patients. The prognosis is excellent with most patients becoming pain-free by 16–24 months after disease onset.

Proximal motor neuropathy of the lower extremity in diabetic patients has been described under the term of diabetic amyotrophy. It occurs in 0.3–1.0% of diabetics and is more common in type II diabetes (8). Diabetic amyotrophy occurs under circumstances similar to diabetic truncal neuropathy or radiculopathy (i.e., in the setting of weight loss, poor appetite, and over a wide range of diabetic severity, including mild disease (9). The disease presents over days to weeks with severe, deep-aching pain in the back, hip, groin, and anterior thigh area. This is soon followed by weakness and wasting in the iliopsoas, quadriceps, and adductors of the thigh and, less frequently, in the glutei, hamstrings, and gastrocnemius muscles. Usually, the knee reflex is lost or markedly reduced. Although some authors have reported weakness of only the quadriceps muscles, close examination usually discloses weakness in the hip flexors and adductors. Electrodiagnostic testing typically shows denervation in muscles innervated by the lumbar and sometimes the sacral plexus. The paraspinal muscles may also be affected, implying that diabetic amyotrophy in some patients may reflect any underlying polyradiculopathy, rather than a lumbosacral plexopathy. Fortunately, the prognosis for recovery is good with approximately 60% of patients making a substantial improvement within 30 months (10). Usually pain resolves first, later followed by improvement in motor function. Subramony and Wilbourn have reported that more than half of patients with diabetic amyotrophy have an underlying distal symmetrical polyneuropathy (10). A peculiar and unexplained phenomena in diabetic amyotrophy is the finding of a Babinski sign in approximately 50% of patients on the same side as the weakness and in the absence of other upper motor features. Some authors have reported relapses in approximately 20% of cases of diabetic amyotrophy.

It is generally recognized in the neurological literature that patients with an underlying generalized polyneuropathy are more prone to compression and entrapment mononeuropathies. This pattern is also observed in patients with diabetic symmetrical distal neuropathy. The sites of compression are similar to those observed in patients without generalized neuropathy. For carpal tunnel syndrome, the risk is 2.2–2.5 higher in diabetics compared with patients without an underlying neuropathy. Carpal tunnel syndrome was detected in 22% of patients with diabetes by Dyck et al. using nerve conduction studies, yet the prevalence of symptomatic carpal tunnel syndrome was only 11% (3). Ulnar neuropathy is also more common in diabetics, typically affecting the dominant limb.

2. Electrophysiological Testing

In the evaluation of the neuropathies associated with diabetes, electrophysiological testing (nerve conduction testing and electromyography) is the single most helpful tool to confirm the type of neuropathy present, to determine its severity and duration, and to differentiate neuropathies associated with diabetes from those that mimic it. Electrophysiological testing can inform the referring physician whether the distal polyneuropathy is primarily sensory or motor, and whether the major pathophysiological process is axon loss or demyelinating. Electromyography can differentiate between a lumbosacral plexopathy and polyradiculopathy and is the only electrophysiological test that can confirm a thoracoabdominal neuropathy or radiculopathy. In a diabetic with rapidly progressive weakness and sensory loss, nerve conduction studies are useful in distinguishing diabetic polyneuropathy from a superimposed chronic inflammatory demyelinating polyneuropathy (CIDP). This differentiation is critical because therapeutic implication may arise (i.e., CIDP is often responsive to therapies not usually used for diabetic neuropathy such a corticosteroids, plasma exchange, intravenous immunoglobulin, and immunosuppressants). Electrophysiological testing is crucial for substantiating a clinically suspected mononeuropathy, such as carpal tunnel syndrome, ulnar neuropathy at the elbow, or a superimposed polyradiculopathy.

Nerve conduction studies have inherent limitations because only large myelinated motor and sensory fibers are evaluated. Consequently, diabetics with painful feet and hands may have normal nerve conduction studies despite the presence of a significant polyneuropathy that affects small unmyelinated sensory fibers.

Electrophysiological studies are abnormal in up to 20% of diabetics who do not have symptoms of neuropathy. Abnormalities are detected in 75–80% of patients with symptomatic disease, typically showing changes in the amplitude, distal latency, and conduction velocity of sensory and motor nerves. The needle examination may show features of acute and chronic denervation in distal limb muscles. Some authors, using extensive testing of many nerves and electromyography of numerous muscles, have reported detecting abnormalities in essentially every patient with a distal symmetrical polyneuropathy.

In addition to identifying the presence of neuropathy, nerve conduction studies have been used to monitor its progression. Frequently, the serial changes recorded in patients over time have been minimal and unimpressive, some of which could be attributed to recording technique, limb temperature, or chance. Consequently, many recent pharmacological studies of agents used to slow the progression of diabetic neuropathy have added serial quantitative sensory testing of vibration and pain–temperature to their protocols to assess modalities subserved by small fibers.

3. Pathology

Despite extensive research over many years, our understanding of the pathogenesis of diabetic polyneuropathy remains incomplete. Any attempt to explain this disorder must reconcile hyperglycemia and the metabolic abnormalities it induces to the pathological abnormalities that are observed. Also to be explained are the issues of microvascular disease and ischemia. Commonly observed pathological changes in peripheral nerve are wallerian degeneration, focal axonal swellings containing neurofilaments, axonal atrophy, and primary demyelination (11). In a postmortem study of distal polyneuropathy, Dyck and colleagues analyzed root and proximal and distal sections of large nerves from patients with diabetes and contrasted their findings with those from controls (11). They observed fiber loss at the segmental nerve or between the segmental and proximal nerves. The abnormalities were worse distally than proximally. The authors concluded that the spatial distribution of fiber loss was best explained by multifocal ischemic injury. Other authors have expressed a contrary view that the pathological evidence more favors a metabolic derangement with axon loss representing the major pathological feature.

The relatively good prognosis in the asymmetrical diabetic neuropathies has led to a paucity of postmortem material for clues to the underlying pathophysiology. Consequently, little pathological information is available to explain the pathogenesis of diabetic amyotrophy and truncal neuropathy. Only one thorough autopsy study of proximal lower extremity nerves has been performed in diabetic amyotrophy. The authors described microinfarcts in the obturator, femoral, sciatic, and posterior tibial nerves, and extensive fibrotic thickening of small arterioles and capillary walls. In the same report, the authors commented on absence of pathology in the spinal cord and roots. Given this information, the asymmetrical neuropathies have been ascribed to ischemia. Recently, Said and colleagues described their pathological findings in ten patients with proximal diabetic neuropathy (12). They obtained biopsies of the intermediate cutaneous nerve of the thigh and demonstrated ischemic changes in three patients. In two of those three patients, ischemia was associated with vasculitis and inflammatory infiltration. In the remaining seven patients, the pathological features were those of axon loss and demyelination, findings similar to those observed in distal symmetrical polyneuropathy. In a follow-up article, the authors reported four additional patients, several of whom had inflammatory infiltrates in the endoneurium and nerve fibers in various states of demyelination and axon loss (13).

Neuropathological abnormalities in diabetic oculomotor neuropathy consist of focal demyelination without axon loss of the oculomotor nerve in the intracavernous portion. The location of the demyelination is central, thus explaining the pupillary sparing usually observed in this condition. Because the fibers responsible for pupillary function reside peripherally in the nerve, they are not affected by the central demyelination.

4. Laboratory Evaluation

The laboratory evaluation of patients with diabetic polyneuropathy varies depending on the type of neuropathy under investigation. Patients with cranial mononeuropathies will often require an MRI and MRA scan, a lumbar puncture, and serological testing for infectious and inflammatory conditions. Similar testing is necessary for a thorough evaluation of patients with truncal radiculopathy except for the substitution of a spinal MRI (with gadolinium) or a spinal myelogram for a head MRI. In patients with diabetic amyotrophy who are worsening, imaging studies of the pelvis and coagulation studies are needed to eliminate a space-occupying lesion. As mentioned earlier in this chapter, nerve conduction studies and electromyography are recommended for substantiating a mononeuropathy or plexopathy and for excluding any pathology that they resemble. Table 2 lists a

Table 2 Evaluation of Diabetic Symmetrical Distal Polyneuropathy

CBC	Urinalysis
Fasting blood sugar	Metabolic panel
Serum B_{12}	Erythrocyte sedimentation rate
Serum protein electrophoresis	Thyroid function tests
Nerve conduction studies and EMG	

diagnostic workup for patients with a symmetrical distal polyneuropathy thought to be secondary to diabetes.

In clinical situations for which diabetes does not appear to be the most likely etiology for the neuropathy, the following studies may be helpful for establishing the diagnosis: HIV testing, angiotensin-converting enzyme (ACE) level, rheumatological studies. chest x-ray films or computed tomography (CT) scan, 24-h urine collection for heavy metals, and cerebrospinal fluid (CSF) analysis.

5. Therapy of Diabetic Neuropathy

Table 3, a list of therapies for diabetic neuropathy, is arbitrarily divided into those for systemic and those for autonomic neuropathy.

Because hyperglycemia is the cardinal feature of diabetes, good control of glucose levels would intuitively be considered crucial in the treatment of neuropathy and other complications of diabetes. It is considered good medicine to recommend strict glucose control to all patients with diabetes. Nevertheless, until recently, little proof existed that careful euglycemia prevents the development of neuropathy or retards or reverses the condition when present.

For many years clinicians suspected that poor glucose control was deleterious for diabetic neuropathy. Diabetics with prominent hyperglycemia tended to develop more severe neuropathy and at an earlier age. Institution of insulin therapy was reported to improve nerve conduction velocities and vibratory perception thresholds. The improvement was attributed to changes in the metabolic alteration of myelin induced by hyperglycemia. The recent Diabetes Control and Complications Trial (DCCT) showed that intensive therapy (which included three or more injections of insulin each day or use of an insulin pump to achieve tight control of blood glucose) reduced the development of peripheral neuropathy by 64% after 5 years of follow-up (14). The detection of neuropathy was based on a history or physical examination consistent with a clinical neuropathy, verified by abnormalities in nerve conduction or autonomic nerve testing. Nerve conduction or autonomic nervous system testing abnormalities were reduced by 44% in the group receiving intensive care (14). Further verification of the benefit of intensive insulin treatment was found in the stabilization of nerve conduction velocities in this group. In contrast, significant slowing of nerve conduction velocities was observed in the conventional group.

Common sense dictates that restoration of normal pancreatic function should be the ultimate treatment for diabetes and diabetic neuropathy. Recently, Navarro and colleagues reported their results from 115 patients undergoing pancreatic transplantation compared with 92 patients treated with insulin (15). Patients were followed for 10 years. In the transplant group, significant improvement was recorded in the physical examination and composite indices of motor and sensory nerve conduction studies at all intervals (1,2,3.5, 5,7, and 10 years) (15).

Table 3 Therapies for Diabetic Neuropathy

Systemic disease
    Control of hyperglycemia   Pancreatic transplantation
    Daily examination of feet   Nerve growth factor
Pain management
    Ibuprofen
    Tricyclic antidepressants: amitriptyline, imipramine, nortriptyline, doxepin
    Antiepileptic medications: diphenylhydantoin, carbamazepine, gabapentin
    Selective serotonin-reuptake inhibitors: fluoxetine
    Antipsychotics: thorazine
    Benzodiazepines: clonazepam
    Topical capsaicin cream
    Cardiac antiarrythmic agents: mexiletine
    Tramadol HCl
    Epidural spinal cord stimulation
Autonomic dysfunction
    Orthostatic hypotension
        Hydration   Elastic stockings
        Increased dietary salt 9α-Fludrocortisone
        Midodrine
    Gastric atony
        Metoclopramide   Erythromycin
        Domperidone   Cisapride
    Constipation
        Hydration   Increased dietary fiber
        Exercise   Bulking agents
        Enemas
    Urinary dysfunction
        Oxybutynin   Tricyclic antidepressants
        Bethanechol   Pseudoephedrine
        Phenylpropanolamine   Phenoxybenzamine
        Prazocin
    Impotence
        Vacuum devices   Inflatable penile prostheses
        Sildenafil

Autonomic testing results improved only after year 1 in the transplantation group. The neuropathy worsened in the control group. Thus, the restoration of normoglycemia from transplantation of insulin islet cells improves the symptoms and signs of peripheral neuropathy for up to 10 years.

    Animal studies have shown that the concentration of *myo*-inositol, an important constituent of cell membranes, is diminished in peripheral nerves of experimentally-induced diabetic rats. Diet supplementation of *myo*-inositol in these animals has slowed the decline of nerve conduction velocities. Unfortunately, as substantiated by several studies, the addition of *myo*-inositol to the diet of humans with diabetes has not reversed or slowed the progression of neuropathy.

In the setting of hyperglycemia, the polyol pathway is accentuated in many tissues, including peripheral nerves. Glucose is converted by an aldose reductase to sorbitol and, in animal studies, evidence exists that excess sorbitol is toxic to peripheral nerves. To reduce nerve sorbitol, efforts have been made to block this conversion to sorbitol using aldose reductase inhibitors. Numerous studies have been performed, several showing no benefit, whereas others have demonstrated improvement in sensory impairment, deep tendon reflexes, motor and sensory nerve conduction studies, and sensory discrimination (16). Other investigators have shown improvement in some parameters and deterioration in other parameters in the same patients. Aldose reductase inhibitors may have a role in the management of early mild diabetic neuropathy. Guiliano et al. showed that tolrestat improved orthostatic hypotension, sinus arrythmia, lying-to-standing heart rate ratio, and vibration perception, compared with a placebo group in patients with mild diabetic neuropathy (17). Adverse effects appear to be common with aldose reductase inhibitors, with rash, fever, photosensitivity, lymphadenopathy, and abnormal liver function studies predominating.

No conclusive evidence, backed by controlled studies, exists to support the prescription of vitamins for the treatment of diabetic neuropathy. Gangliosides have been tried in diabetic neuropathy, based on the premise that their use might stimulate nerve growth. Several controlled trials of gangliosides have been completed that showed slight improvement in symptoms and increases in nerve conduction velocities after treatment. The results were not considered sufficiently robust to warrant their use in diabetic neuropathy.

6. Symptomatic Treatment

One of the most serious complications of diabetic neuropathy is the insensitive or insensate foot. Patients lacking sensation in the feet are unable to feel the pain caused by stones, nails, or tacks penetrating the skin as well as skin fissures and ulcerations. Consequently, the skin is prone to acute and chronic infection, often unbeknownst to the patient who cannot easily examine the soles of his or her feet. Chronic infection may lead to osteomyelitis, cellulitis, phlebitis, and sepsis. The distal limbs of diabetics are more prone to infection because of poor blood flow and ischemia related to large and small blood vessel disease.

The primary goal of treatment is prevention, prompt removal of foreign bodies, and early treatment of infections. The patient or caregiver should examine the foot, especially the sole, several times each day. Fissures, ulcers, and infections should be treated early and aggressively with careful removal of dead tissue, bed rest, and antibiotics. Mechanical injury can be minimized by the selection of supportive, yet comfortable, footwear.

One of the most common indications for patient referral to a neurologist is management of pain and sensory symptoms. Treatment of neuropathic pain is often a frustration for the patient and treating physician. The pain may be difficult to describe. Patients often use descriptions such as burning, knife-like, stabbing, and ice pick, words which neurologists interpret as indicating neuropathic pain. The pain is typically worse at night and may delay initiation of sleep for hours. Patients may report worsening of the pain when sheets and bed covers contact the skin. Other patients complain of worsening of the pain after prolonged standing and walking. Some patients prefer to wear sandals, even during cold weather, insisting that the tight binding of a regular shoe and heat intensifies their discomfort.

Rarely are simple analgesics, such as aspirin or acetaminophen, helpful for long-term treatment of neuropathic pain. Surprisingly, an occasional patient will report good pain relief when taking ibuprofen 400–600 mg (18). Most patients referred to neurologists require treatment with long-term agents. Helpful medications for the treatment of diabetic neuropathy include tricyclic antidepressants, antiepileptic drugs, selective serotonin-reuptake inhibitors, antipsychotics, and benzodiazepines. Narcotics may occasionally be necessary for breakthrough pain, but should be avoided as the primary analgesic because of their propensity to induce taxiphylaxis and dependency.

Amitriptyline is a popular first-line therapy because of its efficacy, low cost, ease of use (at bedtime), and predictable side effect profile. Patients may respond to doses as low as 25 mg at night, but usually amounts between 50 and 150 mg are needed to achieve acceptable analgesia. A dose–benefit relations exists for amitriptyline, with higher dosages producing greater pain relief. A starting dose of 10 mg is advisable in elderly patients because of their sensitivity to tricyclic antidepressants and potential interaction with other drugs prescribed for coexisting conditions. Common side effects reported by patients taking tricyclic antidepressants are drowsiness, dry eyes and mouth, constipation, weight gain, and increased appetite. The efficacy of amitriptyline for neuropathic pain appears to be separate from its effect on depression (19). Max et al. reported that amitriptyline-induced analgesia was similar in patients with diabetic neuropathy who were depressed or nondepressed and the benefit was not associated with mood improvement (19). The same authors showed that desipramine was equally as effective as amitriptyline in the treatment of painful diabetic neuropathy, yet the selective blocker of serotonin reuptake, fluoxetine, was no more effective than placebo for the relief of pain (20). Of interest, 41% of subjects in that study receiving placebo reported pain relief. Other tricyclic antidepressants that have been used with success include imipramine, nortriptyline, and doxepin (21).

Antiepileptic medications have been prescribed for decades to control the pain of diabetic neuropathy (22). In an uncontrolled study published in 1968, Ellenberg reported excellent pain relief in 68% of patients with diabetic polyneuropathy and fair relief in another 10% who were prescribed diphenylhydantoin (23). If improvement was likely to occur, pain relief was achieved within the first 4 days. The dosage used was 100 mg three or four times daily.

Carbamazepine has been studied in several neuropathic conditions, including trigeminal neuralgia, facial pain, thalamic pain, and diabetic neuropathy (22). Patients typically respond to doses of 200–300 mg twice, three or four times daily.

Gabapentin has recently gained favor as a popular treatment for all types of neuropathic pain, including painful diabetic neuropathy. Although developed as an antiepileptic medication, its excellent patient tolerance profile, infrequent interaction with concomitant medications, and efficacy make it a good choice. A recently published controlled study of gabapentin in diabetic neuropathy showed clear superiority compared to placebo in producing pain relief (24). Patients were titrated to a dose of 3600 mg/day by the fourth week of the study. Drug tolerance was good with 67% of patients achieving the maximum dosage. Side effects included dizziness and somnolence.

Thus far, no studies have been conducted comparing the efficacy of one anticonvulsant with another.

In painful diabetic neuropathy, topical treatment of areas of intense pain has been tried with good results. Capsaicin is the active ingredient in hot pepper. Research has shown that capsaicin applied to the skin eventually leads to a reduction of substance P in the subcutaneous nerve endings and in the dorsal root ganglion subserving the area of pain. A multicenter, placebo-controlled study of topical capsaicin applied four times per day showed statistical significance in the areas of pain relief, reduction of pain intensity, and pain improvement using a physician's global evaluation scale (25). Unfortunately, many patients abandon capsaicin within the first week of treatment because of the adverse effects of burning and erythema. Patients who persevere and continue to apply capsaicin often achieve good pain relief by the second week of treatment.

Because of their capacity to stabilize cell membranes, antiarrhythmic medications are logical choices to treat diabetic neuropathy. Deijgard and colleagues, in a randomized, double-blind crossover trial showed that mexiletine, given in a dosage of 10 mg/kg produced statistically beneficial reduction of pain, dysesthesia, and paresthesia in 16 of 19 patients with painful diabetic neuropathy (26).

Tramadol HCl is a centrally acting analgesic the mechanism of which includes inhibition of norepinephrine and serotonin reuptake and low-affinity binding to μ-opioid receptors. Tramadol HCl has been marketed in Germany for over 2 decades with excellent results and a very low incidence of drug dependency. In a recently published study, tramadol was superior to placebo in the areas of pain intensity reduction and improvement of pain relief in a group of patients with painful diabetic neuropathy (27). Patients receiving tramadol scored better in the categories of physical and social functioning. The average dosage used was 210 mg/day. The most commonly experienced side effects were nausea, constipation, headache, and somnolence.

Patients who do not respond to conventional therapies may benefit from more invasive approaches. Epidural spinal cord stimulation of the thoracic or lumbar area led to greater pain relief in eight of ten patients with painful diabetic neuropathy who had not responded to more conventional treatment (28). The authors reported significant improvement of both background and peak neuropathic pain at 3, 6, and 14 months. Exercise tolerance was better at 3 and 6 months. Six of the patients were able to control their pain using the stimulator as the only source of pain relief.

Similar to gangliosides, agents that promote nerve fiber growth have an appeal as a long-term treatment and ultimately as a potential cure for diabetic neuropathy. Apfel and the NGF Study Group recently reported their results from 250 patients with symptomatic diabetic polyneuropathy who were relegated to the placebo arm or one of two doses of recombinant nerve growth factor (NGF) for 6 months (29). Patients receiving NGF improved in the sensory component of the neurological examination, two quantitative sensory tests, and subjective impression (29). Injection site reactions were the most common adverse effects. Currently, a larger phase III protocol is underway that will study the effect of NGF over 12 months.

7. Treatment of Autonomic Dysfunction in Diabetic Neuropathy

The management of autonomic dysfunction in patients with diabetes does not differ from the treatment of autonomic symptoms stemming from other disorders. Orthostatic hypotension may arise from advanced diabetic neuropathy or as an adverse effect of medications. Drugs that commonly produce or exacerbate orthostatic hypotension include diuretics, β-adrenergic blockers, tricyclic antidepressants, drugs containing L-dopa, anxiolytics, and phenothiazines. Simple symptomatic treatment for orthostatic hypotension begins with adequate hydration, increased use of dietary salt (if not medically contraindicated), and elevation of the head of the bed. Tight elastic stockings help prevent the pooling of blood in the lower extremities that often occurs after prolonged sitting. The physician should prescribe stockings that extend to the upper thighs, rather than the more popular and patient-compliant type that extend only to the knee. Unfortunately, patient tolerance for elastic stockings is poor because the hose are uncomfortable, hot in the summer, aesthetically unappealing, and sometimes require the purchase of larger shoes to accommodate the thick stockings. Even if used properly, elastic stockings frequently do not reverse orthostasis, leading to patient frustration and discontinuation. Often patients benefit from counseling to avoid rapid changes of position, particularly early in the day. When first arising from bed in the morning, patients with orthostatic hypotension should sit on the side of the bed for 1–2 min before standing. Before standing up from the sitting position, they should be encouraged to exercise their legs to increase blood return to the heart.

Two pharmacological treatments can be effective for orthostatic hypotension. For decades, 9α-fludrocortisone has been the drug of choice for increasing intravascular volume and sensitizing adrenergic receptors to circulating catecholamines. The usual dosage is 0.1–0.5 mg twice a day. Once treatment with 9α-fludrocortisone is initiated, careful monitoring is necessary to screen for supine hypertension, hypokalemia, and congestive heart failure. Recently, midodrine, an α-adrenergic agonist that selectively stimulates vasoconstriction, has been prescribed for the treatment of orthostatic hypotension (30). The starting dose is 5 mg three times a day. Depending on the clinical response, the dosage can be advanced to 10 mg three times a day. Wright et al. reported in a recently published, double-blind, placebo-controlled, four-way crossover trial that patients with neurogenic orthostatic hypotension receiving midodrine, 10 mg twice or three times daily, experienced increased standing systolic blood pressure and an improvement of a global assessment of orthostatic symptoms (30). There was a significant linear relation between the dose of midodrine and mean systolic blood pressure. Common adverse effects of midodrine are supine hypertension, paresthesia, pruritus, urinary urgency, and gastrointestinal complaints.

The gastrointestinal autonomic complaint for which diabetics often seek medical management is gastric stasis and bloating. A highly effective agent for gastric atony is metoclopramide, prescribed as 10 mg 1/2 h before meals. After prolonged use, some patients have developed drug-induced parkinsonism or tardive dyskinesias. Other agents that can be prescribed for bloating are erythromycin, domperidone, and cisapride.

Constipation in diabetic neuropathy is managed using the time-proved remedies of hydration, augmentation of dietary fiber, increasing mobility, bulking agents, laxatives, and enemas. Simple but effective treatments of diarrhea include over-the-counter diphenoxylate hydrochloride and loperamide hydrochloride.

Proper management of urinary dysfunction requires information available only through appropriate urological and urodynamic testing. Those studies are needed to determine whether decreased or increased bladder contractility is the primary problem and whether the bladder outlet is over- or undercontracted. Blind prescription of pharmacological agents often results in the wrong drug for the underlying pathology. If urodynamic testing confirms a spastic bladder, the most commonly prescribed agent is oxybutynin, 5-mg three times daily. Occasionally, patients with diabetic neuropathy will comment on improved bladder control after taking tricyclic antidepressants for neuropathic pain. This improvement is attributed to the anticholinergic properties of tricyclic antidepressants which, in the case of bladder function, decrease contractility and increase bladder outlet resistance. Bethanechol chloride, a muscarinic cholinergic agonist, is prescribed for an underactive bladder.

Because the bladder outlet is innervated by adrenergic fibers, treatment to increase bladder outlet resistance can begin with over-the-counter adrenergic agonists, such as pseudoephedrine or phenylpropanolamine. To decrease bladder outlet resistance, α-adrenergic antagonists, phenoxybenzamine and prazosin, may be prescribed.

Impotence is extremely common in men with diabetes and is a major source of frustration. Once nonorganic causes are excluded, treatment can be mechanical or pharmacological. Some men can attain a satisfying erection using a vacuum device and rubber bands. Other mechanical therapies that can be tried are semirigid and malleable or the inflatable penile prostheses.

Unquestionably, the pharmacological agent receiving the greatest fanfare and publicity for the treatment of impotence has been sildenafil (31). It functions by inhibiting hydrolysis of cyclic guanosine monophosphate in the corpus cavernosum, leading to an accentuated penile response to sexual stimulation. Two sequential studies demonstrated the efficacy of sildenafil in men with impotence from organic, psychogenic, and mixed causes (31). Sixty-nine percent of all attempts at sexual intercourse were successful in the men taking sildenafil compared with a 22% success rate in the placebo group. Higher doses of sildenafil (50 and 100 mg) were more effective in producing an erection than the 25-mg dose. The most common side effects were headache, flushing, and dyspepsia, occurring in 6–18% of men. Postmarketing experience has uncovered a higher than anticipated incidence of cardiovascular adverse events, including myocardial infarction, arrythmia, stroke, transient ischemic attacks (TIAs), and death. Most of these occurred in patients with preexisting cardiovascular risk factors.

In summary, diabetic neuropathy has many clinical presentations, ranging from acute to chronic and focal to symmetrical. Identification of the type of neuropathy is based on a high degree of clinical suspicion and, usually, confirmation by a carefully planned electrophysiological study. Many therapeutic options are available for the management of neuropathic pain and autonomic complications. The future appears to be promising for therapies that hold the potential for arresting and potentially reversing nerve fiber loss.

REFERENCES

1. J Pirart. Diabetes mellitus and its degenerative complications: a prospective study of 4400 patients observed between 1947 and 1973. Diabetes Care 1978; 1:168–188.
2. PJ Dyck, J Karnes, PC O'Brien. Diagnosis, staging and classification of diabetic neuropathy and associations with other complications. In: PJ Dyck, PK Thomas, AK

Asbury, AI Winegard, D Porte, eds. Diabetic Neuropathy. Philadelphia: WB Saunders, 1987:36–44.

3. PJ Dyck, KM Kratz, JL Karnes, WJ Litchy, R Klein, JM Pach, DM Wilson, PC O'Brien, LJ Melton III. The prevalence by staged severity of various types of diabetic neuropathy, retinopathy, and nephropathy in a population-based cohort: the Rochester Diabetic Neuropathy Study. Neurology 1993; 43:817–824.

4. JA Cohen, BW Jeffers, D Faldut, M Marcoux, RW Schrier. Risks for sensorimotor peripheral neuropathy and autonomic neuropathy in noninsulin-dependent diabetes mellitus (NIDDM). Muscle Nerve 1998; 21:72–80.

5. LS Hakin, I Goldstein. Diabetic sexual dysfunction. Endocrinol Metab Clin North Am 1996; 25:379–400.

6. O Saito, M Aoyagi, H Tojima, Y Koike. Diagnosis and treatment for Bell's palsy associated with diabetis mellitus. Acta Otolaryngol Suppl 1994; 511:153–155.

7. NA Brandenburg, JF Annegers. Incidence and risk factors for Bell's palsy in Laredo, Texas. Neuroepidemiology 1993; 12:313–325.

8. JA O'Hare, F Abuaisha, M Geoghegan. Prevalence and forms of neuropathic morbidity in 800 patients. Ir J Med Sci 1994; 163:132–135.

9. MK Pascoe, PA Low, AJ Windebank, WJ Litchy. Subacute diabetic proximal neuropathy. Mayo Clin Proc 1997; 72:1123–1132.

10. SH Subramony, AJ Wilbourn. Diabetic proximal neuropathy. Clinical and electromyographic studies. J Neurol Sci 1982; 53:293–304.

11. PJ Dyck, JL Karnes, P O'Brien, H Okazaki, A Lais, J Engelstad. The spatial distribution of fiber loss in diabetic polyneuropathy suggests ischemia. Ann Neurol 1986; 19:440–449.

12. G Said, C Goulon-Goeau, C Lacroix, A Moulonguet. Nerve biopsy findings in different patterns of proximal diabetic neuropathy. Ann Neurol 1994; 35:559–569.

13. G Said, F Elgrably, C Lacroix, V Plante, C Talamon, D Adams, M Tager, G Slama. Painful proximal diabetic neuropathy: inflammatory nerve lesions and spontaneous favorable outcome. Ann Neurol 1997; 41:762–770.

14. The Diabetes Control and Complications Trial Research Group. The effect of intensive diabetes therapy on the development and progression of neuropathy. Ann Intern Med 1995; 122:561–568.

15. X Navarro, DER Sutherland, WR Kennedy. Long-term effects of pancreatic transplantation on diabetic neuropathy. Ann Neurol 1997; 42:727–736.

16. AAF Sima, V Bril, V Nathaniel, TAJ McEwen, MB Brown, SA Lattimer, DA Greene. Regeneration and repair of myelinated fibers in sural-nerve biopsy specimens from patients with diabetic neuropathy treated with sorbinil. N Engl J Med 1988; 319:548–555.

17. D Guigliano, R Marfella, A Quatraro, N De Rosa, T Salvatore, D Cozzolino, A Ceriello, R Torella. Tolrestat for mild diabetic neuropathy: a 52-week, randomized, placebo-controlled trial. Ann Intern Med 1993; 118:7–11.

18. KL Cohen, S Harris. Efficacy and safety of nonsteroidal anti-inflammatory drugs in the therapy of diabetic neuropathy. Arch Intern Med 1987; 147:1442–1444.

19. MB Max, M Culnane, SC Schafer, RH Gracely, DJ Walther, B Smoller, R Dubner. Amitriptyline relieves diabetic neuropathy pain in patients with normal or depressed mood. Neurology 1987; 37:589–596.

20. MB Mitchell, SA Lynch, J Muir, SE Shoaf, B Smoller, R Dubner. Effects of desipramine, amitriptyline, and fluoxetine on pain in diabetic neuropathy. N Engl J Med 1992; 326:1250–1256.

21. B Kvinesdal, J Molin, A Froland, LR Gram. Imipramine treatment of painful diabetic neuropathy. JAMA 1984; 251:1727–1730.

22. H McQuay, D Carroll, AR Jadad, P Wiffen, A Moore. Anticonvulsant drugs for management of pain: a systemic review. Br J Med 1995; 311:1047–1052.

23. M Ellenberg. Treatment of diabetic neuropathy with diphenyhydantoin. NY State J Med 1968; 68:2653–2655.

24. M Backonja, A Beydoun, KR Edwards, SL Schwartz, V Fonseca, M Hes, L LaMoreaux, E Garofalo for the Gabapentin Diabetic Neuropathy Study Group. Gabapentin for the symptomatic treatment of painful neuropathy in patients with diabetes mellitus: a randomized controlled trial. JAMA 1998; 280:1831–1836.

25. The Capsaicin Study Group. Treatment of painful diabetic neuropathy with topical capsaicin: a multicenter, double-blind, vehicle-controlled study. Arch Intern Med 1991; 151:2225–2229.

26. A Dejgard, P Petersen, J Kastrup. Mexiletine for treatment of chronic painful diabetic neuropathy. Lancet 1998; 2:9–11.

27. Y Harati, C Gooch, M Swenson, S Edelman, D Greene, P Raskin, P Donofrio, D Cornblath, R Sachdeo, CO Siu, M Kamin. Double-blind randomized trial of tramadol for the treatment of the pain of diabetic neuropathy. Neurology 1998; 50:1842–1846.

28. S Tesfaye, J Watt, SJ Benbow, KA Pang, J Miles, IA MacFarlane. Electrical spinal-cord stimulation for painful diabetic peripheral neuropathy. Lancet 1996; 348: 1696–1701.

29. SC Apfel, JA Kessler, BT Adornato, WJ Litchy, C Sanders, CA Rask, NGF Study Group. Recombinant human nerve growth factor in the treatment of diabetic polyneuropathy. Neurology 1998; 51:695–702.

30. RA Wright, HC Kaufmann, R Perera, TL Opfer-Gehrking, MA McElligott, KN Sheng, PA Low. A double-blind, dose–response study of midodrine in neurogenic orthostatic hypotension. Neurology 1998; 51:120–124.

31. I Goldstein, TF Lue, H Padma-Nathan, RC Rosen, WD Steers, PA Wicker. Oral sildenafil in the treatment of erectile dysfunction. N Engl J Med 1998; 338: 1397–1404.

30

The Diagnosis and Management of Lipoprotein Disorders

Ernst J. Schaefer and Leo J. Seman
New England Medical Center and Tufts University, Boston, Massachusetts

I. INTRODUCTION

Coronary heart disease (CHD) is a major cause of death and disability in the United States. Although the age-adjusted mortality rate of CHD is on the decline, on an annual basis CHD still kills about 500,000 Americans. It is estimated that nearly 70% of all Americans have some degree of atherosclerotic narrowing of their coronary arteries. Approximately 14 million Americans suffer from CHD and one-third of these individuals have limited activity as a result. In addition, each year about 1.5 million Americans will suffer a myocardial infarction, about 1 million will undergo cardiac catheterization, about 500,000 will die of CHD, about 400,000 will have coronary artery bypass grafts, and another 350,000 will have an angioplasty procedure performed.

A primary contributing factor to CHD is an elevated blood cholesterol level owing to an increased level of low-density lipoprotein (LDL) cholesterol. Other significant risks include age, gender, hypertension, smoking, diabetes, family history of premature CHD, and decreased high-density lipoprotein (HDL) cholesterol. About 50% of all U.S. adults (95 million persons) have cholesterol levels over 200 mg/dL, and about 37 million adults have values over 240 mg/dL. Many of these persons (approximately 60 million) are candidates for medical advice and intervention.

II. PLASMA LIPOPROTEINS

Cholesterol and triglyceride, which are insoluble in water, are transported in blood within lipoproteins. Serum lipoproteins have been classified on the basis of their density, electrophoretic mobility, and relative lipid and protein content. Interest in plasma lipoproteins stems from their role in the development of atherosclerosis.

A. Chylomicrons

Chylomicrons are secreted by the intestine and are large triglyceride-rich lipoproteins with more than 90% triglyceride (by weight) and 1% protein. These particles allow the transport of dietary fat (triglyceride), cholesterol, and fat soluble vitamins and nutrients from the intestine to the bloodstream and then to various tissues in the body, and are usually not present in the serum of fasting subjects. Elevated chylomicron levels in the fasted state can cause markedly elevated serum triglyceride values (> 1000 mg/dL or 11.3 mmol/L) and are associated with an increased risk of pancreatitis. Chylomicrons are metabolized in the bloodstream by the action of lipoprotein lipase, which removes much of their triglyceride and phospholipid. During this process, chylomicrons pick up cholesterol from other lipoproteins, and lose triglyceride and phospholipid, becoming cholesterol-enriched chylomicron remnants. A new direct measure of chylomicron and very low density lipoprotein (VLDL) remnants is now available. Remnant-like lipoprotein cholesterol and triglyceride may increase two to fourfold after a meal rich in fat and cholesterol. In our view, these particles are atherogenic.

Chylomicron remnants are taken up by the liver by specific remnant receptors. The binding protein or ligand for these receptors is apolipoprotein E (apo E). This protein may be present in plasma in three forms: apo E-III, apo E-IV, and apo E-II: apo E-III is a 299-amino acid protein that has a cysteine at residue 112 and an arginine at residue 158; apo E-IV has an arginine at both locations; and apo E-II has a cysteine at both locations. apo E-III is the normal form of apo-III: about 60% of the population have the apo E-III/III genotype, about 20% have apo E-IV/III, about 15% have apo E-III/II, about 3% have apo E-IV/IV, about 1% have apo E-IV/II, and about 1% have apo E-II/II. The apo E-II-containing lipoprotein remnants appear to be taken up more slowly by the liver than those containing apo E-III. Therefore, having the apo E-II allele, especially being an apo E-II/II, results in increased levels of chylomicron and VLDL remnants, upregulation of the liver LDL receptor, and decreased LDL cholesterol. Having the apo E-IV allele appears to result in enhanced remnant uptake, down-regulation of the liver LDL receptor and higher LDL cholesterol levels. An elevated level of chylomicron remnants is thought to be a CHD risk factor.

B. Very Low Density Lipoproteins

The VLDLs are synthesized in the liver and are the major vehicle for plasma triglyceride transport in the fasting state. VLDL allow the transport of lipids from the liver to other tissues. VLDL are triglyceride-rich, and contain about 12% of total plasma cholesterol, and are precursors for LDL. Similar to chylomicrons, VLDL are metabolized by the action of lipoprotein lipase. During this process much of the triglyceride and phospholipid is removed, and cholesterol ester is picked up from other lipoproteins. VLDL remnants are then formed that may be taken up by the liver by the same mechanism as chylomicron remnants, or converted to form LDL by further lipolysis. An elevated level of VLDL remnants is a probable CHD risk factor.

C. Low-Density Lipoproteins

The LDLs are cholesterol-enriched, triglyceride-depleted products of VLDL catabolism. LDLs contain and transport about 60% of total plasma cholesterol and function to deliver cholesterol to peripheral tissues in the body, where it is used for the synthesis of cell membranes and steroid hormones. The major protein constituent of LDL is apo B. An LDL receptor that recognizes apo B allows the liver and other tissues to catabolize LDL. Modified or oxidized LDL can also be taken up by scavenger receptors on macrophages in various tissues including within the arterial wall.

When there is an excess level of LDL in the blood, it can be deposited in the blood vessel wall and becomes a major component of atherosclerotic plaque lesions. According to the recommendations of the National Cholesterol Education Program's (NCEP) Adult Treatment Panel (ATP), LDL cholesterol levels should be used as the basis for initiating and monitoring treatment of patients with elevated blood cholesterol (6–8).

D. Lipoprotein(a) or Lp(a)

Lipoprotein(a) is an LDL particle with an additional apolipoprotein known as apo(a) attached to it. Some apo(a) in serum is also attached to VLDL. Lp(a) carries about 3% of the cholesterol in plasma. Apoprotein(a) is attached to apo B by a disulfide bond: apo(a) has protein domains with significant homology to kringle 4 and kringle 5 domains within plasminogen. Lp(a) may interfere with clot lysis as well as being deposited in the artery wall similar to LDL. Elevated serum Lp(a) levels (> 30 mg/dL for the total particle or ≥ 10 mg/dL for Lp(a) cholesterol) have been associated with premature CHD and stroke in most studies. Significant issues remain relative to Lp(a) measurement, especially with immunoassays. A reliable assay for Lp(a) cholesterol is now available, and can be run in any routine clinical chemistry laboratory. Lp(a) can be reduced with niacin or estrogen replacement therapy.

E. High-Density Lipoproteins

The HDLs are synthesized in the liver and intestine, and they are responsible for transporting about 25% of the total serum cholesterol. HDLs are rich in protein and phospholipid. They act as a vehicle for reverse cholesterol transport from tissue to the liver. Levels of HDL cholesterol are inversely correlated with the risk for CHD; HDL is commonly referred to as "good" cholesterol: apo A-I is the major protein of HDL.

The liver is the major site of HDL catabolism, and HDL appears to be a major source of liver cholesterol. HDL uptake by the liver, the adrenals, and the ovaries is modulated by the scavenger receptor B1. In the liver, cholesterol can be either excreted directly into bile, converted to bile acids, or reutilized in lipoprotein production. Most gallstones are formed from cholesterol that precipitates if present in amounts in excess of that which can be solubilized by bile acids and phospholipids.

III. RATIONALE FOR TREATMENT OF LIPID DISORDERS

A. Intervention Studies

Human populations on high-saturated fat, high-cholesterol diets have elevated LDL cholesterol levels, and a significantly higher rate of CHD caused by atherosclerosis than populations on low saturated fat–low cholesterol diets. High-saturated fat, high-cholesterol diets delay LDL clearance, resulting in serum LDL cholesterol elevation. Elevated LDL cholesterol levels, as well as decreased HDL cholesterol levels, are independent risk factors for premature CHD in our society. Women have higher HDL cholesterol levels than men, owing to increased production of HDL constituents, and a lower age-adjusted risk of CHD. Prospective studies indicate that lowering of LDL cholesterol through diet treatment or diet and drug therapy can reduce subsequent CHD morbidity and mortality. Studies indicate a benefit in CHD risk reduction both from lowering LDL cholesterol and increasing HDL cholesterol with diet only or diet and modification. Moreover, aggressive lipid modification can result in stabilization of existing coronary atherosclerosis as well as some regression of this process (21). One of the largest trials, the Lipid Research Clinics Coronary Primary Prevention Trial (LRC-CPPT), which compared the cholesterol-lowering drug cholestyramine with a placebo, produced statistically significant reductions in LDL cholesterol levels and in the incidence of CHD (19,22,23).

The 1984 Consensus Development Conference on Lowering Blood Cholesterol to Prevent Heart Disease concluded, based on LRC-CPPT Trial that "It has been established beyond a reasonable doubt that lowering definitively elevated blood cholesterol levels, specifically, blood levels of low-density lipoprotein (LDL) cholesterol, will reduce risk of heart attacks caused by coronary artery disease (11)."

Recent large prospective primary and secondary intervention studies using hydroxymethylglutanyl coenzyme A (HMGCoA) reductase inhibitors, specifically simvastatin, pravastatin, and lovastatin (Scandinavian Simvastatin Survival Study or 4S, the West of Scotland Coronary Prevention Study or WOSCOPS, the Cholesterol and Recurrent Events Trial or CARE, AFCAPS/TEXCAPS and LIPID) have documented significant reductions in total mortality (4S, WOS-COPS, LIPID), CHD mortality (4S, WOSCOPS, LIPID), CHD morbidity (all studies), stroke (4S, CARE, LIPID), need for coronary artery bypass surgery (all studies), and angioplasty (all studies), as well as hospitalizations for CHD (all studies) (14,17,24,30–32).

The greatest benefit has been observed in patients with established CHD and hypercholesterolemia, not only in reduction in CHD, but also stroke risk. No benefit was noted in CHD patients with baseline LDL cholesterol values less than 125 mg/dL in the CARE trial; however, this latter conclusion was based on a subset analysis. The efficacy, tolerability, and significant benefit noted in large placebo-controlled, randomized, and blinded clinical trials with HMGCoA reductase inhibitors now make these agents the drugs of choice for cholesterol lowering in asymptomatic subjects as well as those with CHD. Moreover, results from these trials support the NCEP guidelines. Diabetic patients have benefited as much, or more so, than other patients.

B. Epidemiological Evidence

A large body of epidemiological evidence supports a direct relation between the level of serum total and LDL cholesterol and CHD risk. This association is continuous throughout the range of cholesterol levels in the population and is curvilinear. The data indicate the greatest benefit in risk reduction would be obtained in those with the highest cholesterol values. According to results from the third National Health and Nutrition Examination Survey (NHANES), the average LDL cholesterol level of U.S. adults is about 130 mg/dL. At higher levels of total and LDL cholesterol, the direct relation between CHD risk and cholesterol levels becomes particularly strong; for persons with cholesterol values in the top 10% of the population distribution, the risk of CHD mortality is four times as high as the risk in the bottom 10% of the population.

C. Genetic and Physiological Evidence

Premature CHD can result from high LDL cholesterol levels even in the absence of other risk factors. This is most clearly demonstrated in patients with the rare homozygous familial hypercholesterolemia, which is characterized by the absence of the specific cell-surface receptors that normally remove LDL from the circulatory system. LDL cholesterol levels can be as high as 1000 mg/dL (26 mmol/L), and severe atherosclerosis and CHD often develop before age 20. Patients with the more common heterozygous form of familial hypercholesterolemia and partial deficiencies of LDL receptor function generally develop premature CHD in the middle decades of life.

D. Animal Model Evidence

Animal models have demonstrated a direct relation between LDL cholesterol and atherosclerosis. Animals consuming diets high in saturated fat and cholesterol develop LDL cholesterol elevation and atherosclerosis. Such diets also increase HDL cholesterol; this latter effect may be compensatory. These hypercholesterolemic animals develop intimal lesions that progress from fatty streaks to ulcerated plaques resembling those of human atherosclerosis. In laboratory trials, severe atherosclerosis in monkeys regresses when blood cholesterol is lowered through diet or drug therapy. Such studies support a causal relation between LDL cholesterol and atherosclerosis, and suggest reversibility of the process with the reduction of LDL cholesterol in serum.

E. Summary

This combined evidence supports the concept that lowering total and LDL cholesterol levels will reduce the incidence of CHD events, and the death rate caused by myocardial infarction. Moreover, the pooled analysis of clinical trial findings suggests that intervention is as effective in preventing recurrent myocardial infarction and mortality in patients experiencing a recurrent attack as it is in primary prevention. The complete set of evidence strongly supports the concept that reducing elevated total and LDL cholesterol levels will reduce CHD risk in men and women, both in asymptomatic subjects and those with established CHD.

It is important to recognize the magnitude of CHD reduction associated with lowering of serum cholesterol levels. For individuals with serum cholesterol initially in the 250–300 mg/dL (6.5–7.8 mmol/L) range, each 1% reduction in serum cholesterol level yields approximately a 1–2% reduction in CHD rates. Thus, it is reasonable to estimate that a 35% reduction in serum cholesterol level would reduce CHD risk by as much as 60% in this group. More modest reduction in risk could be expected in those with lower values. Moreover, studies indicate that aggressive lipid modification can result in stabilization of existing coronary atherosclerosis, as well as some regression.

IV. EVALUATION AND TREATMENT OF PATIENTS

A. The NCEP Guidelines

The 1984 Consensus Development Conference on Lowering Blood Cholesterol to Prevent Heart Disease (11) developed plans for a National Cholesterol Education

Program (NCEP). The NCEP's continuing mandate is to develop guidelines that improve the detection of hypercholesterolemia, and therapeutic guidelines that affect its treatment. The NCEP enlists participation by and contributions from interested national, state, and local organizations. Its purpose is to educate physicians, other health professionals, and the general public on the significance of elevated blood cholesterol levels and the importance of treatment.

An National Institutes of Health (NIH)-sponsored consensus conference on triglycerides and HDL and the Adult Treatment Panel II of the NCEP in 1993 recommended identification of individuals at risk for CHD by total serum cholesterol and HDL cholesterol levels, and that they further be classified for treatment based on LDL cholesterol levels if indicated (7,8,12).

B. Total Cholesterol and HDL Cholesterol

The classification system begins with the measurement of total cholesterol and HDL cholesterol levels as a screen for the general population in the fasting or nonfasting state (Table 1). Accurate fingerstick methodology is available for both cholesterol and HDL cholesterol for screening purposes in the office setting. More recently, an accurate home cholesterol test that can be self-administered by the patient has become available. Total cholesterol levels below 200 mg/dL have been classified as "desirable," those between 200 and 239 mg/dL have been classified as "borderline-high," and those 240 mg/dL or higher as "high risk" (Table 2). Levels of HDL cholesterol less than 35 mg/dL have been classified as low, and those 60 mg/dL or more have been classified as high and protective for CHD (see Table 2).

Table 1 Screening for Lipid Abnormalities[a]

Step 1 Measure serum total cholesterol and HDL cholesterol fasting or nonfasting.
Step 2 Do fasting (12-h) serum lipid profile (cholesterol, triglyceride, HDL cholesterol) if:
1. Total cholesterol $\geq$ 240 mg/dL (6.2 mmol/L)
2. HDL cholesterol $\leq$ 35 mg/dL (0.9 mmol/L)
3. Total cholesterol $\geq$ 200 mg/dL (5.2 mmol/L) and the patient has two or more CHD risk factors
4. Patient has CHD
Step 3 Calculate LDL cholesterol as below:

$$LDL\text{-}C = total\ cholesterol - (HDL\text{-}C + TG/5)$$

provided patient is fasting and TG < 400 mg/dL.

[a] Alternative is nonfasting or fasting direct LDL-C, HDL-C, and TG.

Table 2 Classification of Lipid Values

Lipid	Optimal	Borderline	High-risk
Total cholesterol	< 200 mg/dL	200–239 mg/dL	≥ 240 mg/dL
LDL cholesterol	< 130 mg/dL	130–159 mg/dL	≥ 160 mg/dL
HDL cholesterol	≥ 60 mg/dL	35–59 mg/dL	< 35 mg/dL
Triglyceride	< 200 mg/dL	200–399 mg/dL	≥ 400 mg/dL

Approximately 25% of the entire adult population (more than 40 million people) in the United States (20 years of age and older) fall into the high-risk blood cholesterol classification, whereas another 54 million persons have borderline-high blood cholesterol levels. About 20% of males and 5% of females have low HDL cholesterol levels.

All patients who are screened should receive information about a step 1 diet and CHD risk factors. According to the NCEP Adult Treatment Panel (ATP) guidelines, patients who have desirable total cholesterol and normal HDL cholesterol values should have their values checked again within 5 years. If the patient has a borderline-high value, information about other CHD risk factors should be given (Table 3).

If the patient has a cholesterol value in the borderline-risk category (200–239 mg/dL) and a normal HDL cholesterol level of 35 mg/dL or higher in the absence of CHD (prior myocardial infarction, angina) or two or more of the CHD risk factors in Table 3 (male ≥ 45, female ≥ 55, smoking, diabetes,

Table 3 NCEP CHD Risk Factors[a]

Positive	Negative
Male ≥ 45 years	HDL-C ≥ 60 mg/dL
Female ≥ 55 years	
Family history of premature CHD	
HDL-C < 35 mg/dL	
Smoking	
Diabetes	
Hypertension	

[a] Subtract a risk factor if the HDL C ≥ 60 mg/dL.
Family history of premature CHD has been defined as the presence of CHD in a male first-degree relative younger than 55 and younger than 65 in a female first-degree relative.

hypertension, or family history of premature CHD), the dietary information discussed later should be provided and the cholesterol value checked within the next year.

If the patient has a borderline-high value (200–239 mg/dL) with a history of CHD or two or more CHD risk factors, or has a high-risk total cholesterol value (≥ 240 mg/dL) or has a low HDL cholesterol value (< 35 mg/dL), or has CHD, LDL cholesterol levels need to be assessed so that an appropriate treatment regimen can be determined. A controversial issue is whether apo A-I, apo B, LDL size, or Lp(a), should be measured for CHD risk assessment. None of these parameters has been shown to be an independent risk factor after smoking, blood pressure, diabetes, LDL cholesterol, and HDL cholesterol have been taken into account in prospective studies, except for Lp(a). In our view, Lp(a) or Lp(a) cholesterol should be part of CHD risk assessment in patients with established CHD as well as all subjects who are candidates for drug therapy for LDL cholesterol lowering, or have a strong family history of CHD. Measurement of the other parameters cannot be recommended at this time.

C. LDL Cholesterol

The NCEP Adult Treatment Panel has developed guidelines for the diagnosis and treatment of individuals older than age 20 with elevated blood cholesterol levels associated with an increase in LDL cholesterol levels. Levels of LDL cholesterol requiring the initiation of diet and drug therapy, as well as the goals of therapy, are dependent on the presence or absence of CHD or two or more of the CHD risk factors in Table 3. LDL cholesterol decision points for initiating diet and drug therapy are given in Table 4. The presence of secondary causes of elevated LDL cholesterol levels (≥ 160 mg/dL or 4.1 mmol/L) must be ruled

Table 4 Treatment Guidelines for Patients with Elevated LDL Cholesterol

	Initiate diet therapy	After diet therapy initiate drug therapy	Goal of therapy
Less than two CHD risk factors	≥ 160 mg/dL (4.1 mmol/L)	≥ 190 mg/dL (4.9 mmol/L)	< 160 mg/dL (4.1 mmol/L)
Two or more CHD risk factors	≥ 130 mg/dL (3.4 mmol/L)	≥ 160 mg/dL (4.1 mmol/L)	< 130 mg/dL (3.4 mmol/L)
CHD	≥ 100 mg/dL (2.6 mmol/L)	≥ 130 mg/dL (3.4 mmol/L)	< 100 mg/dL (2.6 mmol/L)

LDL, low-density lipoprotein; CHD, coronary heart disease.

Table 5 Secondary Cause of Hypercholesterolemia

Hypothyroidism
Obstructive liver disease
Nephrotic syndrome
Diabetes mellitus
Progestins
Anabolic steroids

out (Table 5). The NCEP guidelines have been accepted by all major U.S. medical organizations, including the American College of Physicians, the American Heart Association, and the American Medical Association. Guidelines for the general population and children and adolescents have also been developed.

The recommendation that LDL cholesterol values be used as the primary criterion for treatment decisions in patients with elevated cholesterol levels makes the need for accurate measurement a national public health imperative.

If a patient has an LDL cholesterol level of 160 mg/dL, it represents approximately the 75th percentile for middle-aged Americans. It is important to confirm the presence of abnormalities by repeat determinations. Hospitalization or acute illness including myocardial infarction can markedly lower lipid values; therefore, lipid determinations should generally be carried out in the free-living state. An elevated or borderline high triglyceride level ($\geq$ 200 mg/dL) has not clearly been shown to be an independent risk factor for premature heart disease in men. However, an elevated triglyceride level is inversely associated with a low level of HDL cholesterol, which is a significant risk factor for CHD. If possible, these factors should be screened for and treated before initiating diet or drug treatment. Screening should include evaluation of glucose, albumin, liver transaminases, alkaline phosphatase, creatinine, thyroid-stimulating hormone (TSH), and urinalysis, as well as asking about alcohol intake and use of progestins and anabolic steroids (see Table 5).

D. The American Diabetes Association Guidelines

The treatment goals for persons with diabetes mellitus (Table 6) underwent minor modification in the Clinical Practice Recommendations from the American Diabetes Association in the January 1999 Supplement to *Diabetes Care* (1). The optimal recommended LDL cholesterol is less than 100 mg/dL for all adults with diabetes because of the very high incidence of coronary disease. Medical nutrition therapy is initiated above this level followed by pharmacological therapy with the current recommendation for drugs when the LDL cholesterol is higher than 130 mg/dL

Table 6 Treatment Decisions Based on LDL Cholesterol Level in Adults with Diabetes

	Medical nutrition therapy		Drug therapy	
	Initiation level	LDL goal	Initiation level	LDL goal
With CHD, PVD, or CVD	> 100 mg/dL	≤ 100 mg/dL	> 100 mg/dL	≤ 100
Without CHD, PVD, or CVD	> 100 mg/dL	≤ 100 mg/dL	> 130 mg/dL[a]	≤ 100

[a] For diabetic persons with multiple CHD risk factors (low HDL [< 35 mg/dL], hypertension, smoking, family history of CVD, or microalbuminuria or proteinuria) some authorities recommend initiation of drug therapy when LDL levels are between 100 and 130 mg/dL. Caveats: (a) medical nutrition therapy should be attempted before starting pharmacological therapy; (b) because diabetic men and women are considered to have equal CHD risk, age and sex are not considered "risk factors."
Source: Ref. 1.

in adults without known coronary or peripheral vascular disease and more than 100 mg/dL in those with known CHD or PVD. However, many experts are recommending an LDL cholesterol treatment goal of less than 100 mg/dL in all adults with diabetes.

E. LDL Cholesterol Measurement

There are now approved and validated methods for the direct measurement of LDL cholesterol. Accurate measurement depends first on the separation of LDL particles in serum from other lipoproteins; namely, chylomicrons, VLDL, and HDL. Options for measuring LDL cholesterol include ultracentrifugation, the Friedewald calculation for estimating LDL cholesterol levels, or new direct methods for measuring LDL cholesterol that remove non-LDL lipoproteins from serum or plasma by immunoprecipitation or binding to polyanions.

Ultracentrifugation involves the separation of lipoproteins based on their density differences following an 18-h spin at 109,000 *g*. The procedure has been adopted by the Lipid Research Clinics, other lipoprotein research laboratories, and some clinical laboratories as a means of directly measuring LDL cholesterol in the research setting and serves as the current standard. Ultracentrifugation is poorly suited to the routine clinical laboratory for several reasons: it requires cumbersome procedures, it is extremely labor-intensive and technique-dependent, and it requires expensive instrumentation.

Currently, most clinical laboratories use the equation known as the Friedewald formula to estimate a patient's LDL cholesterol concentration. The formula uses the following calculation: LDL cholesterol = total cholesterol − HDL cholesterol − triglyceride/5. It estimates the LDL cholesterol concentration by subtracting the cholesterol associated with the other classes of lipoproteins from total cholesterol and involves three independent lipid analyses, each contributing a potential source of error. It also involves an often inaccurate estimate of VLDL cholesterol. Because no direct VLDL cholesterol assay is available, it is calculated from the triglyceride value divided by a factor of 5. All of these factors add error to LDL cholesterol estimates, especially in individuals with elevated triglyceride levels. In addition, clinical laboratories use automated enzymatic analyses for cholesterol and triglyceride quantitation within serum or plasma, and HDL cholesterol is measured after precipitation of other lipoproteins in serum or plasma with either heparin manganese chloride, dextran magnesium sulfate, or phosphotungstic acid.

The drawbacks of using the Friedewald formula for determining levels of LDL cholesterol are that it is estimated by calculation; it requires multiple assays and multiple steps, each adding a potential source of error; it is inaccurate as triglyceride levels increase; it requires that patients fast for 12–14 h before specimen collection to avoid a triglyceride bias; and it is not standardized. Moreover, LDL cholesterol concentrations cannot be calculated in individuals with elevated triglyceride levels (> 400 mg/dL). In addition, it has been reported that the formula becomes increasingly inaccurate at borderline triglyceride levels (200–400) misclassifying more than 25% of subjects in terms of LDL-cholesterol cutpoints.

Inadequacies in these methods have resulted in the development of direct methods by which clinical laboratories may accurately, practically, and precisely assess LDL cholesterol concentrations in patient samples. These tests involve separation technology utilizing affinity-purified goat polyclonal antisera to specific human apolipoproteins coated to latex particles that facilitate the removal of chylomicrons, VLDL, and HDL in nonfasting or fasting specimens or removal of these particles with polyanions. LDL is not removed by these procedures, and the LDL cholesterol concentration is obtained by performing an enzymatic cholesterol assay.

Direct LDL cholesterol methods allow (a) direct quantitation of LDL cholesterol from one measurement; (b) use of fasting and nonfasting samples; and (c) LDL cholesterol measurement in the presence of elevated triglyceride levels. Studies in fasting or nonfasting subjects who are either normal or hyperlipidemic indicate that LDL cholesterol results obtained with this direct assay correlate very highly with ultracentrifugation analysis. Subjects with LDL cholesterol levels of 160 mg/dL or higher by ultracentrifugation were correctly classified 94% of the time. Between-run and within-run coefficients of variation of less than 3% have been observed. This assay has been approved, and is currently commercially available to laboratories. It is especially useful for the practicing physician who sees patients in the afternoon. In addition, newer on-line direct LDL cholesterol and HDL cholesterol assays are now available, permitting rapid automated analysis of lipoprotein cholesterol levels. In the future, physicians will also use measurements of Lp(a) and remnant-like lipoprotein cholesterol values.

V. DIET THERAPY

Low-density lipoprotein cholesterol levels requiring dietary intervention are shown in Tables 4 and 6. Secondary causes of hypercholesterolemia shown in Table 5 also need to be ruled out and treated. The cornerstone of the treatment of lipid disorders is diet therapy. Approximately 50% of saturated fat and 70% of cholesterol in the U.S. diet comes from hamburgers, cheeseburgers, meat loaf, whole milk, cheese, other dairy products, including ice cream, beef steaks, roasts, hot dogs, ham, lunch meat, doughnuts, cookies, cakes, and eggs. These foods should be restricted. Instead, it is recommended that poultry (white meat) without skin, fish, skimmed or low-fat milk, nonfat or low-fat yogurt, and low-fat cheese be eaten. The use of fruits, vegetables, and grains is encouraged. Oils that can be used are unsaturated vegetable oils containing polyunsaturated fat and monounsaturated fatty acids, such as canola, soybean, olive, or corn oil. However, such oils should be used only in moderation because they are rich in calories. Consumption of hydrogenated vegetable oils rich in *trans*-fatty acids such as stick margarine should also be kept to a minimum. Soft margarine is a better alternative than stick margarine or butter. Alternatively, vegetable oil can be placed on directly bread.

Excellent patient dietary pamphlets are available from the American Heart Association. The step 1 diet is recommended for the entire U.S. population; for patients with elevated LDL cholesterol, the step 2 diet is used if an adequate response to the step 1 diet is not achieved (Table 7). Patients who fail to obtain an adequate response with diet after being given pamphlets and counseled by the physician and office nurse should be referred to a registered dietitian for instruction on the step 2 diet. In most cases, diet therapy should be tried for at least 6 months before initiating drug therapy, and a regular exercise program and control of other risk factors should also be encouraged. In patients with established CHD, drug therapy can be instituted almost immediately, to obtain benefit as soon as possible. Dietary fat restriction to approximately 20% of calories, along with exercise, appears to be very important to prevent the age-related weight gain and obesity that so often is associated with dyslipidemia, hypertension, and diabetes in our society. Information about the U.S. dietary guidelines are provided in Table 8.

Table 7 National Cholesterol Education Program Guidelines on Dietary Therapy[a]

Nutrient	Average U.S. diet[b]	Step 1 diet	Step 2 diet
Total fat	34%	≤ 30%	≤ 30%
Saturated fat	12%	< 10%	< 7%
Monounsaturated fat	13%	< 15%	< 15%
Polyunsaturated fat	7%	< 10%	< 10%
Total energy calories	To achieve and maintain desirable body weight		

[a] Percentage of total energy calories.
[b] Total population data from National Health and Nutrition Examination Survey (NHANES) III, excluding children younger than 2 years of age.

Table 8 Daily Food Intake Recommendations

I.   6–11 servings of bread, cereal, rice, or pasta
     One serving is 1 slice of bread, 1 ounce of ready-to-eat cereal, or a ½ cup of cereal, rice, or pasta.
     Emphasis should be placed on whole-grain foods prepared with little or no fats or sugars.
II. 3–5 servings of vegetables
     One serving is 1 cup of leafy vegetables; ½ cup of other vegetables (cooked or chopped raw); or ¾ cup of vegetable juice.
III. 2–4 servings of fruit
     One serving is 1 apple, banana, or orange; ½ cup of chopped, cooked, or canned fruit; or ¾ cup of fruit juice.
     Use items with little or no added sugar.
IV. 2–3 servings of milk, yogurt, or cheese
     One serving is 1 cup of milk or yogurt; 1 ½ ounces of natural cheese; or 2 ounces of processed cheese.
     Use nonfat or low-fat items such as skimmed or low-fat milk, or cheeses made from these products.
V.   2–3 servings of meat, poultry, fish, dried beans, or nuts
     One serving is 2–3 ounces of lean meat, poultry (white meat without skin), or fish, or 1 cup of beans or nuts.
VI. Use fats, oils, and sugars (including syrup) sparingly.

Eggs have been deleted because of their high cholesterol content (210 mg/egg); however, egg whites are an excellent source of dietary protein.

Thirty minutes per day of exercise is strongly recommended, using both aerobic and strength-building exercises.

Step 2 diets can be effective in significantly lowering LDL cholesterol and reducing CHD risk. Moreover, such diets with sufficient fat restriction may promote weight loss because low-fat diets are less calorically dense than high-fat diets. Information about the USDA Diet Pyramid is provided in Table 8.

Benefit in terms of CHD risk reduction with dietary intervention using restriction of dietary saturated fat and cholesterol often accompanied by increased polyunsaturated fat intake has clearly been shown. Benefit has also been noted with fish oil and vitamin E supplementation, and with diets rich in α-linolenic acid. No benefit has been noted with β-carotene supplementation.

Responsiveness to dietary therapy is related to compliance and specific genetic factors (apo E and apo A-IV phenotype), and should be monitored using LDL cholesterol levels. USDA food pyramid guidelines for the prevention of chronic disease are shown in Table 8. A myriad of dietary intervention studies support the concept of restricting total fat, saturated fat, cholesterol, and sugars, and increasing the intake of cereals, grains, fruits, and vegetables. Diet therapy is often ineffective in the outpatient setting because of decreased compliance and lack of intensive therapy. Often patients are seen only once or twice by the dietitian with little efficacy in lipid lowering. More intensive group approaches or multiple follow-up visits are often required.

VI. DRUG THERAPY GUIDELINES

Levels of LDL cholesterol requiring drug therapy after diet treatment are shown in Tables 4 and 6. Lipid-lowering medications can be divided into two general classes: drugs effective in lowering LDL cholesterol (greater than 15% reduction), and drugs effective in lowering triglyceride levels (greater than 15% reduction). There are currently three classes of agents that meet the LDL cholesterol-lowering criteria: (a) hydroxymethylglutaryl-coenzyme A (HMGCoA) reductase inhibitors (lovastatin, pravastatin, simvastatin, fluvastatin, atorvastatin, and cerivastatin); (b) anion-exchange resins (cholestyramine and colestipol); (c) niacin. Of these three types of drugs, patient compliance with resins and niacin is often poor, whereas with the HMGCoA reductase inhibitors it is generally excellent, as is their efficacy.

Safety and efficacy in CHD risk reduction in large-scale, long-term, placebo-controlled randomized and blinded trials with HMGCoA reductase inhibitors has now been documented in both primary and secondary CHD prevention studies. Angiographic studies also indicate significant benefit with HMGCoA reductase inhibitors in preventing progression of coronary atherosclerosis and CHD risk reduction. Therefore, HMGCoA reductase inhibitors are now the drugs of choice for lowering LDL cholesterol in all subjects because of efficacy, safety, and tolerability.

There are currently four agents that lower triglyceride levels by more than 15%: niacin, gemfibrozil, HMGCoA reductase inhibitors, and fish oil capsules. Niacin and HMGCoA reductase inhibitors also significantly lower LDL cholesterol levels, and all agents raise HDL cholesterol levels modestly. All of these agents also lower CHD risk prospectively. In patients with severe hypertriglyceridemia, gemfibrozil is the drug of choice because of efficacy, tolerability, and because such patients often have diabetes, which can be exacerbated by niacin.

A. Patients with Only Elevated LDL Cholesterol

For all patients with only increased LDL cholesterol, the drugs of choice are HMGCoA reductase inhibitors. If patients cannot tolerate these agents, anion resins, then niacin, or a combination of resins and niacin, should be used. The combination of an HMGCoA reductase inhibitor with an anion-exchange resin is very effective. In postmenopausal women, estrogen replacement is quite effective in lowering LDL cholesterol and raising HDL cholesterol, but estrogens should not be used in patients with hypertriglyceridemia because they raise triglyceride levels. In these cases the estrogen patch can be used, and the hypertriglyceridemia treated with other medications. Estrogen use has been associated with a significant reduction in CHD mortality in postmenopausal women. In postmenopausal women with an intact uterus, estrogen must be combined with progesterone. A dose of either 0.625 mg or 0.3 mg of conjugated equine estrogen and 2.5 mg of progesterone given continuously is generally well tolerated. However, in a recent study in postmenopausal CHD patients, no significant benefit in CHD risk reduction was noted using this regimen versus placebo. In contrast, HMGCoA reductase inhibitors have been very effective in decreasing CHD risk in postmenopausal women.

B. Patients with Elevated LDL Cholesterol and Elevated Triglycerides

For patients with elevations in both LDL cholesterol and triglycerides ($>$ 200 mg/dL or 2.3 mmol/L), the drugs of choice are HMGCoA reductase inhibitors. For patients who cannot tolerate these agents, niacin or fibric acid derivatives can be considered.

C. Patients with Hypertriglyceridemia and Normal LDL Cholesterol

For patients with hypertriglyceridemia ($>$ 200 mg/dL) and normal LDL cholesterol levels, there are as yet no clear medication guidelines. However, diet, exercise, and weight control, as well as elimination of secondary causes of elevated triglycerides are encouraged. In patients with triglycerides in excess of 1000 mg/dL while on a restricted diet, gemfibrozil to reduce the risk of pancreatitis is recommended. The physician should make sure that these patients are not taking oral estrogens, thiazides or β-adrenergic blockers, using alcohol, or have uncontrolled diabetes mellitus. Caloric and fat restriction is also important in these patients. The drug of choice in such patients is generally gemfibrozil because most have glucose intolerance. In the absence of glucose intolerance, niacin can be tried. In patients in whom these agents are not effective, or if additional triglyceride reduction is needed, fish oil capsules (1 g) at a dose of three to five capsules twice daily may be effective in lowering triglycerides.

D. Patients with Moderate Hypertriglyceridemia or Low HDL Cholesterol

In patients with moderate hypertriglyceridemia ($\geq$ 200 mg/dL), especially in those with HDL cholesterol deficiency, lifestyle changes, including weight reduction and an exercise program, are very helpful, as are cessation of smoking and β-adrenergic blockers. Control of blood glucose concentration is very important because these patients are often diabetic. If patients have established CHD, the use of either an HMGCoA reductase inhibitor, niacin, or gemfibrozil should be considered to normalize their lipid levels. The goal of therapy in CHD patients is to lower their LDL cholesterol value below 100 mg/dL. Some experts also recommend reduction of triglycerides to less than 200 mg/dL, and increasing their HDL cholesterol to over 40 mg/dL if possible, and decreasing their total cholesterol/HDL cholesterol ratio to less than 5.0. In the absence of heart disease, only lifestyle modification (diet and exercise) is currently recommended in patients with hypertriglyceridemia or HDL cholesterol deficiency. It has also been suggested that the goal of therapy in such patients with diabetes should be to lower the LDL cholesterol to less than 100 mg/dL, and in this setting atorvastatin is the drug of choice, because of its LDL and triglyceride-lowering effects.

VII. DRUGS

A. HMGCoA Reductase Inhibitors

These drugs inhibit HMGCoA reductase, the rate-limiting enzyme in cholesterol biosynthesis, decrease LDL apo B production, and decrease plasma LDL cholesterol by 25–60% at maximal doses. These agents can also enhance LDL clearance and are now the drugs of choice of lipid management because of efficacy, safety, and tolerability.

1. Lovastatin

Lovastatin therapy is usually started at 20 mg daily at suppertime, and can be increased to 40 mg daily, 20 mg twice daily, or even 40 mg twice daily. Reductions in LDL cholesterol of up to 40% have been reported at maximal doses. It is a fungal metabolite, and is produced by fermentation. It was approved in the United States in 1988. CHD risk reduction of 25% was documented in the Monitored Atherosclerosis Regression Study (MARS) and the Canadian Coronary Athero-sclerosis Intervention Trial (CCAIT) (13,33). In the AFCAPS/TEXCAPS Trial, lovastatin at either 20 or 40 mg/day lowered CHD risk 35% prospectively in 6605 men older than 45 and women older than 55, with LDL cholesterol of 130–190 mg/dL and HDL cholesterol values less than 50 mg/dL (17).

2. Pravastatin

Pravastatin therapy is usually started at 10 or 20 mg daily at bedtime, and can be increased to 40 mg. Its structure is similar to lovastatin, except it is given as the open acid form and has a hydroxyl group attached to it, making it a more polar compound with greater liver selectivity. It is a fungal metabolite, and is produced by fermentation. It was approved in the United States in 1991. It has been successfully given in combination with gemfibrozil as well as with cyclospo-rine. Pravastatin at 40 mg/day has been reported to lower LDL-C 28%, total mortality 46%, fatal and nonfatal CHD 62%, and stroke 62% in over 1800 patients with atherosclerosis (PLAC I, PLAC II; REGRESS, KAPS) (14). Pravastatin at 40 mg/day reduced LDL-C 26%, total mortality 22%, fatal and nonfatal myocardial infarction (MI) 31%, and need for angioplasty or bypass surgery 37% in middle-aged men with moderate hypercholesterolemia without documented CHD in the large ($n = 6595$) prospective West Scotland Study (32). Pravastatin at 40 mg/day lowered LDL-C 26%, fatal and nonfatal MI 24%, bypass 26%, angioplasty 23%, fatal MI 37%, and stroke 31% in post-MI patients with LDL cholesterol values in the range of 115–174 mg/dL, (mean 137 mg/dL) in the Cholesterol and Recurrent Events (CARE) trial ($n = 4159$) (30). This study also indicated no significant benefit if baseline LDL-C values were less than 125 mg/dL, with no significant benefit on total mortality. In the large prospective Australian LIPID trial, 9013 men and women with CHD with total cholesterol values between 155 and 271 mg/dL were randomized to pravastatin 40 mg/day or placebo. Total, CHD, and stroke mortality were significantly reduced by 23, 24, and 20% in the drug group versus the placebo group (24).

3. Simvastatin

Simvastatin therapy is usually started at 10 mg at suppertime, and can be increased to 20 or 40 mg. Its structure is similar to lovastatin, except that it has an additional methyl group. It is a fungal metabolite, and is produced by fermentation. Simvastatin at a dosage of 20–40 mg/day has been shown to decrease LDL-C 35%, total mortality 30%, nonfatal and fatal CHD 34%, stroke 37%, and PTCA or CABG 37% in CHD patients with moderate hypercholesterolemia in the large (n = 4444) prospective Scandinavian Simvastatin Survival Study (4 S Study; 31).

4. Fluvastatin

Fluvastatin is structurally different from the other agents, and was the first synthetic HMGCoA reductase inhibitor. It is available in 20 and 40 mg tablets, and treatment is usually started at 20 mg/day and can be increased to the maximal dose of 40 mg. Fluvastatin lowered LDL-C by 22% at 20 mg/day and 25% in familial hypercholesterolemic patients at 40 mg/day. Fluvastatin was evaluated in the recent Lipoprotein and Coronary Atherosclerosis Study (LCAS) in which 429 men and women were placed on placebo or 20 mg twice daily of fluvastatin. LDL-C was reduced by 27%, triglyceride by 10%, and HDL-C was increased by 6%, as compared with baseline. There was significantly less angiographic progression in coronary arteries in the fluvastatin group than in the control group (20).

5. Atorvastatin

Atorvastatin is a synthetic HMGCoA reductase inhibitor, available in 10-, 20-, and 40-mg tablets, with reductions in LDL-C of 39, 43, and 50%, respectively. The starting dosage is 10 mg/day. The maximal dose is 80 mg, with LDL-C reductions of 60% and triglyceride reductions of 40% being observed at this dose. This new agent also appears to be quite effective in lowering triglyceride levels in hypertriglyceridemic patients. In the recent AVERT trial, CHD patients with one to two vessel disease, randomized to atorvastatin 80 mg/day versus angioplasty, experienced a 36% reduction in CHD endpoints over 1.5 years, indicating great benefit from very aggressive lipid lowering.

6. Cerivastatin

Cerivastatin is a new synthetic HMGCoA reductase inhibitor available in 0.2, 0.3 mg, and 0.4 mg tablets, resulting in LDL cholesterol reductions of 25–37%.

The key with all HMGCoA reductase inhibitors is to begin with a low dosage regimen (10–20 mg/day) and gradually titrate the dosage upward, as the effect may be maximized at 20 mg of any of these agents, instead of 40 mg. These drugs are generally well tolerated, but may occasionally cause liver enzyme elevation (1–2%); significant creatine phosphokinase (CPK) elevation, with myaglias and myositis (0.1%); and gastrointestinal side effects. Carefully controlled studies indicate these agents do not cause cataracts, sleep problems, or daytime performance disturbances. Pravastatin use may be associated with less myositis, and should be considered in patients who have developed this problem with other statins. Fluvastatin is the least expensive of these compounds, but only 25% reductions in LDL cholesterol have been reported at a dosage of 40 mg/day. Atorvastatin appears to be the most potent in terms of LDL cholesterol lowering, with a 60% reduction being noted at 80 mg/day, and also is quite effective in lowering triglyceride levels. Pravastatin has been the best-studied agent, with large-scale primary and secondary prevention studies documenting 39% reductions at 10 mg/day. Large-scale studies are now also available for lovastatin and simvastatin documenting significant benefit in CHD risk reduction and efficacy.

B. Anion-Exchange Resins

Cholestyramine and colestipol are anion-exchange resins that bind bile acids, increase conversion of liver cholesterol to bile acids, and up-regulate LDL receptors in liver. This results in an increase in LDL catabolism, and a decrease in plasma LDL cholesterol by about 20%. Side effects include bloating and constipation, elevation of triglycerides, and interference with the absorption of digoxin, tetracycline, thyroxine, phenylbutazone, and warfarin (Coumadin) (give drugs 1 h before or 4 h after resin). Cholestyramine (4 g packets or scoops) or colestipol (5 g scoops) treatment can be started at one scoop or packet twice per day and gradually increased to two scoops twice per day (the scoops are half the price of the packets) or two scoops three times daily. Colestipol is available in 1-g tablet form as well, and a standard dosage is four to eight tablets twice daily. Constipation may require treatment. Cholestyramine (6 scoops/day) lowered LDL cholesterol by 12.5% and reduced CHD risk prospectively by 19% over 7 years in middle-aged, asymptomatic, hypercholesterolemic men in the large (n = 3806) prospective, randomized, placebo-controlled Lipid Research Clinics Coronary Primary Prevention Trial (LRC-CPPT; 22,23). Total mortality was reduced by 6%, angina by 20%, and need for bypass by 21%. Most subjects receiving the active medication took far less than the dose prescribed. The resins are now second-line drugs.

C. Niacin

Niacin decreases VLDL and LDL production and raises HDL cholesterol values by 20%. Niacin therapy should be started at 100 mg twice daily with meals and gradually increased to 1 g two or three times per day with meals (some authorities recommend doses as high as 9 g/day). Side effects include flushing, gastric irritation, and elevations of uric acid, glucose, and liver enzymes in some patients. Niacin should not be used in patients with liver disease, a history of an ulcer, or in diabetic patients not receiving insulin, and is now a second-line drug. Niacin lowers total cholesterol levels by 10% and reduces the recurrence of myocardial infarction by 20% after a 5-year period of administration in men with CHD in the Coronary Drug Project involving 8341 subjects randomized to placebo, niacin, clofibrate, *d*-thyroxine, or estrogen (16). The use of niacin was also associated with an 11% reduction in all-cause mortality 10 years after cessation of niacin. No significant benefit and, in some cases, excess mortality was associated with the other therapies. Niacin in combination with clofibrate reduced total mortality 26% and CHD mortality 36% in CHD patients ($n = 555$) as compared with usual care in the Stockholm Ischemic Heart Disease Study over a 5-year period (15). A new long-acting once-daily niacin product (Niaspan) is now available with 375-, 500-, 750-, and 1000-mg tablets, with the starting dosage being 375 mg/day and the standard dosage being 2 g/day.

D. Gemfibrozil

Gemfibrozil is given at a dosage of 600 mg twice daily, and is generally well tolerated. The drug is very effective in lowering triglycerides and VLDL cholesterol by 35%, by decreasing production and enhancing breakdown of VLDL. It usually lowers LDL cholesterol by 5–15% and increases HDL cholesterol by 5–15%. Rarely, patients may develop gastrointestinal symptoms, muscle cramps, or intermittent indigestion. It should not be used in patients with renal insufficiency, and is also known to potentiate the action of warfarin (Coumadin). The drug may raise LDL cholesterol levels in hypertriglyceridemic patients. Gemfibrozil has reduced CHD risk (fatal and nonfatal MI) prospectively by 34% over 5 years in middle-aged, asymptomatic, (non-HDL cholesterol > 200 mg/dL) hypercholesterolemic men ($n = 4081$) as determined in the prospective, randomized, placebo-controlled Helsinki Heart Study (18,25,26). CHD risk reduction was associated with a rise in HDL cholesterol and a lowering of LDL cholesterol, but not that of triglycerides. No reduction in total mortality was noted, and there were nonsignificant increases in deaths from hemorrhagic stroke, accidents, and violence (homicide and suicide). In the recent Veterans Administration High-Density Lipoprotein Intervention Trial (VA HIT), 2531 men with CHD and an HDL cholesterol less than 40 mg/dL, triglycerides less than 300 mg/dL, and LDL cholesterol less than 140 mg/dL were randomized to gemfibrozil 600 mg twice daily versus placebo. Of those patients, 25% were diabetic and 50% had elevated insulin levels. Use of gemfibrozil was associated with a 22% reduction (p < 0.000) in CHD events over a 5-year period, associated with a 7% increase in HDL cholesterol and a 34% reduction in triglyceride levels relative to placebo (29).

E. Fenofibrate

Fenofibrate micronized is a fibric acid derivative that has recently been made available in the United States for the treatment of triglycerides above 1000 mg/dL (type V hyperlipidemia). It is as effective as gemfibrozil in lowering triglycerides and raising HDL. Fenofibrate has also been shown to lower LDL cholesterol by 15% in type IIB hyperlipidemia. Presently fenofibrate is being evaluated in the Diabetes Atherosclerosis Intervention Study, an angiographic study to determine if there is a benefit to using fenofibrate as an intervention for coronary heart disease in a diabetic population. The standard dose is 201 mg (three 67 mg capsules given with food) daily. If there is significant renal insufficiency, fenofibrate should be given at a reduced rate and is also known to potentiate the action of warfarin (Coumadin).

F. Probucol

Probucol is an antioxidant given at a dosage of 500 mg twice daily, and is a second-line drug that lowers LDL cholesterol 10–15%. It can be used in familial hypercholesterolemia for increasing nonreceptor LDL catabolism. It may cause gastrointestinal side effects. The drug also lowers HDL cholesterol by 15–25% by decreasing its production. Long-term safety and efficacy in CHD risk reduction has not been established. A recent prospective angiographic study did not demonstrate significant benefit with probucol. However, probucol may have significant benefit in reducing restenosis after angioplasty.

G. Combination Therapies

The use of HMGCoA reductase inhibitors and resins together are very effective, as are niacin and resins in lowering LDL cholesterol (50–60% reduction). The combination of gemfibrozil and reductase inhibitors is not recommended because myositis incidence is quite high with the lovastatin–gemfibrozil combination. If this combination is used, it should be used with caution, and CPK levels should be monitored. However, pravastatin and gemfibrozil in combination have been efficacious in lipid lowering and well tolerated. Niacin and reductase inhibitors are also effective, but the incidence of significant liver enzyme elevation is about 10%, so this combination should be used with caution. Gemfibrozil with either fish oil capsules or niacin can be used to lower triglycerides. The new HMGCoA reductase inhibitor atorvastatin obviates the need for combination therapy for additional LDL cholesterol lowering or triglyceride lowering in many patients because of its striking efficacy.

VIII. FAMILIAL LIPOPROTEIN DISORDERS

A. Familial Combined Hyperlipidemia

By far the most common of these disorders is familial combined hyperlipidemia in which affected kindred members may have elevated LDL cholesterol alone (> 190 mg/dL or 4.9 mmol/L), elevated triglycerides alone (> 200 mg/dL or 2.3 mmol/L), or elevations of both parameters. Both abnormalities must be present in the family to make the diagnosis. These patients overproduce VLDL apo B-100, but not triglyceride. They also often have decreased HDL cholesterol values owing to enhanced HDL degradation. The apo E-IV genotype is a predisposing genotype for this disorder. Approximately 15% of patients with premature CHD have this disorder. Treatment consists of diet, and if necessary, use of reductase inhibitors, niacin, gemfibrozil, or combinations of these medications with anion-exchange resins. Sporadic or polygenic hypercholesterolemia is also quite common.

B. Familial Hypercholesterolemia

Isolated elevations of LDL cholesterol are found in patients with a disorder known as familial hypercholesterolemia, often associated with tendinous xanthomas. These patients generally have marked hypercholesterolemia (in excess of 350 mg/dL or 9.1 mmol/L) with normal triglyceride values and may have defects at the LDL receptor locus or abnormalities of the apo B protein. The major metabolic abnormality in these individuals is an impaired ability to catabolize LDL. Approximately 3% of patients with premature CHD have this disorder. Treatment generally consists of diet and a combination of medications (HMG CoA reductase inhibitors, resins, and niacin).

C. Familial Dysbetalipoproteinemia (Type III Hyperlipoproteinemia)

A much rarer form of combined elevations of cholesterol and triglyceride is familial dysbetalipoproteinemia (type III hyperlipoproteinemia) in which affected subjects have accumulations of chylomicron remnants and VLDL in the fasting state. These patients usually are homozygous for a mutation in the apo E protein (apo E-II/II phenotype) or rarely have apo E deficiency, resulting in defective hepatic clearance of chylomicron and VLDL remnants as well as increased VLDL production. They may also have tuboeruptive and planar xanthomas. Precise diagnosis requires quantitation of lipoprotein cholesterol values following ultracentrifugation and apo E genotyping. Treatment consists of diet, niacin, gemfibrozil, or an HMGCoA reductase inhibitor. These patients are also very responsive to gemfibrozil or niacin. Patients with both familial combined hyperlipidemia and familial dysbetalipoproteinemia often have obesity, glucose intolerance, and hyperuricemia.

D. Familial Hypertriglyceridemic States

By far the most common of these disorders is familial hypertriglyceridemia (triglycerides > 200 mg/dL), an autosomal dominant disorder in which obesity, glucose intolerance, hyperuricemia, and HDL cholesterol deficiency are often present. The disorder is associated with overproduction of hepatic VLDL triglyceride but not VLDL apo B-100. Some patients may have defects in VLDL clearance as well. CHD risk appears to be increased in those kindreds in whom HDL cholesterol deficiency is also present. Approximately 15% of patients with premature CHD appear to have this disorder. HDL cholesterol levels are usually low in these subjects because of enhanced degradation. Treatment with diet, exercise, and abstinence from alcohol and estrogens is recommended. In patients with CHD, niacin, gemfibrozil, or reductase inhibitors can be used to optimize lipid values.

E. Severe Hypertriglyceridemia

Severe hypertriglyceridemia (triglyceride values > 1000 mg/dL) is occasionally observed in middle-aged or elderly individuals who are obese and have glucose intolerance and hyperuricemia. These subjects usually have familial hypertriglyceridemia or familial combined hyperlipidemia that is exacerbated by other factors, such as obesity and diabetes mellitus. These patients generally also have HDL cholesterol deficiency and may develop lipemia retinalis and eruptive xanthomas. They are at increased risk for developing pancreatitis owing to triglyceride deposition in the pancreas and may have paresthesias and emotional lability. These patients often have delayed chylomicron and VLDL cholesterol clearance and excess VLDL production. Treatment consists of a calorie-restricted step 2 diet. In patients with diabetes mellitus, blood glucose is controlled as tightly as possible. Medications that are effective in lowering the triglycerides to less than 1000 mg/dL in these patients, to reduce their risk of pancreatitis, include gemfibrozil or fish oil capsules (six to ten capsules per day).

Patients who have severe hypertriglyceridemia in childhood or early adulthood and who are not obese often have a deficiency of the enzyme lipoprotein lipase or its activator protein (apo C-II), resulting in markedly impaired removal of triglyceride. These patients are at increased risk for recurrent pancreatitis; it is important to restrict their dietary fat to less than 20% of calories. Niacin or gemfibrozil, or both, are generally ineffective in these patients. However, fish oil capsules (six per day) may occasionally be helpful in certain patients to keep their triglyceride levels below 1000 mg/dL and minimize the risk of pancreatitis.

F. Lipoprotein(a) Excess

Elevated Lp(a) levels (> 30 mg/dL for total mass or > 10 mg/dL for cholesterol) have been associated with premature CHD in most studies. Lp(a) is a highly heritable trait, not lowered by diet or standard cholesterol-lowering medications except niacin or hormonal replacement therapy. Familial Lp(a) excess is common in patients with premature CHD. In such patients, treatment with niacin is warranted to lower Lp(a), as it reduces CHD morbidity and mortality. Routine screening in the general population cannot be recommended at this time.

G. Familial Hypoalphalipoproteinemia

Isolated deficiency of HDL cholesterol (below the tenth percentile of normal) can be genetic, and it is then known as familial hypoalphalipoproteinemia. This disorder is found in approximately 4% of patients with premature CHD. Treatment consists of diet, weight reduction if indicated, and an exercise program. In patients with CHD, treatment with HMGCoA reductase inhibitors to optimize LDL cholesterol levels is the current treatment of choice.

IX. CONCLUSIONS

Treatment directed at lowering elevated LDL cholesterol with diet and, if necessary, with HMGCoA reductase inhibitors has been effective in reducing CHD morbidity and mortality, especially in patients with CHD with an LDL cholesterol level of 130 mg/dL or higher. In this setting, reduction in stroke risk has also been noted. The cornerstone of diet remains restriction of saturated fat to less than 7% of calories and cholesterol to less than 200 mg/day. Diets enriched in α-linolenic acid or fish oil also appear to be quite beneficial. β-Carotene supplementation has not been beneficial in CHD risk reduction, and one study suggests benefit from vitamin E supplementation, the data are very limited. A new HMGCoA reductase inhibitor, atorvastatin, has recently been introduced and appears to have great promise because of greater efficacy in lowering both LDL cholesterol and triglyceride levels than the other "statins." The goal of therapy in CHD patients and diabetes, in addition to control of other CHD risk factors, is to keep the LDL cholesterol level less than 100 mg/dL. A recent trial indicates benefit of gemfibrozil in male CHD patients with low HDL cholesterol and normal LDL cholesterol. Goals for HDL cholesterol-raising and triglyceride- and Lp(a)-lowering await the results of present and future prospective studies. In patients with established CHD or diabetes it would not be unreasonable to try to lower triglycerides to less than 200 mg/dL and Lp(a) cholesterol to less than 10 mg/dL.

REFERENCES

General

1. American Diabetes Association. Management of dyslipidemia in adults with diabetes. Diabetes Care 22(suppl 1):S56–S59, 1999.
2. American Heart Association. Heart and Stroke Facts. Statistical Supplement. Dallas, TX: AHA, 1998:1–22.

3. Fredrickson DS, Levy RI, Lees RS. Fat transport in lipoproteins—an integrated approach to mechanisms and disorders. N Engl J Med 276:34–44, 94–103, 148–156, 215–225, 273–281, 1967.

4. Genest JJ Jr, Martin-Munley SS, McNamara JR, Ordovas JM, Jenner JL, Myers RH, Silberman SR, Wilson PWF, Salem DN, Schaefer EJ. Familial lipoprotein disorders in patients with premature coronary artery disease. Circulation 85:2025–2033, 1992.

5. Schaefer EJ, Levy RI. The pathogenesis and management of lipoprotein disorders. N Engl J Med 312:1300–1310, 1985.

Panels and Recommendations

6. Expert Panel. Report of the National Cholesterol Education Program Expert Panel on Detection, Evaluation, and Treatment of High Blood Cholesterol in Adults. Arch Intern Med 148:36–69, 1988.

7. Expert Panel. Summary of the second report of the National Cholesterol Education Program (NCEP) Expert Panel on Detection, Evaluation, and Treatment of High Blood Cholesterol in Adults (Adult Treatment Panel II). JAMA 269:3015–3023, 1993.

8. Expert Panel. Second report of the Expert Panel on Detection, Evaluation, and Treatment of High Blood Cholesterol in Adults (Adult Treatment Panel II). Circulation 89:1329–1445, 1994.

9. Expert Panel. Blood cholesterol levels in children and adolescents. National Institutes of Health Publication No. 91-2732, 1-119, Washington DC: US Government Printing Office, 1990.

10. Expert Panel. Population strategies for blood cholesterol reduction. National Institutes of Health Publication No. 90-3046, I-39, Washington, DC: U.S. Government Printing Office, 1990.

11. NIH Consensus Conference. Lowering blood cholesterol to prevent heart disease. JAMA 253:2080–2086, 1985.

12. NIH Consensus Conference. Triglycerides, HDL cholesterol, and coronary heart disease. JAMA 269:505–510, 1993.

Trials

13. Blankenhorn DH, Azen SP, Kramsch DM, Mack WJ, Cashin-Hemphill L, Hodis HN, DeBoer LW, Mahrer PR, Mosteller MJ, Vailas LI, Alaupovic P, Hirsch LJ. Coronary angiographic changes with lovastatin therapy. The Monitored Atherosclerosis Regression Study (MARS). Ann Intern Med 1119:969–976, 1993.

14. Byington RP, Jukema JW, Salonen JT, et al. Reduction in cardiovascular events during pravastatin therapy: pooled analysis of clinical events of the Pravastatin Atherosclerosis Intervention Program. Circulation 92:2419–2425, 1995.

15. Carlson LA, Rosenhamer G. Reduction of mortality in the Stockholm Ischemic Heart Disease Study by combined treatment with clofibrate and nicotinic acid. Acta Med Scand 223:405–418, 1988.

16. Coronary Drug Project Research Group. Clofibrate and niacin in coronary heart disease. JAMA 231:360–381, 1975.

17. Downs JR, Clearfield M, Weis S, Whitney E, Shapiro DR, Beere PA, Langendorfer A, Stein EA, Kruyer W, Gotto AM Jr, for the ARCAPS/TexCAPS Research Group. Primary prevention of acute coronary events with lovastatin in men and women with average cholesterol levels. Results of AFCAPS/TexCAPS. JAMA 279:1615–1622, 1998.

18. Frick MH, Elo O, Haapa K, Heinonen OP, Heinsalmi P, Helo P, Huttunen JK, Kaitaniemi P, Koskinen P, Manninen V, Maenpaa H, Malkonen M, Mantari M, Norola S, Pasternak A, Pikkaranen J, Romo M, Sjomblom T, Nikkila EA. Helsinki Heart Study: primary prevention trial with gemfibrozil in middle-aged men with dyslipidemia. N Engl J Med 317:1237–1245, 1987.

19. Gordon DJ, Knoke J, Probstfeld JL, Superko R, Tyroler HA. High density lipoprotein cholesterol and coronary heart disease in hypercholesterolemic men. The Lipid Research Clinics Coronary Primary Prevention Trial. Circulation 74:1217–1225, 1986.

20. Herd JA, West MS, Ballantyne CM, et al. The Lipoprotein and Coronary Atherosclerosis Study (LCAS): design, methods, and baseline data of a trial of fluvastatin in patients without severe hypercholesterolemia. Am J Cardiol 80:278–284, 1997.

21. Jukema JW, Bruschke AVG, van Boven AJ, et al, on behalf of the REGRESS Study Group. Effects of lipid lowering by pravastatin on progression and regression of coronary artery disease in symptomatic men with normal to moderately elevated serum cholesterol levels: the Regression Growth Evaluation Statin Study (RE-GRESS). Circulation. 91:2528–2540, 1995.

22. The Lipid Research Clinics Program. The Lipid Research Clinics Coronary Primary Prevention Trial. I. Reduction in incidence of coronary heart disease. JAMA 251:351–364, 1984.

23. The Lipid Research Clinics Program. The Lipid Research Clinics Coronary Primary Prevention Trial. II. The relationship of reduction in incidence of coronary heart disease to cholesterol lowering. JAMA 251:365–374, 1984.

24. Lipid Study Group. Prevention of cardiovascular events and death with pravastatin in patients with coronary heart disease and a broad range of initial cholesterol levels. N Engl J Med 339:1349–1357, 1998.

25. Manninen V, Elo O, Frick MH, Haapak K, Heinonen OP, Heinsalmi P, Helo P, Huttunen JK, Kaitanceim P, Koskinen P, Maenpaa H, Malkonen M, Mantari M, Norola S, Pasternak A, Pikkaranen J, Romo V, Sjomslom T, Nikkila K. Lipid alterations and decline in the incidence of coronary heart disease in the Helsinki Heart Study. JAMA 260:641–651, 1988.

26. Manninen V, Tenkanen L, Koskinen P, Huttunen JK, Martarri M, Heinonen OP, Frick MH. Joint effects of triglyceride, LDL cholesterol, and HDL cholesterol concentrations on coronary heart disease risk in the Helsinki Heart Study. Implication for treatment. Circulation 85:37–45, 1992.

27. MAAS Investigators. Effect of simvastatin on coronary atheroma: the Multicentre Anti-Atheroma Study (MAAS). Lancet 344:633–638, 1994.

28. Pitt B, Mancini GBJ, Ellis SG, Rosman HS, Park J-S, McGovern ME, for the PLAC I Investigators. Pravastatin Limitation of Atherosclerosis in the Coronary Arteries

(PLAC I): reduction in atherosclerosis progression and clinical events. J Am Coll Cardiol 26:1133–1139, 1995.

29. Rubin HB, Robins SR, et al. Results of the Veterans Administration High Density Lipoprotein Intervention Trial (HIT) with gemfibrozil. Circulation II:328, 1998.

30. Sacks FM, Pfeffer MA, Moye LA, et al., for the Cholesterol and Recurrent Events Trial Investigators. The effect of pravastatin on coronary events after myocardial infarction in patients with average cholesterol levels. N Engl J Med 335:1001–1009, 1996.

31. Scandinavian Simvastatin Survival Study Group. Randomized trial of cholesterol lowering in 4444 patients with coronary heart disease: the Scandinavian Simvastatin Survival Study (4S). Lancet 344:1383–1389, 1994.

32. Shepherd J, Cobbe SM, Ford I, et al. Prevention of coronary heart disease with pravastatin in men with hypercholesterolemia. N Engl J Med 333:1301–1307, 1995.

33. Waters D, Higginson L, Gladstone P, et al. Effects of monotherapy with an HMGCo-A reductase inhibitor on the progression of coronary atherosclerosis as assessed by serial quantitative arteriography: the Canadian Coronary Atherosclerosis Intervention Trial. Circulation 89:959–968, 1994.

34. Watts GF, Lewis B, Brunt JNH, Lewis ES, LoHart DJ, Smith LDR, Mann JI, Swan AV. Effects on coronary artery disease of lipid lowering diet, a diet plus cholestyramine in the St. Thomas Atherosclerosis Regression Study (STARS). Lancet 339: 563–569, 1992.

31
Hypoglycemia

Patrick J. Boyle
University of New Mexico Health Sciences Center, Albuquerque, New Mexico

I. INTRODUCTION

Hypoglycemia is a common limiting factor that may prevent patients with either type 1 or type 2 diabetes from achieving tight metabolic control over their disease. The mechanisms leading to low glucose concentrations diverge somewhat between the two types of the disease, but the net result is that during critical deficits of glucose provision to the brain, the patient falls into a coma or experiences a seizure.

II. GLUCOSE COUNTERREGULATION

The critical problem with systemic glucose concentrations falling below the normal range is that the brain, an obligate glucose consumer, is ultimately unable to conduct its fundamental functions. Under normal conditions, the brain imports roughly three times more sugar than it needs from the circulation across the blood–brain barrier. At some critical glucose concentration, however, the brain receives inadequate glucose to support its metabolic needs. Centers in the hypothalamus are likely responsible for sensing the fall in systemic glucose concentration, and when a critical glucose threshold is reached (approximately 70 mg/dL), a release of epinephrine and glucagon is triggered. Thus, minimal perturbations in glucose homeostasis lead to the release of hormones that initiate physiological countermeasures that prevent worsening hypoglycemia and restore normal glucose concentrations (so-called counterregulatory hormones). Epinephrine release causes many of the classic symptoms of hypoglycemia: shakiness, trembling, nervousness, tachycardia, and such. Additionally, epinephrine has two other important functions in responding to hypoglycemia: (a) it drives glycogen breakdown to glucose and stimulates gluconeogenesis in the liver, thereby increasing the delivery of glucose to the circulation; and (b) it decreases peripheral glucose uptake by muscle, further preserving brain glucose uptake. Under normal conditions, increased glucagon release is the dominant counterregulatory hormone in terms of restoring glucose homeostasis so that epinephrine release is not crucial. However, in patients with either type 1 or type 2 diabetes, glucagon secretion in response to hypoglycemia is defective, and in this setting epinephrine secretion becomes the critical counterregulatory factor.

A. Type 1 Diabetes

Glucagon responses to hypoglycemia are markedly impaired in type 1 diabetes. The reason is not totally clear, but appears to be an acquired defect that is related to the loss of beta-cell function. Hypoglycemia normally begets a raised glucagon level through attenuation of the local (paracrine) regulatory effect of intraislet insulin to inhibit glucagon secretion; the hypoglycemia-induced lowering of insulin release thus results in increased glucagon secretion. In type 1 diabetes, beta cells are obliterated by a selective autoimmune process that leaves the glucagon-producing alpha cells of the islet relatively intact. The absent glucagon response to hypoglycemia results from loss of the paracrine influence of intraislet insulinemia; in these patients, insulinemia results totally from exogenously injected insulin, which is unaffected by hypoglycemia so that alpha cells remain under tonic inhibition by the high systemic insulin concentration that is causing the hypoglycemia.

B. Type 2 Diabetes

Patients with type 2 diabetes do not appear to have as substantial a risk of hypoglycemia as type 1 diabetes. Several clinical trials that have attempted to achieve near-normalization of glucose concentrations in patients with type 2 diabetes have noted remarkably few hypoglycemic events. Two factors are relevant to this phenomenon. First, these studies generally failed to normalize the hemoglobin A_{1c}; thus, it remains to be determined whether or not hypoglycemia is a serious problem in very tightly controlled patients. Second, and likely more important, the average patient with type 2 diabetes is quite insulin resistant with insulin secretory responses that are reasonably intact because substantial numbers of functioning beta cells are present in this form of diabetes. Under these circumstances, patients with type 2 diabetes hypersecrete endogenous insulin to compensate for the insulin resistance, and a fall in the glucose concentration to the normal range or slightly below leads to a feedback decrease in endogenous insulin release, causing glucagon secretion, although in quantitative terms the response is not fully normal (relative defect in the glucagon response as opposed to no response in type 1 diabetes). This is not to say that persons with type 2 diabetes are fully resistant to hypoglycemia, especially if a sulfonylurea is used alone or in combination with any of the other active glucose-lowering compounds. In that case, the insulinotropic effect of sulfonylureas drives beta cells to release insulin despite the hypoglycemia. Still, a large study performed in patients with type 2 diabetes in Veterans Administrations Hospitals which extensively use sulfonylureas, observed a frequency of severe hypoglycemia that was less than 1% of that seen in the Diabetes Control and Complications Trial (intensive insulin treatment trial done in patients with type 1 diabetes, which is discussed in Chap. 21). Furthermore, hypoglycemia was also relatively uncommon in the recently released United Kingdom Prospective Diabetes Study (intensive treatment trial in type 2 diabetes patients', see Chap. 9). Once again, the glycemic control in these studies was not pushed into the normal range, hence, it remains to be seen if these patients would have been more prone to hypoglycemia had normoglycemia been achieved.

C. Hypoglycemic Unawareness

Besides the loss of an appropriate glucagon response to hypoglycemia, there are other issues that contribute to the increased propensity for hypoglycemia in type 1 diabetes. When recurrent hypoglycemia is present for a multitude of reasons, such as imprecise insulin regimens or doses, fluctuating eating habits, alcohol, exercise, or whatever, the brain is faced with a special dilemma. Because it must have an adequate glucose supply to function, it has developed the functional capacity to enhance its efficiency of glucose uptake from the circulation in response to recurrent hypoglycemia. Glucose is transported from the circulation across the blood–brain barrier by the insulin-independent glucose transport protein, GLUT1. The ambient glucose concentration plays a key role in determining the amount of this protein that is present on the capillary endothelial surface. Isolated brain capillary cells demonstrate an increased amount of this protein when they are glucose-starved. As a result, animals that are exposed to chronic hypoglycemia have an increased ability to extract glucose from the circulation into the brain. In healthy humans, brain glucose uptake is augmented by recurrent hypoglycemia in as little as 56 h. Moreover, in patients with type 1 diabetes, the lower the glycosylated hemoglobin, the greater is their efficiency to extract glucose from the circulation so that at glucose concentrations that would normally induce epinephrine release, sufficient glucose is transported into the brain by the increased number of transporters so that brain energy metabolism is maintained.

Clinically, this increased ability to extract glucose is associated with the development of an unawareness to hypoglycemia—the patient now tolerates subnormal glucose concentrations without any of the standard autonomic symptoms of sweating and shaking because the brain is not really hypoglycemic and has no reason to signal for epinephrine release. Thus, the hypoglycemia is no longer "perceived" by the patient. Likewise, cognitive abilities are relatively well preserved, and the patient functions as though his or her glucose concentration were normal. As such, this increased ability to extract glucose from the circulation into the brain is useful, given that hypoglycemia is likely to happen again. However, from the standpoint of patient safety, there is only a narrow window of hypoglycemia before a critically low concentration is reached that shuts down normal brain function, and their loss of the perception of hypoglycemia often becomes a crucial disabling feature of their disease. Patients can be retrained to recognize subtle warning signs that hypoglycemia is developing, such as minor tingling around the lips or becoming more emotional. However, one disturbing issue is that often by the time the patient realizes they are hypoglycemic, insufficient time remains between their treating the insulin reaction and for adequate food absorption before the critical reduction in systemic glucose concentration is reached that results in loss of consciousness. Often a spouse or significant other becomes the best judge of hypoglycemia and may simply note a distant look in the patient's eye or the onset of typical idiosyncratic behaviors (blinking, loss of word choice, agitation, deeper breathing). The risk of hypoglycemia in susceptible persons must be viewed cautiously in terms of how it affects daily living tasks, such as driving, operating heavy equipment, flying airplanes, and such. An important observation here is that patients with well-controlled diabetes who monitor frequently during more-demanding activities are often able to troubleshoot hypoglycemia before it occurs.

Fortunately, the development of hypoglycemia unawareness is not necessarily permanent. Just as the brain is able to increase the production of the GLUT1 transport protein during repeated hypoglycemia, it is sometimes able to reverse this alteration if patients carefully avoid hypoglycemia. Patients may regain their ability to appreciate low glucose concentrations at a point when treatment can be successful. However, a fear of some patients is that a lessening of glycemic control may lead to a rise in glycosylated hemoglobin and thus their risk of complications. They should be reminded that hemoglobin A_{1c} represents the average glycemia concentration over several weeks and that a desirable number often represents a substantial number of low glucose concentrations balancing a number of highs. The strategy in these patients is to smooth out the blood glucose control so that less hypoglycemia and hyperglycemia is attained and hemoglobin A_{1c} remains relatively unchanged. A critical issue for patients and physicians to remember is that optimal control of diabetes is not only to achieve a near-normal hemoglobin A_{1c} concentration, but also to condense the range of the glucose excursion, thereby minimizing the number of low glucose concentrations to an acceptable frequency.

III. INTENSIFIED DIABETES MANAGEMENT: SPECIAL ISSUES

The risks of hypoglycemia in terms of mortality are relatively small; therefore, intensified diabetes management should be the standard of care for most patients, with the proviso they are taught ways to minimize significant hypoglycemia, including learning precipitating events and the times in their days that pose the greatest risk. Many insulin-taking patients are on split-mixed NPH or Lente regimens. One common and effective strategy is to have the patient split the evening dose to give the fast-acting insulin with the evening meal and the NPH at bedtime. By doing so, the NPH peaks during the early morning hours (so-called dawn time, which is the greatest time of insulin resistance because of nocturnal growth hormone release). Although this maintains appropriate liver glucose production by having sufficient insulin in the portal vein when the patient awakens, it can also produce excessive insulinization during the middle of the night. Patients who select this treatment regimen with their team generally should eat a bedtime snack. The quantity of bedtime carbohydrate that is required to prevent nocturnal hypoglycemia is small—perhaps 25 g of starch (a half sandwich, some yogurt, cottage cheese, or half cup of cereal with skin milk). Undoubtedly, going to bed with a normal glucose concentration and using bedtime NPH is part of the explanation of why midnight to 4 AM is a peak time for the occurrence of severe hypoglycemia in intensively treated patients.

Sliding scales of rapid-acting insulin can lead to a tremendous amount of instability in glucose concentrations. The rate of fall in glucose concentration is no more rapid after giving a larger dose of insulin than with a smaller dose. Instead, the higher dose leads to excessive reductions in the glucose concentration that can persist for hours after the injection. We prefer to match the dose of insulin to the meal (often by carbohydrate counting) that will be consumed and add perhaps 10% to that which normally would be taken. Furthermore, we have the patient build in a greater interval between the insulin injection and when they begin to eat to permit liver glucose production to be shut down and insulin-mediated glucose uptake to be enhanced. There are no concrete rules of thumb for how long is long enough—each patient is different and the amount of time that needs to pass depends on whether regular or Humalog insulin has been used. We generally teach patients how long to wait by having them measure their glucose concentrations every 20 min after the injection. Once a glucose concentration of about 150 mg/dL has been reached, we have them begin eating.

Exercise is another potential factor that can increase hypoglycemia. Although no one would argue that exercise is a critical element of every diabetes prescription, it leads to enhanced insulin sensitivity for up to 36 h after each exercise bout. Thus, insulin needs following exercise continue to be reduced during this period, as muscle continues to have an elevated rate of glucose uptake in the "cool-down period." Additionally, we generally coach patients to add slightly more starch to their bedtime snack after a day that has had substantial exercise or heavy labor.

It is important to formally educate all patients about hypoglycemia-promoting factors, such as exercise, skipping meals, or snacks, and alcohol intake. On the other hand, it is well worth noting that these risk factors explained only 7% of the severe hypoglycemia in the Diabetes Control and Complications Trial, and we now believe that the development of hypoglycemia unawareness through repeated episodes of hypoglycemia is the most important precipitating factor that accounts for the bulk of severe events.

IV. TREATMENT OF HYPOGLYCEMIA

A. Oral Glucose

Hypoglycemia is one of the greatest urges to open the refrigerator and inhale everything there. The average insulin reaction with a glucose concentration near 50 mg/dL is easily dealt with by having the patient take in 20–30 g of starch. Eating more does not accelerate the rate of recovery and, instead, likely causes hyperglycemia in the hours following the reaction. Thus, it is essential that patients be taught not to panic and to use fingerstick glucose concentrations to reassure themselves that their glucose concentration is on the rise after an oral treatment has been completed. The choice of the carbohydrate depends on where the patient is at the time of the low glucose concentration. We have found that drinking a 6- to 8-oz glass of milk will restore the glucose concentration to normal as rapidly as juice. Milk has the advantage that, because of the protein and fat that go along with the sugar, there is a slowed and prolonged duration of the rate of absorption of starch. The glucose concentration quickly returns to normal, but rather than dropping again several hours later (especially common occurrence when treating nighttime insulin reactions), the glucose can be stabilized for several hours after the reaction. Milk is not generally available when patients are at work or in school. In that case, we recommend boxed juices that do not require refrigeration (each contain 15–20 g of starch). Prepackaged boxes of juice also take the guess work out of treating the reaction because decision making and logic relative to how much oral sugar is needed to overcome the reaction are regularly lost as hypoglycemia deepens. Consequently, we advise against patients drinking part of a can of regular soda to treat a reaction, as they are likely to guzzle the entire can and will then end up too high with a glucose level within the hour. Overtreatment of insulin reactions leads to a yo–yo-like effect in which the patient then overcompensates with extra insulin after overtreating a prior insulin reaction. Still, in some instances, we do advise that when patients regain their mental faculties and are aware they overdid the treatment of the reaction, that they take a small supplementary dose of insulin. The object of intensified diabetes management is to prevent hyperglycemia and not put the patient in the position of constantly chasing the glucose concentration back down into the normal range.

B. Glucagon

Families or significant others of patients with type 1 diabetes should be educated in the use of glucagon treatment of severe hypoglycemia. Glucagon is supplied in a 1-mg vial as the lyophilized powder which must be reconstituted with a diluent that either comes preloaded in a syringe or must be drawn up from a separate bottle with a syringe. It should be administered only when the patient has lost consciousness, or is so close to this that they have lost the ability to coordinate swallowing. Therefore, the spouse, parent, or significant other, not the patient, is the person who must be trained to administer the injection. It can be given subcutaneously or intramuscularly; the onset of action is not greatly different between these two injection methods. Often, this hormone is given when the patient is seizing from a low glucose concentration and any convenient limb muscle group (deltoid or gluteus) is appropriate. Furthermore, the full milligram that is provided in the ampule is more than enough to raise the glucose concentration to well above normal; thus, repeated injections are unnecessary. The person giving the dose must understand that sufficient time needs to elapse for the dose to be absorbed and for it to mobilize glycogen from the liver to normalize the glucose concentration. The usual time to improvement in glucose concentration is about 10 or 15 min and the duration of action of this peptide is 1 or 2 hours. The major side effect of using glucagon is a change in gut motility; therefore, most patients experience some nausea. Because this treatment causes only a transient increase in glucose concentration, we recommend that patients eat some starch (crackers are generally best tolerated) after recovery to prevent recurrence of the hypoglycemia several hours later. This is especially important when the severe hypoglycemia occurs during the early part of the night and the patient hopes to sleep safely for the remainder of the night. By training patients to use this therapy, many 911 calls and subsequent emergency room visits can be averted. Indeed, patients are typically very upset to find a complete stranger in their bedroom restraining them as their glucose level returns to normal and they opens their eyes for the first time after the severe low. Emergency room visits after such events are generally not required. If persistent neurological sequela of the hypoglycemia are noted by the patient or the person providing assistance, then further evaluation is obviously indicated.

V. SULFONYLUREA OVERDOSE

Intravenous glucose is the traditional recommendation for the management of hypoglycemia induced from an intentional or accidental overdose of a sulfonylurea. These agents in some patients generate hypoglycemia by excessively potentiating insulin release when beta cells are exposed to glucose concentrations above normal. The *Physician's Desk Reference* recommends that treatment of repeated boluses of hypertonic glucose be used followed by intravenous infusion of dextrose as required. Such therapy creates repeated pulses in glucose concentration that are well above normal, thus the beta cells (potentiated by sulfonylurea) continue to release more insulin. The net result is a transient increase in glucose concentration, followed by repeated hypoglycemia.

Even when intravenous infusions are used, the amount of glucose that must be continuously given slowly edges up if the infusion rate even slightly exceeds the amount needed to maintain a glucose level of 90–100 mg/dL. Finally, because of the hypertonicity of the solutions being infused, a long arm intravenous line or central line is suggested, and because of the amount of free water that will be given to patients by 20 or 50% dextrose administration, the elderly patient should be carefully watched for signs of volume overload or hyponatremia.

Alternatively, diazoxide, an antihypertensive agent that inhibits insulin release can be given intravenously. In our own studies, this therapy was only partially successful, and dextrose supplementation was still required. We also noted that the drug solubility is reduced when it is mixed with dextrose; thus, it must be given through its own intravenous line. Hypotension was not a problem in our experimental overdose situation in which young volunteers participated, although care should obviously be used in the patient receiving concomitant antihypertensive agents.

The preceding two methods for dealing with what can be a protracted event are not optimal, especially if the overdose is from long-acting agents, in particular chlorpropamide. Our best treatment success is seen with octreotide administration. Octreotide is a somatostatin derivative that inhibits the secretion of many hormones and is usually used to reduce tumor-induced hypersecretion syndromes, such as growth hormone, in patients with acromegaly. It also inhibits insulin and glucagon release. We have observed in normal subjects taking upward of 100 mg of glipizide that octreotide caused the dextrose infusion requirements to regularly fall to zero. Octreotide can be given subcutaneously and we have anecdotally found that 50 μg every 6–8 h provides much the same result as a continuous infusion of the drug. The major side effect of octreotide therapy is fat malabsorption, thus we generally recommend low-fat meals while this medication is being administered.

VI. RARE CAUSES OF HYPOGLYCEMIA

Multiple hormones counteract the effects of insulin after hypoglycemia to produce a normal glucose concentration (counterregulatory hormones). Deficiencies of any of these can induce hypoglycemia. Classically, patients presenting with cortisol deficiency from Addison's disease may have hypoglycemia owing to diminished hepatic glucose production and heightened insulin sensitivity (adults and children). Children with panhypopituitarism from a combination of growth hormone and corticotropin (ACTH) deficiency present in the first weeks of life with hypoglycemia. With restoration of only the cortisol deficiency, hypoglycemia is resolved, thus isolated growth hormone deficiency is not generally sufficient to cause hypoglycemia. The concomitant absence of any of these hormones in type 1 diabetes, such as occurs in the polyendocrine syndromes (see Chap. 42) can promote significant hypoglycemia that can be misdiagnosed as simply compliance difficulty on the part of the patient.

Alcohol consumption is a common precipitating factor for emergency room visits for hypoglycemia in patients using insulin. Alcohol inhibits hepatic glucose production by pathways similar to those that are affected by insulin. Thus, any patient using insulin in an intensified treatment schedule should be advised about the increased risk of hypoglycemia with alcohol, plus that the risk does not generally occur during the time when the alcohol is being consumed, but many hours afterward. Additionally, alcohol consumption is often associated with extra snacking and so the patient may measure a higher than desirable glucose concentration at bedtime and be tempted to take supplementary fast-acting insulin before sleep only to wake up in the middle of the night with a low glucose concentration. When asked for a specific recommendation, I prefer that patients consume lite beer as opposed to hard liquor because of the lower carbohydrate and alcohol contents.

Hypoglycemia is said to occur with a higher frequency in the setting of cirrhosis. I have seen a multitude of cirrhotic adults, the vast majority of whom do not have hypoglycemia despite significant impairment in synthetic function, as assessed by prothrombin time or albumin concentration. However, in the setting of infection with cirrhosis, hypoglycemia is not uncommon. A typical example is the patient with ascites, spontaneous bacteroperitonitis, and cirrhosis, who without any glucose-lowering medication presents with hypoglycemia. Such a presentation may seem counterintuitive because infection is a time of tremendous insulin resistance. However, under these conditions, hepatic glucose production is low and peripheral utilization by white cells can be quite high. In this setting, treatment of the infection can lead to a dramatic normalization of the glucose concentration.

Patients with renal insufficiency present a significant challenge to the diabetes care team. The kidney is a significant site of glucose production (yes, it is not just the liver). As renal parenchymal mass shrinks, the patient is less capable of gluconeogenesis plus the renal mechanism for insulin clearance is lost. The liver can increase the clearance of insulin, however, and the most likely defect that leads to hypoglycemia in azotemic patients is the loss of glucose production. Further exacerbating this problem is the average patient with end-stage renal disease is under significant protein restriction and so the conversion of alanine to glucose through gluconeogenesis is limited by the substrate intake. Thus, prevention of hypoglycemia as renal function deteriorates by reducing the insulin dosage is of paramount concern. Philosophically, the major complication of diabetes has already occurred, and the potential benefits from near-normalization of glucose concentrations are passed. This is not to say that persons with modest renal insufficiency and microalbuminuria would not benefit from intensified glycemic management, as the Diabetes Control and Complications Trial unequivocally demonstrated that both early retinopathy and early renal disease are slowed in progression by intensive glycemic control.

VII. SUMMARY

Hypoglycemia is a common consequence of diabetes treatments. The more intensive the treatment, its propensity to cause swings in glycemia, and how the underlying pathophysiology affects the counterregulation system, all influence the risk of this significant morbidity. With appropriate care and education of the patient, tight glycemic control can be achieved in most patients in tandem with an acceptable frequency of relatively mild hypoglycemia.

BIBLIOGRAPHY

Boyle PJ, Schwartz NS, Shah SD, Clutter WE, Cryer PE. Plasma glucose concentrations at the onset of hypoglycemic symptoms in patients with poorly controlled diabetes and in nondiabetics. N Engl J Med 318:1487–1492, 1988.

Boyle PJ, Justice K, Krentz AJ, Nagy RJ, Schade DS. Octreotide reverses hyperinsulinemia and hypoglycemia induced by oral sulfonylurea overdose. J Clin Endocrinol Metab 76:752–755, 1993.

Boyle PJ, Nagy RJ, O'Connor AM, Kempers SF, Yeo RA, Qualls C. Adaptation in brain glucose uptake following recurrent hypoglycemia. Proc Nat Acad Sci USA 91: 9352–9556, 1994.

Boyle PJ, Kempers SK, O'Connor AM, Nagy RJ. Brain glucose uptake and hypoglycemia unawareness in patients with insulin dependent diabetes mellitus. N Engl J Med 333:1726–1731, 1995.

Cranston I, Lomas J, Maran A, Macdonald I, Amiel SA. Restoration of hypoglycaemia awareness in patients with long-duration insulin-dependent diabetes. Lancet 344: 283–287, 1994.

Cryer PE. Does central nervous system adaptation to antecedent glycemia occur in patients with insulin-dependent diabetes mellitus? Ann Intern Med 103:284–286, 1985.

Dagogo-Jack S, Rattarasarn C, Cryer PE. Reversal of hypoglycemia unawareness, but not defective glucose counterregulation, in IDDM. Diabetes 43:1426–1434, 1994.

Fanelli CG, Epifano L, Rambotti AM, et al. Meticulous prevention of hypoglycemia normalizes the glycemic thresholds and magnitude of most of neuroendocrine responses to, symptoms of hypoglycemia in intensively treated patient with short-term IDDM. Diabetes 42:1683–1689, 1993.

32

Skin Changes Associated With Diabetes

John R. T. Reeves
University of Vermont College of Medicine, Burlington, Vermont

I. INTRODUCTION

There are no skin changes that are absolutely diagnostic of diabetes or invariably accompany it, but there are many skin changes that may be seen in diabetes. Insulin affects the utilization of glucose in the skin, and levels of insulin and glucose are reflected in the skin as they are in other tissues. However, how the insulin and glucose specifically affect the skin and whether and how they contribute to any of the skin changes are not completely understood.

Diabetes, particularly if it is long-standing, is accompanied by increasing disease of small vessels, which is responsible for many of the worst complications of diabetes involving, for example, the eye and the kidney. Blood vessels in the skin, particularly those of small caliber, are similarly affected and may lead to or contribute to skin changes. Some of the changes from vascular insufficiency of the skin are probably exacerbated by the frequent neuropathy that occurs in diabetes. Interestingly, the origin of this neuropathy may be from gradual obliteration of the tiny vessels that serve large nerves in the extremities.

Type I diabetes is an autoimmune disease. Autoimmune diseases tend to appear in clusters, with an increased risk of skin autoimmune diseases, including vitiligo and alopecia areata, in persons with type I diabetes.

The gross metabolic changes that may occur in diabetes also occasionally have manifestations on the skin, such as in the form of xanthomas resulting from blood lipid disturbances. Finally, one may see skin complications from the drugs and medications that are used to treat diabetes.

539

II. DIABETIC SKIN CHANGES OF UNKNOWN CAUSE

A. Necrobiosis Lipoidica Diabeticorum

1. Clinical Features

Necrobiosis lipoidica diabeticorum (NLD) starts as shiny usually slightly elevated, fairly sharply demarcated plaques often 1–3 cm in size, but sometimes up to 25 cm. They begin as slightly dusky or pink, but may become darker red or even reddish-brown as they slowly progress over weeks and months. Eventually, they become atrophic, with very thinned shiny wax-paper-like skin, often slightly hyperpigmented at the periphery and yellowish in the center (Fig. 1). The term *lipoidica* is from the earlier belief that the yellow color was deposits of fat in the lesions, but the yellow color may be from the loss of collagen fibers with retention of yellowish elastin fibers, or from such severe thinning that the color of the subcutaneous fat begins to show through. Sometimes small plaques occur

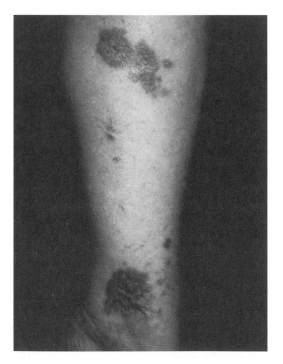

Fig. 1 Necrobiosis lipoidica diabeticorum: fully developed lesions; shiny atrophic yellowish plaques.

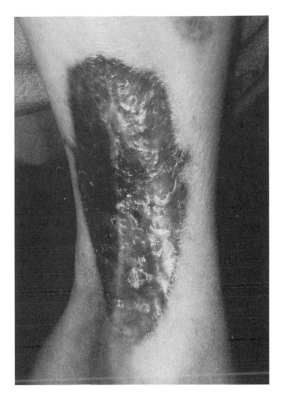

Fig. 2 Necrobiosis lipoidica: burned out, atrophic scar.

close to one another and, as they grow, merge into a large plaque. Over a passage of months or years these patches become so thinned and atrophic that they may ulcerate, particularly with minor trauma, and remain as painful ulcers for prolonged periods. Not all lesions progress to this extreme atrophic or ulcerative stage (Figs. 2 and 3).

In 90% of patients, NLD is on one or both shins, but it may occur on the extensor arms, the trunk, face, or even the scalp. Women are three times more likely than men to be afflicted by NLD.

Classically, it has been reported that 70% of cases of NLD occur in persons with active diabetes, about 20% occur in persons in whom diabetes or glucose intolerance later develops, and about 10% occurs in persons in whom diabetes never develops. In general, the association is more common with severe, long-standing diabetes than with mild or early diabetes. However, a very recent report has failed to confirm these long-held beliefs. Of 65 patients with NLD, only 11%

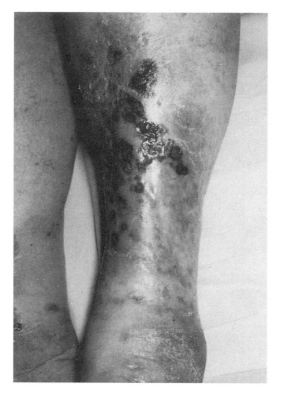

Fig. 3   Necrobiosis lipoidica: ulcerating.

had diabetes at diagnosis and an only 11% more developed impaired glucose or diabetes over a 15-year follow-up period, leaving 78% of patients in whom diabetes was not associated. In some literature, the skin lesion is now referred to as ''necrobiosis lipoidica'' without the added ''diabeticorum,'' to reflect the frequent lack of association with diabetes.

The onset of NLD is usually in the 40s or 50s, but can be seen even in childhood, particularly in severe diabetes. Spontaneous resolution occurs in at least 15% of patients after 6–12 years. Progression or regression of lesions does not appear to be related to the activity of the diabetes itself.

2. Pathology

The early pathological changes are in the mid- to lower-dermis where in focal areas the collagen swells, becomes basophilic, and the collagen bundles become broken and wavy. This constellation of pathological changes is called necrobiosis. Histochemical stains show that there is also loss and fragmentation of elastic fibers. As the lesions progress, the collagen and elastin fibers become atrophic and begin to disappear, correlating with the thinning of the skin. There may be a variable number of histiocytes present containing foamy fat globules. Examination of the vasculature always shows changes, primarily with endothelial proliferation and occlusion of the lumina of venules and arterioles, as well as thickening of capillary walls. However, somewhat similar changes can be seen in normal skin near the lesions, probably as a consequence of degenerative changes of diabetes, and it is not known if these vascular changes result in the clinical lesions or are a parallel change that are not responsible for the lesions.

3. Therapy

If NLD is suspected, referral to a dermatologist is recommended. If the dermatologist feels that NLD is possible or likely, based on the clinical appearance, then a biopsy should be performed to confirm the diagnosis. Other patches on the shin, such as eczema or fungal infections, may be diagnosed clinically and treated without biopsy, thus sparing the patient a surgical procedure which might heal with difficulty in diabetic skin.

Once the diagnosis is established the most effective therapy is injection of corticosteroid, usually triamcinolone acetonide, into the lesions, particularly at the edges, which often stops the activity and progress of the disease. The injections have a therapeutic effect lasting at least 6 weeks, and they can be repeated periodically if necessary. Superpotent topical corticosteroid creams may also be helpful in early cases, but prolonged use of these can lead to superficial atrophy, which can be clinically confusing in a disease that itself is atrophic.

Many other therapies have been tried aside from corticosteroids, usually with negative results. Several years ago there were some positive reports of response to oral aspirin and dipyrimidole, acting as vasodilators and reducing platelet aggregation, but later studies were much less favorable.

Treatment of very advanced ulcerative lesions is unsatisfactory. These lesions are frequently painful and debilitating, and the patients are very anxious for effective therapy. However, because of the severe atrophy and vascular compromise, healing is extremely slow and grafts often do not "take" in the relatively hypoxic wound base. Symptomatic relief can be achieved by constant placement of synthetic hydrocolloid dressings. Dermatologists often refer these patients to highly specialized wound care clinics where sometimes artificial skin substitutes, or even skin cultures from the patient's own skin, are used to try to resurface these areas.

B. Granuloma Annulare

Granuloma annulare (GA) are asymptomatic dermal plaques that often occur over extensor joints in children to young adults. As these papules and plaques enlarge they heal in the center giving an elevated ring-like border and a depressed center, hence *annulare* (ring). Biopsy shows the same peculiar "necrobiosis" changes seen in NLD. This has led to a search for a connection between GA and diabetes, which has been unfruitful in the children or young adults who have single or few lesions. However, there is a rare generalized type of GA that occurs with dozens to hundreds of small lesions in middle-aged to older adults, in whom some studies have shown a possible association of this condition with diabetes, although other studies have not seen such an association. When the diagnosis of this rare form of GA is made, it is not unusual for dermatologists to at least draw a fasting glucose level as a screen for diabetes.

Single or few lesions of GA may enlarge for 1 or 2 years, and then slowly involute without therapy. Very potent topical corticosteroids or intralesional injection of depot corticosteroid will stop their growth and hasten resolution. Generalized GA may progress slowly or remain steady for years. No highly effective therapy is available, but it occasionally responds to such varied agents as dapsone, niacinamide, hydroxychloroquine, and isotretinoin.

C. Acanthosis Nigricans

1. Clinical Manifestations

Acanthosis nigricans is a peculiar brown to grayish-brown pigmentation occurring in the fold areas (axilla, submammary, groin, sides of neck) with a velvety soft ridged thickening of the skin (Fig. 4). These changes resemble lichenification, a result of chronically rubbing the skin, but lichenification is hard and rough to the touch and itches, and AN is soft and does not itch.

There are several clinical associations with AN. In very rare instances, it may be familial and start at an early age and last throughout life. If there is a sudden onset after the age of 40 there is a high correlation with the presence of an internal malignancy, particularly a solid malignancy of the gastrointestinal or genitourinary systems. If AN is seen in this setting, vigorous and repeated workup for internal malignancy is warranted. The most common association with AN is marked obesity, and the condition may improve or disappear if weight is lost. Recent studies, however, have shown that AN is particularly associated with insulin-resistant diabetes, with or without associated obesity. It has been hypothesized that insulin resistance leads to hyperinsulinemia that may compete for insulin growth factor receptors on keratinocytes, thus stimulating growth of epidermal cells.

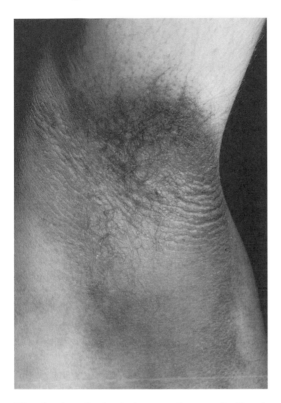

Fig. 4 Acanthosis nigricans: velvety, soft, dirty-brown thickening of skin in fold area.

2. Pathology

Histopathological changes reflect the clinical changes: The epidermal cell layer is thicker than normal and thrown into folds. There is no inflammation. There probably is not increased activity of pigment cells, but rather, just an increased number of epidermal cells that are capable of holding pigment, thus giving the darker color.

3. Treatment

Diagnosis is clinical, and once the practitioner is familiar with the appearance referral to a dermatologist is not necessary. Biopsies are rarely required to confirm diagnosis. There is no effective treatment of the skin changes of acanthosis nigricans, but reversal of obesity and control of blood insulin levels may lead to gradual resolution. Be aware that if this condition occurs in an older individual in the absence of diabetes or insulin resistance, a vigorous search for internal malignancy is warranted.

D. Vitiligo

1. Clinical Findings

Vitiligo is the sudden appearance of patches of complete loss of pigment, resulting in chalk-white lesions. They often occur in children or young adults, but may occur much later in life. The most common locations are over extensor joints (elbows, knees, knuckles), and around orifices (periocular, perioral, perianal). They are asymptomatic but may be disfiguring, particularly in darker-skinned people.

Vitiligo is known to be an autoimmune disease, causing lymphocytes to attack melanocytes in the skin. The incidence of vitiligo is higher in persons with other autoimmune diseases such as alopecia areata, autoimmune thyroiditis, and Addison's disease. It occurs in 0.2–1.0% of the normal population, but close to 5% of patients with diabetes. The association with diabetes is an inexact one, and it may precede or follow the onset of symptoms of diabetes.

Therapy of autoimmune diseases accompanying vitiligo never has an effect on the vitiligo itself, because the autoantibodies and autoimmune responses are separate. Therapy of vitiligo itself is difficult, for melanocytes multiply with reluctance, although spontaneous improvement occurs in a small percentage of cases. Benefit can be induced with potent topical cortosteroids and with certain types of ultraviolet light therapy, but complete resolution occurs in less than 30% of cases.

III. SKIN CHANGES OF CHRONIC DEGENERATIVE DISEASE

A. Diabetic Dermopathy

1. Clinical Findings

Also called shin spot, or pigmented pretibial patch, diabetic dermopathy is seen on the shins as scattered, fairly sharply demarcated, slightly depressed, slightly pigmented lesions, often with a slight scale (Figs. 5–7). These are identical with lesions seen on the shins, often in older individuals, resulting from minor trauma (such as striking the shin on the edge of a coffee table), but they occur at a much younger age and in much larger numbers in some diabetics, particularly those with severe long-standing disease. In that setting, they may be seen to appear spontaneously as scattered small red or reddish-brown macules that slowly evolve

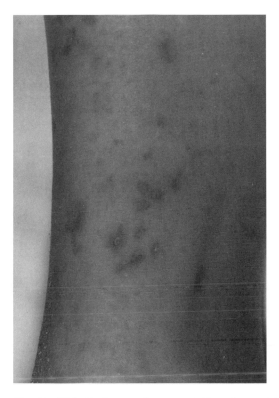

Fig. 5 Diabetic dermopathy: new, inflamed, punctate macules, becoming atrophic.

into the atrophic pigmented lesions. One study has shown that local heat and cold injury, experimentally performed in diabetics, causes the appearance of these lesions in over 75% of patients who already have diabetic dermopathy, but occur in no control patients and in very few diabetic patients who do not already have the dermopathic lesions. There have been some studies showing that they occur more commonly in persons with retinopathy, nephropathy, neuropathy, but other studies have not found this association.

2. Pathology

Biopsies often show obliterative endarteritis of small- and medium-sized arterioles, but this change can be seen in long-standing diabetes without the lesions. The etiology of this condition is unknown, but there are none of the collagen changes that are seen in necrobiosis lipoidica diabeticorum.

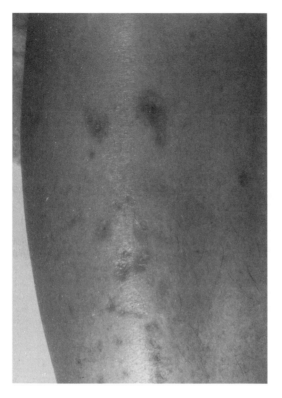

Fig. 6 Dermopathy: long-standing "shin spots," are hyperpigmented, atrophic, and slightly scaly.

3. Treatment

There is no satisfactory treatment for what are essentially scars. In general, diabetics should take care not to injure their lower extremities because of the susceptibility they have to exaggerated tissue responses and debilitating wounds. Moving furniture out of the way and changing some habits, such as not leaving the door down on a dishwasher, can help minimize these injuries. In a rare case where an individual might be occupationally exposed to injury, thick boots, clothing or even shin guards might be recommended.

B. Skin Atrophy and Ulceration

1. Clinical Manifestations

As in many other organs, small- to medium-sized arterials of the skin often suffer diminished blood-carrying capacity and occlusion, leading to decreased perfusion.

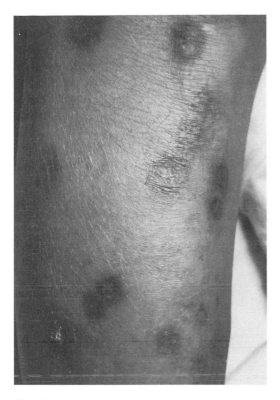

Fig. 7   Severe dermopathy: hypertrophic and scaly.

This vascular change occurs in small vessels feeding nerves in the skin, contributing to neuropathy and numbness of the skin, even though muscular activity is retained.

As a result of diminished nerve innervation and blood supply, the skin of the lower extremities often becomes slightly atrophic appearing, shiny and perhaps even hairless and cool. The skin is easily wounded and heals with difficulty. The most severe complication of these changes is the neurotropic (or mal perforans) ulcer. This is essentially an ambulatory bed sore where repeated pressure or trauma in the absence of pain sensation results in liquefaction of subcutaneous fat, with subsequent erosion through the dermal layer of skin, resulting in a sudden appearance of a large deep ulcer that is frequently bigger at the base than it is through the perforating superficial defect. These typically occur in bedridden diabetics on the lower Achilles area, where the foot rests against the mattress, or across the ball of the foot in ambulatory diabetics. Prevention and management of leg and foot ulcers is discussed in the Chap. 28.

C. Thick Skin

It has been reported that as many as one-third of diabetics have thickened, tight, waxy skin, particularly over the dorsae of the hands. Sometimes there are tiny "pebbles" of small flesh-colored confluent papules on the dorsae of the knuckles and around the fingernails. A possible associated change is a slight contracture in the fingers, making it difficult to completely extend them. This can be demonstrated by having the patient place his or her palms together and try to straighten the fingers, but a small gap can be seen between the fingers of the opposing hands where they cannot be straightened against each other.

A more well-defined entity is scleredema (not scleroderma) adultorum (Fig. 8). This is manifested as a thickening and inflexibility of the skin predominately

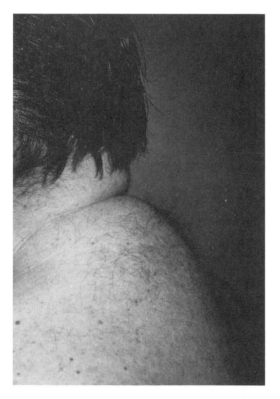

Fig. 8   Scleredema: skin of the upper back and nape of neck thick and woody; inhibits tilting the head back, creates a bulge in the skin.

at the nape of the neck and extending down the upper back, but in extreme cases, it can proceed across the shoulders down the anterior and posterior thorax as well as down the arms, and even rarely involve the abdomen, arms, and hands. The skin is very firm and can actually restrict movement of the neck, but retains its normal texture. In contrast, scleroderma predominately involves the distal extremities, the skin becomes very hard, shiny, and cool.

Most cases of this rare condition, scleredema adultorum, are preceded by a febrile illness, often streptococcal. The condition develops slowly over a period of weeks to months, reaches a peak and then gradually recedes over a period of months. However, the condition can be seen in association with diabetes, usually in obese diabetics with severe long-standing disease. The etiology of thick skin and scleredema is unknown, but may be related to the effect of hyperglycemia and hyperinsulinemia on the metabolism of collagen and ground substance in the dermis. There is sometimes an associated paraproteinemia, in which there is a monoclonal gammopathy of IgG, IgM, or IgA. Paraproteinemias have occasionally been associated with thickening of skin, with deposits of mucin, but biopsies of scleredema usually show no increase or only slight increase in dermal mucin, the predominate finding being swollen collagen bundles and increased hyaluronic acid.

Unfortunately, no effective treatment exists for scleredema. In one patient in whom it was accompanied by a paraproteinemia, there was improvement with prednisone and melphalan.

D. Bullous Lesions

Although a rare complication of diabetes, the apparent spontaneous appearance of large blisters (bullae) in diabetics is reported regularly. It is sometimes referred to as bullosus diabeticorum (Fig. 9). It occurs most commonly on the feet, particularly the dorsae of the feet, but may occur on the fingers and dorsae of the hands and forearms. Strikingly, they occur as dramatic blisters with no accompanying redness. They are fairly thick-roofed and so last for several days before they deflate and heal without scarring.

In general, they occur in persons with fairly advanced long-standing insulin-dependent diabetes and neuropathy, but can occur in fairly recent-onset mild diabetics. Some have hypothesized that the sensory neuropathy seen in diabetes leads patients to inadvertently overheat or apply friction to their feet, resulting in blisters, but careful studies have failed to confirm this. A pathophysiological mechanism for this blister formation is not known, but one study showed that insulin-dependent diabetics have a decreased threshold to the formation of suction blisters on their forearms. Biopsy shows separation in the basement membrane between the epidermis and dermis, but the pathological appearance is not diagnostic. Treatment should be similar to that for friction blisters, for which the blister

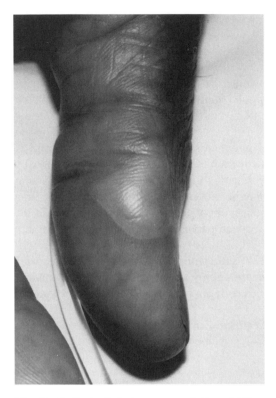

Fig. 9 Bullosis diabeticorum: noninflamed blister on the extremity.

is carefully drained with a sterile needle and then the deflated blister is treated with bathing, topical antibiotics, and dressings.

IV. SKIN CHANGES FROM SEVERE METABOLIC ABNORMALITIES

A. Xanthomas

Diabetes is often accompanied by hyperlipidemia, particularly with triglyceride being more elevated than cholesterol. With the sudden onset of diabetic ketoacidosis there may be a dramatic sudden rise of triglycerides to levels five to ten times higher than normal, which can bring about the appearance of *eruptive xanthomas.*

Eruptive xanthomas are seen so rarely in the absence of diabetes that in the distant past they were called "xanthoma diabeticorum."

Eruptive xanthomas appear suddenly over the extensor surfaces of the arms, legs, and buttocks. In the first few days they may be small red slightly itchy papules, but they rapidly become an orange-red and eventually yellowish color (Fig. 10). They usually stay smaller than a centimeter and sometimes small yellowish papules will form a "rosette," which is a circular cluster similar to daisy petals. Biopsy will show lipid-laden macrophages in the middermis. Serum triglyceride levels are often higher than 800 ng/dL and may exceed 1500 or 2000 ng/dL.

Control of diabetes results in rapid correction of gross lipid abnormalities, and eruptive xanthomas can be expected to gradually resolve in a few weeks.

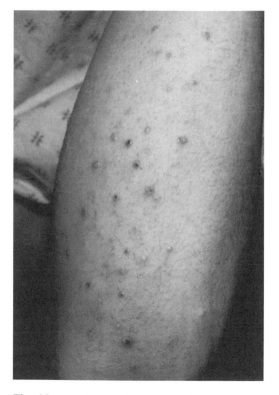

Fig. 10 Eruptive xanthoma ("xanthoma diabeticorum"): sudden appearance of numerous yellow papules on the extensor extremities; initially itchy, some of these are excoriated.

B. Infections

Diabetics are probably no more likely to become infected than nondiabetics, but when diabetes is poorly controlled, skin infections tend to be more severe and more difficult to control. The aggressive behavior of infections in diabetics may be attributed to numerous immunological dysfunctions found in diabetes, including abnormalities of leukocyte function, decreased ability of leukocytes to migrate through thickened capillary walls, effect of decreased insulin on interleukins, and hyperosmolality. Some of these factors may also account for poor wound healing in diabetes, and because infections are a "wound" in the skin, their healing may be delayed. Importantly, "trivial" infections of the skin, such as athletes foot (tinea pedis) create a break in the cutaneous barrier that may allow more significant deeper infections to occur.

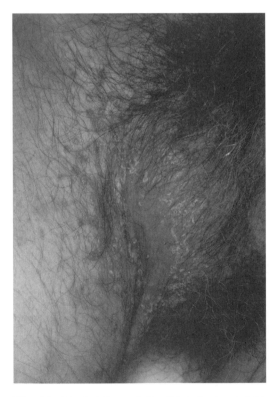

Fig. 11 Typical flexural *Candida* infection: bright red patch in fold, with punctate satellite lesions; may occur in normal persons or in diabetics.

Among infections that occur with more vigor in diabetics are staphylococcal folliculitis (furunculosis), and bacterial cellulitis of the feet and lower extremities. Dermatophyte (tinea) infections, frequently of the feet or groin, may be more widespread and resistant to therapy. Candida infections of the vagina, anogenital area, submammary, and axillae tend to be recurrent and severe (Figs. 11 and 12), and because they occur more often in obese persons, are particularly a problem in adult-onset obese diabetics.

At this point it should be noted that in the past diabetes was listed as a cause of generalized itching of no apparent cause. This observation has not stood up to modern scrutiny, but there is an increased incidence of perianal itching, and possibly vulvar itching, probably owing to the increased prevalence of *Candida* found in those areas.

A, fortunately, rare complication of diabetes is mucormycosis, a saprophytic fungal infection of the paranasal sinuses. The outcome of this infection is often

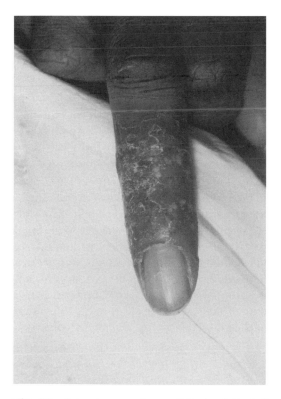

Fig. 12 Extensive pustular candidiasis of distal finger, extending from a routine yeast paronychia: dramatic extent of infection suggests diabetes or immunosuppression.

catastrophic, as the infection can expand around the eyes, and extend deeper into the skull and, eventually, into the brain. It can also invade vascular channels, producing thrombosis. It presents as discomfort in the sinus area, often with inflammation around the eyes and possibly even with bulging of the eyes and restriction of eye movement. Mucormycosis occurs in the setting of severe ketoacidosis, and so now is rarely seen in the era of modern diabetic management. If this infection is suspected, immediate referral to an otorhinolaryngologist is essential.

V. REACTIONS TO DIABETIC THERAPY

A. Insulin

Repeated injections of insulin into the same site may result in lipoatrophy, or gradual depressions in the skin, or, more rarely, lipohypertrophy, which are large lipoma-like fatty masses in the subcutaneous tissue. These abnormalities will return to normal if the sites are no longer injected, and they can be avoided by constantly rotating sites of insulin injection.

B. Oral Hypoglycemics

The modern oral medications for diabetes are not especially likely to cause cutaneous drug reactions, but the sulfonylureas (tolbutamide) are in the "sulfa" family and can result in allergies in up to 7% of individuals who take them. This is particularly true in patients who are infected with the human immunodeficiency virus (HIV), when 40–80% of individuals become allergic to sulfa drugs.

Most drug reactions are of the uncomfortable, but relatively harmless, morbilliform ("measles-like") variety, but erythema multiforme and even Stevens-Johnson syndrome have been reported. Unfortunately, there is no reliable test for determining if a rash appearing in a person taking these drugs is due to the drug, and a clinical judgment must be made. If the eruption is of the morbilliform type, the drug could be discontinued and restarted later as a trial, as it is unlikely that the eruption will progress to a more severe reaction when the patient is rechallenged. If allergy to sulfonylurea is strongly suspected, then the patient should be warned about taking other drugs in this family, such as sulfa antibiotics, phenothiazines (e.g., chlorpromazine), and thiazines (e.g., hydrochlorothiazide).

BIBLIOGRAPHY

Brik R, Berant M, Verdi P. The scleroderma-like syndrome of insulin-dependent diabetes mellitus. Diabetes Metab Rev 1991; 7:121–128.

Cole GW, Headley J, Skowsky R. Scleredema diabeticorum: a common and distinct cutaneous manifestation of diabetes mellitus. Diabetes Care 1983; 6:189–192.

Cruz P Jr, Hud J Jr. Excess insulin binding to insulin-like growth factor receptors: proposed mechanism for acanthosis nigricans. J Invest Dermatol 1992; 98:82s–85s.

Feingold KR, Elias PM. Endocrine-skin interactions. J Am Acad Dermatol 1987; 17: 921–940.

Haim S, Freidman-Birnbaum R, Shafrif A. Generalized granuloma annulare: relationship to diabetes as revealed in 8 cases. Br J Dermatol 1970; 83:303–305.

Lowitt MH, Dover JS. Necrobiosis lipoidica. J Am Acad Dermatol 1991; 25:735–748.

Lugo-Somolinos A, Sanchez JL. Prevelance of dermatophytosis in patients with diabetes. J Am Acad Dermatol 1991; 26:408–410.

O'Tode EA, Kennedy U, Nolan JJ, Young MM, Rogers S, Barnes L. Necrobiosis lipoidica: only a minority of patients have diabetes mellitus. Brit J Dermatol 1999; 140: 283–286.

Perez MI, Kohn SR. Cutaneous manifestations of diabetes mellitus. J Am Acad Dermatol 1994; 30:519–531.

Toonstra J. Bullosis diabeticorum. J Am Acad Dermatol 1985; 13:799–805.

33

Psychosocial Complications of Diabetes

Alan M. Jacobson and Katie Weinger
Joslin Diabetes Center and Harvard Medical School, Boston, Massachusetts

I. INTRODUCTION

Type 1 and type 2 diabetes mellitus are prototypical chronic illnesses for which there are no known cures. Treatment is dependent on a set of complex therapeutic decisions that involve titration of pharmaceuticals and lifestyle changes addressing dietary intake and exercise, and that demand careful education of the patient and his or her family to take on these challenges. There is often an extended period during which the patient's treatment is preventive (i.e., the patient is essentially asymptomatic, and the treatment is designed to prevent the development of complications). Motivation may be difficult to maintain during this period. Finally, when and if complications develop, there are profound implications for the patient's quality and length of life. Not surprisingly, these aspects of diabetes have led to an array of studies about the psychological, behavioral, and quality of life aspects of the illness.

This chapter will address four elements of relevance to the practicing clinician: (a) an understanding of the psychological effects of diabetes; (b) a general approach to the incorporation of psychological methods in the treatment of diabetes; (c) identification and treatment of common coexisting psychiatric illnesses; and (d) psychoeducational interventions of specific relevance to the diabetic patient.

II. PSYCHOLOGICAL EFFECTS OF THE DIABETES

From a psychosocial perspective, diabetes can be broken into four stages, each initiated by a crisis period. Given the course of type 1 versus type 2 diabetes

Table 1 Psychosocial Stages of Diabetes

1. Onset: adaptive crisis linked to realization that I am ill
2. Preventive therapy: the challenge of learning and following a complex and demanding therapy when the benefit is distant
3. Development of early medical complications: the frightening facts embed themselves
4. Complications dominate the illness: "new" illnesses change the patient's view of self

these stages vary, but they may be considered together. Table 1 summarizes these stages.

A. Onset

Each phase carries with it specific psychological implications for both the patient and the family. For the patient with type 1 diabetes, onset is often abrupt and may involve an immediate need for intense medical care and education. Consequently, the onset is almost always experienced as a major adaptive challenge (i.e., a crisis in the lives of the patient and family). Sudden and rapid changes are required, and the family must mobilize its resources to make this adaptation. Commonly, patients and families go into a survival mode, in which the basics are learned and therapy initiated. During this phase, both patients and family members will often experience a period of grief and mourning of the loss associated with development of an illness of the magnitude of type 1 diabetes. The shock and emotional adjustment will be obvious to friends as well as to the clinical team. Prior experience with diabetes has an important influence on the patient and family's initial view and experience of the illness. For example, prior knowledge of a family member or friend who died of diabetes or developed major complications will color the experience differently from prior exposure to someone who has been living an apparently "healthy" life with diabetes. Thus, psychological and social issues can influence an individual's response to both diagnosis and treatment (Table 2). An understanding of these key issues should be used to guide treatment and education planning through the course of diabetes.

For the patient with type 2 diabetes, the crisis of onset is often delayed to a later phase of illness. If the patient is identified and placed on a successful diet and exercise program, this may be seen as a variant of a need for a healthier lifestyle, and the perception of the onset of illness delayed to the beginning of therapy with an oral agent. To some patients, beginning to take a pill in midlife may also be seen as normative (i.e., similar to the use of an antihypertensive or lipid-lowering drug) and simply one more aspect of aging instead of a true illness.

Table 2   A General Approach to the Incorporation of Psychological Methods in the Treatment of Diabetes: Psychosocial Issues Relevant to Diabetes Care

---

The patient's and family members' expectations, attitudes, and goals for treatment
Past experiences with illness in general and diabetes in particular
Current affective state
Extent of grief or acceptance of the diagnosis
Readiness to learn and make behavioral changes
Extent and sources of current stress
Emotional reactions to key issues related to diabetes (e.g., ideals for weight, intolerance
  of regularity, fear of needles, fears about hypoglycemia, fear of complications)
Psychiatric illness, especially depression and eating disorders
Key people in the patient's life
Reactions to and relationships with members of the health care team
Cultural factors affecting the perception of the meaning of illness and its treatment
Financial issues, especially insurance coverage

Source: Jacobson, 1996.

It may be years before the patient is suddenly confronted with the self-perception of being sick (i.e., when the oral agent is no longer sufficient and insulin therapy is recommended). The type 2 patient may go through a gradual period of awakening, rather than an abrupt crisis of onset. Thus, the phases of onset and preventive treatment are frequently blurred for patients with type 2 diabetes.

B.   Preventive Therapy

For both the type 1 and type 2 patients there may be a considerable period of time in which the treatment focus is on the prevention of complications, living a healthy lifestyle, and incorporating lifestyle changes into family life. As with any chronic illness, the patient with diabetes has entered a new world, filled with altered life experiences, demanding the acquisition of a new identity. The patient taking insulin has a pronounced sense that his or her world includes greater regularization of habits, need for intrusive checking of blood sugar levels, and the prospect of unavoidable, sudden, and frightening hypoglycemic events.

Because this is an identity that was not sought, but was forced on the patient, it may be met with much denial, periods of resistance to recommended treatment, and testing to see whether the treatment is actually required by lowering or stopping insulin administration. Although typical patients struggle with their identity, the illness is handled with a remarkable degree of equanimity by most persons. Indeed, studies of children and adolescents have indicated that most patients and families, while experiencing more emotional stress, do not demonstrate decreased self-esteem or increased psychopathology. For the clinician, it is important to realize that taking on a chronic illness is a process of becoming acculturated. Physicians, nurses, and other key clinicians are the guides to this new culture and have key roles to play in minimizing both medical and psychosocial "complications."

C. The Onset of Medical Complications

Although type 2 diabetes may be diagnosed when a complication is already present, commonly patients go through some period of time before the first micro- or macrovascular complications develop. Typically, the educational process has included information about these complications through formal talks, medical visits, laboratory testing, patient-to-patient contact, and a wide variety of "data" from pamphlets, news articles, television, and the Internet. Thus, the onset of a complication should come as no surprise; nonetheless, its occurrence can lead to enormous anxiety and fear. Moreover, some complications may not be adequately discussed because they are uncommon or embarrassing (e.g., impotence); hences knowledge may be very imprecise. Prior experiences of family and friends can also have powerful effects on patient comprehension of complications.

Many visits to the physicians include some test or evaluation that involves the identification of a complication. Thus, for the patient, each visit can become an anxiety-provoking experience, resulting in either relief or confirmation of fears. Even the smallest sign of a complication can have profound meaning for a patient: mild background retinopathy, the first report of microalbuminuria, a decreased ankle reflex, a decreased sensation in the feet on formal testing. All of these are harbingers of a cascade of later frightening possibilities. Although the patient may not overtly show any signs of fear, it should be assumed, until proved otherwise, that every visit contains some amount of anticipatory concern. Visits to the ophthalmologist, because blindness is universally described as the most frightening disability that humans anticipate, can be especially evocative.

As complication identification becomes more sophisticated, and the interventions are applied earlier, patients may be informed of "complications" because of a laboratory value. Although these may seem of minor emotional importance to clinicians, they can have serious personal implications for the patients. Thus, the presentation of even the earliest findings related to a potential serious complication should be provided with an understanding that the patient may have surprisingly powerful reactions to the information. As one patient described it, when informed that he had some initial signs of diabetic retinopathy on an ophthalmological examination, he noted he had been "waiting for this time bomb to explode" all his diabetic life. We all need order and control in our lives. Disorder and lack of control dominate at times of change, such as the diagnosis of a complication. As noted earlier, patients will use the experiences of other people they know with diabetes to organize their assumptions. Patients who have known someone that has had a particular course of illness will tend to assume that they will follow the same path. Therefore, it is useful to ask patients periodically what they have heard about and seen of diabetes. These will be among the more dominating influences of how patients come to understand the meaning of a particular new complication or its evolution. If siblings, parents, grandparents, or other close relatives have had diabetes, assume that your patient will benchmark his or her condition against this course. For example, one patient assumed she would die at age 40 because that was the age her diabetic father had died with end-stage renal disease. For that reason she was afraid to have children.

D. Complications Dominate

This stage typically develops when one or more of the complications take on such seriousness that regular treatment or intervention is required. However, for each patient this stage may occur at a different point in the course of complications. Almost certainly, patients with end-stage renal disease or requiring laser treatment for proliferative retinopathy, experiencing persistent pain from neuropathy, or with impotence or other autonomic neuropathies will be influenced, if not dominated, by the complications of illness as much as by its original characteristics. Patients will experience a double burden (i.e., they still must take care of the illness, yet they now must adhere to new, complex therapeutic regimens in concert with new clinicians and new implications). Surprising reactions can occur. Intense focus on receiving a living relative's kidney may be so great that the patient will anticipate a sense of being cured once the kidney transplant has occurred. After the transplant, the patient will still have to treat the diabetes, however, and also be scrutinized for the danger of rejection. Thus, there can be unexpected disappointment, sadness, and repeated grieving, even while remarkable treatments have addressed progressive complications.

E. Behavioral and Psychiatric Effects

Although the process of diabetes changes the words and themes and shapes the experience of life, this does not mean that all patients with diabetes are inevitably going to be more depressed, more anxious, or susceptible to more psychiatric illnesses than their friends without a chronic illness.

Numerous studies have examined these issues and indeed suggest that the population of diabetic patients, as a whole (especially type 1 patients), have an increased risk of depression, possibly anxiety, and eating disorders. This increased risk of common psychiatric disorders found in diabetes has also been found in patients with other chronic medical illnesses. From a theoretical perspective, however, it is interesting that depression, in particular, may often develop before the onset of complications. Thus, there has been considerable speculation about possible biological and psychosocial linkages between diabetes and depression. These include speculation about the effects of diabetes on the hypothalamic–pituitary axis, the role of recurrent hypo-4 and hyperglycemia affecting areas of the brain that regulate affect, and the social psychological effect of a difficult chronic illness in children. However, the mechanism by which the increased prevalence of depression occurs in diabetic patients has not been worked out. What is clear is that the presence of psychiatric conditions, particularly depression, anxiety disorders, and eating disorders, bring with them greater likelihood of adherence difficulties and, consequently, chronic poor glycemic control. Both cross-sectional and longitudinal studies have suggested that psychosocial factors, such as family adjustment, presence of eating disorders, and depression, all may increase the risk of later microvascular complications because of an associated problem with glycemic regulation and chronic hyperglycemia.

There have been a few studies that have examined the possibility that diabetes can influence central nervous system (CNS) functioning and cause dementia. Evidence exists for type 2 patients who are older and type 1 patients with disease onset before the age 5, suggesting that subtle detriments in cognitive functioning may occur over time. However, the role of recurrent hypoglycemia during the course of diabetes in adolescents and adults causing brain damage is still unclear. For example, the Diabetes Control and Complications Trial (DCCT) failed to demonstrate an effect of recurrent hypoglycemia on cognitive functioning.

III. A GENERAL APPROACH TO PSYCHOLOGICAL METHODS

The centerpiece of medical care is the clinician–patient relationship. Understanding how to strengthen and use these relationships to influence, motivate, listen to, and treat patients is the point of departure for any broad understanding of incorporating psychological issues in the care of patients with diabetes. The therapeutic relationship is often strengthened by an approach that has been termed "patient centered." This approach focuses on the patient as an active collaborator with the clinician. It involves shared decision making and responsibility for setting the care plan. Thus, a powerful method for both strengthening the relationship and identifying those elements of treatment and education that the patient is most eager to address involves encouraging patients to actively participate in the setting of goals for each encounter and for the treatment overall. Elucidating patient goals can be accomplished in multiple ways. These include the use of questionnaires that patients fill out before a visit, a brief discussion of possible goals with an appropriate ancillary health provider such as an office nurse or a discussion at the start of a clinical visit. Open-ended questions are an extremely valuable way to gather information about patient goals because they are most likely to capture patient requests that are hidden because of patient discomfort. A key step in any treatment plan is negotiating differences between patient and clinician goals. This can be done briefly and quickly in the course of each visit. Thus, jointly developed goals become the equivalent of an active, strategic, and practical plan, one that is adaptable, readily changed, and the starting point of each encounter. Patients who actively participate in the establishment of therapeutic goals are more likely to adhere to treatment recommendations for their diabetes. Thus, adherence is actually maximized by an approach that shares the power in this relationship. In addition, rapport between patient and clinician is enhanced by open discussion of differences in goals, if the clinician responds in a nonjudgmental manner.

Some patients will initially be reluctant to participate in this form of encounter because they have adapted to a more circumscribed and formatted visit. When patients are hesitant, simple preambles such as "some of my patients are concerned about . . ." may assist patients in opening up areas of concern. It is also quite useful at the end of each visit to briefly summarize what the clinician has heard of the patient's concerns and objectives and the plan that they have jointly established for review at the next visit.

In some instances, differences in objectives lead to therapeutic impasses when patients are not able or willing to carry out a planned treatment. These impasses can be associated with intensified emotional reactions. An approach in which the clinician listens, tolerates, and acknowledges the patient's expressed feelings will help maintain rapport and enhance the likelihood in the future that the patient and clinician will be more effective in their shared planning and therapy implementation.

IV. IDENTIFICATION AND TREATMENT OF COMMON PSYCHIATRIC ILLNESSES

As noted in Sec. II, there is growing literature suggesting that depressive disorders occur at increased rates among patients with diabetes leading to an increased risk for complications. More limited literature exists evaluating the relation of eating disorders with diabetes outcomes. These studies suggest that eating disorders lead to likelihood of diabetic retinopathy. Clearly, the accurate identification and successful treatment of such disorders could have important medical as well as quality of life benefits for patients with diabetes.

A. Depressive Disorders

Depressive disorders are among the most common psychiatric conditions found in general populations. The age of greatest risk is the young-adult years. Although many patients may experience only a single episode of depression that remits with treatment and does not recur, there is some suggestion that among diabetic patients there is an increased likelihood of recurring depression. Moreover, in the general population, there is substantial minority of patients for whom depression recurs periodically throughout the life span.

Depressive disorders can be difficult to diagnose because of the array of possible presenting symptoms and because the common symptoms of depression mimic those of diabetes and other medical ailments. As shown in Table 3, depression can present with physical, cognitive, or affective symptoms, or a combination thereof. Most patients experience only a subset of these symptoms. When physical symptoms, such as fatigue, dominate the presentation, distinguishing depression from poorly controlled diabetes may be very difficult. However, when affective symptoms, such as pessimism, guilt, and suicidal ideation, are clearly present, it is quite unlikely that poorly controlled diabetes would account for this syndrome. Because diabetes is associated with a greater risk of other endocrinopathies, patients with diabetes who present with depressive symptoms should be carefully screened for thyroid and parathyroid disease. Both parathyroid and thyroid disease can lead to secondary depressions that are indistinguishable from primary depressive disorder. When physical symptomatology dominates the presentation and the patient is not actively suicidal, a period of diabetic treatment designed to improve metabolic control may be a useful first step in the treatment process. If fatigue does not improve with better metabolic control and other medical causes of fatigue have been ruled out, then depression should be entertained as a likely diagnosis.

Most depressive disorders are very responsive to treatment. In the last 10 years several antidepressants have arrived on the market. The differential benefit of one antidepressant over another is minimal for the typically depressed patient.

Table 3 Common Symptoms of Depression

Sadness
Crying spells
Pessimism
Increased sense of guilt or worthlessness
Recurrent thoughts of death or suicide attempts
Decreased concentration
Fatigue; loss of energy
Loss of interest or pleasure
Social withdrawal
Significant weight (appetite) loss or gain
Insomnia (especially early morning awakening or hypersomnia)

The difference between antidepressants used to treat depressive disorders derives mainly from their varying side effect profiles. Some side effects warrant special attention in patients with diabetes. The older tricyclic antidepressants have sometimes been associated with elevations in blood glucose levels, and the newer selective serotonin-reuptake inhibitors (SSRIs) have been associated with hypoglycemia. These side effects are not usually troubling, but should be explained to the patient. Depressive disorders are often associated with changed eating patterns, so symptomatic improvement of the depression may lead to either more or less of an appetite. Therefore, changes in glycemic control associated with treatment, may not be related to pharmacological effects of antidepressants, but may be related to the alleviation of the core syndrome. Other side effects of particular note for diabetic patients include the frequent side effect of impaired erectile functioning found with SSRIs; possible aggravation of gastroparetic symptoms by both SSRIs and tricyclic antidepressants; and the increased risk of arrhythmia in patients taking tricyclics who have coexisting cardiac disease.

Several issues and problems need to be kept in mind when treating depressed patients:

1. Underrecognition and failure to diagnose.
2. The failure to carefully identify the target symptoms of the depressed patient and follow the symptom response to treatment over time: Because there are no biological markers that can be used to follow depressive symptoms reliably, and symptoms vary between patients, careful notation of each patient's symptom cluster is important for follow-up.
3. Failure to follow patients with sufficient frequency: Depressive disorders are a common and important risk factor for suicide. Suicide risk may increase as symptoms begin to remit because the patient's energy level increases before the degree of pessimism and ability to deal with any underlying stresses has occurred.
4. Underdosing: Even with the new antidepressants such as fluoxetine, titration of the dose upward may be important to obtain full response. The most common reason for treatment failure in a patient who has been started on an antidepressant regimen is an insufficient dose of medication.
5. Use of adjunctive medication is often required: For example, SSRIs typically do not assist with the insomnia of depression and may themselves aggravate it, even when taken in the morning. Therefore, initial treatment may require a sedative, hypnotic, or sedating antidepressant at night. Trazadone is commonly used for this purpose because of its sedation qualities and because it does not lead to addiction. Moreover, concomitant anxiety may require mild tranquilizers until the benefits of the antidepressant are experienced.

6. The length of treatment: Typically it takes 2–6 weeks to evaluate the effect of initial antidepressant therapy. In patients with a first or isolated depressive episodes, the antidepressants should be maintained at the same dose for a 4- to 6-month period. Gradual reduction in the therapeutic dose can be initiated. Some patients will require maintenance, over extended periods.

Even though antidepressants are now the most common approach to the treatment of depression, there are well-described psychotherapeutic methods that have efficacy equivalent to that of antidepressants. Cognitive behavioral therapy is the most widely tested and used of these methods. This short-term approach focuses on the well-recognized negative cognitive distortions (e.g., pessimism) that are embedded in the depressive syndrome. Therapy that addresses their negative distortions has been a useful treatment for depression. Moreover, cognitive behavioral therapy may be useful in preventing relapse of depression, thereby lessening the need for long-term antidepressant therapy. Cognitive behavioral therapy should be undertaken only by mental health professionals who have been carefully trained in this method. Other forms of psychotherapy have also been tested and are useful treatments for depression.

B. Eating Disorders

Among women, the desire to be as thin as possible has become the dominant ideal of beauty. This view of the body is also increasing in frequency among young men. A substantial minority of women patients with type 1 diabetes report of purposely underdosing with insulin to maintain or lose weight on at least some occasions. Successful intervention of patients having this set of attitudes and behaviors is often exceedingly difficult because of the profound cultural attitudes that support the drive for thinness. It takes only a glance at an old painting or even a picture of Marilyn Monroe to realize that the body weight ideals at the end of the 20th century have shifted remarkably from those of even 40 years ago. Moreover, purging, vomiting, laxative use, diuretics, and insulin underdosing are often considered shameful and embarrassing and, therefore, will be hidden from the treating physician. The keystone for successful treatment of eating disorders involves nonjudgmental questioning, acceptance, and a focus on the quality of life issues from the patient's perspective, rather than an intense focus on diabetes control. Pharmacological interventions can be useful adjuncts to treatment. For example, antidepressants may be useful for associated depressive disorders and neuroleptic medications, such as risperidone, may be helpful for intense cognitive distortions around body weight ideals. However, the primary focus of intervention is on social psychological behavioral therapies. Often group setting will be useful and family involvement required. With mild bulimia, short interventions can be helpful, but for more serious bulimic and anorexic syndromes, long-term and persistent therapies are often required. For the diabetic patient, it is important that the reinstitution of therapeutic levels of insulin is often associated with fluid shifts and sudden weight gain that is frightening to the eating-disordered patient. The patient will commonly be unable to distinguish weight gain caused by fluid from that caused by fat. Weight is weight; size is size; it does not matter the source of the change. Therefore, reinitiation of insulin may require hospitalization and may lead to a resurgence in attempts to purge by multiple methods.

V. SPECIFIC PSYCHOEDUCATIONAL INTERVENTIONS

Use of group psychoeducational programs for the treatment of psychosocial complications in diabetes has become more common in recent years. Programs that incorporate advances in applying cognitive and behavioral techniques are helpful when teaching patients how to cope with specific aspects of rigorous and demanding treatment programs. In addition, the use of groups not only provides a cost-effective approach, but also the group interaction actually supports and enhances patient behavior change. We present three psychoeducational intervention methods that can help patients cope with problems arising from diabetes and its treatment, specifically recognition of glucose fluctuations, adjusting to intensive treatment, and problems with adhering to complex treatment regimens: (a) Blood Glucose Awareness Training; (b) coping skills training for adolescents; and (d) cognitive behavioral approaches to adherence problems.

A. Blood Glucose Awareness Training

Blood Glucose Awareness Training (BGAT) provides a structured format for patients to learn how to recognize early or to anticipate the occurrence of fluctuations in blood glucose levels. Although BGAT teaches recognition of individualized warning signs of both hypoglycemic and hyperglycemic shifts in glucose level, it is particularly useful for addressing several of the barriers to diabetes self-care management that hypoglycemia fosters. These barriers include the following:

1. Fear of hypoglycemia: Fear of hypoglycemia may motivate individuals to maintain glucose levels higher than their target ranges and stimulate these individuals to overtreat low blood glucose episodes.
2. Inappropriate treatment of hypoglycemia: Overtreatment of hypoglycemia is a common problem that can aggravate glucose fluctuations. Although sometimes caused by fear of hypoglycemia, overtreatment may also be simply due to lack of knowledge and reinforced behavior

that becomes that person's accepted way of treating low blood glucose levels.

3. Individual differences in hypoglycemic warning symptoms: Warning symptoms of hypoglycemia vary among individuals, yet, many of the tools commonly used for teaching about hypoglycemia do not include or emphasize this point. In addition, hypoglycemic symptoms may change with increased frequency of hypoglycemia and with prolonged duration of diabetes.

4. Hypoglycemia unawareness: Some individuals may completely lose their ability to detect hypoglycemia, placing them at increased risk of loss of consciousness, seizures, and coma. The presence of neuropathy or frequent antecedent hypoglycemia may make those with insulin-treated diabetes more susceptible to the inability to detect hypoglycemia.

Through the identification of individualized early-warning symptoms and the development of an understanding about the interrelations of food, insulin, and exercise, patients begin to develop skills in actually recognizing and treating hypoglycemia earlier when it does occur and in predicting and, thereby, preventing its occurrence. These newly acquired skills enhance patients' sense of self-efficacy for managing diabetes and may reduce some of the frustration surrounding these complications of diabetes treatment. However, it is important to note that BGAT is not designed to help patients specifically improve glycemic control.

BGAT consists of a series of classes that employ in-class activities and extensive homework records designed to help patients recognize which neurogenic symptoms (symptoms based on counterregulation) or neuroglycopenic symptoms (symptoms resulting from decreased blood supply to the brain) they actually experience, rather than relying on lists of symptoms identified as those that may occur in the general diabetic population during glucose shifts. In addition, participants learn how insulin, exercise, and food actually affect their blood glucose level throughout the day. BGAT employs behavioral techniques along with extensive recording of glucose levels and graphing of the effects of exercise, insulin and food to emphasize the individual differences in physiological responses and to help individuals identify personalized early-warning signs of blood glucose fluctuations.

B. Coping Skills Training

Another psychoeducational program has been used to teach small groups of two to three adolescents to develop more positive-coping styles and behaviors that will allow them to cope with the stresses of the diabetes and its treatment. By using techniques drawn from behavioral modification, social skills training, and conflict resolution, coping skills training (CST) employs scenarios and role-playing to help adolescents develop life skills that will allow them to cope with their demanding diabetes treatment and may even translate to other stresses that challenge the average adolescent with or without diabetes. Coping skills training completed by adolescents who were undergoing intensification of their diabetes management was associated with a greater improvement in glycemic control, better diabetes self-efficacy, fewer problems coping with diabetes, and less negative influence of intensive diabetes management on quality of life. Thus CST can be an important and effective adjunct to medical and educational management during adolescence, a period of life that is often associated with poor glycemic control.

C. Cognitive Behavioral Approaches to Treatment Adherence Problems

Additional programs that deal with important treatment psychosocial problems, such as nonadherence to treatment regimen, are currently under development and evaluation. Because diabetes self-care involves demanding lifestyle adaptations, adherence to prescribed self-care behaviors is challenging at best. Psychoeducational programs that employ cognitive behavioral therapy techniques have great potential for helping patients resolve and overcome some of the behavioral and attitudinal treatment barriers to improved glycemia. The focus of these 6- to 8-week courses is to help patients set realistic, achievable personal goals, learn to manage stress, examine personal assumptions and beliefs that underlie their current behavior, and reevaluate their automatic thought habits that reinforce nonadherence to their prescribed diabetes treatment plan. By learning how to recognize and challenge negative thought habits that interfere with their diabetes self-care, patients are better able to both carry out their self-care and utilize health care services more appropriately.

These group psychoeducational programs may have a synergistic effect with traditional and intensive medical and educational approaches to improving glycemic control. These programs can help overcome some of the complex psychosocial complications associated with diabetes and its treatment that impede an otherwise successful approach to treatment.

BIBLIOGRAPHY

Anderson BJ, Rubin RR, eds. Practical Psychology for Diabetes Clinicians. Alexandria, VA: American Diabetes Association, 1996.

Blackburn IM, Moore RG. Controlled acute and follow-up trial of cognitive therapy and pharmacotherapy in out-patients with recurrent depression. Br J Psychiatry 171: 328–334, 1997.

Cox DJ, Gonder-Frederick LA, Polonsky W, Schlundt D, Julian D, Clarke W. A multicenter evaluation of Blood Glucose Awareness Training II. Diabetes Care 18:523–528, 1995.

Gavard JA, Lustman PJ, Clouse RE. Prevalence of depression in adults with diabetes. An epidemiological evaluation. Diabetes Care 16:1167–78, 1993.

Goodnick PJ, Henry JH, Buki VM. Treatment of depression in patients with diabetes mellitus. J Clin Psychiatry 56:128–136, 1995.

Grey M, Boland EA, Davidson M, Yu Chang, Sullivan-Bolyani S, Tamborlane WV. Short-term effects of coping skills training as adjunct to intensive therapy in adolescents. Diabetes Care 21:902–908, 1998.

Heller SR, Clarke P, Daly H, Davis I, McCulloch DK, Allison SP, Tattersall RB. Group education for obese patients with type 2 diabetes: greater success at less cost. Diabetic Med 5:552–446, 1988.

Jacobson AM. The psychological care of patients with insulin-dependent diabetes mellitus. N Engl J Med 334:1249–1253, 1996.

Jacobson AM, Weinger K. Treating depression in diabetic patients: Is there an alternative to medications? Ann Intern Med 129:656–657, 1998.

Lazare A, Putnam SM, Lipkin M. Three functions of the medical interview. In: Lipkin M Jr, Putnam SM, Lazare A, eds. The Medical Interview: Clinical Care, Education, and Research. New York: Springer-Verlag, 1995:3–19.

Lustman PJ. Anxiety disorders in adults with diabetes mellitus. Psychiatr Clin North Am 11:419–432, 1988.

Lustman PJ, Griffith LS, Freedland KE, Kissel SS, Clouse RE. Cognitive behavior therapy for depression in type 2 diabetes mellitus. A randomized control trial. Ann Intern Med 129:613–621, 1998.

Sank LI, Shaffer CS. A Therapist's Manual for Cognitive Behavioral Therapy in Groups. New York: Plenum Press, 1984.

Tattersall RB, McCulloch DK, Aveline M. Group therapy in the treatment of diabetes. Diabetes Care 8:180–188, 1985.

Vasile RG. Depressive disorders. In: Jacobson JL, Jacobson AM, eds. Psychiatric Secrets. Philadelphia: Hanley & Belfus, 1996:261–269.

Wulsin LR. Depressive disorders. In: Jacobson JL, Jacobson AM, eds. Psychiatric Secrets. Philadelphia: Hanley & Belfus, 1996:74–79.

34
Hypertension and Diabetes

James R. Sowers and Bharat Raman
Wayne State University School of Medicine, Detroit, Michigan

I. INTRODUCTION

Diabetes mellitus and hypertension both increase with advancing age in western-ized societies. Current estimates suggest that 15 million Americans are affected by diabetes mellitus, 90% of whom have type 2 diabetes or non–insulin-dependent diabetes mellitus. The prevalence is about 20% in non-Hispanic whites older than age 65 and is higher in African Americans and Hispanics. Obesity and a sedentary lifestyle are also contributors to the increasing incidence of diabetes mellitus in industrialized nations.

Hypertension is twice as common in persons with diabetes than in those without this metabolic disorder. Eighty percent of the premature mortality associated with diabetes and hypertension is related to cardiovascular disease (CVD) and hypertension is a major contributor to CVD in diabetes mellitus. Whereas, 40% of the overall mortality in the United States can be attributed to CVD, 80% of the deaths in elderly diabetics are related to its complications, such as sudden death, congestive heart failure, cerebrovascular and peripheral vascular disease. More than half the patients with newly diagnosed type 2 diabetes mellitus have hypertension at the time of presentation.

Obesity appears to be an important factor contributing to the increased prevalence of diabetes mellitus and hypertension. Central obesity is an especially powerful risk factor for the development of type 2 diabetes mellitus, hypertension, dyslipidemia, insulin resistance, and premature CVD. Visceral fat is thought to be the factor predisposing to this association. Although the body mass index is a relatively potent determinant of blood pressure, especially systolic blood pressure, a visceral distribution of fat is an even more powerful risk factor for the development of hypertension. Two characteristic abnormalities of visceral obesity, fasting hyperinsulinemia and elevated apolipoprotein β were the strongest independent risk factors for CVD.

Hypertension and coexistent diabetes are often associated with lipid and coagulation abnormalities. Persons with clinical diabetes as well as those with impaired glucose tolerance and hypertension manifest a characteristic dyslipidemia with low high-density lipoprotein (HDL), high very low density lipoprotein (VLDL), and a phenotypically small, dense LDL. This small, dense LDL is associated with a threefold increase in CVD risk, and this risk is further enhanced in the presence of elevated apolipoprotein β levels. Disturbances in the fibrinolytic system have been reported in hypertensives and especially in those with lipid and glucose abnormalities and vascular disease. There is a tendency toward increased coagulability and decreased fibrinolysis. This is caused by an increase in several components of the coagulation cascade (endothelial-derived von Willebrand's factor, factor VIII fibrinogen) and deficiencies of endogenous factors that normally inhibit clot generation (factors C, S, and antithrombin III). Lipoprotein a(Lpa) levels are often elevated in diabetes mellitus, and by inhibiting fibrinolysis, this contributes to plaque progression. Elevated levels of plasminogen activator inhibitor-1 (PAI-1) have been observed in untreated essential hypertension and in men with prior myocardial infarction and increased risk of reinfarction. Elevated PAI-1 levels are associated with abdominal obesity, and insulin resistance–hyperinsulinemia and associated dyslipidemia.

Essential hypertension and diabetes mellitus are both associated with increased levels of intracellular platelet calcium. Elevated levels of intracellular calcium appear to be key determinants of enhanced platelet activation, aggregation, and adhesion to the endothelium. Dysfunction of the vascular endothelium appears to play a major role in the accelerated atherosclerosis in persons with hypertension and associated metabolic abnormalities. Hyperglycemia results in decreased endothelial nitric oxide production. This combined with activation of protein kinase C, results in a constellation of changes that lead to an increase vasomotor tone and vascular growth.

Insulin resistance and hyperinsulinemia are often present in persons with hypertension. High levels of insulin stimulate mitogenic activity and synthesis of atherogenic factors (endothelial and plasminogen activator inhibitor). Much of the effect of insulin on cardiovascular growth is likely mediated through the actions of insulin on an insulin-like growth factor I (IGF-1) receptor in endothelial and vascular smooth-muscle cells. Unlike insulin, which is not produced by cardiovascular tissue, IGF-1 is and is more likely to function in an autocrine–paracrine role. There is increasing evidence that IGF-1 synthesis and expression plays an important role in mesangial hyperplasia and left ventricular hypertrophy, both manifestations of diabetes mellitus and hypertension.

The contribution and association of hypertension and diabetes mellitus to CVD in women is just as, if not more, dramatic. CVD is a leading cause of morbidity and mortality in women in the United States. Although CVD is less common in premenopausal women than in men, this difference begins to disappear after menopause, presumably owing to reduced production of female sex hormones. A similar pattern occurs with hypertension. Men have higher blood pressures than women, until approximately age 50–65, after which blood pressure, especially systolic, is higher in women. Diabetes mellitus removes the normal gender differences in the prevalence of CHD. Evidence exists for the role of high insulin levels as a potential cause for the absence of the sex-related differences in atherosclerotic vascular disease (ASVD).

The onset of hypertension is markedly different in type 1 and type 2 diabetes mellitus. Whereas 50% of persons with type 2 diabetes mellitus are hypertensive at presentation, blood pressure is usually normal in newly diagnosed type 1 disease and remains so for the first 5–10 years. The onset of nephropathy and renal disease precede the development of hypertension in type 1 diabetes mellitus. As a corollary, many newly diagnosed patients with type 2 diabetes mellitus have preexisting nephropathy. With the existence of overt albuminuria (proteinuria values higher than 300 mg/24 h) hypertension occurs in three-fourths of type 2 diabetics. If they also have a serum creatinine value higher than 1.4 mg/dL the majority will be found to have coexisting hypertension. Increased urinary albumin excretion as microalbuminuria also occurs in poorly treated essential hypertensives without diabetes mellitus. Microalbuminuria is a predictor of early mortality in type 2 diabetes mellitus and in the general population. Elevated blood pressure is a common factor in both groups and, at least in the diabetic group, early detection and treatment result in decreased mortality. It appears important to control hyperglycemia in part because this makes it easier to control blood pressure. Several of the newer oral agents for treatment of diabetes mellitus have potentially positive effects on diabetic cardiovascular disease. Thiazolidinediones decrease vascular smooth muscle cell (VSMC) proliferation and decrease vascular contractility; metformin promotes VSMC glucose uptake. However, prospective controlled trials of morbidity and mortality with these agents need to be conducted to determine if they affect CVD in diabetes mellitus (Fig. 1).

II. DIAGNOSIS AND TREATMENT GOALS

The goal of lowering blood pressure in persons with diabetes is to prevent hypertension associated death and disability. Diabetics frequently have more labile blood pressures and are more susceptible to postural hypotension, in part, because of reduced baroreceptor sensitivity. They also, often, do not have the normal nocturnal dip in blood pressure.

Thus, the diagnosis of hypertension requires multiple blood pressure measurements obtained in a standardized fashion on at least three occasions. Standing

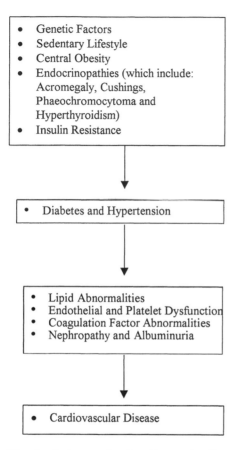

Fig. 1 Pathogenesis of cardiovascular disease in diabetes and hypertension.

blood pressure should also be measured on each office visit because of the propensity to orthostatic hypotension. With very high blood pressures, (systolic ≥ 210 mmHg, diastolic ≥ 120 mm Hg) the diagnosis can be made at the first visit. Because of the variability of blood pressure in diabetics, ambulatory and home blood pressure recordings may be particularly important, and valuable information may be obtained to (a) identify white coat hypertension, (b) monitor response to therapy, (c) improve patient compliance, and (d) potentially decrease cost. Validated aneroid or electronic devices may be used for home monitoring with an appropriately sized cuff. Finger monitors tend to be inaccurate. Periodic comparison of the patients device with a mercury sphygmomanometer and auscultatory readings should be performed to determine accuracy of the home monitors.

The consensus blood pressure goal in diabetics with hypertension is less than 130/85 mmHg. While evaluating diabetics with hypertension, the following should be addressed: (a) Is this a surgically curable form of hypertension? (b) Is there target organ involvement (cerebral, ocular, cardiac, renal, peripheral vasculature)? (c) Are there other cardiovascular risk factors (smoking, family history)? (d) What is the current level of control of diabetes and hypertension?

Medications used by the patient should be reviewed as many medications can raise blood pressure and interfere with treatment, some of these include:

1. Sympathomimetics
2. Decongestants
3. Appetite suppressants
4. Cocaine and other illicit drugs
5. Caffeine
6. Oral contraceptives
7. Steroids
8. Licorice (chewing tobacco)
9. Erythropoietin
10. NSAIDS
11. Antidepressants

During the physical examination, special attention needs to be paid to target organs.

1. Fundii: For evidence of diabetic and hypertensive retinopathy: A periodic eye examination by an opthalmologist is recommended even if the patient is asymptomatic.
2. Neck: Check for bruits, thyromegaly, distended veins.
3. Cardiac: Signs of LVH (e.g., sustained PMI, murmurs, arrhythmias, additional heart sounds).
4. Abdomen: Bruits, enlarged bladder.
5. Extremities: Diminished or absent pulses, edema.
6. Neurological: Especially sensory examination.

Laboratory tests recommended before initiation of therapy are the following:

1. Hemoglobin and hemocrit valve
2. Urinalysis complete: Albumin/creatinine ratio or microalbumin excretion rate if urine dipstick protein is negative or quantitative urine protein measurement with a positive dipstick.
3. Serum creatinine, K^+, Mg^{2+}, blood glucose levels.

Table 1   Checklist for a Diabetic with Hypertension

1. Measure blood pressure on each visit.
2. Check for orthostatic changes.
3. If new onset, confirm elevated blood pressure on at least two other occasions unless blood pressure > 210/120 mmHg.
4. Evaluate medications.
5. Look for surgically treatable causes of hypertension (e.g., renal artery stenosis, hyperaldosteronism secondary to an adenoma).
6. Evaluate target organs.
7. Begin therapy to achieve goal blood pressure of 130/85 mmHg.

    4.   Glycosylated Hb or HbA_{1C} levels.
    5.   Fasting lipid profile (Table 1).

Two groups of patients with diabetes and hypertension need special mention:

1. Pregnant Patients. Screening is recommended between the 24th and 28th weeks of gestation in women who meet any one of the following criteria:

$\geq$ 25 years of age.
< 25 years of age and obese ($\geq$ 20% over desired body weight or BMI $\geq$ 27 kg/m^2).
Family history of diabetes mellitus in first-degree relative
Patient belongs to an ethnic group with a high prevalence of diabetes mellitus (e.g., African American, Native American, Asian American, or Hispanic American).

It is unclear whether patients with gestational diabetes have a higher incidence of hypertension. Therapy for hypertension should begin when blood pressure is 140/90 mmHg or higher. The presence of proteinuria mandates a more aggressive therapeutic approach, and consultation with a perinatal specialist should be considered. Pharmacological treatment with methyldopa is preferred. β-Adrenergic blockers appear safe in the second and third trimester. Angiotensin-converting enzyme inhibitors (ACEI) are contraindicated.

2. Children. Diabetes mellitus in childhood is usually type 1. When hypertension develops it usually suggests the onset of nephropathy, but it may also represent essential hypertension. The diagnosis of hypertension in children requires that they have blood pressure levels repeatedly above the 95th percentile for age and sex, as defined by the Task Force on Blood Pressure Control in Children. The

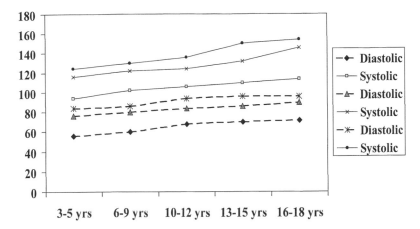

Fig. 2 Childhood blood pressure distribution for the 50th, 95th, and 99th percentiles. (From Ref. 3, JNC-VI.)

figure provides blood pressure values for 50th, 95th, and 99th percentiles in Childhood Blood Pressure Distribution (Fig. 2).

A reasonable goal of treatment is to lower blood pressure to the 90th percentile or less. Drug treatment is similar to that in adults.

III. TREATMENT

The least intrusive means of managing these diseases should be sought. Lifestyle modifications are an integral part of therapy and should include

Weight reduction
Regular aerobic physical activity
Reduction of sodium intake
Smoking cessation
Moderation of alcohol intake
Dietary interventions to control hyperglycemia and dyslipidemia

Some authorities recommend initiation of pharmacological therapy simultaneously with lifestyle modification for patients with high normal blood pressure (systolic 130–139 mmHg and diastolic 85–89 mmHg) and diabetes mellitus. The use of ACEI, α-adrenergic blockers, calcium channel antagonists, and diuretics are preferred because of fewer adverse effects, specifically those related to glycemic control, dyslipidemia, and renal function. β-Adrenergic blockers constitute the fifth class of drugs used to treat diabetic hypertensives. Each class will be discussed individually. They are listed in alphabetical order.

A. α-Adrenergic Blockers

The α-adrenergic blocking drugs do not have an adverse effect on glucose metabolism or the lipid profile. During short-term therapy they have shown benefit on lipids with increased HDL and decreased TG. They may also decrease insulin resistance. Postural hypotension frequently is the limiting factor in their use, and titration of dosage should be cautious.

B. ACE Inhibitors

The ACE-inhibiting agents are preferred, especially in patients with nephropathy. In diabetics, various studies have shown a beneficial effect of ACEI on mortality from CVD. The cardiovascular protection is even more compelling than the well-known renoprotective effects. Cough is sometimes a cause for a change in therapy and much more rare is angioedema. Renal function and potassium values should be followed closely with initiation of therapy and for a few weeks subsequently. Sudden worsening of renal function with ACEI may occur in patients with bilateral renal artery stenosis. Life-threatening hyperkalemia is possible and is more likely to occur in the presence of hyporeninemic hypoaldosteronism (type IV RTA).

C. β-Adrenergic Blockers

The β-adrenergic blockers are the drugs of choice in postinfarction therapy in both diabetics and nondiabetics, and are good choices as adjunctive antihypertensive therapy in this scenario. However, their adverse effects on glucose homeostasis, prolonged hypoglycemia, and hypoglycemia unawareness should be borne in mind. Combinations of an ACEI or calcium antagonist (dihydropyridine) and a β-blocker may be preferable.

D. Calcium Channel Antagonists

The calcium channel antagonists are useful adjuncts in treating hypertension and, in combination with an ACEI, may have a greater benefit in decreasing CVD mortality than either agent alone. The combination of a nondihydropyridine calcium antagonist and an ACEI have also decreased proteinuria to a greater extent than the individual agents used separately. Further studies, however, are required to elucidate this.

Treatment Goal < 130/85 mm Hg

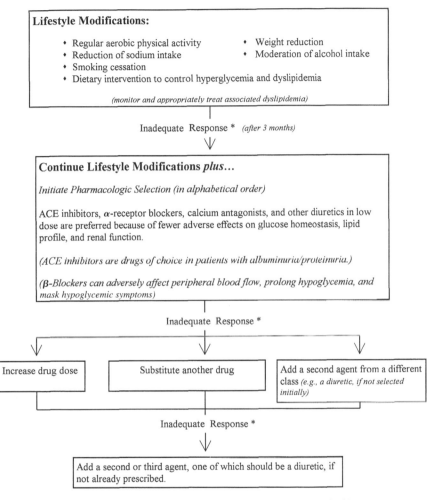

Lifestyle Modifications:

- Regular aerobic physical activity
- Reduction of sodium intake
- Smoking cessation
- Dietary intervention to control hyperglycemia and dyslipidemia
- Weight reduction
- Moderation of alcohol intake

(monitor and appropriately treat associated dyslipidemia)

Inadequate Response * *(after 3 months)*

Continue Lifestyle Modifications *plus...*

Initiate Pharmacologic Selection (in alphabetical order)

ACE inhibitors, α-receptor blockers, calcium antagonists, and other diuretics in low dose are preferred because of fewer adverse effects on glucose homeostasis, lipid profile, and renal function.

(ACE inhibitors are drugs of choice in patients with albuminuria/proteinuria.)

(β-Blockers can adversely affect peripheral blood flow, prolong hypoglycemia, and mask hypoglycemic symptoms)

Inadequate Response *

Increase drug dose

Substitute another drug

Add a second agent from a different class *(e.g., a diuretic, if not selected initially)*

Inadequate Response *

Add a second or third agent, one of which should be a diuretic, if not already prescribed.

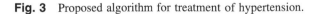

* An adequate response means goal blood pressure achieved or considerable progress

Fig. 3 Proposed algorithm for treatment of hypertension.

E. Diuretics

In low doses (25 mg or less of chlorthalidone or hydrochlorothiazide; HCTZ), diuretics are effective antihypertensives in diabetics, especially in the elderly with isolated systolic hypertension. The low dose of the diuretic is not often associated with electrolyte (hypokalemia and hypomagnesia) abnormalities nor with adverse effects on carbohydrate metabolism. A synergism exists with ACEI and with it a tendency for orthostatic hypotension. Care must be used when adding either agent to the other.

Treatment of hypertension in diabetics is a challenging task and multiple drugs (an average of three to five) may be required to achieve the goal of reducing blood pressure to less than 130/85 mmHg (Fig. 3).

BIBLIOGRAPHY

Clinical Practice Recommendations. Diabetes Care 1998; Suppl 1.

National High Blood Pressure Education Program Working Group Report on Hypertension in Diabetes. (Chair: James R. Sowers, MD). Hypertension 1994; 23:145–158.

Sixth Report of the Joint National Committee on Prevention, Detection, Evaluation and Treatment of High Blood Pressure. Arch Intern Med 1997; 157:2413–2446.

Sowers JR, Epstein M. Diabetes mellitus and associated hypertension, vascular disease and nephropathy: an update. Hypertension 1995; 26:869–879.

Sowers JR. Diabetes mellitus and cardiovascular disease in women. Arch Intern Med 1998; 158:617–621.

35
Diabetes and Aging

Caroline S. Blaum and Jeffrey B. Halter
University of Michigan, Ann Arbor, Michigan

I. INTRODUCTION

Diabetes mellitus is a common chronic disease among older adults. It is present in up to 18% of persons older than 65, comprising more than 40% of all persons with diabetes in the United States (1,2). Because such a sizable proportion of diabetes patients are 65 and older, it is important to consider both the similarities and differences between older and younger diabetes patients. In both groups, type 2 diabetes is the most common form of diabetes, and the macrovascular complications of diabetes are the major causes of morbidity and mortality in all diabetes patients. As with younger diabetes patients, most older patients with diabetes are highly functional and active, and deserve the same attention to diabetes management as younger patients. However, older patients are different in several important ways: (a) Because of their numbers and prevalence of complications, older patients have a large influence on health service utilization and costs. Therefore, even minor successes of management interventions in preventing or mitigating complications can potentially have a large effect on the health status of the older population and health care utilization. (b) Older patients are heterogeneous, often with comorbidities and disabilities that must be considered for their influence on the patient's clinical status; therefore, the physician must perform a detailed evaluation to determine appropriate management goals and inventions. (c) Some older patients may be more symptomatic from hyperglycemia than younger patients, but they are also more prone to complications of treatment. (d) Special evaluation and treatment goals must be devised for the "frail" elderly. Table 1 summarizes some of these differences.

Table 1 Differences Between Older and Younger Diabetic Patients

Older patients extremely heterogeneous
More complications, comorbidities, and disability
More symptomatic from hyperglycemia and hypoglycemia
Special considerations for frail elderly

II. EFFECTS OF DIABETES

Diabetes has a major influence on the health of older Americans, and as such has a major effect on health care utilization and costs. It is the seventh leading cause of visits to primary care physicians; 60% of diabetes patients are on Medicare, and Medicare has been estimated to pay 45.5% of office visits for diabetes (3). The total per capita annual health care expenditures for patients with diabetes have been estimated as four times greater than for persons without diabetes, and direct diabetes health care costs were estimated at $91.8 billion in 1992.

III. EPIDEMIOLOGICAL ASPECTS OF DIABETES AND AGING

The NHANES III study found that about 18% of people 60 and older have diabetes, about one-third of whom have undiagnosed diabetes, and about 14% have impaired fasting glucose (1). Most older patients have type 2 diabetes. Type 2 is a heterogeneous syndrome owing to abnormalities of pancreatic islet function and insulin action. Although insulin is not required for survival, many patients with type 2 diabetes are treated with insulin to control hyperglycemia. Only 5–10% of older patients have type 1 diabetes, which is due to an autoimmune destructive process in the islet cells.

The prevalence of impaired fasting glucose (IFG) increases with age. *Impaired fasting glucose* is defined as a fasting glucose value of 110 or higher and less than 126 mg/dL (4). Impaired fasting glucose is an independent risk factor for increased atherosclerotic disease in older persons. Because of the recent redefinition of diabetes and IFG by the American Diabetes Association, more information is available about impaired glucose tolerance (IGT), defined by abnormal postchallenge hypoglycemia. IGT increases the risk for the development of frank diabetes mellitus, although much variability has been reported in different populations relative to the risk of development of diabetes mellitus (5).

Older patients with diabetes are heterogeneous in the characteristics of their diabetes. In some it may be newly diagnosed; NHANES III suggests an age-stable incidence rate of 2.7 : 1000 new diabetes cases per year. However, a "new" diabetes patient may have had years of undiagnosed diabetes or impaired fasting glucose, and thus have increased risk or clinical evidence for diabetic complications. Alternatively, older patients may have had diagnosed diabetes for years, with varying clinical burdens from microvascular and macrovascular complications.

Older patients are also at increased risk for many of the conditions that add to the morbidity and mortality of diabetes. Hypertension, especially systolic, increases with age; 60% of older patients with diabetes also have hypertension, which independently increases risk for both macrovascular and microvascular diabetic complications (6). Sixty percent of older patients have hyperlipidemia, also conferring increased risk for atherosclerotic disease. Although not as many older diabetes patients are obese as younger ones (7), obesity is still a significant problem for many older diabetic patients. Similarly, fewer older diabetic patients smoke cigarettes, but those who do are at greatly increased risk for increased morbidity and mortality.

Recent findings from the United Kingdom Prospective Diabetes Study (UKPDS) showed that baseline (at the time of known diagnosis) increased low-density lipoprotein (LDL) cholesterol, decreased high-density lipoprotein (HDL) cholesterol, level of hyperglycemia, increased systolic blood pressure, and smoking conferred increased risk for coronary artery disease in type 2 diabetic patients. In this study, older age also increased risk independently from other risk factors (8). Established macrovascular complications of diabetes, cerebrovascular disease, cardiovascular disease, and peripheral vascular disease, are from 1.5 to 2 times more prevalent in the older diabetic populations than in the older nondiabetic population (9).

Older persons with diabetes have a greater prevalence of disability and functional impairment than those without diabetes (10,11). Older adults with diabetes are about 1.5 times more likely to have physical limitations and activities of daily living (ADL) disability than those without. This excess disability is a direct result of complications of diabetes, such as eye disease, increased strokes and cardiovascular disease, and increased neuropathy and peripheral vascular disease. The presence of functional impairments also has implications for diabetes self-management in some older patients. For example, some older patients may not be able to go to the store or the physician, handle their own medications, or make their own meals.

The fastest-growing segment of the rapidly growing older population in the United States are those 80 years of age and older. Epidemiological data suggests that diabetes incidence and prevalence level-off or decrease in persons older than 75 (1), but the numbers are still substantial, ranging from a 6.7 to 13.3% prevalence of self-reported diabetes in persons older than 85 in the Established Populations for the Epidemiological Study of the Elderly (EPESE) studies (11).

This oldest segment of the population also has the highest disability rates, resulting in an increased need for personal assistance and caregiver attention. Approximately one-third of persons older than 85 years of age live in nursing homes. These trends result in a substantial number of functionally disabled elderly, either in the community or in nursing homes, who have diabetes, and their numbers will increase. Data from the Medical Expenditure Survey II shows that from 10 to 14.5% of nursing home patients have diabetes, and these patients have higher levels of comorbid diseases, diabetic complications, and disability than nursing home patients without diabetes (12).

The most important point to remember about older patients with diabetes is that they represent an extremely heterogeneous population. This heterogeneity involves not only their diabetes, but also their disease burden, functional status, and social situation. Most older diabetic patients, even those with complications of diabetes and cormorbid conditions, do not have major functional impairments. Many older patients are very active, traveling, volunteering, and even continuing to work, whereas others, even of the same chronological age, are disabled and frail. A diabetic patient in her 70s may be truly a newly diagnosed diabetic; may be newly diagnosed, but with many years of undiagnosed diabetes; or may have had diabetes for 10 years or longer, with or without complications and comorbidities. If she is generally healthy and truly newly diagnosed, her median life expectancy is another 14 years (13), and management decisions geared toward preventing diabetic complications make sense. On the other hand, if she has had diabetes for many years, and has atherosclerotic, visual, and other comorbidities and resultant functional impairments, a more basic management strategy would be appropriate.

IV. DIABETES AND THE PHYSIOLOGY OF AGING

Many physiological changes associated with diabetes accelerate age-related physiological changes. In women, the presence of diabetes has long been known to negate the protective effect of estrogen on atherosclerotic disease, conferring on diabetic women a risk of cardiovascular disease equal to that of men at the same age (14). Some of the mechanisms presumed to underlie this accelerated vascular aging include diabetes' effects on platelets, increased glycosylation of vascular tissues, and lipoprotein alterations associated with diabetes (15–17).

Physiological changes with diabetes that occur at the cellular level may also simulate age-related changes. Diabetes, as aging, is associated with thickening of the basement membranes of cells, with decreased cell density of skin fibroblasts, and with increased cellular doubling time (18).

Age-related changes in body composition and cellular proteins may also be related to glucose intolerance. Aging is associated with increased proportion of fat tissue, which is relatively insulin-resistant. Available evidence suggests that aging is not associated with a decrease in insulin receptors at the cellular level, but that a postreceptor defect associated with insulin resistance is more common in aging individuals. Research also suggests a decrease in phase 2 insulin secretion response to glucose, leading to a relative insulin deficiency in some persons (19).

Changes that occur with diabetes and changes that occur with aging may interact with each other. This is especially true for the general age-related decrease in physiological reserve in many organ systems. Although most physiological systems (cardiovascular, renal, pulmonary, CNS) function appropriately under normal stable conditions, in older persons, they may be unable to cope with increased demands posed by acute illness or injury. Diabetic complications leading to end-organ damage may further accelerate this loss of physiological reserve. In addition, the clinical manifestations of diabetes may stress physiological systems even in the absence of frank pathology. For example, even a mild increased urine volume in an older diabetic patient may exacerbate bladder dysfunction and lead to urinary incontinence. Glycosuria, even without polyuria, can lead to electrolyte imbalance and cardiac arrhythmias.

V. DIAGNOSIS

A redefinition of the diagnosis of diabetes, in both older and younger persons, that is based on the fasting blood sugar has recently been endorsed by an expert committee of the American Diabetes Association (20). Based on these criteria, diabetes would be present if the fasting blood sugar value is 126 mg/dL or higher for all ages. Increased fasting blood glucose was defined as fasting glucose values of 110 mg/dL or more to less than 126 mg/dL. These definitions hold for all ages, and produce a prevalence of diabetes that is somewhat different for older persons when compared with the previous World Health Organization (WHO) diagnostic criteria (21). Although this approach to diagnosis seems reasonable, the implications for older persons have not yet been fully defined and have generated some controversy (22).

VI. SYMPTOMS OF DIABETES IN OLDER PATIENTS

Hyperglycemia can lead to symptoms in all diabetes patients, but changes of aging and comorbid conditions present in many older patients can worsen symptoms. Polyuria associated with hyperglycemia can be confused with urinary infection and incontinence, which are also common in older persons, and can worsen incontinence caused by comorbid diseases. Osmotic diuresis associated with persistent hyperglycemia may predispose the patient to volume depletion and resultant orthostatic hypotension, increasing the likelihood of falls and fatigue. In addition, impaired central thirst response in older persons may contribute to the volume depletion caused by osmotic diuresis from hyperglycemia.

Weight loss secondary to uncontrolled hyperglycemia can be a significant problem. Such patients may be in a constant catabolic state, which leads to loss of muscle mass, weakness, and potentially falls and injury. Older patients may not perceive increased hunger, and their lack of polyphagia may delay diagnosis of this problem and exacerbate their poor nutritional status.

Older persons may also be at increased risk for trace nutrient depletion from osmotic diuresis. Potassium, zinc, chromium, and magnesium deficiencies may be present. Magnesium and potassium deficiencies can have deleterious effects on cardiac conduction. Glycosuria can also increase phosphate excretion, which can accelerate calcium loss from bone (2).

An increased concentration of glucose or its metabolites in the lens and aqueous humor of the eye can lead to visual problems. Hyperglycemia may increase the perception of pain (23) and predispose patients to bacterial and fungal infection. It may alter platelet adhesiveness, worsening intermittent claudication. Lipid abnormalities also worsen with poor glycemic control, and high triglyceride levels can predispose to pancreatitis. A careful search for such symptoms of hyperglycemia is clearly indicated in elderly diabetic patients.

In many older patients, symptoms associated with diabetes and hyperglycemia may be atypical. For example, hyperglycemia does not usually lead to dramatic polyuria and polydipsia; more often there will be increased incontinence, or a urinary tract infection, or increased lethargy or mental confusion. Similarly, undiagnosed or unmanaged diabetes may manifest as increased bacterial or fungal infections of the skin, unexplained weight loss, increased fatigue, or slow wound healing. Increased paresthesias and weakness, orthostatic hypotension with falls, or decreased vision should also raise suspicion for undiagnosed or inadequately managed diabetes.

VII. COMPLICATIONS OF DIABETES IN OLDER PATIENTS

Elderly diabetic patients have a substantial number of diabetic complications, comorbid diseases, and functional disabilities owing to both an age-related increase in chronic disease prevalence and the longer duration of their diabetes (24). The macrovascular complications of diabetes, which lead to coronary vascular, cerebrovascular, and peripheral vascular diseases, are the major cause of morbidity and mortality in elderly diabetic patients. Older patients with diabetes are 1.5–4 times more likely to have atherosclerotic disease than older patients without diabetes (14). The risk is particularly increased in older women with diabetes.

Peripheral vascular disease leading to foot ulcers, gangrene, and amputations is also highly associated with age (25).

Several major issues are pertinent for macrovascular complications of older diabetic patients, and type 2 diabetes patients in general. Accumulated clinical knowledge from clinical trials, outcome studies, and clinical experience suggests that clinical and behavioral interventions can decrease mortality and morbidity from atherosclerotic disease. Evidence is also accumulating to suggest that such interventions are equally, if not more, effective in persons with diabetes, but often studies demonstrating these effects did not include older diabetic patients. An even more controversial question in type 2 diabetes is whether strict control of hyperglycemia will decrease macrovascular complications. The DCCT clearly showed benefit of tight control of diabetes for the prevention and decrease in microvascular complications for type 1 patients, but it did not demonstrate, even for type 1 patients, clear benefit for prevention or decrease of macrovascular complications (26). Similar conclusions were drawn from the recently completed UKPDS in patients with type 2 diabetes, but this study excluded persons over age 65 (27,28).

Microvascular complications are related to the duration of diabetes, regardless of age (29,30). The relation has been most clearly defined in diabetic retinopathy, for which diabetes duration is related to extent of retinopathy in type 2 diabetes. However, elderly patients more often have macular edema than proliferative retinopathy, and are less likely to go blind from diabetic retinopathy. However, older patients have increased prevalence of age- and diabetes-related medical eye diseases other than diabetic retinopathy. Both cataracts and glaucoma are increased in older patients with diabetes, and older patients with diabetes have a 60% increase in visual impairments compared with older persons without diabetes (31).

There is little specific information on diabetic renal disease in older patients with diabetes. Older diabetic patients could potentially be exposed to multiple insults to their renal function. Age-related changes in renal functioning could interact with changes in renal function caused by diabetes. Also, increased prevalence of atherosclerotic disease and hypertension in older patients can also add to increased prevalence of renal dysfunction. Finally, older diabetic patents with multiple diabetes-related and other chronic diseases may be taking multiple medications that can also adversely affect kidney function.

VIII. MANAGEMENT OF DIABETES IN OLDER PATIENTS

Diabetes mellitus is the most complicated disease regularly managed by primary care physicians. Because a high proportion of diabetic patients in the United States are 65 and older, the primary care physician is often doubly challenged to combine principles of geriatric medicine with diabetic management decisions. In addition, as changes in the health care delivery systems emphasize chronic disease management and population-based care, physicians may confront diabetes management guidelines and protocols and need to consider whether such guidelines fit their older patients.

A. Goals of Diabetes Management in Older Patients with Diabetes

The goals of diabetic management in older patients are not substantially different from goals in other diabetic patients and, as with other diabetic patients, include far more than just treatment of hyperglycemia. These goals are summarized in Table 2.

There is accumulating evidence of systematic undertreatment of older patients with diabetes, both relative to risk factor detection and treatment and management of hyperglycemia (32). The heterogeneous older diabetic population includes persons who have advanced disability or dementia or preterminal disease. For such individuals, preventative treatment may not be a priority. However, the vast majority of older patients are highly functional, have a life expectancy of several to many years, and are highly motivated to avoid disability and continue an active lifestyle as long as possible. Even highly disabled or preterminal patients require basic diabetes management to optimize function, prevent distressing symptoms, and potentially improve caregiver burden. The development of an individualized management plan that fits the goals and health status of each older patient is an essential component of diabetic care in the elderly.

B. Assessment of the Older Patient with Diabetes

The key to developing an appropriate treatment plan for older diabetic patients is comprehensive assessment of health status. Signs and symptoms related to

Table 2 Goals of Diabetes Management in Older Patients with Diabetes

Alleviation of symptomatic hyperglycemia
Treatment of risk factors for atherosclerotic disease
Identification and treatment of diabetic complications and related comorbid disease
Improvement of general health status by attention to nutrition, physical conditioning, and
    functional status
Diabetes self-management education and counseling
Possible prevention of the development or worsening of diabetic complications by lowering
    glucose levels

Table 3 Components of Comprehensive Assessment of Older Diabetes Patients

---

History and physical
Function
Cognition and affect
Nutritional status
Medication use and possible inappropriate polypharmacy
Social situation and social support

---

hyperglycemia and diabetic complications should be carefully assessed. Evaluation for hyperlipidemia, hypertension, and other risk factors for atherosclerosis is important. The history and physical examination will provide evidence of local atherosclerotic disease as well as co-occurring conditions.

However, health status involves issues beyond those considered in the traditional medical history and physical examination. It is important to evaluate the patient's medications; dietary and exercise habits; nutritional, functional, and cognitive status; attitudes toward his or her health; and financial and social status. In many functional diabetic patients, this can be accomplished by the primary care physician. In patients with multiple chronic diseases and disabilities who may also face problems with financial or social support, assessment by a geriatrician and multidisciplinary team may be necessary. Subspecialty consultation may also be necessary for ophthalmological, neurological, podiatric, and other complications. Without a thorough evaluation, a safe and effective treatment plan cannot be developed. Table 3 lists the components of the comprehensive assessment of an older diabetes patient.

1. Treatment of Symptomatic Hyperglycemia

Treatment of symptomatic hyperglycemia is always indicated. In older persons these symptoms may be similar to symptoms of other conditions, or may exacerbate symptoms from other conditions. Symptoms may be atypical, and could include cognitive changes, anorexia, falls, and incontinence. As discussed later, there are many therapeutic options for hyperglycemia treatment.

2. Prevention and Treatment of Risk Factors for Atherosclerotic Disease

In younger diabetic patients, whether type 1 or type 2, identification and treatment of risk factors for atherosclerotic disease improve both morbidity and mortality (33). In older persons, the evidence is not as extensive. However, the most significant morbidity and mortality in older diabetic patients is attributable to atherosclerotic disease, and many other risk factors for atherosclerosis also increase with age.

Smoking confers a markedly increased risk of atherosclerotic complications and worsening atherosclerotic disease in all population groups. Although fewer older than younger diabetic patients smoke, those that do should be strongly urged to quit. Studies show that older patients are potentially more likely than younger to be successful in smoking cessation programs (34), and recent data have verified that, in general, stopping smoking improves both morbidity and mortality in older former smokers.

Treatment of hypertension in patients with diabetes has been demonstrated to lower risk of atherosclerotic events (33), including coronary artery disease and stroke. In older diabetic patients with isolated systolic hypertension, a subgroup analysis of the diabetic patients participating in the original trial suggested that treatment significantly decreased atherosclerotic events and mortality (35). The UKPDS study also showed that blood pressure control in type 2 diabetes significantly decreased diabetes complications and mortality related to diabetes (36). Angiotensin-converting enzyme (ACE) inhibitors are a good choice for hypertension treatment in older patients because of their protective effect on renal function in diabetes. Clinical experience in the elderly does suggest that side effects, especially cough, are more common in older than younger patients. In addition, older patients have a higher prevalence of peripheral vascular disease and renal artery stenosis, and are more likely be taking other medications, such as NSAIDs, that could add to potential hyperkalemia, decreased renal function, or accelerated hypertension when an ACE inhibitor is added. Therefore, any older diabetic patients in whom an ACE inhibitor is contemplated must be carefully evaluated for potential drug–drug interactions and the presence of renal vascular disease.

The Systolic Hypertension in the Elderly Trial (SHEP) demonstrated that hypertension treatment in older patients, including diabetes patients, using low-dose thiazides and cardioselective β-adrenergic blockers, could be accomplished with minimal side effects (35). Although higher-dose thiazides could increase hyperglycemia, and β-blockers may be problematic in some diabetic patients by decreasing hypoglycemia awareness, increasing triglycerides and decreasing HDL, accumulating evidence suggests that, in general, their use is well tolerated. If a β-blocker is used, it should be cardioselective.

A high proportion of older diabetic patients also have hyperlipidemia. The presence of both older age and diabetes clearly confers high risk, and because of the high prevalence of CAD in these patients, they should be screened and treated for hyperlipidemia, regardless of age, unless there is severe functional or cognitive disability, or a preterminal state. Here also, clinical experience suggests that older patients may experience an increased frequency of side effects with HMGCoA reductase inhibitors, especially muscle symptoms, so they must be monitored. Increased triglycerides are an independent risk factor for atherosclerotic disease in persons with diabetes (37). In older as well as younger patients, diet, exercise, and improved glycemic control are first-line therapy for hypertriglyceridemia. If these are ineffective, pharmacological treatment is indicated. Gemfibrizole is preferred, as nicotinic acid worsens hyperglycemia and may cause increased side effects in older patients.

Persons with diabetes derive the same cardiovascular protection from aspirin (ASA) as persons without diabetes (38). A recent metanalysis of studies suggests that older patients may have an even greater benefit (39). Research has shown that, in both type 1 and type 2 diabetes patients with diabetic retinopathy, ASA is not associated with an increased incidence of ocular bleeding (38). Therefore, ASA therapy is recommended for older diabetic patients. The vast majority of older patients can tolerate low-dose, coated ASA.

3. Prevention and Treatment of Microvascular Complications

Diabetic peripheral neuropathy, especially that which results in foot ulcers and amputations, is a particular problem for older diabetes patients. Multiple studies have shown that both foot ulcers and amputations increase in the older-aged group, as well as with a longer duration of diabetes. Amputations, which result from both macrovascular and microvascular diabetes complications, are most prevalent in older diabetic patients (25), and foot ulcers are one of the major causes of hospitalization in these patients. Research suggests that early detection of diabetic neuropathy results in fewer hospital admissions for foot ulcers and amputation (40). All older diabetic patients should have foot care education emphasized and the foot examination prioritized by their primary care physician.

Yearly dilated retinal examinations lower the incidence of blindness in both type 1 and type 2 diabetic patients by early detection and treatment of diabetic retinopathy (31). In older patients, however, there are some differences from younger patients in their experience with diabetic eye disease. First, older patients tend to have less progression of diabetic retinopathy, and it is more often macular edema than proliferative retinopathy (41). Photocoagulation therapy can also prevent visual loss caused by macular edema. Second, older diabetic patients have a higher frequency of other diabetes-related eye diseases, such as glaucoma and cataracts, than younger patients. Although diabetic retinopathy is not the major cause of blindness in older diabetic patients, as it is with younger diabetic patients, older patients have a higher prevalence of visual impairment than younger patients (11). Older diabetic patients would clearly benefit from yearly ophthalmological evaluations.

In patients with type 2 diabetes, both adequate systemic blood pressure control (38,39) and use of ACE inhibitors (44,45) reduce the rate of progression of early renal disease. Testing for microalbuminuria is an appropriate screen for early renal disease and decreases progression of such disease in type 1 diabetes. Little information is available specifically in older diabetic patients, although, based on the weight of evidence in other population groups, it is reasonable to check urinary microalbuminuria, use ACE inhibitors when possible, and obtain renal evaluation if there is evidence of renal disease. In older diabetic patients, it is important to remember that there are many other causes of microalbuminuria, such as urinary tract infections, hematuria owing to prostate disease, and intercurrent illness. In addition, there is a higher prevalence of other causes of renal insufficiency, including most commonly, hypertensive renal disease or reaction to medications.

4. Improvement of General Health Status by Attention to Functional Status

In older patients, it is important to assess how their chronic diseases and comorbid conditions affect their ability to function. Many older patients may have a long list of medical diagnoses, but will be completely functional and active. Others may have few medical diagnoses, but may have functional limitations or even require assistance in complex or basic functioning. Older patients who have diabetes may also have coexisting problems, related or unrelated to their diabetes, that impair their ability to function. Patients may have poor nutritional status, sensory deficits, especially vision, depression, mobility impairment, and cognitive decline. Some may have social problems, such as recent bereavement or social isolation; many live alone. All these problems have a much higher prevalence in older diabetic patients than in similar middle-aged or younger patients, and many of these problems can be overlooked if the physician does not consider them. Management plans can often be developed to address these problems. For example, poor nutritional status can be handled by nutritional referral, attention to caregiver status, and careful monitoring; depression can be appropriately diagnosed and treated; mobility impairments may respond to physical therapy. Older diabetic patients with functional problems and multiple comorbidities are discussed in more detail later. In general, if a physician suspects multiple complex problems in an older patient with diabetes, referral for geriatric assessment may be indicated.

5. Diabetes Self-Management Education and Counseling

Diabetes is primarily a disease of self-management. Metanalysis of diabetes education studies has shown that education in self-management of diabetes can improve many important outcomes, such as diabetes knowledge and self-care behaviors (41). Diabetes self-management and improved self-care behaviors are also associated with improved metabolic control (42,43).

There is no evidence that older patients derive less benefit from self-management education than younger patients. In fact, because older patients are usually retired and have more time to spend on self-management behaviors, and because they may have other diseases requiring attention to lifestype changes and self-education, they may be very receptive to educational interventions and highly compliant with self-management techniques.

There are two extremely important components of self-management education that should be particularly emphasized in older patients: hypoglycemia awareness education, because of the risk of hypoglycemia in older patients, and medication teaching, because older patients are likely to be taking multiple medications. They must be educated to inform prescribing physicians about their various medications, and to inquire about potential drug–drug and drug–diabetes interactions.

6. Control of Hyperglycemia in Older Diabetic Patients: Targets and Rationale

The heterogeneity of diabetes and general clinical status of older diabetic patients affects the targeted level of glycemic control, the types of dietary and exercise programs, and the choice of pharmacological agent to assist management. Clinicians must consider a multitude of factors and, along with the patient and family, decide on a glycemic target.

Although there is currently no conclusive evidence that achieving near-normal glucose levels can prevent or decrease the complications of diabetes in older patients with type 2 diabetes, recent results from the UKPDS provide some evidence. In that trial, patients younger than 65 with type 2 diabetes, treated with any intensive regimen, had decreased microvascular complications and, with an intensive metformin regimen, had decreased diabetic complications in general (27,28). In addition, observational studies and clinical trials in other populations have added to the accumulating evidence that tight control may be beneficial, particularly for prevention of microvascular and neuropathic complications. For example, observational evidence suggests that diabetic retinopathy is highly related to degree of hyperglycemia, and may slow progression or even improve with glycemic control (30). These studies did not specifically deal with older diabetic patients.

In older diabetic patients, however, the major issue is the effect of diabetes on morbidity and mortality from macrovascular complications, especially cardiovascular disease and strokes. Recent observational studies in Europe have linked better glycemic control with decreased mortality rates, decreased cardiovascular disease, and decreased strokes over an 8-year period in persons 70 years of age and older (44–46). Although such findings must be explored in other studies, they strengthen the argument that for some older patients who are healthy and motivated, tight glycemic control is a reasonable therapeutic goal.

The development of microvascular complications is linked to the duration of diabetes, and many older diabetic patients have a long duration of disease. As life expectancy continues to increase, this problem will worsen. Furthermore, if diabetic complications add to or intensify the aging process, it will become even more important to explore ways of preventing or mitigating these complications. As evidence accumulates that control of hyperglycemia can decrease the rate of progression of complications, intensive antihyperglycemic therapy may become more strongly indicated in some older patients. In this context, intensive therapy means a target value for glycosylated hemoglobin within 1% of the upper limit of normal.

Some older diabetic patients are obvious candidates for intensive antihyper-glycemic therapy (i.e., those who are relatively healthy, functional, and motivated to comply with an intensive regimen). Table 4 suggests characteristics of older patients who might benefit from tight glycemic control. Even relatively advanced age should not be a contraindication to intensive therapy. The median life expectancy of a 75-year-old white woman in 1980 was 12 years (half would be expected to live longer), plenty of time to develop complications of diabetes. In contrast, those with a limited life expectancy, multiple chronic diseases and medications, functional or cognitive impairments, and poor social support are candidates for less aggressive hyperglycemic management, geared to preventing symptoms. Some older diabetic patients fall in between these two extremes, and would benefit from lowering glucose levels to nearly normal range, and education about their options. Older diabetic patients should not be denied intensive hyperglycemic therapy on the basis of age alone.

A recent article concerning evidence-based diabetes management guide-lines suggested that useful way of conceptualizing the decision on tight glycemic control was to consider whether there would be no benefit or high risk (42). For older patients, characteristics such as frequent hypoglycemia or cognitive impairment, would suggest high risk, whereas a preterminal state or advanced disability would suggest that there would be no benefit. Table 5 suggests characteristics of older diabetic patients that would confer high risk or no benefit from tight glycemic control.

The therapeutic options for treating hyperglycemia in older patients are the same as with younger patients. Because 40% of older diabetic patients are obese

Table 4 Characteristics of Older Patients Who Might
Benefit from Near-Normal Glycemic Control[a]

Minimal or no functional impairments
Few comorbidities
Early or no diabetes complications
High motivation
Relatively long life expectancy
Good social support

[a] Glycosylated hemoglobin within 1% of upper limit of normal.

Table 5 Older Patients Who Are Less Likely to Benefit from Tight Glucose Control

High risk
  Frequent hypoglycemia requiring assistance
  Severe cardiac or cerebrovascular disease
  Severe autonomic neuropathy
  Cognitive impairment
  Impaired self-care ability
  Unsafe environment
Not likely to benefit
  Preterminal
  Extreme old age
  Advanced disability
  Advanced cognitive decline
  Advanced diabetes complications already present

Adapted from Vijan S, et al. J Gen Intern Med 12:574 (1997) by permission of Blackwell Science, Inc.

(47), a trial of caloric restriction in these patients makes sense. If pharmacological therapy becomes necessary, dietary therapy will remain an important part of the patient's diabetes self-management program. Even if ideal body weight is not attained, glycemic control may be substantially improved with a modest weight loss.

Elderly diabetic patients who are thin or of normal body weight should not restrict their caloric intake. In some older patients, weight loss may be a manifestation of poorly controlled diabetes. In addition, homebound, poor, or disabled elderly may have poor nutritional status, which must be addressed by increased caloric intake and management of subsequent hyperglycemia to improve their catabolic state and allow improvement of nutritional status.

An exercise program can be an important part of the regimen of some older diabetic patients, although it may not significantly affect hyperglycemia. However, an exercise program is not suitable for all patients in this group. As either symptomatic or asymptomatic coronary heart disease may preclude rigorous exercise, clinical cardiac evaluation, in some cases including stress testing, is indicated before an exercise regimen is begun. Some older patients may also be limited from implementing an exercise regimen by other comorbidities, such as cerebrovascular disease, peripheral vascular disease, diabetic foot disease, or arthritis. Recent evidence suggests, however, that many older diabetic patients can benefit from exercise and even achieve improved metabolic control, but the major barrier is adherence to an exercise regimen (48).

7. Pharmacological Therapy of Hyperglycemia

Several factors must be considered in choosing pharmacological therapy of hyperglycemia for elderly patients. These include efficacy of the chosen agent and potential adverse effects. At the same time, the target level of glycemic management, the comorbidities of the patient, the patient's potential for compliance and self-management, and the patient's risk of hypoglycemia will need to be considered in the choice of the exact agent.

Sulfonylureas have been available for many years, and there is wide experience with their use. In older patients, there is an advantage to the second-generation agents because they are nonionically protein-bound, which could theoretically lessen drug–drug interactions with such acidic drugs as warfarin (Coumadin) or salicylates (49). All sulfonylurea drugs are rapidly absorbed from the gastrointestinal tract. All are metabolized to some degree by the liver and excreted, at least partly, by the kidneys. Thus, these drugs should be used with caution when significant liver or kidney disease is present. Half-lives vary in this drug class. Although compliance may be improved by using longer-acting agents that allow once-daily dosing, the risk of prolonged hypoglycemia is also greater with such drugs.

Metformin has a potential advantage in some older patients because it is not associated with hypoglycemia when used alone. When combined with a sulfonylurea agent, however, it can precipitate hypoglycemia. Older patients are more likely to have comorbid diseases or other medications that would interact with metformin. These include renal insufficiency, and cardiac or hepatic failure. Metformin appears to be most useful in obese patients, and recent results from the UKPDS' study suggest that in obese diabetic patients, it may decrease diabetic complications and have fewer side effects than insulin and sulfonylureas (28). However, fewer older diabetes patients are obese, and multiple dosing and gastrointestinal side effects may decrease compliance in older patients. Metformin has a clear role in the treatment of older diabetic patients, especially those who are obese and without significant comorbidities. However, many older diabetic patients will be more appropriately treated with other medications.

$1,3\alpha$-Glucosidase inhibitors are newer agents for treating diabetes. These drugs do not cause hypoglycemia when used as single agents, and appear to have few side effects other than gastrointestinal symptoms, such as flatulence and diarrhea. Although information on their use in older patients is sparse, a recent study suggested significant reductions in hyperglycemia and few side effects in older patients treated with miglitol (50).

Another newer drug class for treating hyperglycemia are the 1,4-thiazolidinediones; several are now available. These medications work by increasing insulin sensitivity through a postreceptor mechanism. These drugs would appear to be most useful in obese, insulin-resistant patients. Troglitazone, the first one available in the US, has been effective as both monotherapy and in combination.

Because it is relatively new, there is little information about its use in older patients. In addition, rare severe hepatic damage has been reported, so it should not be used in patients with hepatic problems, and all patients using it should be monitored for the development of hepatic abnormalities.

The issue of combination drug therapy for type 2 diabetes, analogous to the long-established idea of stepped therapy for hypertension, is of particular importance for older patients. As new classes of medications become increasingly available, the issue of combining medications from different classes for complementary effects, or combining them with insulin therapy, will be one of the major therapeutic concepts for research. There are potential pitfalls of this approach with older patients, including increased risk of hypoglycemia, unknown tolerance for the adverse effects of newer medications, compliance problems with multiple drug regimens, and affordability. On the other hand, older patients also have problems with insulin, including minor impairments that may make it difficult to draw the correct amount into syringes, increased risk of hypoglycemia, and older patients, similar to younger ones, prefer to take pills rather than injections. Physicians caring for older patients will need to monitor effectiveness information as it is published, and use their own growing clinical experience with combination regimens to assess whether older patients will truly benefit without undue risk.

Patients who are not appropriate for oral antihyperglycemic therapy, either because of persistent, marked hyperglycemia or failure to achieve or maintain the target for glycemic control, will need to take insulin. It is important to remember that there are distinct advantages of insulin therapy in older patients with diabetes. It has no medical contraindications, and does not interact with other medications or disease states. Insulin use is very flexible, and precise dosing is possible. Insulin use encourages increased diabetes education and care participation by the patient and family.

Insulin therapy also has disadvantages. Patient disability may hamper safe use, especially among frail elderly, and caregivers may need to be actively involved. Some patients have a psychological barrier to insulin administration. In addition, there is added complexity and cost of insulin use, including the need for frequent blood glucose monitoring, increased patient education and hypoglycemia education. The risk of hypoglycemia is also increased, although serious episodes are rare (49).

C.   Diabetes Management of Frail Elderly

Most older diabetic patients, along with most older Americans, are "successfully aging." Although they may have some diabetic complications or comorbid diseases, and may take several medications, by and large they remain active and are very interested in maintaining their health, and avoiding disability. However, among older diabetic patients, there is a group with severe disabilities and multiple comorbidities, a poor quality of life and diminished life expectancy. Many of these patients live in nursing homes, although they may also live in the community, generally with extensive help from caregivers. In these patients, sometimes referred to as the "frail elderly," some have suggested that there is no role for preventative interventions, self-management techniques, or management of hyperglycemia. However, it is precisely in this group of patients that appropriate basic diabetes management can improve patient symptomatology, prevent or slow functional deterioration, and assist caregivers in their difficult job.

There is no clear clinical definition of *frail elderly*. In general, however, frail elderly can be considered those patients with limited physiological reserve who have significant functional impairments and multiple comorbid conditions. Such patients have one or often several additional problems, such as dependency in ADLs, cognitive impairment, sensory impairment, depression, and malnutrition. They may experience falls and urinary incontinence. Very little empirical information exists about diabetes and diabetes management in this group of patients. The few research articles available suggest "laissez-faire" diabetes management in nursing home residents with diabetes (51,52).

Basic diabetes management is appropriate for this group of patients. As listed in Table 6, this consists of (a) treatment of symptomatic hyperglycemia; (b) attention to nutritional status; (c) social support; and (d) prevention and treatment of diabetes complications to optimize functional status and decrease caregiver burden. Many frail elderly patients with multiple other comorbid problems and functional disabilities along with their diabetes will benefit from referral for comprehensive geriatric assessment (53).

Frail elderly diabetic patients can be extremely symptomatic from uncontrolled hyperglycemia. Because of an impaired thirst response, or an inability to take care of themselves, they are at risk for volume depletion. Incontinence, urinary tract infections, volume depletion, falls and increased mental confusion, can all result from polyuria. Even without recognized polyuria, uncontrolled hyperglycemia can result in confusion, lethargy, decreased vision, increased malnutrition, and a catabolic state, and increased risk for infections. Although tight control is not a goal in this group, poor control can be harmful. Expert opinion suggests that an average glucose level of about 200 mg/dL (11 mmol/L) is a reasonable target that is not associated with hyperglycemic symptoms (49).

Table 6 Basic Diabetes Management

Treatment of symptomatic hyperglycemia
Attention to nutritional status
Attention to social support
Prevention and treatment of diabetes complications that might threaten functional status
    and increase caregiver burden

Nutritional problems are common in frail elderly patients with diabetes. A large proportion of these patients have undernutrition, rather than obesity, and may be in a continuous catabolic state owing to poor metabolic control, which will exacerbate malnutrition. Significant morbidity, such as increased pressure ulcers and increased infectious complications, can be linked to malnutrition (54). Such complications are both distressing to the patient and costly to the health care system. Nutritional problems, which can include murasmus, protein–calorie malnutrition, and micronutrient deficiency, must be evaluated and treated. The first step is to reverse the catabolic state by achieving an appropriate measure of glycemic control. Appropriate caloric intake and micronutrient supplementation must be instituted, and consultation with a nutritionist is generally necessary.

Frail elderly diabetic patients, whether in the community or in a nursing home, may be dependent on caregiver support for basic ADLs, and often need assistance with dressing, bathing, or even eating. Their mobility is often impaired, and they require assistance with preparing meals, taking medications, and maintaining a household. Diabetes "self-managment" will actually be diabetes management by the caregiver. As such, the physician, often with the help of a social worker or geriatric nurse practitioner, will need to identify and work closely with the caregiver to develop, implement, and monitor a diabetes management plan. If an appropriate caregiver can be identified and educated, a basic diabetes management plan can be safely and successfully implemented.

Finally, unless a true preterminal state exists, a major goal of management of the frail elderly patient is to maintain functional status, or at least slow the rate of decline. This approach minimizes patient morbidity, organizes clinical interventions in a way that constantly assesses their relevance to functional status, and supports the caregiver, whose job becomes much more difficult as a patient declines. This approach can help the clinician assess the cost–benefit of diabetic management interventions. For example, basic foot care is very easy and inexpensive to implement, and preventing foot ulcers or catching them before they become complex and require specialized care is an extremely reasonable approach. A cerebrovascular accident (CVA) will increase disability, can worsen cognitive function, increase patient depression, and vastly increase caregiving resources. As far as is known, continuing to treat hypertension and use of aspirin in a frail elderly patient still prevents strokes. Similarly, medical eye disease associated with diabetes should be treated when possible, because impaired vision is a major reason for increased disability and depression. Finally, poor glycemic control not only increases the symptom burden of frail elderly patients, but also saddles the caregiver with the consequences of the patient's increased incontinence, infections, confusion, and even falls. Such additional morbidity in a frail elderly patient is distressing and will also increase caregiver burden.

In summary, although morbidity and mortality from atherosclerotic diseases has continued to decrease in the United States, at least partly related to lifestyle changes and preventative medical interventions, the incidence and prevalence of diabetes in this country has continued to rise. In addition, the continued increase in average life expectancy and the increasing numbers of the older population will result in increasing numbers of diabetic patients in their 70s and older. However, empirical information about diabetes in the elderly is still very limited. In fact, the major unanswered question in diabetes: "Does glycemic control influence the development and progression of macrovascular complications in type 2 diabetes?" is arguably most relevant to elderly diabetic patients. Other unanswered questions about diabetes in the elderly include questions about the epidemiology and clinical characteristics of diabetes diagnosed later in life, self-management compliance and success in older patients, the relation of diabetes and disability in the oldest age groups, and outcomes of diabetes management in the elderly. Fortunately, the next few years will see a substantial increase in our knowledge of clinical characteristics and appropriate management of diabetes in our growing elderly population.

REFERENCES

1. Harris MI, Flegal KM, Cowie CC, Eberhardt MS, Goldstein DE, Little RR, Wiedmeyer H-M, Byrd-Holt DD. Prevalence of diabetes, impaired fasting glucose, and impaired glucose tolerance in U.S. adults. Diabetes Care 21:518–525, 1998.
2. Morely JE, Kaiser FE. Unique aspects of diabetes mellitus in the elderly. Clin Geriatr Med 6:693–719, 1990.
3. Aubert RE, Geiss LS, Ballard DJ, Cocanougher B, Herman WH. Diabetes-related hospitalization and hospital utilization. In: Harris MI, Cowie CC, Stern MP, Boyko EJ, Reiber GE, Bennet PH, eds. Diabetes in America. 2nd ed. Bethesda, MD: National Institute of Diabetes and Digestive and Kidney Diseases, 1995:553–570.
4. American Diabetes Association. Report of the Expert Committee on the diagnosis and classification of diabetes mellitus. Diabetes Care 7:1183–1197, 1997.
5. Edelstein SL, Knowler WC, Bain RP, et al. Predictors of progression from impaired glucose tolerance to NIDDM: an analysis of six prospective studies. Diabetes 46: 701–710, 1997.
6. Wingard DL, Barrett-Connor E. Heart disease and diabetes. In: Harris MI, Cowie CC, Stern MP, Boyko EJ, Reiber GE, Bennet PH, eds. Diabetes in America. 2nd ed. Bethesda, MD. National Institute of Diabetes and Digestive and Kidney Diseases. 1995:429–448.
7. Reed RL, Mooradian AD. Nutritional status and dietary management of elderly diabetic patients. Clin Geriatr Med 6:883–889, 1990.
8. Turner RC, Holman RR. The UK Prospective Diabetes Study. Ann Med 28:439–444, 1996.
9. Blaum CS, Halter JB. Diabetes in the elderly. Drug Ther 24:18–30, 1994.

10. Songer TJ. Disability in diabetes. In: Harris MI, Cowie CC, Stern MP, Boyko EJ, Bennet PH, eds. Diabetes in America. 2nd ed. Bethesda, MD: National Institute of Diabetes and Digestive and Kidney Diseases, 1995:259–283.

11. Moritz DJ, Ostfeld AM, Blazer DI, Curb D, Taylor JO, Wallace RB. The health burden of diabetes for the elderly in four communities. Public Health Rep 109: 782–790, 1994.

12. Mayfield JA, Deb P, Potter DEB. Diabetes and long-term care. In: Harris MI, Cowie CC, Stern MP, Boyko EJ, Reiber GE, Bennett PH, eds. Diabetes in America. 2nd ed. Bethesda, MD: National Institute of Diabetes and Digestive and Kidney Diseases, 1995:571–589.

13. Hazzard WR. The sex differential in longevity. In: Hazzard WR, Bierman EL, Blass JP, Ettinger WH, Halter JB, eds. Principles of Geriatric Medicine and Gerontology. New York: McGraw-Hill, 1994:37–47.

14. Vokonas PS, Kannel WB. Diabetes mellitus and coronary heart disease in the elderly. Clin Geriatr Med 12:69–78, 1996.

15. Betteridge DJ. Diabetic dyslipidemias. Am J Med 96(suppl 6A):25S–31S, 1994.

16. Brownlee M, Cerami A, Vlassara H. Advanced glycosylation end products in tissue and the biochemical basis of diabetic complications. N Engl J Med 318:1315–1321, 1988.

17. Lyons TJ. Lipoprotein glycation and its metabolic consequences. Diabetes 41(suppl 2):67–73, 1992.

18. Minaker KL. What diabetologists should know about elderly patients. Diabetes Care 13:34 46, 1990.

19. Silver AJ, Guillen CP, Kahl MJ, Morley JE. Effect of aging on body fat. J Am Geriatr Soc 41:211–213, 1993.

20. American Diabetes Association: ADA Position Statement: Report of the Expert Committee on the Diagnosis and Classification of Diabetes Mellitus. Diabetes Care 20(suppl 1):S5–S19, 1997.

21. WHO. WHO Expert Committee on Diabetes Mellitus. Second report. (Tech Rep Serv no 646). Geneva: WHO, 1980.

22. Wahl PW, Savage PJ, Psaty BM, Orchard TJ, Robbins JA, Tracy RP. Diabetes in older adults: comparison of 1997 American Diabetes Association classification of diabetes mellitus with 1985 WHO classification. Lancet 352:1012–1015, 1998.

23. Morley JE, Mooradian AD, Levine AS, et al. Why is diabetic peripheral neuropathy painful? The effect of glucose on pain perception in humans. Am J Med 77:79–83, 1984.

24. Harris MI. Epidemiology of diabetes among the elderly in the United States. Clin Geriatr Med 6:703–719, 1990.

25. Palumbo PJ, Melton LJ III. Peripheral vascular disease and diabetes. In: Harris MI, Cowie CC, Stern MP, Boyko EJ, Reiber GE, Bennett PH, eds. Diabetes in America. 2nd ed. Bethesda, MD: National Institute of Diabetes and Digestive and Kidney Diseases, 1995:401–408.

26. DCCT Research Group. The effect of intensive treatment of diabetes on the development and progression of long-term complications in insulin-dependent diabetes mellitus. N Engl J Med 329:977–986, 1995.

27. UKPDS Group. Intensive blood-glucose control with sulphonylureas or insulin compared with conventional treatment and risk of complications in patients with type 2 diabetes (UKPDS 33). Lancet 352:837–853, 1998.

28. UKPDS Group. Effect of intensive blood-glucose control with metformin on complications in overweight patients with type 2 diabetes (UKPDS 34). Lancet 352: 854–865, 1998.

29. Porte D, Kahn SE. What geriatricians should know about diabetes mellitus. Diabetes Care 13:47–54, 1990.

30. Klein R, Klein BEK, Moss SE. Relation of glycemic control to diabetic microvascular complications in diabetes mellitus. Ann Intern Med 124:90–96, 1996.

31. Klein R, Klein BEK. Vision disorders in diabetes. In: Harris MI, Cowie CC, Stern MP, Boyko EJ, Reiber GE, Bennett PH, eds. Diabetes in America. 2nd ed. Bethesda, MD: National Institute of Diabetes and Digestive and Kidney Diseases, 1995: 293–338.

32. Weiner JP, Parente ST, Stephen T, et al. Variation in office-based quality: a claims-based profile of care provided to Medicare patients with diabetes. JAMA 273: 1503–1508, 1995.

33. Vijan S, Hofer TP, Hayward RA. Estimated benefits of glycemic control in microvascular complications in type 2 diabetes. Ann Intern Med 127:788–795, 1997.

34. The Smoking Cessation Clinical Practice Guideline Panel and Staff. The Agency for Health Care Policy and Research Smoking Cessation Clinical Practice Guideline. JAMA 275:1270–1280, 1997.

35. Curb JD, Pressel SL, Cutler JA, et al. Effect of diuretic-based antihypertensive treatment on cardiovascular disease risk in older diabetic patients with isolated systolic hypertension. JAMA 276:1886–1892, 1996.

36. UKPDS Group. Tight blood pressure control and risk of macrovascular and microvascular complications in type 2 diabetes: UKPDS 38. Br Med J 317:703–713, 1998.

37. Koskinen P, Mantarri M, Manninen V, Huttunen JK, Heinonen OP, Frick MH. Coronary heart disease incidence in NIDDM patients in the Helsinki Heart Study. Diabetes Care 15:820–825, 1992.

38. Antiplatelet Trialists Collaboration. Collaborative overview of randomized trials of antiplatelet therapy, I: prevention of death, myocardial infarction, and stroke by prolonged antiplatelet therapy in various categories of patients. Br Med J 308: 81–106, 1994.

39. ETDRS Investigators. Aspirin effects on mortality and morbidity in patients with diabetes mellitus: Early Treatment Diabetic Retinopathy Study Report 14. JAMA 268:1292–1300, 1992.

40. Bresater L-E, Welin L, Romanus B. Foot pathology and risk factors for diabetic foot disease in elderly men. Diabetes Res Clin Pract 32:103–109, 1996.

41. Wang F, Javitt JC. Eye care for elderly Americans with diabetes mellitus. Ophthalmology 103:1744–1750, 1995.

42. Vijan S, Stevens DL, Herman WH, Funnell MM, Standiford CJ. Screening, prevention, counseling, and treatment for the complications of type II diabetes mellitus. J Gen Intern Med 12:567–580, 1997.

43. Blaum CS, Velez L, Hiss RG, Halter JB. Characteristics related to poor glycemic control in NIDDM in community practice. Diabetes Care 20:7–11, 1997.

44. Kuller LH. Stroke and diabetes. In: Harris MI, Cowie CC, Stern MP, Boyko EJ, Reiber GE, Bennett PH, eds. Diabetes in America. 2nd ed. Bethesda, MD: National Institute of Diabetes and Digestive and Kidney Diseases, 1995:449–456.
45. Kuusisto J, Mykkanen L, Pyorala K, Laakso M. NIDDM and its metabolic control predict coronary heart disease in elderly subjects. Diabetes 43:960–967, 1994.
46. Kuusisto J, Mykkanen L, Pyorala K, Laakso M. Non–insulin-dependent diabetes and its metabolic control are important predictors of stroke in elderly subjects. Stroke 25:1157–1164, 1994.
47. Morley J, Mooradian AD, Rosenthal MJ. Diabetes mellitus in elderly patients—is it different? Am J of Med 83:533–541, 1987.
48. Clark DO. Physical activity efficacy and effectiveness among older adults and minorities. Diabetes Care 20:1176–1182, 1997.
49. Mooradian AD. Drug therapy of non–insulin-dependent diabetes mellitus in the elderly. Drugs 51:931–941, 1996.
50. Johnston P, Lebovitz H, Coniff R, Simonson D, Raskin P, Munera C. Advantages of alpha-glucosidase inhibition as monotherapy in elderly type 2 diabetic patients. J Clin Endocrinol Metabol 83:1515–1522, 1998.
51. Benbow SJ, Walsh A, Gill GV. Diabetes in institutionalized elderly people: a forgotten population? Br Med J 314:1868–1869, 1997.
52. Funnell MM, Herman WH. Diabetes care policies and practices in Michigan nursing homes, 1991. Diabetes Care 18:862 866, 1995.
53. Stuck AE, Siu AL, Wieland GD, Adams J, Rubenstein LZ. Comprehensive geriatric assessment: a meta-analysis of controlled trials. Lancet 342:1032–1036, 1993.
54. Panel on the Prediction and Prevention of Pressure Ulcers in Adults. Pressure ulcers in adults: prediction and prevention. Quick reference guide for clinicians. AHCPR Publication No. 92-0050. Rockville, MD: Agency for Health Care Policy and Research, Public Health Service, U.S. Department of Health and Human Services. May 1992.

36
Weight Management in Patients with Type 2 Diabetes Mellitus

Jorge Calles Escandón
University of Vermont College of Medicine, Burlington, Vermont

I. INTRODUCTION

Obesity is the most important risk factor for type 2 diabetes, and is found in 80% of affected persons in the United States. Moreover, successful control of excess adiposity is of great help in the glycemic management of these patients. This chapter presents strategies for weight control in obese patients.

II. MULTIDISCIPLINARY TEAM

Weight loss is best achieved under the guidance of a team of experts with experience in defining achievable goals for weight control and how to attain them. The team is ideally composed of a physician, dietitian, and psychologist. The team functions to

1. Identify patients who need to lose weight based on a comprehensive medical and psychological evaluation, with special emphasis on the weight history, body fat distribution, cardiovascular risk profile, family history of diseases associated with obesity, such as type 2 diabetes mellitus or insulin resistance, and previous attempts by the patient to lose weight. Current guidelines state that the most important indicator of the severity of obesity is the *body mass index* (BMI), which is defined as the ratio of body weight in kilograms to the height in meters squared. Individuals with a BMI of more than 25 should be encouraged to lose

weight, in particular when there is an upper body distribution of obesity, which is defined as a waist/hip ratio of 0.8 or higher in women and 1 or higher in men, or a waist circumference of more than 100 cm.

2. Define the readiness of the patient to participate in a structured weight loss program, including promoting strategies and operating procedures that help maximize the patient's possibility of success.

3. Define appropriate and achievable goals not only for weight loss, but also for other relevant parameters such as glycosylated hemoglobin (HbA_{1C}) for patients with diabetes, lipid values, blood pressure, and so on. Of great importance, the loss of even a few pounds can markedly improve the HbA_{1C} in some patients. Glycemic control is thus sometimes achieved when weight loss goals are not met, which should be viewed by the team and patient as a success because the purpose of weight loss in patients with type 2 diabetes is first and foremost to control the disease to minimize the risk of macro- and microvascular complications.

4. Bring out the patient's best efforts. Weight loss is a frustrating experience for the patient and physician, with great effort required and few tangible rewards. Experience has shown that many patients' motivation mirrors the enthusiasm they perceive from the weight loss team. It is crucial that all staff be cognizant of the key role they play in this and to the importance of maintaining a positive attitude. Even small successes in terms of weight loss should be acknowledged and met with celebration, as this can motivate the patient to go farther.

5. Be knowledgeable about community resources and weight loss services so that the patient is directed to the program that best meets their financial, social (ethnic, language, or other), and medical needs.

III. ELEMENTS OF THE WEIGHT LOSS PROGRAM

General elements of a comprehensive weight loss program are its being located in a patient-friendly environment with proper-sized furniture, and with congenial staff who are trained in how to deal socially and medically with overweight individuals. The workings of the weight loss program at the University of Vermont are described in the following as an example of a formal coordinated program (see Fig. 1).

A. Initial Evaluation

Self-referred or physician-referred patients undergo a comprehensive clinical evaluation. Areas of special emphasis are:

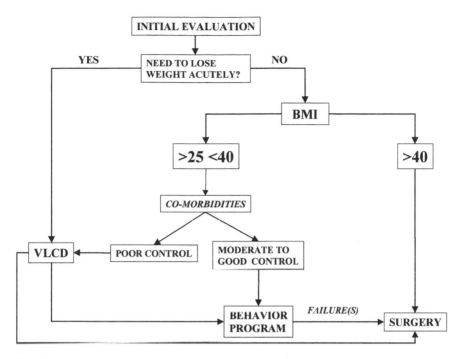

Fig. 1 Flowdiagram of the treatment strategy to select treatment in patients with obesity and type 2 diabetes. See the text for details.

1. Family history of obesity and comorbidities.
2. Previous attempts by the patient to lose weight that may include commercially available programs, medications, or surgery.
3. Metabolic and clinical parameters of comorbidities, including hemoglobin A_{1C}, lipid profile, blood pressure, microalbuminuria, and atherosclerotic vascular disease risk profile.
4. Evaluate and screen where appropriate for medical causes of obesity, such as endocrinopathies, genetic syndromes, or other.
5. Evaluate the readiness of the patient for a weight loss program and whether they are a candidate for a behavior-based program or a more drastic approach that may include a very low calorie diet, pharmaceuticals, gastrointestinal surgery, or any combination of these approaches.

B. Behavioral-Based Weight Loss Program

A behavioral-based program emphasizes lifestyle change without the use of medications or surgery. The most appropriate patients for this "conservative approach'' have moderate obesity as defined by a BMI of 26–39; if type 2 diabetes is present, moderate to excellent glycemic control on current treatment; and no psychological barrier that prevents their participation. The initial screening entails being interviewed by a PhD psychologist with specialty training in this area who concurs with the choice of therapy and recommends a group or individual program.

The group approach entails 15 members that stay together throughout the program. Groups can be homogeneous or differ substantially in gender, age, weight, or severity of diabetes. Meetings are weekly for the first 16 weeks, last 1.5–2.5 h, and are held in the early evening for the patients' convenience. They meet every-other-month thereafter, and if needed, individuals are followed more intensively by the weight loss team. A psychologist with training in behavioral modification and prior experience in weight control programs leads the meetings in tandem with a nutritionist or exercise physiologist. Meetings begins with a private weight-in, which is entered in the patient's personal record, followed by review of their eating and exercise diaries. Next, behavioral skills are taught in a seminar style, using a curriculum that is based on the LEARN Program for Weight Control of Kelly Brownell. A participant discussion then follows with the team leader keeping the discussion relevant to the topic and directing it toward specific issues that were raised in prior sessions or in response to participants' questions. The main skills focused on in the program are how to (a) decrease caloric intake, (b) decrease fat consumption, and (c) increase physical activity. For the latter, diabetic retinopathy, neuropathy, or cardiovascular complications sometimes mandate limitations in physical activity; in that event, exercise goals must be individualized. Those patients are often enrolled in a cardiovascular rehabilitation program.

A fundamental tenet of behavioral modification is to make the patients an integral part of the program and teach them how to manage their own behavior; self-assessment and self-monitoring techniques are emphasized, with the goal that the participants self-direct and control the behavioral changes. Team leaders help primarily in setting the goals for both weight loss and its metabolic effect. The aim is not to foster the concept of ideal body weight. Instead, emphasis is placed on making goals appropriate and achievable. Families and relatives of the participants are frequently involved because behavioral changes rarely are maintained without changing the patient's daily environment. In summary, the program is intended to sensitize patients and those around them to the need for a changed lifestyle, and to teach the skills to enact the change.

C. Very Low Caloric Diet Programs

The very low caloric diet (VLCD) programs were popular in the 1980s, but fears over an association with increased cardiovascular death resulted in a dramatic decrease in use. However, there remains a role for a drastically reduced caloric intake in selected patients. Suggested circumstances include

1. Hospitalized patients with massive obesity complicated by cardiovascular or respiratory failure who are in urgent need of decreased body weight to improve oxygenation and diminish fluid retention.
2. In preparation for gastric bypass surgery in patients with a high surgical risk related to the massive obesity.
3. For short periods in selected persons with type 2 diabetes to render them more responsive to oral hypoglycemic agents or insulin therapy. Moreover, a VLCD program can be repeated without diminution of its effectiveness so that some patients achieve and maintain their target glycemic control through periodic, limited periods of VLCD.
4. Massively obese (BMI > 40) persons who refuse gastric bypass surgery.

My general recommendation is not to go below 800 kcal/day because no advantage was demonstrated between programs of 400 kcal/day and 800 kcal/day, whereas cardiovascular morbidity is higher with a caloric intake below 800 kcal. Supplementation with a multivitamin preparation is always recommended, as is regular monitoring of body weight, blood pressure, and self-monitoring of blood glucose because adjustments in diabetes and blood pressure medications are frequently noted and can occur rapidly. Serum electrolytes are monitored on a weekly basis for the first month and every 2 weeks thereafter with potassium supplements added if the serum level becomes subnormal. Commercially available VLCD formulas are expensive. As such, my general outpatient approach is to prescribe 800–1000 kcal/day of supermarket yoghurt (fat-free, Aspartame-sweetened, 8–10 yoghurts per day) for patients without lactose intolerance, which has the advantages of being easily available, cheap, and not needing calcium or vitamin supplementation. Patients are followed in conjunction with a dietitian who adds food items as the program evolves to offer diversity of choices.

Even in patients who have success with this approach, it must be recognized by the patient and physician that VLCD is a temporary measure. Whatever weight is lost often returns rapidly unless an adjunctive behavioral-based program or gastrointestinal surgery is added. The goal of any therapy for obesity must be life-long, sustainable weight control so that VLCD is most useful as a prelude to other therapies, rather than as an obesity "quick fix."

D. Gastrointestinal Surgery

The 1992 NIH Consensus Conference on the role of gastrointestinal surgery in the treatment of obesity agreed with clinical experience which has shown that the only available treatment that is proved to induce sustained weight loss (> 5 years) in patients with massive obesity, with or without comorbidities, is gastric surgery. The major indications for gastrointestinal surgery are

1. Patients with a BMI higher than 40, especially those who have failed other therapies.
2. Patients with a BMI of 35–39; medical problems or comorbidities attributable to obesity as well as holding a significant chance for improvement with weight loss, such as type 2 diabetes, cardiovascular failure, respiratory failure, sleep apnea; failed to achieve sustained weight loss using other weight loss modalities.
3. Patients who have experienced repeated failures with nonsurgical approaches to weight loss in the past.

The preferred surgical approach is gastric stapling with a gastrojejuno anastomosis (Y-en-Roux reconstruction). Surgery should be performed in institutions that have a combined medical and surgical obesity program, with substantial experience with the surgical procedure and follow-up of these patients, including the presence of a multidisciplinary team (surgeon, psychologist, and dietitian) that is involved in the initial evaluation of candidates.

E. Drug Treatment

The recent debacle of fenfluramine alone or in combination with phenformin in terms of inducing cardiac valvular dysfunction demonstrates the need to go cautiously. Sibutramine was recently approved for use in promoting weight loss. This medication shares some mechanistic properties with the combination of fenfluramine and phentermine and has the potential of inducing hypertension. A second agent is xenical (Orlistat), which is an inhibitor of pancreatic lipase and diminishes gastrointestinal fat absorption on an average of 30% at the doses used in the initial trials plus inducing a 10% weight loss after 2 years of treatment. This medication has thus far proved safe; and the FDA has given final approval for its use. My overall recommendation for physicians and patients is that drug treatment should be considered in a controlled environment after a fair trial of behavior modification has failed.

BIBLIOGRAPHY

Brownell KD. The LEARN Program for Weight Control. Dallas, TX: American Health Publishing, 1991.
Dvorak R, Starling RV, Calles-Escandón J, Sims EA, Poehlman ET. Drug therapy for obesity in the elderly. Drugs Aging 11:338–351, 1997.

NIH Consensus Statement Conference. Role of gastrointestinal surgery in the treatment of obesity. Am J Clin Nutr 55(suppl 2), 1992.

Wadden TA, Foster GD, Letizia KA. One year behavioral treatment of obesity: comparison of moderate and severe caloric restriction and the effects of weight maintenance therapy. J Consult Clin Psychol 62:165–171, 1994.

Wadden TA, Berkowitz RI, Silvestry F, Bogt RA, St John Sutton MG, Stunkard AG, Foster GD, Aver JL. Fen-Phen finale: study of weight loss and valvular heart disease. Obesity Res 6:278–284, 1998.

Williams KD, Mullen ML, Kelley DE, Wing RR. The effect of short periods of caloric restriction on weight loss and glycemic control in type 2 diabetes. Diabetes Care 21:228, 1998.

Wing RR. Use of very low calorie diets in the treatment of obese persons with non–insulin dependent diabetes mellitus. J Am Diet Assoc 95:569–572, 1995.

Wing RR, Vendittie, Jakicic JN, Pollay BA, Lang W. Lifestyle intervention in overweight individuals with a family history of diabetes. Diabetes Care 21:350–359, 1998.

37
Inpatient Management of Diabetes

Suzanne S. P. Gebhart
Emory University School of Medicine, Atlanta, Georgia

I. INTRODUCTION

Diabetes is a common, although underreported, concurrent medical problem in many patients admitted to the hospital. The rate of hospitalization for persons with diabetes is about three times higher than the general population. Diabetes management is often unaggressive in the hospital and opportunities for education are missed. In addition, hyperglycemia is often unrecognized, untreated, and unrecorded in ill patients not known to have diabetes. Physicians should be wary of making the diagnosis of diabetes during the stress of hospitalization. The diagnostic criteria are based on ambulatory glucose values. However, given present concern about the role of chronic hyperglycemia in the development of diabetic complications, it is justifiable to view hospitalization as a metabolic stress test. Hyperglycemia in this setting certainly warrants correction and further outpatient evaluation. An elevated hemoglobin A_{1C} (HgA_{1C}) suggests a duration of hyperglycemia of at least 2 months. It is estimated that half the persons with diabetes are not aware that they have the disease. Often the diagnosis is made when severe complications have already developed. Identification of hyperglycemia during a hospital stay, even if glucose tolerance is normal at later testing, is an opportunity for intervention that should not be overlooked.

Individuals known to have diabetes may be hospitalized for a myriad of reasons, sometimes coincident with their disease, sometimes unrelated. It is important to realize that therapeutic choices during a hospital stay will have little or no effect on long-term management unless the patient is aware of the problems being addressed and is an active participant in determining the discharge recommendations. This is especially true if outpatient care is to occur under another physician.

II. INITIAL EVALUATION

Three issues need to be addressed for each hospitalized patient with diabetes. These are the type of diabetes, nutritional status and requirements, and glycemic goals.

A. Type of Diabetes

Type 1 diabetes, also called insulin-dependent diabetes, is an autoimmune disease of beta-cell destruction, whereas type 2 diabetes, non–insulin-dependent diabetes, represents a disorder of insulin action in combination with inadequate production. In the past many physicians defined the type of diabetes by the treatment (i.e., patients taking insulin had insulin-dependent diabetes). Not only was this inaccurate, as most patients taking insulin have type 2 diabetes, but also it failed to delineate the critical distinction of insulin production between type 1 and type 2 diabetes. If insulin is withheld or discontinued in individuals with type 1 diabetes, ketosis will ensue. On the other hand, type 2 patients who are likely insulin-resistant may have improvement in glucose concentrations during fasting, and insulin administration may be unnecessary.

The decision about the type of diabetes can often be made based on classic features at the time of diagnosis. Type 1 diabetes, for the most part, is a disease of youth that presents most commonly during the teen years or young adulthood. Presentation is usually abrupt, patients are usually lean at the time of diagnosis, and there is often a history of ketoacidosis. Most cases occur sporadically with no other family members affected. Type 2 diabetes is commonly a disease of middle-age, with gradual onset. Obesity is often present, and there is usually a family history of the disease. People with type 1 diabetes are usually begun on an insulin regimen from the time of diagnosis; however, it is often observed that after initiation of treatment, insulin requirements decrease. Called the "honeymoon phase," this transient period of metabolic compensation usually lasts less than 6 months and may permit temporary discontinuation of insulin. Ultimately the pancreatic insulin production is lost, and insulin administration becomes a life-sustaining requirement. This history of the honeymoon phase, however, can lead to some confusion over whether the individual has type 1 or type 2 diabetes. People with type 2 diabetes often are begun on a diet or oral therapeutic regimen, but can be started on insulin treatment at the onset of their diagnosis, especially if glucose levels are very high at the time. After several years of therapy, at least 50% of individuals with type 2 diabetes will have insulin added to their therapy to achieve better glycemic control. Therefore, the treatment is often the least helpful part of the patient's diabetes history in determining the underlying pathophysiology of the disease. If the diabetes type is unclear, it is safer to assume endogenous insulinopenia and continue insulin throughout the hospitalization than to withhold insulin.

B. Nutritional Status and Requirement

During illness or following surgery, most patients will be catabolic. If the stressful interval is short, this is of little physiological consequence; however, with more severe stress, adequate nutrition either orally or parenterally becomes an important issue. Initial evaluation should include an assessment of nutritional status. Comparing the patient's ideal body weight (IBW) with his or her present weight is a useful beginning. Given the height and body frame, it is possible to consult insurance tables for ideal weight. Another simple method of estimation of IBW is shown in Table 1.

There are several methods of varying complexity to estimate caloric requirements. The Harris–Benedict equation is, perhaps, the most commonly referenced (Table 2). It uses the parameters of sex, weight (kg), height (cm), and age (yr) to estimate basal energy expenditure (BEE) (kcal).

A reasonably accurate alternative estimate is 25–30 kcal/kg body weight (which includes about 400–800 kcal above basal requirements to account for activity; (Table 3). It is important to remember that these formulas are based largely on ambulatory caloric requirements, and in a hospital setting, severity of illness may be the most important predictor of energy need. An additional 10% increase in calories for mild illness, 25% increase for moderate illness, and 50–100% increase for severe illness is reasonable.

C. Glycemic Goals

The glycemic goals for long-term management of diabetes have been established and are widely disseminated. Approximation of normal glycemia as closely as safety allows offers the benefit of reducing the risk of chronic complications. In the hospital setting, outpatient glycemic goals may or may not be appropriate.

Table 1 Estimation of Ideal Body Weight (Hamwi)

For medium frame adults:
For women: 100 lb for first 60 in. in height
5 lb for each additional inch in height
For men: 106 lb for first 60 in. in height
6 lb for each additional inch in height
Add 10% for large frame, subtract 10% for small frame

Table 2   Harris–Benedict Equation

For women:

$$BEE = 655 + 9.6\ W + 1.8\ H - 4.7\ A$$

For men:

$$BEE = 66.5 + 13.7\ W + 5.0\ H - 6.8\ A$$

> BEE = basal energy expenditure (cal)
> W = weight (kg)
> H = height (cm)
> A = age (yr)

$$\text{Total caloric need} = BEE \times \text{activity factor} \times \text{injury factor}$$

Activity factor:
   Bed rest = 1.2; ambulatory = 1.3

Injury factor:
   Surgery, minor = 1.1; major = 1.2
   Infection, mild = 1.2; moderate = 1.4; severe = 1.8
   Trauma, skeletal = 1.35; head = 1.6; blunt = 1.35
   Burns, 40% surface area = 1.35: 100% surface area = 1.95

Hyperglycemia during a limited hospital stay would not be expected to adversely affect diabetic complications, but energy balance and wound-healing would benefit from normoglycemia. To a large extent, the determining factors in setting glycemic goals are patient safety and the skill and interest of the medical staff in managing diabetes. Although this certainly varies from one hospital to another, it can also vary by nursing unit or hospital service or even by duty shifts within a single unit. Most physicians are well aware of the strengths and weaknesses of their hospital setting. It can either serve as a source of continual frustration, or an opportunity for ongoing professional education, or a little of both. Hospitalization

Table 3   Simple Estimation of Caloric Needs

30 kcal/kg body weight
+ additional 10% increase in calories for mild illness
      25% increase for moderate illness
      50–100% increase for severe illness

provides greater opportunity for patient observation, increased therapeutic options, and control of diet and exercise, which may permit achievement of lower glycemia with greater safety during a hospital stay than achieved as an outpatient. On the other hand, in the critically ill patient or one with altered mental function, hypoglycemia may pose so significant a hazard that it warrants a somewhat higher glycemic goal. Other examples of situations for which acceptable glycemic levels as an inpatient may not coincide with acceptable outpatient levels are initiation of insulin therapy in preparation for discharge and evaluation of home management skills. The desired glycemic range largely determines the therapy. The therapy should not determine the glycemic range.

III. NUTRITION

The nutritional requirements of patients with diabetes do not differ from patients without diabetes; however, unless insulin is adequate, utilization of calories received will be suboptimal. Most well-nourished persons, including those with diabetes, can tolerate several days of fasting, providing intravascular volume and electrolyte balance are maintained. Five percent dextrose intravenously provides 200 kcal/L, far less than minimal caloric needs even at a rate of 3 L/day. If a fast of more than 5 days is likely, parenteral nutrition should be considered. In malnourished patients, not tolerant of enteral feeding, parenteral nutrition should be initiated early.

Liquid meals as substitution for solid food, as supplements, or as tube feedings, come in a variety of formulations. Most offer 1 kcal/mL with 50–75% of calories as carbohydrate. The protein, fat, fiber, and electrolyte proportions vary with the formulation. Preparations offering 1.5–2 kcal/mL are also available.

The recommended carbohydrate load for enteral or parenteral feeding is 3–5 mg of glucose per kilogram per minute. If hyperglycemia ensues, initiating or adjusting insulin therapy is more appropriate than reducing the infusion rate or changing the feeding formula. It is safe to add insulin to the parenteral nutrition mixture at an initial dose of 0.1 U regular insulin per gram of carbohydrate per day. This usually results in an underestimate of insulin requirement, but may be adequate in individuals with good endogenous insulin production. A preferable approach in individuals already requiring insulin is to titrate a variable insulin infusion simultaneously, using the parenteral preparation as steady-state substrate (see discussion of intravenous insulin in Sec. V). Once the insulin requirement is determined, the dose may be added to the parenteral mixture eliminating the need for the additional infusion.

In patients who are resuming oral intake after a fast, it is common to begin with clear liquids. Individuals with diabetes often have a calorie level specified with the liquid diet followed by ''ADA'' indicating the diet recommended by the

American Diabetes Association. This produces a dilemma for nutrition services in that although there is no specific American Diabetes Association diet per se, the ADA diet implies avoidance of simple sugars. A clear liquid diet eliminates inclusion of fats and complex carbohydrates; therefore, a strict interpretation of an ADA clear liquid diet would permit only soluble protein (which has limited palatability) to achieve the desired calorie content. Most often the prescribed calorie requirement is deferred and artificially sweetened gelatin and drinks are sent. Occasionally, the ADA portion of the diet prescription is ignored and sugared nutrition is sent. The thoughtful physician should consider for what purpose the diet is being ordered. If it is a test of enteral tolerance, then the caloric content is irrelevant and, especially if an insulin/dextrose infusion is part of the diabetes regimen, a noncaloric oral liquid trial would serve. On the other hand, if resumption of oral intake is expected to be smooth, full liquids that include complex carbohydrates as well as protein offer a better initial diet choice.

The estimated caloric needs of the diet prescription are derived from the initial evaluation. In most hospitals, the ADA prescriptive implies three isocaloric meals and usually a bedtime snack. Sometimes midmorning and midafternoon snacks are also considered part of the ADA diet. It is wise to clarify with nutrition services exactly how an ADA diet order is interpreted. Meals are composed of approximately 50–60% carbohydrate, 15–20% protein, and no more than 30% fat, with only 300 mg or less cholesterol. Foods grouped by composition and size allow "exchanges" or substitutions within a group. Because the meals are isocaloric, this diet offers a larger breakfast and a smaller supper than is the habit of most Americans. Isocaloric meals are helpful in optimizing endogenous insulin effectiveness in type 2 diabetes, but the ADA and many endocrinologists now favor a more flexible outpatient diet, and the exchange system is becoming less used. In the hospital setting, the exchange system offers some decided benefits in prescribing a subcutaneous insulin dose. Meal size and composition are standardized, and simple sugars are eliminated. However, food may be more bland and less attractive to many patients. Hospital "special diets" are usually prepared in bulk with low salt and spice content. Meal trays are adjusted to include or eliminate sugar or salt packets or specific foods based on the particular dietary restriction. A regular diet with "no concentrated sweets" may provide an acceptable alternative.

Some individuals with diabetes are accustomed to calculating their insulin dose based on the carbohydrate content of the meal. A hospital tray is particularly amenable to "carb counting," as this technique is called, because single-serving packages have the carbohydrate content plainly on the label. If the patient is not too ill, having the patient continue to calculate the premeal insulin dose is reasonable. The nursing staff should confirm and document the dose given. This is an excellent opportunity to review and reassess the patient's carbohydrate-counting technique under the supervision of the hospital registered dietitian.

IV. BLOOD GLUCOSE MONITORING

Self-monitoring of blood glucose (SMBG) has become the standard of care for all individuals with diabetes, although in reality, monitoring is often too infrequent. The hospital setting provides an opportunity to assess the patient's SMBG habits and to reinforce the advantages of good data gathering and interpretation. Most hospital units rely on bedside glucose meters for premeal and symptomatic glucose testing, but often laboratory glucose determinations are also done. Laboratory glucose determinations reflect plasma glucose, which is 10–15% higher than whole-blood glucose used for bedside meters. This is particularly important to remember when interpreting asymptomatic "hypoglycemia," as detected by meter. Most hospital bedside meters measure glucose by reflectance based on glucose oxidase-containing strips that generate peroxide in a linear response on contact with glucose. Accuracy is extremely operator- and instrument-dependent. Hospitals should record frequent quality control checks and have periodic refresher inservice staff training for meter use. Handheld bedside meters should not be used for diagnostic purposes and severe asymptomatic hypoglycemia should be confirmed by laboratory plasma glucose testing. Given the limitations of the handheld meter, the purist might well question its usefulness in the hospital setting. The important advantage of the bedside glucose meter is that it permits frequent glucose determinations, with reasonable accuracy, thereby allowing titration of intravenous insulin to glucose level and examination of the glycemic pattern that is so helpful in the hospital management of diabetic patients.

The frequency of glucose determinations should be based on the therapeutic intervention, the glycemic pattern (or lack of pattern), and the glycemic goal, determined at the time of initial evaluation. For patients eating predictably, four checks daily, before meals and at bedtime, is the standard monitoring pattern. For patients taking intermediate-acting insulin before supper, an additional 3:00 AM glucose check is useful because this time point captures the insulin peak effect. Although a 3:00 AM check interrupts sleep, it is much easier to obtain in the hospital than at home, and it gives very important information that is applicable after discharge. Asymptomatic nocturnal hypoglycemia is much more common than was originally believed, especially when intermediate-acting insulin, NPH or Lente, is given before supper, rather than at bedtime.

When bedside glucose determinations are performed, it is important to share the result with the patient. Patients should be encouraged to continue their SMBG record in the hospital if their health permits and to discuss insulin dose or pattern variation with their nurse or physician. Much of outpatient diabetes education aims to achieve patient autonomy and good decision making. It makes sense to reinforce this in the hospital setting as much as possible.

V. ORAL ANTIDIABETIC AGENTS IN THE HOSPITAL SETTING

Oral antidiabetic medication is often discontinued at the time of hospital admission. In general this is a reasonable approach. It is certainly recommended for the insulin-sensitizing drug metformin because acute alterations in glomerular filtration may predispose to life-threatening lactic acidosis. During acute illness or in the perioperative period, stress hormones are high and insulin requirements increase. Although sulfonylurea drugs or repaglinide are not definitely contraindicated if oral medication is tolerated, they are not as likely to be effective in lowering glucose during acute illness as in a less stressful ambulatory setting. Acarbose, an α-glucosidase inhibitor, is probably contraindicated in the hospital setting except in patients who are already taking the drug and in whom therapy will be uninterrupted during hospitalization. Brief discontinuation of a thiazolidinedione will have little effect on insulin sensitivity, but it should be resumed as soon as possible. Most antidiabetic drugs are partially or wholly metabolized by the liver or have the potential for inducing liver enzyme elevation and, therefore, should not be used if there is serious hepatic dysfunction.

VI. INSULIN

Hyperglycemia can substantially add to the morbidity of acute illness and should be treated aggressively. Insulin is the drug of choice in the hospital setting because it is flexible, rapid in onset, and physiological.

Intravenous insulin has the advantage of immediate onset of action and easy titratability. In the perioperative or intensive care setting, it provides the most responsive mode of delivery. There are many good algorithms for insulin infusion. Two are outlined in Table 4. Important components of any protocol for intravenous insulin are as follows:

1. Subcutaneous insulin is discontinued before initiating intravenous insulin.
2. Blood glucose is measured at 1- to 2-h intervals at the bedside.
3. There is a continuous source of glucose, either as a dextrose infusion or as part of a parenteral or enteral nutrition mixture. Intravenous infusions of either 5% dextrose or 10% dextrose may be given as peripheral infusions by an infusion pump. The higher concentration of dextrose may be used to minimize the infusion volume. Potassium may be added to the dextrose in patients with normal renal function to compensate for insulin-induced hypokalemia.
4. Insulin as regular insulin in saline is infused by an infusion pump independently from the dextrose.

Table 4 Insulin Infusion Algorithms

Continuous dextrose infusion by an infusion pump (5% dextrose at 100 mL/h)
Regular insulin 125 U/250 mL 9% saline by infusion pump (1 U = 2 mL)
Glucose checks (BG) every 2 h
Steady-state infusion:
    Begin insulin at ___ (example: 1.5 U/h or 3 mL/h)
    BG 110–160 mg/dL = no change in rate
    BG 161–220 mg/dL = increase insulin rate by 0.5 U/h (1 mL)
    BG > 220 mg/dL = give 8 U iv regular insulin + increase rate by 0.5 U/h
    BG 80–110 mg/dL = decrease rate by 1.0 U/h (2 mL)
    BG < 80 mg/dL = decrease rate by 1 U/h and give 25 mL 50% dextrose iv
Dynamic infusion:
(BG − #) × f = U/h
where # = nadir BG where infusion rate stops (usually 60)
f = sensitivity factor 0.01–0.05 (average 0.03)
Physician should be notified if BG < 80 or > 220 mg/dL on two consecutive checks
    with either protocol

With the "steady-state" insulin infusion protocol, an initial infusion rate is selected with incremental increases of 0.5 U/h or decreases of 1.0 U/h based on the glucose response to the current rate until a desirable glycemic range (usually 100–150 mg/dL in a hospital setting) is reached. Adjustments are made at 2-h intervals. If there is an underestimate of the insulin rate initially, it may take a long time to achieve the goal range. In a study of 24 postoperative patients followed for 24 h on this protocol, goal glycemia was achieved in an average of 8 h and maintained within goal after that without hypoglycemia for the remainder of the observation period. The advantage of this protocol is that the patient's insulin sensitivity determines the ultimate steady-state dose. The disadvantage of this protocol is that the incremental change is small, and is not designed to respond to situations that produce large perturbations in insulin requirements, such as concurrent titration of a catecholamine infusion or steroid administration.

The "dynamic" insulin protocol is useful for a more rapid increase or decrease in insulin rate. In this protocol, the rate of infusion is calculated with each glucose measurement and is independent of the previous rate. The formula is (BG − #) × f = units insulin per hour, where BG is current blood glucose in mg/dL, # is the BG nadir at which infusion rate will equal zero, and f is an insulin sensitivity factor that may be chosen empirically, based on the clinical setting, and it usually ranges from 0.01 to 0.05. If f is too low, the BG will not fall into desired range. If f is too high, the rate of fall will be too rapid. In choosing #, consideration must be given to whether or not it is desirable to totally stop the infusion. If # = 100 in a patient with type 1 diabetes, the protocol would dictate interrupting insulin for 2 h at a blood glucose level of 100 mg/dL and might result in accelerated hyperglycemia and ketosis. In a patient with type 2 diabetes, this interruption might be quite appropriate. A # value of 60, i.e., $(BG - 60) \times f$ = units insulin per hour is commonly used in patients with type 1 diabetes (and works equally well with type 2 diabetes) with the modification that the physician be called for a BG of less than 80 mg/dL so that f can be reduced.

Although hourly glucose checks are often recommended, checks every 2 h using a bedside meter appear equally safe and provide a sufficient interval between checks to effect a glucose response for each dose change. Glucose checks at 2-h intervals also permit using intravenous insulin in a variety of hospital settings, both intensive and general care.

Hypoglycemia is rare as long as a steady source of glucose is maintained, either as a dextrose infusion or enteral or parenteral feeding. However, if the glucose infusion or tube feeding is suspended, even if the insulin infusion is also stopped, plasma glucose levels will fall rapidly because the insulin effect will extend at least 30 min beyond circulating plasma insulin levels.

Neither insulin algorithm provides an anticipatory insulin peak to correspond to postprandial glucose excursions. The "dynamic" formula will respond better to meals, but either formula may be modified by specifying an increase of an additional 1–2 U/h in the insulin infusion rate when the meal tray arrives at the bedside with further insulin rate adjustments to be based on the algorithm. This immediate insulin increase also assists in reducing the degree of postprandial hyperglycemia; however, if the patient is able to eat, subcutaneous insulin is more appropriate.

The transition from intravenous to subcutaneous insulin requires some consideration. All too often intravenous insulin is stopped as part of the transfer orders from intensive care in patients with no subcutaneous insulin reservoir and with no thought given to whether the patient is capable of producing basal insulin. Patients with type 1 diabetes are incapable of producing sufficient insulin to provide even low levels required to inhibit lipolysis and will develop ketoacidosis if circulating insulin levels become undetectable. This will begin within 30 min of discontinuing intravenous insulin unless the discontinuation has been preceded by a subcutaneous insulin injection.

For simplicity, it is easiest to make the transition from intravenous insulin to subcutaneous insulin at mealtime. The subcutaneous insulin injection is given 30 min before the meal with the intravenous insulin (and companion dextrose infusion) continued until about 1–2 h after the meal, when both infusions are stopped together. This allows some insulin absorption from the subcutaneous site before the intravenous insulin is interrupted.

Deciding on the subcutaneous insulin dose is largely empiric. In patients who had been previously taking insulin it may be logical to resume their previous dose. The hospital setting, however, rarely corresponds to normal life, and other factors should be considered. Was the patient's glucose well-controlled before admission? Is appetite back to normal, and does the hospital diet approximate the home diet? Are the stressors of hospitalization subsiding, or is the patient still very ill or in a lot of pain? Ultimately, most physicians make an educated guess at the total requirement and then proportion to doses to achieve a physiological pattern.

It is possible to estimate an insulin requirement based on the intravenous insulin infusion rate. If only minimal calories are being provided (as with 5% dextrose at 100 mL/h), one can assume the total insulin infused over 24 h approximates basal insulin needs or about 40–50% of the insulin daily requirement once the patient starts eating. The total may be divided into equal 12-h doses and given as Ultralente insulin. The remaining 50–60% total insulin dose (assuming good oral intake) may be given as regular or lispro insulin before each meal. If intravenous insulin has been titrated to support continuous tube feeding, the transition to subcutaneous insulin is the same total daily dose divided equally as NPH or Lente insulin every 8 h or Ultralente every 12 h.

Drugs that increase insulin requirements, such as steroids, growth hormone, or catecholamines, often given in an intensive care setting on a tapering dose schedule, must be considered in anticipating insulin requirements. Dexamethasone given daily and hydrocortisone given two or more times daily will result in a fairly stable pattern of insulin resistance. Prednisone, however, typically shows a peak effect on insulin requirements at about 8–12 h after the oral dose. Insulin resistance begins to decrease thereafter. Patients taking a morning dose of prednisone often show a clear diurnal variation in insulin need, with a peak in the early evening and a nadir before the next morning dose.

The many different insulin preparations designed to achieve different peak effects are discussed in Chap. 18. In the hospital setting it is important to be facile in using two or three different combinations. More complicated regimens, if needed, can be explored in the outpatient setting. The premixed combination NPH–regular insulin offers few advantages in the hospital setting. Simplicity of administration is hardly an issue, and the loss of flexibility in dosing insulin is a sizable disadvantage. In preparation for discharge premixed insulin can be resumed in selected patients who have used premixed insulin with good effect in the past or it can be initiated in patients who for various reasons are not likely to be successful with individualized insulin mixing at home. If a presupper dose of NPH–regular insulin is given, a 3:00 AM glucose level should be checked at least once before discharge. If hypoglycemia is detected, splitting the evening insulin dose to regular before supper and NPH at bedtime (with a lower dose) may provide a safer regimen.

Supplemental or "sliding-scale" insulin is probably the most frequently ordered insulin therapy in the hospital setting. At the same time, it is the most likely to elicit pejorative comments from diabetes specialists. The discrepancy lies in the application. In principle, it is reasonable to assume that in the hospital setting perturbations in insulin requirement occur that are not always predictable and that a flexible dosing regimen based on glycemic level would be beneficial. Common errors in application occur when scheduled insulin doses are arbitrarily discontinued without considering the underlying diabetes pathology and when supplemental insulin doses are relied on exclusively for glycemic management despite clear evidence of a sustained insulin requirement. In patients with type 1 diabetes, it is essential that insulin be continued on a regular basis to prevent ketosis. Some patients with type 2 diabetes taking insulin at home may not need insulin in the hospital, but it is likely, given the stress associated with hospitalization, that insulin requirements will be higher, not lower, in the hospital. Because it is never advantageous to produce marked hyperglycemia, discontinuing insulin until hyperglycemia ensues is generally unwise. The following guidelines maximize the benefits of supplemental insulin:

1. If it is certain the patient will require insulin, anticipate a modest requirement with a scheduled dose, supplement with additional insulin.
2. Set the glycemic level for supplement at the upper 30% of desirable range (i.e., BG > 140 mg/dL).
3. The greater the BG deviation from the supplemental level, the greater the insulin dose should be.

    The formula $BG - 100/f =$ units insulin is often used. BG equals current blood glucose in mg/dL, 100 is nadir below which the insulin dose equals zero, f is a sensitivity factor. The smaller the denominator f, the larger the supplement for any given blood glucose. Initial calculation of f may be based on the total daily dose of insulin: $f = 1500$/total U insulin daily. The usual range for f is between 20 and 60; however, modifications should be made if the resultant fall in glucose is too large or too small. The sensitivity factor formula does not take into account the effects of drugs or illness during hospitalization. Use of a fixed dose of insulin per glucose level can be equally effective although the orders written must reflect an appreciation of the individual patient's insulin sensitivity, rather than a standard order for all patients receiving insulin.

4. Given the desirable glycemic range, the standing insulin dose and the formula for supplement should be modified on a daily basis, with the goal that the requirement for supplemental insulin will be reduced, but the effectiveness of the supplement in restoring desirable glycemia will be increased.

The critical issue in determining insulin therapy in the hospital setting is to change the focus from the mode of therapy to the effectiveness of glycemic control. Too often it is reported that the patient is hyperglycemic despite insulin therapy, which translates into the patient is hyperglycemic because the insulin therapy is inadequate.

Some patients may enter the hospital with insulin pumps. Buffered regular insulin or lispro insulin is administered by continuous infusion at rates that may be programmed to change hourly and boluses of insulin may be delivered manually. If the patient is alert and comfortable, it may be reasonable to continue pump administration throughout the hospitalization. If this course is decided, it is important to give the nursing service and the patient clear guidelines of responsibility. The nursing service should be responsible for inspecting the infusion site and tubing, confirming that the current basal dose of insulin and that each bolus dose is as prescribed. The patient's responsibility is to operate the pump. If the patient uses carbohydrate counting to determine premeal boluses, calculations can be recorded on the meal menu for review by a nutritionist. The patient's nurse should confirm the premeal blood glucose level and that the calculated bolus was delivered. This shared responsibility provides a reasonable patient autonomy, relieves the nursing service from the unreasonable expectation of being able to operate equipment they do not frequently use and, at the same time, provides sufficient supervision for safety.

In the intensive care unit or perioperative setting, it is usually advisable to discontinue subcutaneous infusion in favor of intravenous infusion. The transition back to subcutaneous infusion is usually at the same or slightly lower hourly rate, with a 1-h overlap between initiation of subcutaneous infusion and discontinuation of intravenous infusion.

VII. WHEN TO CALL A SPECIALIST

There are many advantages to setting up a clinical pathway with specialist support in managing patients with diabetes in the hospital. Not only is diabetes a common disease that may be incidental to a full spectrum of causes of hospitalization, but also it has disease-associated morbidity, increasing the likelihood of hospitalization. Several studies have shown that a specialized approach to diabetes management can improve glycemic control and shorten hospital stay. A team may be composed of a diabetes nurse specialist, a nutritionist and a social worker, although a physician, usually an endocrinologist, is extremely helpful, not only to chart the therapeutic course for diabetes but also to act as ombudsman for the team with medical staff and hospital administration. In addition to short-term glycemic management, the diabetes team focuses on early planning for discharge. Glucose monitoring or insulin administration skills can be reviewed, and problems addressed. Taking the opportunity to observe how the patient draws up and injects insulin can be extremely important. Even patients who have injected insulin for years can benefit from having a professional review their technique. Some patients have been observed to draw up half a syringe of air without realizing the error, or may have such poor eyesight that they only crudely approximate the dose. If it is clear that the patient will not be able to master glucose monitoring or insulin, discussing the home situation, talking to and teaching family members, or anticipating the need for home help will prevent these problems from delaying discharge once the immediate medical problem is resolved.

VIII. EDUCATION IN A HOSPITAL SETTING

Diabetes education during hospitalization is best understood in terms of its limitations and opportunities. Ill patients have short attention spans and are not likely to retain a large amount of information given in a short amount of time. Diagnostic tests and procedures necessarily take precedence and may fragment the education process. At the same time, hospitalization offers a singular opportunity to observe and demonstrate skills such as insulin administration, glucose monitoring, and carbohydrate counting. Problems can be addressed, and there is repetitive opportunity for practice under expert guidance. Education techniques that require active patient participation are more successful than films or didactic sessions and allow the educator to temper the education to patient receptiveness. Written material is helpful for family members and provides a source of reference after discharge; however, patients are rarely able to concentrate on written material while they are ill. Making the education process between hospital, home, and outpatient clinic seamless is a challenge. Hospital diabetes educators should communicate with home health services and the primary physician to identify problem areas that need special attention and to make sure that the educational approach is clear and consistent.

IX. COMPLICATION SURVEILLANCE

Most persons with diabetes are aware that diabetes can produce tissue damage in the general sense, but in the personal sense they may have no notion of whether they are developing complications or whether their primary physician is maintaining complication surveillance. Some patients rarely see physicians except when acute illness necessitates. Consequently, it is useful to consider performing those evaluations recommended as part of routine surveillance while patients are in the hospital. These tests include a fasting lipid profile, glycated hemoglobin, and urine albumin, if no proteinuria is present on routine urine analysis. If proteinuria or abnormal albuminuria is present, a quantitative 24-h urine collection should be performed if appropriate given the medical circumstances. Abnormalities in blood pressure or sensory deficits noted on examination should be discussed with the patient. The patient needs to be aware of all of the surveillance tests performed and the implications. When and how to impart this information requires some appreciation for the patient's hospital course and tolerance for new information. Discharge instructions should include a recapitulation of complication surveillance tests checked with results and a recommendation for outpatient follow-up. A patient's experience in the hospital may significantly alter his or her view of diabetes and his or her own role in its management.

BIBLIOGRAPHY

American Diabetes Association. Medical management of insulin-dependent (type 1) diabetes. 2nd ed. Alexandria, VA: American Diabetes Association, 1994.

Davidson PC. Bolus and supplemental insulin. In: Fredrickson L, ed. The Insulin Pump Therapy Book. Los Angeles: MiniMed, 1995:58–71.

Genuth SM. The automatic (regular insulin) sliding scale or 2,4,6,8- call H.O. Clin Diabetes 12:40–42, 1994.

Hamwi GJ. Therapy: changing dietary concepts. In: Danowski TS, ed. Diabetes Mellitus: Diagnosis and Treatment, vol 1. New York: American Diabetes Association, 1964: 73–78.

Hirsch IB, McGill JB. Role of insulin in management of surgical patients with diabetes mellitus. Diabetes Care 13:980–991, 1990.

Hirsch IB, Paauw DS, Brunzell J. Inpatient management of adults with diabetes. Diabetes Care 18:870–878, 1995.

Koproski J, Pretto Z, Poretsky L. Effects of an intervention by a diabetes team in hospitalized patients with diabetes. Diabetes Care 20:1553–1555, 1997.

Levetan CS, Passaro M, Jablonski K. Unrecognized diabetes among hospitalized patients. Diabetes Care 21:246–249, 1998.

Marhoffer W, Stein M, Maeser E, Federlin K. Impairment of polymorphonuclear leukocyte function and metabolic control of diabetes. Diabetes Care 15:256–260, 1992.

Masson EA, MacFarlane IA, Power E, Wallymahmed M. An audit of the management and outcome of hospital inpatients with diabetes: resource planning implications for the diabetes care team. Diabetic Med 9:753–755, 1992.

McClellan WM, Knight DF, Karp H, Brown WW. Early detection and treatment of renal disease in hospitalized diabetic and hypertensive patients: important differences between practice and published guidelines. Am J Kidney Dis 29:368–375, 1997.

Meyer GR, Gates GE. Evaluation and comparison of the nutrition care process for persons with diabetes among inpatient and outpatient dietitians. Diabetes Educator 19: 403–408, 1993.

Page CP, Hardin TC. Nutritional Assessment and Support: A Primer. Baltimore, MD: Williams & Wilkins, 1989.

Shagan BP. Does anyone here know how to make insulin work backwards? Why sliding-scale insulin coverage doesn't work. Pract Diabetol 9:1–4, 1990.

Watts NB, Gebhart SSP, Clark RV, Phillips LS. Postoperative management of diabetes mellitus: steady-state glucose with bedside algorithm for insulin adjustment. Diabetes Care 10:722–728, 1987.

38

Perisurgical Management of the Patient with Diabetes

Burritt L. Haag
Baystate Medical Center, Springfield, Massachusetts

I. INTRODUCTION

Patients with diabetes are more likely to require surgery than the general population throughout their lifetime. This is true because of the accelerated macrovascular disease they have, and that patients with diabetes are living longer lives. Specifically, they may have to undergo vascular surgery at some time in their life. There is an increased frequency of coronary artery bypass grafts, peripheral vascular disease surgery, amputations, and carotid artery bypass surgery in the diabetic population. Renal transplantation surgery is also increased because of end-stage diabetic nephropathy. Diabetes by itself is not a risk factor for postoperative morbidity and mortality when adjusted for other comorbidities that occur more frequently in diabetes, such as atherosclerosis.

This chapter is a practical approach that is useful for most routine surgeries whether performed at a rural hospital or the world's greatest hospital, for the management of the patient with diabetes who is undergoing surgery. The approach contains some old tried and true treatment concepts as well as newer techniques for good control of the diabetes throughout the perioperative period, and is useful for all surgeries whether they are early-morning admissions or daystay surgeries.

There are four general principles that are important to understand and apply to all patients with diabetes who are undergoing surgery.

1. Know your patient.
2. Anesthesia and surgery are a stress to metabolic control in diabetes.
3. Good control of diabetes is important in the perisurgical period.
4. All patients with diabetes can be managed in a similar way.

II. GENERAL PRINCIPLE 1: KNOW YOUR PATIENT

The preoperative evaluation of the patient with diabetes must begin with an understanding of what type of diabetes the patient has. Does the patient have type 1, insulin-dependent, diabetes or does the patient have type 2 diabetes? Is the type 2 insulin-requiring or not? This is important because of the implications of the perisurgical management of the patient. For example, the type 1 diabetic secretes no insulin so that the lack of the administration of insulin on a regular schedule in the postoperative period can result in rapid deterioration of metabolic control.

The patient with diabetes who is to undergo a surgical procedure must have a carefully history and physical examination preoperatively. The complications of diabetes need to be carefully assessed, including both the microvascular complications (retinopathy, neuropathy, and nephropathy), as well as the macrovascular complications (coronary artery disease with an anginal syndrome, past history of myocardial infarction, peripheral vascular disease with intermittent claudication, or a history of a prior transient ischemic attack or cerebral vascular accident).

The microvascular complications are related to the duration of the diabetes and the quality of long-term metabolic control. A careful assessment of the presence of autonomic neuropathy is important preoperatively. Cardiovascular autonomic neuropathy presents with orthostatic hypotension and a lack of increase in pulse rate on assuming the upright position, and patients with cardiovascular autonomic neuropathy have an increased risk of cardiovascular lability during anesthesia. A history of impaired gastric emptying indicating the presence of diabetic gastroparesis is important because anesthesia may result in an exacerbation of underlying gastroparesis and make postoperative resumption of oral intake of food very difficult. The presence of diabetic nephropathy needs to be evaluated by obtaining urine for a microalbumin/creatinine ratio and a serum creatinine level. Microalbuminuria is a predictor of the progression to clinical diabetic nephropathy and is a risk factor for cardiovascular mortality in type 2 diabetes. The presence of diabetic nephropathy is important to determine preoperatively because of the risks that occur with the use of contrast medium and the resultant acute deterioration of renal function that may occur following its use. The physician is also alerted to potential fluid and electrolyte problems that may occur postoperatively as well as the danger that postoperative dehydration, with hypovolemia and hypotension, could further deteriorate renal function in patients with diabetic nephropathy.

The physical examination should include a careful evaluation for both microvascular and macrovascular complications. The pupils of the eyes should be dilated for a proper evaluation of the presence of diabetic retinopathy. A careful neurological examination should be performed to include the patient's blood pressure and pulse responses to the recumbent and upright positions. Remember that patients with underlying autonomic neuropathy usually have a well-established peripheral neuropathy that is easily quantitated by a careful neurological examination. The physical examination should include a careful evaluation for macrovascular disease, with examination of the heart, peripheral pulses, the presence of vascular bruits, and the presence of atrophic skin changes of the feet.

Finally, if the surgical procedure is elective and the patient is not in good metabolic control, then time should be taken to improve the control of the diabetes preoperatively to get the patient into an anabolic state and to correct any existing fluid or electrolyte abnormalities.

A. Emergency Surgery

If the patient requires emergency surgery and is in hyperosmolar nonketotic coma or diabetic ketoacidosis, the surgery should be delayed at least long enough to stabilize the diabetes and correct the fluid and electrolyte losses.

III. GENERAL PRINCIPLE 2: ANESTHESIA AND SURGERY ARE A STRESS TO METABOLIC CONTROL IN DIABETES

Anesthesia and surgery both cause hyperglycemia. In bygone days when the anesthetics were ether and chloroform, the anesthesia itself induced significant hyperglycemia, but in current times the employed anesthetics cause much less difficulty, and most of the hyperglycemia that results is due to the surgery. Surgery induces a catabolic state, the severity of which is dependent on the surgical procedure and the severity of the postoperative complications. Metabolically, it is easy to think of what happens in terms of a children's seesaw. On one side of the seesaw there is the anabolic hormone insulin, and on the other side are the catabolic counterregulatory hormones: glycogen, epinephrine, norepinephrine, cortisol, and growth hormone. In a person who does not have diabetes these opposing hormones are balanced so that glucose homeostasis is maintained. With anesthesia and surgery there is an increase in the catabolic counterregulatory hormones that results in hyperglycemia unless insulin secretion is increased to counterbalance the increase in the counterregulatory hormones. These counterregulatory hormones cause hyperglycemia by several mechanisms, including stimulation of glycogenolysis and gluconeogenesis, inhibition of insulin secretion, and impairment of insulin action in the periphery. A nondiabetic individual has the ability to increase insulin secretion and, thereby, maintain glucose homeostasis throughout the surgical procedure and postoperatively, whereas the patient with diabetes is unable to do so. The severity of the hyperglycemia and the catabolic state that results is dependent on the type of surgery, its inherticant stress, and the severity of the postoperative complications that may occur. If the surgical stress is severe enough, then either hyperosmolar nonketotic coma or diabetic ketoacidosis may occur. The patient who is undergoing an uncomplicated laparoscopic cholecystectomy represents a low-grade surgical stress, whereas the patient who is undergoing open heart surgery represents a severe surgical stress. Thus, the physician needs to know what to expect as far as the response of his patient with diabetes to surgery. It must be appreciated that the more stressful the surgery and the more severe the complications postoperatively, the more severe the hyperglycemia will be. The patient will be more resistant to insulin because of the persistent higher levels of the counterregulatory hormones.

IV. GENERAL PRINCIPLE 3: GOOD CONTROL OF DIABETES IS IMPORTANT IN THE PERISURGICAL PERIOD

Good control of the blood glucose is important throughout the perisurgical period. The goal is the avoidance of hyperglycemia and hypoglycemia. *Hyperglycemia,* defined as a blood glucose level greater than 250 mL/dL, may result in an increased osmotic diuresis with resultant loss of body water and electrolytes leading to fluid and electrolyte problems. Dehydration, hypovolemia, and hypotension, resulting in a deterioration of renal function in a patient with underlying diabetic nephropathy, may result. It has been shown experimentally that hyperglycemia of more than 250 mL/dL inhibits normal leukocyte functions by mechanisms including a decrease in phagocytosis and chemotaxis, and bacterial kill. These are corrected by maintaining a blood glucose level of less than 250 mL/dL. Serious infections in the postoperative period occur with increased frequency in patients with diabetes. There is experimental evidence that wound healing is impaired in the presence of hyperglycemia owing to an interference with collagen synthesis and a decrease in the tensile strength of incisional wounds. Hyperglycemia results in an increase in plasminogen activator inhibitor and in abnormal platelet function with increased platelet aggregation. These changes result in an increased risk of abnormal coagulation. Hyperglycemia may exacerbate ischemic brain damage in the elderly. Finally, hyperosmolar nonketonic coma or diabetic ketoacidosis may occur if the surgical stress and the postoperative complications are severe enough.

Hypoglycemia is likewise to be avoided in the perisurgical period. Patients with diabetes with their increased cardiovascular disease are at risk of sustaining a myocardial infarction or a postoperative cerebral vascular accident as a result of hypoglycemia. The risk of having a hypoglycemic seizure is always present and certainly needs to be avoided in the perisurgical period.

Although blood glucose levels in the perisurgical period up to 250 mg/dL have not been shown to be harmful, the goals for good control of the blood glucose throughout the perisurgical period are a range of 120–180 mL/dL, and the goal blood glucose is 150 mL/dL.

V. GENERAL PRINCIPLE 4: ALL PATIENTS WITH DIABETES CAN BE MANAGED IN A SIMILAR WAY

A. Problem Areas

Most physicians do not have a good understanding of normal insulin secretory dynamics. This is a very important concept to understand so that it can be applied to insulin management in patients with diabetes during the perioperative period. The normal pancreas in an adult secretes 35–40 U of insulin per day. Of this total, 24 U is secreted as a basal rate at 1 U of insulin per hour. Insulin secretion with meals typically might be 6 U with breakfast, 3 U with lunch, 5 U with supper, and 2 U with a bedtime snack. Patients with type 1 diabetes are not insulin-resistant and their 24-h insulin requirement usually follows the normal secretory pattern unless they are obese. On the other hand, type 2 insulin-requiring diabetics are insulin-resistant, most being obese, and hence, require much more insulin over a 24-h time period for good metabolic control.

The second problem area is in the use of bolus intravenous insulin. The half-life of insulin in the blood is 4–8 min. The effect of a bolus of insulin injected intravenously (iv) lasts approximately 1 h. A single bolus of 10 U of regular insulin injected iv will saturate the insulin receptors and is the most effective way to rapidly lower the blood glucose level. However, bolus iv insulin must be combined with insulin administered by another route (subcutaneously, intramuscularly, or by continuous iv infusion) to provide a more lasting effect.

The third problem area is the use of sliding-scale insulin coverage in the traditional manner. This technique taught to you by your Chief Medical Resident, of writing for fixed sliding-scale insulin coverage in the recovery room for patients with diabetes and then walking away from it is not acceptable. Sliding-scale insulin coverage written in this manner is particular dangerous for patients with type 1 diabetes. They can often end up receiving no insulin for 12 h postoperatively as the sliding-scale dictates coverage q6h only for blood glucoses of 200 mL/dL or higher, a commonly written sliding scale order. By the time the problem is recognized the patient may be well on the way to diabetic ketoacidosis. Patients with type 1 diabetes need to be given insulin every 4–6 h even if their blood glucose levels are within target range.

The physician must observe the patient's blood glucose response to the chosen amount of insulin coverage and adjust the insulin dosage algorithm based on the degree of insulin resistance that is present. The proper use of insulin dosage algorithms postoperatively must involve the use of bedside glucose monitoring with a glucose meter. This is now called point-of-care blood glucose testing and is an essential requirement for good metabolic control in the perioperative period. The use of the central laboratory results in an unacceptable delay in obtaining blood glucose results and, therefore, timely insulin administration.

What follows is an approach for most routine surgeries. Special problems will be discussed separately.

1. Day of Surgery Management of Patients with Type 1 Diabetes

1. Obtain a fasting point-of-care blood glucose.
2. Start iv 5% glucose in 0.5 normal saline at 100 mL/h.
3. Give 50% of the usual intermediate insulin dosage (NPH or Lente insulins) and a small amount of regular insulin (2–4 U) subcutaneously.
4. Obtain a STAT point-of-care blood glucose in the recovery room and begin regular insulin coverage at that time and then q4–6h administered subcutaneously. Adjust the q4–6h regular insulin coverage based upon the observed blood glucose response.
5. Resume the patient's usual morning intermediate and regular insulin dosage as soon as the patient is able to take oral feedings.

2. Day of Surgery Management of Patients with Type 2 Diabetes, Insulin-Requiring

1. Obtain a fasting point-of-care blood glucose.
2. Start iv 5% glucose in 0.5 normal saline at 100 mL/h.
3. Give 50% of the usual intermediate insulin dosage (NPH or Lente insulin) and a small amount of regular insulin (2–4 U) subcutaneously.
4. Obtain a STAT point-of-care blood glucose in the recovery room and begin regular insulin coverage at that time and then q4–6h administered subcutaneously. Adjust the q4–6h regular insulin coverage based upon the observed blood glucose response.
5. Resume the patient's usual morning intermediate and regular insulin dosage as soon as the patient is able to take oral feedings.

3. Day of Surgery Management of Patients with Type 2 Diabetes Taking an Oral Hypoglycemic Agent

1. Discontinue the oral hypoglycemic agent the day of surgery and do not resume until the patient is taking oral feedings postoperatively. The sulfonylureas can result in hypoglycemia that persists well after the medication has been discontinued. This is particularly true in the case of chlorpropamide. Metformin does not need to be discontinued 48 h before surgery, but because of its dependence on renal excretion and

the danger of lactic acidosis, it should not be resumed postoperatively until the patient is taking oral feedings and renal function has returned to baseline. Monotherapy of diabetes with metformin, troglitazone, rosiglitazone, or acarbose does not cause hypoglycemia.

2. Obtain fasting point-of-care blood glucose.
3. Start iv 5% glucose in 0.5 normal saline at 100 mL/h.
4. Obtain a STAT point-of-care blood glucose in the recovery room and begin regular insulin coverage at that time and then continue q4–6h administered subcutaneously.
5. Resume the oral hypoglycemic agent when the patient is able to take oral feedings.

4. Day of Surgery Management for Patients with Type 2 Diabetes: Diet-Controlled

1. Obtain a fasting point-of-care blood glucose.
2. Start iv normal saline at 100 mL/h.
3. Obtain a STAT point-of-care blood glucose in the recovery room and begin regular insulin coverage at that time and then q4–6h administered subcutaneously as needed. Remember that a patient with type 2 diet-controlled diabetes is likely to require insulin coverage postoperatively.

B. Special Problems

1. Patients Who Undergo an Extended Operation

Patients whose surgery lasts longer than 4 h may require a more intensive approach. In this situation it is best to obtain a STAT blood glucose at 4 h and begin regular insulin coverage at that time and then q4h administered subcutaneously.

2. Patient With Diabetes Who Are Undergoing Open Heart Surgery

Patients undergoing open heart surgery have severe insulin resistance intraoperatively and postoperatively. The intraoperative management of the diabetes varies from institution to institution. Continuous intravenous insulin administered by an infusion pump is a popular method for good control. Whatever the intraoperative management approach is at your hospital, the postoperative management of these patients is best done with continuous intravenous insulin administered by an infusion pump.

1. Mix 100 U of regular insulin diluted in 100 mL of normal saline (this results in a concentration of 1 U of insulin per milliliter.

2. Flush out the infusion tubing with 25 mL because insulin will adhere to the infusion tubing wall.
3. Begin the insulin infusion at a rate of 10 U/h and expect the range to be 4–20 U/h of insulin. Patients after open heart surgery with mediastinitis may require as much as 100 U/h of insulin to maintain good blood glucose control.
4. Obtain a point-of-care blood glucose q1h initially and decrease as indicated to q2–q4h. An insulin dosage algorithm should be written for adjustment of the insulin infusion rate based on the patient's observed blood glucose response. Remember that when the adrenergic drug therapy is discontinued the insulin requirement will decrease dramatically. Finally, when converting back to subcutaneous insulin coverage from a continuous insulin infusion, always continue the intravenous insulin infusion for 1 h after the injection of the subcutaneous regular insulin because it takes time for the subcutaneous insulin to have its hypoglycemic effect.

3. Patients Who Are Unable to Resume Oral Feedings Postoperatively

Those patients who are unable to resume normal feedings after surgery and require total parenteral nutrition are best treated with continuous intravenous insulin by an infusion pump. This situation occurs in diabetics who have an exacerbation of gastroparesis postoperatively, have undergone gastrointestinal surgery, who are too lethargic to resume oral feedings, or who have suffered a postsurgical cerebral vascular accident.

1. Mix 100 U of regular insulin diluted in 100 mL of normal saline that results in a concentration of 1 U of insulin per milliliter.
2. Flush out the infusion tubing with 25 mL because insulin is very sticky and will adhere to the infusion tubing wall.
3. Begin the insulin at a rate of 2 U/h.
4. Obtain a point-of-care blood glucose q1h initially and decrease as indicated to q2–q4h. It may be necessary to go to a lower concentration (i.e., 50 U of regular insulin diluted in 100 mL of normal saline providing a concentration of 0.5 U of insulin per milliliter as the patient's sensitivity to insulin improves.

4. Induction of Labor

Labor induction is best managed by continuous intravenous insulin administered by an infusion pump. Labor is intense muscular exercise that increases insulin sensitivity.

1. Obtain a point-of-care blood glucose.
2. Start 5% glucose in 0.5 normal saline at 100 mL/h.

3. Mix 50 U of regular insulin diluted in 100 mL of normal saline providing a concentration of 0.5 U of insulin per milliliter.
4. Begin insulin infusion at a rate of 1 U of insulin per hour.
5. Obtain a point-of-care blood glucose q1h and adjust the insulin infusion rate as needed.
6. Continue the intravenous insulin until delivery and then discontinue. Once the placenta has been delivered, insulin resistance decreases dramatically owing to the loss of the counterregulatory hormones of the placenta.
7. Obtain a STAT point-of-care blood glucose in the recovery room and begin regular insulin coverage q4–6h administered subcutaneously. It may take several hours before any insulin is required at all because of the marked improvement in insulin sensitivity that occurs following delivery.

5. Problems with Subcutaneous Regular Insulin Coverage

If problems develop with subcutaneous regular insulin coverage then convert the patient to continuous intravenous insulin by an infusion pump. This method is the safest for the patient and provides the best metabolic control of any of the treatment regimens.

VI. FINAL COMMENT

Resume the patient's usual intermediate and regular insulin schedule as soon as the patient resumes oral feedings. Convert the point-of-care blood glucose testing to 1 h before meals and bedtime snack. Administer additional regular insulin subcutaneously 30 min before meals and bedtime snack as needed. This approach prevents an unwanted extra day of hospitalization because the patient is still receiving regular insulin coverage the day the surgeon decides to discharge the patient. Remember, the insulin dosage that the patient goes home on following surgery may be very different then the prehospitalization insulin dosage.

A number of excellent reviews of the perisurgical management of the patient with diabetes follows.

BIBLIOGRAPHY

Alberti KG, Marshall SM. Diabetes and surgery. In: Alberti KG, Krall LP, eds. Diabetes Annual, vol 4. Amsterdam: Elsevier Science, 1988:248.
Marks JB, Hirsch IB. Surgery and diabetes mellitus. In: DeFronzo RA, ed. Current Management of Diabetes Mellitus. New York, Mosby, 1998:247–254.
Palmisano JJ, Surgery and diabetes. In: Kahn CR, Weir GC, eds. Joslin's Diabetes Mellitus. 13th ed. Lea & Febiger, 1994:955–961.
Schade DS. Surgery and diabetes. Med Clin North Am 1988; 72:1531–1543.

39
Nutritional Support in the Diabetic Patient

M. Molly McMahon
Mayo Clinic and Mayo Foundation, Rochester, Minnesota

I. INTRODUCTION

Diabetes mellitus is a metabolic disorder caused by an absolute (type 1; previously called insulin-dependent diabetes mellitus) or a relative (type 2; previously called non–insulin-dependent diabetes mellitus; and stress diabetes mellitus) lack of insulin. Because of the prevalence of diabetes mellitus and the comorbidity of the disease, most diabetologists will manage hospitalized diabetic patients receiving nutritional support. This chapter will review nutritional support and the importance of glucose control.

The homeostatic mechanisms that maintain euglycemia in the postabsorptive state and buffer the postprandial glycemic excursion in nondiabetic subjects are impaired in patients with diabetes mellitus. These patients have both preprandial and postprandial hyperglycemia owing to excessive hepatic glucose release, impaired glucose uptake, and decreased insulin secretion or action (1).

Severe stress can cause hyperglycemia in patients without an antecedent diagnosis of diabetes mellitus. Severe stress (as during a serious illness) is accompanied by significant increases in the plasma concentration of counterregulatory hormones (i.e., glucagon, epinephrine, cortisol, and growth hormone) that increase hepatic glucose release and decrease peripheral glucose uptake (2). Stress causes an even greater derangement in glucose metabolism in patients with diabetes because they cannot increase insulin secretion as a compensatory response. The exaggerated glucose response following a stress dose counterregulatory hormone infusion in healthy subjects with diabetes, in comparison with nondiabetic subjects, is one explanation for the deterioration in glucose control that occurs in stressed diabetic patients. Cytokines may also profoundly affect carbohydrate metabolism. Typically, the interleukins cause hyperglycemia. Endotoxin can cause hyperglycemia or hypoglycemia.

II. NUTRITIONAL ASSESSMENT

The nutritional assessment, indications for nutritional support, and estimate of nutritional needs for critically ill diabetic patients are similar to those of the nondiabetic patient (12,13). However, diabetes can affect the entire gastrointestinal tract. Significant diabetic gastroparesis is typically observed in patients with type 1 diabetes. This diagnosis is strongly suggested if patients experience bloating, early satiety, nausea, and postprandial vomiting (especially partially digested food retained from earlier meals). It is important to accurately diagnose diabetic gastroparesis to avoid attributing the gastrointestinal symptoms to tube feeding alone or to other factors capable of affecting gut motility. Review of the patient's medication list is important to determine if any of the prescribed medications may delay gastric emptying. These medications include α_2-adrenergic agonists, anticholinergic (tricyclic antidepressants, antihistamines), β-adrenergic blockers, calcium channel blockers, and narcotics. Acute hyperglycemia can decrease gastric emptying. Constipation, diarrhea, and fecal incontinence may also develop with long-standing diabetes.

Protein catabolism (with eventual depletion of body protein) can be a consequence of starvation or severe illness. In the classic sense, malnutrition results from starvation. Nevertheless, either severe illness or illness superimposed on starvation is by far the more common cause of protein catabolism in hospitalized patients.

An understanding of the cytokine and hormonal milieu of sickness enhance interpretation of the nutritional assessment of critically ill patients. Anorexia is common in patients with severe illness. Cytokine infusion causes a significant reduction in food intake. It is important to recognize that illness and cytokines can lead to an abrupt decrease in plasma albumin. This decrease can be attributed to altered capillary permeability (allowing albumin to move from the intravascular to the extravascular space) and to an increase in catabolism. In addition, cytokines can down-regulate the albumin gene, thereby decreasing the rate of messenger RNA translation. Therefore, during severe illness, hypoalbuminemia is an excellent marker of the stress response, but a poor marker of nutritional status. Transferrin, prealbumin, and retinol-binding protein are also negative acute-phase proteins, the concentrations of which fall during the early systemic response to illness. Accordingly, we do not measure these parameters to assess the nutritional status of stressed, hospitalized patients. The prognostic importance of hypoalbuminemia as a marker of stress is supported by data that hypoalbuminemia at hospital admission is associated with increased morbidity and mortality rates.

Hypoalbuminemia can also affect interpretation of plasma trace metal levels and drug pharmacokinetics. Because circulating calcium, magnesium, and zinc are all bound to albumin, a low plasma trace-metal level may be appropriate for a decreased serum albumin level. Albumin is also a major plasma protein responsible for the binding of acidic drugs. A decrease in plasma albumin can significantly alter the distribution of highly protein-bound drugs (e.g., phenytoin) and increase the fraction of the unbound, active drug. Finally, although weight is often a key anthropometric marker, the weight of hospitalized patients must be carefully interpreted. Many critically ill patients have increased total body water and salt owing to the underlying illness (e.g., cardiac, renal, or hepatic diseases), the treatment (e.g., crystalloid or colloid infusion), or the hormonal milieu of critical illness and refeeding. Thus, weight loss alone is not a requisite for initiation of nutritional support.

The nutritional assessment aims to identify malnourished patients or patients at risk for its development. Malnutrition adversely affects respiratory muscle structure and function, cardiac function, gastrointestinal tract architecture, musculoskeletal strength, wound healing, and immune function. In general, a recent (previous 3- to 6-month interval) weight loss in excess of 10% from usual weight necessitates a more thorough nutritional assessment, as this is a good prognosticator of clinical outcome. In addition to the magnitude of recent weight loss, it is the adequacy of recent food intake, the presence or absence of clinical markers of stress, and the anticipated time that the patient will be unable to eat that determine the need for nutritional intervention (Table 1). Usually, a weight loss of up to 10% of body weight is well tolerated and, in the absence of significant stress, the provision of dextrose-containing crystalloid solutions and electrolytes alone is adequate for as long as 7–10 days. Those studies that demonstrated a beneficial influence of nutritional support on clinical outcome administered nutrition for a minimum of 1 week. No data have been established in support of a briefer duration being of clinical benefit.

Avoidance of overfeeding is important because an excess of calories can exacerbate hyperglycemia. The daily energy expenditure of a hospitalized patient

Table 1 Indications for Nutrition Support (Parenteral Nutrition or Tube Feeding)

Unable to meet nutritional needs orally, and
  More than 7–10 days of past or anticipated inadequate nutrition (< 50% of requirements), and
  Severely ill

Table 2   Guidelines[a] for Calories, Protein, and Lipid Requirements

Calories[b]	Basal calories by using the Harris-Benedict (HB) equation to HB plus 20%[c]
Protein	1.0–1.5 g/kg of body weight
Lipid	30% of total calories over 24 h
Harris–Benedict equation:	

Males 66.5 + (13.8 × wt, kg) + (5.0 × ht, cm) − (6.8 × age, yr)
Females 65.5 + (9.6 × wt, kg) + (1.8 × ht, cm) − (4.7 × age, yr)

[a] Guidelines assume normal hepatic and renal function.
[b] Indirect calorimetric measurement of daily caloric needs may be considered for the following groups of patients: severely stressed patients (e.g., closed head injury, multiple trauma, severe burn); volume-overloaded patients in whom the "dry weight" estimate is uncertain; nutritionally supported patients in whom weaning from mechanical ventilation is difficult; or in patients requiring home parenteral nutrition.
[c] If patient weight is more than 120% of estimated "ideal weight"; consider providing 75% of basal caloric requirements based on the obese weight and 1.5 g protein per kilogram based on the estimated "ideal" weight.

can be estimated by using a formula, such as the Harris-Benedict equation, by providing a certain number of kilocalories per kilogram of body weight, or by indirect calorimetry. During the past decade, numerous studies have shown that the actual energy expenditure of most hospitalized patients is between 100 and 120% of predicted caloric expenditure, with use of the Harris-Benedict equation (Table 2). No consensus exists about nutritional requirements of obese patients, and data are limited. Certain investigators recommend that, in obese patients, the weight used to estimate caloric requirements should be the weight halfway between the ideal and the current weight. Our group recommends providing approximately 75% of basal caloric requirements based on the obese weight. Outcome studies are needed to resolve this controversy.

In general, the malnourished patient with normal renal and hepatic function should receive 1.0–1.5 g of protein per kilogram of body weight; the higher end of the range is for more stressed patients. Studies report that no greater sparing of protein occurs when exogenous protein is provided in amounts exceeding 1.5 g/kg per day. Intravenous fat emulsion should be limited to approximately 30% of the total calories and be provided continuously. Most complications (i.e., impairment of the reticulothelial system clearance and immune function) related to the use of intravenous fat occur at higher infusion rates.

The enteral route, rather than the parenteral, is the preferred route for the delivery of nutrition if the gastrointestinal tract is functioning. Advantages of enteral nutrition include lower cost, avoidance of central catheter-related complications, a more physiological route, and its trophic effect on gastrointestinal cells.

III. MANAGEMENT DURING PARENTERAL NUTRITION

1. Dextrose in the parenteral nutrition (PN) is limited to approximately 200 g on the first day of nutrition.

2. Most diabetic patients will require insulin coverage when glucose is infused. For patients previously treated with insulin or oral hypoglycemic agents or for patients with fasting glucose values consistently greater than 200 mg/dL, it is our practice to initially place 0.1 U of regular insulin per gram of dextrose (D) (e.g., 15 U/L of D 15% [150 g/L]). In our experience, this ratio of insulin to dextrose is unlikely to be associated with hypoglycemia and thus minimize the need to waste a bag of PN.

3. It is our practice to initially measure reflectance meter glucose values frequently and to administer supplemental subcutaneous (sq) regular insulin according to a sq insulin algorithm (Table 3). Once glycemic control is acceptable, an alteration in the frequency of glucose monitoring is appropriate.

4. If over a 24-h period, glucose values consistently exceed 200 mg/dL, the PN insulin is increased each day by 0.05 U of regular insulin per gram of dextrose to a maximum of approximately 0.2 U of insulin per gram of dextrose. If the plasma glucose remains higher than 200 mg/dL with insulin coverage of 0.2 U/g of PN dextrose and adherence to the sq insulin algorithm, initiation of an intravenous insulin infusion should be considered. Our group has implemented an order form to standardize the insulin infusion (Table 4).

5. In general, the PN dextrose load should not be increased until the glucose values of the previous 24-h period are consistently less than 200 mg/dL.

Table 3 Guidelines for Subcutaneous Regular Insulin Supplementation[a]

Glucose (mg/dL)	sq regular insulin dose (U)
200–250	2–3
251–300	4–6
301–350	6–9
> 350	8–12

[a] Adjustment of this algorithm may be required for differences in patient weight, response to insulin, and treatment goals. Insulin should not be administered more often than every 4–6 h.

Table 4 Intravenous Insulin Infusion Algorithm

Glucose mg/dL	iv Infusion rate mL/h	Insulin infusion rate U/h
> 400	8	8
351–400	6	6
301–350	4	4
250–300	3	3
200–249	2.5	2.5
150–199	2	2
120–149	1.5	1.5
100–119	1	1
70–99	0	0
<70	0	0

1. Glucose goals should be defined for each patient. In stressed patients, a glucose goal range of 100–200 mg/dL is appropriate. This infusion algorithm is designed for the average 70-kg patient and may require modification for smaller or larger patients. This infusion is not appropriate for the treatment of diabetic ketoacidosis or hyperosmolar states.
2. Glucose should be measured hourly until the glucose concentrations have stabilized in the patient's goal glucose range for 4 h. The frequency of testing may then be decreased to every 2 h, and once the glucose control remains stable, to every 4 h.
3. If hyperglycemia persists, this algorithm may be increased by 50% increments for each glucose range greater than 200 mg/dL. The risk of hypoglycemia may be greater if the algorithm is increased for glucose values less than 200 mg/dL.
4. In patients treated with insulin, plasma potassium, magnesium, and phosphorus concentrations may decrease rapidly and should be monitored.
5. At the time of conversion from intravenous to subcutaneous insulin therapy, the intravenous infusion should be continued for 2–3 h following the administration of the first subcutaneous insulin dose.

6. Insulin in the PN should be proportionally increased or decreased when the PN dextrose content is increased or decreased.
7. The incidence of symptomatic hypoglycemia after discontinuation of PN is uncommon, provided that the patient has not received excessive calories. However, if the patient has a serum creatinine value higher than 2.0 mg/dL or if the PN admixture contains more than 0.2 U of insulin per gram of dextrose, the glucose concentration should be monitored closely during the first hour after discontinuation of PN. If the patient develops hypoglycemia, parenteral dextrose should be administered (Table 5). A substantial (50%) reduction of insulin in the following day's PN admixture should decrease the incidence of recurrent hypoglycemia. Similar reductions in the PN insulin should also be made if there is a significant decrease in the mean glucose concentration over a 24-h period to values below the goal range.

Table 5 Treatment of Hypoglycemia in Hospitalized Adult Patients with Diabetes
Mellitus Receiving Insulin or Oral Agents

I. Presumed symptomatic hypoglycemia should be treated without waiting to check a
plasma or blood glucose level. The unit hypoglycemia tray should be used.

   A. If the patient is able to swallow safely, provide oral administration of glucose.
The patient should ingest approximately 15 g of dextrose. Examples are:

      1. 2 sugar packets or cubes or

      2. 15 g of glucose tablets or gel or

      3. 1/2 cup (4 oz) of fruit juice

   B. If the patient is not able to take oral feeding safely or is NPO for any reason,
do the following:

      1. If intravenous access is available, administer 1/2 ampule (12.5 g) D50W
intravenously.

      2. If no intravenous access is present, administer 1 mg of glucagon by subcuta-
neous or intramuscular injection. Following glucagon treatment, for those
patients who are not NPO, provide a snack in order to prevent subsequent
hypoglycemia.

   C. Contact either the Primary Service or the Diabetes Consulting Service, whichever is responsible for the patient's diabetes management.

II. For treatment of asymptomatic hypoglycemia (glucose less than or equal to 60
mg/dL) follow steps A through C.

III. Glycemic monitoring following treatment:
Obtain a capillary glucose determination in 15 min. If the glucose value is not more
than 80 mg/dL, repeat the treatment outlined above. Recheck the glucose value in
15 min. Repeat further treatment (and glucose checks at 15-min intervals) until the
glucose value is higher than 80 mg/dL.

IV. MANAGEMENT DURING ENTERAL NUTRITION

1. Although insulin administration usually prevents hyperglycemia in patients receiving enteral calories, glycemic control may be difficult to
achieve. Until the patient is able to tolerate tube feeding, intermediate-
acting insulin should be used with caution. Short-acting insulin is preferred to minimize the risk of hypoglycemia that could result from the
continued absorption of insulin from longer-acting insulin preparations
following unexpected discontinuation of tube feeding. Once the tube
feeding infusion rate has reached 30–40 mL/h, the use of intermediate-
acting insulin is generally safe.

2. If tube feedings are to be administered during the day, we frequently
begin by providing one-half of the patient's preadmission morning
insulin dose as intermediate-acting insulin. Increases in the tube-feed-

ing infusion rate should be avoided until adequate glucose control has been achieved. Intermediate-acting insulin should be given in the evening if the tube feeding is administered during the night. Twice daily administration of intermediate-acting insulin may be required if the tube feedings are administered continuously over 24 h.

3. If the feedings are infused by gravity administration, the glucose level should be checked immediately before the feeding is initiated and no sooner than 4 h following the end of the prior feeding. Although some patients receiving this form of feeding can be managed with intermediate-acting insulin alone, others will need combined treatment with intermediate-acting and short-acting insulin.

4. The tube-feeding rate should not be altered until appropriate adjustments have been made in the insulin dosage.

5. Gastroparesis may make tube-feeding tolerance more difficult. In our experience, most patients with diabetic gastroparesis tolerate jejunal feedings when iso-osmolar formulas are started at a low rate (e.g., 20 mL/h) and advanced slowly (e.g., 10- to 20-mL/h–increment increase every 12 h) to the goal infusion rate. Selected patients require gastric decompression. Glucose control can affect gastric emptying, and delayed gastric emptying may make regulation of glucose control difficult. Hyperglycemia may further delay gastric emptying, whereas hypoglycemia may result in patients treated with insulin or oral hypoglycemic agents who do not absorb food normally because of a delay in gastric emptying. Parenteral nutrition should be reserved for those patients who have severe small-bowel dysmotility and who have failed a reasonable trial of nasojejunal tube feeding.

6. A common management error occurs when the health care provider relies on the regular insulin algorithm exclusively for insulin management throughout the hospitalization. Once the patient is medically stable, the preferred management is to review the amount of regular insulin that was required over the preceding 24-h period, and then appropriately adjust the intermediate-acting insulin and short-acting insulin programs.

7. Unexpected discontinuation of tube feeding may cause hypoglycemia in patients who are treated with subcutaneous injections of insulin. Glucose levels should be carefully monitored to determine if intravenous infusion of a dextrose-containing solution is necessary to prevent subsequent hypoglycemia.

8. Oral hypoglycemic agents can be used to treat hyperglycemia in medically stable patients with well-controlled type 2 diabetes and normal renal and hepatic function and may be administered by feeding tube. We do not recommend the use of metformin or rezulin in hospitalized

patients, because lactic acidosis may occur with renal, cardiac, or hepatic dysfunction.
9. In patients with unstable diabetes and significant hyperglycemia, an intravenous insulin infusion may be necessary.

The recent availability of enteral formulas lower in carbohydrate and higher in fat content than standard formulas has prompted studies comparing the glycemic response. Although initial studies suggested that the glycemic response to the lower carbohydrate product was blunted compared with standard formulas, a follow-up study reported that the glycemic response was variable in each patient. The clinical significance of these studies is unclear because the subjects ingested very small amounts of formula over a few hours, a very different pattern from that of continuous tube feeding or gravity administration of the feeding. The high-fat content could impair gastric emptying in patients with gastroparesis. For fiber content, the current American Diabetes Association position statement on nutrition states that, although selected soluble fibers are capable of delaying glucose absorption from the small intestine, the effect of dietary fiber on glycemic control is probably insignificant. Therefore, the fiber intake recommendations for diabetics are probably the same as for the general hospitalized population. During hospitalization, avoidance of overfeeding is likely more important than is the use of a specific enteral formula. Outcome studies will be necessary to address this issue.

V. GLUCOSE GOALS

A major goal in the hospitalized patient is to avoid the extremes of hyperglycemia and hypoglycemia. A reasonable aim is to maintain glucose levels between 100 and 200 mg/dL. Avoidance or minimization of hyperglycemia in hospitalized patients is important. The physician should attempt to identify the cause(s) of hyperglycemia. Illness or infection, overfeeding (nutrition support, dextrose-containing crystalloid, dextrose absorption during peritoneal dialysis, and medications formulated in lipid emulsion, such as propofol), medications (e.g., corticosteroids, sympathomimetic infusion, or cyclosporine), insufficient insulin, or volume depletion can cause hyperglycemia. Because unexplained hyperglycemia may be a harbinger of infection, the central catheter should always be considered a potential source of infection.

During a short time period, hyperglycemia can adversely affect fluid balance and immune function. As the filtered load of glucose increases, it eventually exceeds tubular reabsorptive capacity. As a result, glucose remains in the tubular lumen and acts as an osmotic diuretic, increasing the urinary loss of electrolytes and water. Impaired immune function in diabetic patients has long been recognized (3–8). In vitro studies document that hyperglycemia is associated with abnormalities in granulocyte adhesion, chemotaxis, phagocytosis, and intracellular killing. Most studies report that phagocytosis can be corrected or substantially improved with control of blood glucose levels. Respiratory burst function and superoxide anion production are impaired in patients with non–insulin-dependent diabetes mellitus and are improved by glucose control. Respiratory burst is a critical element in the activation of microbicidal systems because this burst of oxidative metabolism generates toxic products of oxygen. A significant reduction in the respiratory burst also occurs in neutrophils of healthy nondiabetic subjects following exposure to glucose concentrations of more than 200 mg/dL.

Hyperglycemia also adversely affects complement function. The opsonic function of complement is impaired because glucose binds to the biochemically active site of complement, thereby inhibiting complement attachment to the microbial surface. A recent study reported that increased cytosolic calcium levels in polymorphonuclear (PMN) leukocytes of diabetic patients adversely affects immune function. Increased cytosolic calcium in leukocytes of diabetic patients was directly correlated with glucose values and was associated with decreased phagocytosis. Three months of oral hypoglycemic agent therapy resulted in improved glucose control, a reduction in cytosolic calcium levels, and a significant improvement in phagocytosis. Lastly, an association between hyperglycemia and infection with *Candida albicans* has long been recognized. *Candida albicans* expresses a surface protein, which is homologous with the alpha-chain of the neutrophil receptor for complement. There is an abrupt increase in protein expression during hyperglycemia. This protein impairs phagocytosis of the yeast by binding to complement and inhibits adhesion of the yeast to endothelial surfaces. This mechanism may partly explain the increased incidence of candidal infections in diabetic patients.

An appropriate follow-up question is are there clinical studies documenting adverse effects of hyperglycemia? A growing body of clinical evidence has linked hyperglycemia to nosocomial infection in stressed, hospitalized patients. First, the rate of central catheter-related infections was approximately five times higher in diabetic patients receiving central parenteral nutrition compared with nondiabetic patients receiving the same nutrition. Second, as discussed earlier, hyperglycemia was the most common risk factor for infection with *Candida*. Third, a recent metaanalysis summarizing results from prospective, randomized trials comparing parenteral with enteral nutrition in critically ill patients reported that significantly fewer enterally fed patients (compared with parenterally fed patients) experienced septic complications (16 vs. 35%, respectively). Although the authors concluded that the route of administration of nutrients was the key factor in the observed differences, hyperglycemia may have been an additional variable responsible for the increased infection rate. The average glucose at the conclusion of the study was 230 mg/dL in the parenterally fed patients compared with a mean of 130 mg/dL in the enterally fed group. Fourth, the Veterans Affairs Trial was designed to test the hypothesis that perioperative parenteral nutrition decreases the incidence of serious complications following major abdominal or thoracic surgical procedures in malnourished patients. Although there was a reduction in noninfectious complications in the patients receiving parenteral nutrition, the infectious complications were 2.2 times more common.

Although nutritionists would not refute the conclusion that only malnourished patients should receive preoperative nutritional support, it is important that the higher infection rate observed in patients receiving parenteral nutrition may have partly resulted from the severe hyperglycemia. Serum glucose levels higher than 200 mg/dL occurred in 20% of patients receiving parenteral nutrition and in 1% of the control group. Patients receiving parenteral nutrition were also allowed to eat and the combined caloric intake averaged approximately 45 kcal/kg of body weight, which significantly exceeds requirements. Such overfeeding can lead to hyperglycemia. Fifth, a higher incidence of mediastinitis was found in diabetic patients (compared with nondiabetic patients) following coronary artery bypass graft surgery (9). Finally, a recent study suggests that hyperglycemia itself is an independent risk factor for the development of infection. Investigators monitoring perioperative glucose control in 100 previously uninfected diabetic patients undergoing elective surgery and the subsequent development of postoperative infection found that hyperglycemia (glucose level in excess of 220 mg/dL) on postoperative day 1 was associated with a higher rate of infection (10). There was no difference in type or duration of diabetes mellitus, patient age, percentage of ideal body weight, or recent weight loss in excess of 10%, percentage of patients with preoperative length of stay longer than 1 day, or surgical wound classification between the two groups.

Hyperglycemia has also been associated with a higher mortality in diabetic patients than in nondiabetic patients following acute myocardial infarction. Improved outcome was observed in diabetic patients who, following myocardial infarction, were treated with intravenous insulin infusion during the hospitalization or with glucose–insulin infusion during the hospitalization, followed by multiple daily insulin programs (11).

Avoidance or minimization of hypoglycemia is also important. Identifying neuroglycopenic and adrenergic symptoms of hypoglycemia is difficult in severely ill patients who are sedated or dependent on mechanical ventilation. In addition, patients with long-standing diabetes mellitus may have hypoglycemic unawareness, a loss of the ability to recognize the warning symptoms of hypoglycemia. The physician should always attempt to identify the factors responsible for hypoglycemia. Potential causes include unanticipated discontinuation of nutrition support, resolution of severe stress, discontinuation or decreased doses of corticosteroids or sympathomimetic agents, renal dysfunction, severe hepatitis, sepsis, and diabetic gastroparesis.

VI. MONITORING FOLLOWING INITIATION OF NUTRITIONAL SUPPORT

The initiation of nutritional support in a malnourished diabetic patient requires careful monitoring of vital signs, hemodynamic data, weight, fluid balance, plasma glucose and electrolyte levels, and acid–base status. The presence of fever is always significant in a patient with a central catheter. Hemodynamic data, fluid balance, creatinine, urea, and sodium levels should be reviewed to help determine the appropriate volume of nutrition. The presence of high urine output, negative fluid balance, weight loss, or hypernatremia should prompt a review of recent glucose trends to be certain hyperglycemia is not causing an osmotic diuresis. Daily weight should be interpreted in light of the fluid balance. In general, a weight increase in excess of 0.25 kg over a 24-h period should be attributed to fluid gain. Knowledge of the electrolyte and mineral content of gastrointestinal and renal losses allows more appropriate supplementation. Baseline biochemical data should include glucose, electrolytes, creatinine, urea nitrogen, amino transferase, albumin, calcium, and phosphorus. A glycated hemoglobin value is useful to establish recent glucose control and to determine the appropriate diabetes treatment after hospital dismissal. Plasma zinc, copper, and magnesium should also be measured in patients with impaired intestinal absorption or increased gastrointestinal (zinc and copper) or renal (magnesium) output, as requirements may be higher. For selected patients receiving intravenous fat emulsion, triglyceride levels should be checked before and following initiation of fat emulsion. These groups are patients with pancreatitis, poorly controlled diabetes mellitus, or known hypertriglyceridemia. If the triglyceride level is higher than 400 mg/dL, the intravenous fat emulsion should either be decreased or discontinued, for triglyceride uptake appears to be saturated at this level.

Although the extent and frequency of biochemical monitoring following initiation of nutrition support must be individualized, at a minimum plasma glucose, electrolytes, and phosphorus levels should be checked until stable. Because sudden refeeding with hypertonic glucose can lead to an abrupt increase in plasma insulin concentration, it is important to review the effects of hyperinsulinemia on plasma electrolyte levels. The increase in insulin can lead to hypokalemia, hypomagnesemia, and hypophosphatemia if supplementation is inadequate. Hyperinsulinemia shifts potassium and magnesium into skeletal muscle and hepatic cells. Glucose- and insulin-stimulated glycolysis stimulates the cellular uptake and utilization of phosphorus for the phosphorylation of glucose and fructose and for the synthesis of ATP. Therefore, serum potassium, magnesium, and phosphorus concentrations should be monitored until the levels are stable. In addition, because insulin is required for the maintenance of potassium homeostasis, hyperkalemia in the presence of hyperglycemia may be effectively treated by supplemental insulin. We do not follow nitrogen balance studies to assess adequacy of nutrition support. In the absence of overfeeding, critically ill, immobilized patients will not achieve positive nitrogen balance until resolution of the stress.

VII. OUTCOME

Well-designed, prospective, randomized trials are needed to determine the risks, costs, and benefits of achieving glucose control and of providing nutrition support to malnourished patients with diabetes mellitus.

REFERENCES

1. Bell P, Firth R, Rizza R. Assessment of insulin action in insulin-dependent diabetes mellitus using [6-^{14}C]glucose, [3-^{3}H]glucose, and [2-^{3}H]glucose. J Clin Invest 78: 1479–1486, 1986.
2. Shamoon M, Hendler R, Sherwin R. Synergistic interactions among anti-insulin hormones in the pathogenesis of stress hyperglycemia in humans. J Clin Endocrinol Metab 52:1235–1241, 1981.
3. Alexiewicz JM, Kumar D, Smogorzewski M, Klin M, Massry SG. Polymorphonuclear leukocytes in noninsulin-dependent diabetes mellitus: abnormalities in metabolism and function. Ann Intern Med 123:919–924, 1995.
4. Bagdade J, Stewart M, Walters E. Impaired granulocyte adherence: a reversible defect in host defense in patients with poorly controlled diabetes. Diabetes 27: 677–681, 1978.
5. Hostetter M. Perspectives in diabetes: handicaps to host defense: effects of hyperglycemia on C3 and *Candida albicans*. Diabetes 39:271–275, 1990.
6. MacRury SM, Gemmell CG, Paterson KR, MacCuish AC. Changes in phagocytic function with glycemic control in diabetic patients. J Clin Pathol 42:1143–1147, 1989.
7. McMahon M, Bistrian BR. Host defenses and susceptibility to infection in patients with diabetes mellitus. Infect Dis Clin North Am 9:1–9, 1995.
8. Ortmeyer J, Mohsenin V. Glucose suppresses superoxide generation in normal neutrophils: interference in phospholipase D activation. Am J Physiol 264:C402–C410, 1993.
9. Wallace LK, Starr NJ, Leventhal MJ, Fawzy MS, Estafamous FG. Hyperglycemia on ICU admission after CABG is associated with increased risk of mediastinitis or wound infection. Anesthesiology 85:A286, 1996.
10. Pomposelli JJ, Baxter JK, Babineau TJ, Pomfret EA, Driscoll DF, Forse RA, Bistrian BR. Early postoperative glucose control predicts nosocomial infection rate in diabetic patients. J Parenter Enteral Nutr 22:77–81, 1998.
11. Malmberg K, Ryder L, Efendic S, Herlitz J, Nicol P, Waldenstrom A, Wedel H, Welin L, on behalf of the DIGAMI Study Group. Randomized trial of insulin–glucose infusion followed by subcutaneous insulin treatment in diabetic patients with acute

myocardial infarction (DIGAMI Study): effects on mortality at 1 year. J Am Coll Cardiol 26:57–65, 1995.

12. McMahon M. Parenteral nutrition. In: Bennett JC, Plum F, eds. Cecil Textbook of Medicine. 20th ed. Philadelphia: WB Saunders, 1996:1171–1175.

13. McMahon M, Rizza RA. Nutritional support in hospitalized patients with diabetes mellitus. Mayo Clin Proc 71:587–594, 1996.

40

Diabetic Ketoacidosis and Hyperosmolar Coma

Muriel Helene Nathan
University of Vermont College of Medicine, Burlington, Vermont

I. INTRODUCTION

Ketoacidosis and nonketotic hyperosmolar coma are the two most serious acute hyperglycemic emergencies of diabetes mellitus. Insulin-deficient states most typically lead to diabetic ketoacidosis in those with autoimmune diabetes (type 1) or pancreatic disease, whereas nonketotic hyperosmolar coma occurs in the setting of relative, but not absolute, insulin deficiency (type 2 diabetes).

Diabetic ketoacidosis (DKA) is a metabolic derangement in which there is high blood glucose level, ketonemia, and metabolic acidosis. Hyperosmolar coma is characterized by hyperglycemia, dehydration, and an absence of significant ketoacidosis. Few patients actually present in coma ($< 10\%$) during an episode of nonketotic hyperosmolar coma; therefore, many prefer to call this entity nonketotic hyperosmolar syndrome (NKH).

A. Precipitating Factors

Table 1 lists the most frequent causes of hyperglycemic diabetic emergencies. DKA is commonly initiated by infection (30%), omission or inadequate use of insulin (20%), or new onset of diabetes (25%). In 25% of cases, there is no clear precipitating event. For NKH, the precipitant is also most commonly infection (32–60%), usually gram-negative pneumonia (40–60%) or urinary tract infections (16%). Noninfectious causes include cerebral stroke, myocardial infarction, pancreatitis, uremia with nausea and vomiting, burns, heat stroke, and subdural hematoma. About 40% of those with NKH have no prior history of diabetes.

Table 1 Frequent Causes of Diabetic Ketoacidosis and Nonketotic Hyperosmolar Syndrome

Acute illnesses	Thromboembolic disease	Endocrine illnesses	Drugs
Pneumonia	Cerebrovascular	Acromegaly	HIV drugs (didanosine)
Urinary tract	accident	Cushing's	Calcium channel blockers,
infection	Myocardial	syndrome	propranolol
Sepsis	infarction	Thyrotoxicosis	Chlorthalidone
Pancreatitis	Pulmonary	Undiagnosed	Thiazide diuretics
Severe burns	embolus	diabetes	Steroids
Renal failure	Mesenteric		Phenytoin
Heat stroke	thrombosis		Cimetidine
Hypothermia			Total parenteral nutrition
			Antipsychotics (loxapine)
			Omission of insulin

Source: Ennis and Kreisberg, 1996.

Medications, including propranolol, phenytoin, cimetidine, and corticosteroids (see Table 1) that inhibit insulin secretion or block tissue insulin action or do both, can cause glucose intolerance and, if uncorrected, can lead to NKH. Both thiazide and loop diuretics, which act indirectly to inhibit insulin secretion by causing hypokalemia, may unmask diabetes in the predisposed patient. Furthermore, by causing significant volume contraction, decreasing the glomerular filtration rate and increasing counterregulatory hormones, diuretics can precipitate NKH.

NKH may occur in postoperative patients who are bedridden or restrained with restricted access to water, because they are prone to dehydration. Often the patients are drinking sugar-containing fluids (soda, fruit juice) and this exacerbates hyperglycemia. A similar pathogenesis can be invoked to explain the higher rate of NHK in nursing home patients.

B. Incidence and Mortality

In the United States, admissions to hospital in 1987 with a primary diagnosis of DKA was 12.5:1000 and mortality was 0.25:1000. In 1988, there were 454,000 hospital admissions for diabetes and its complications in the United States. Out of these admissions, 18.5% were for DKA. In a European study, 8.6% of 3250 insulin-dependent diabetes mellitus (IDDM) patients were admitted to hospital for DKA one or more times over the previous year. Moreover, the incidence of

DKA is likely underestimated by surveys of hospital admissions, because most cases of mild DKA are treated in emergency rooms or in ambulatory care centers. Although most episodes of DKA occur in children or young adults with type 1 diabetes (autoimmune diabetes), one retrospective study (1987–1993) of adults admitted to hospital with DKA found that 19% of those with no prior history of diabetes were older than 39 years. Another 52% of adults in this age group had a prior diagnosis of type 2 diabetes (non–insulin-dependent diabetes mellitus; NIDDM).

Deaths during episodes of DKA are rarely due to the decompensation of diabetes per se, but rather, occur because of the associated catastrophic illnesses, such as sepsis or cardiovascular events. Patients older than 65 have a much higher risk of death; their mortality rate during DKA is 20% compared with younger individuals, for whom the mortality rate is less than 2%. A rare but often fatal complication of DKA in children and young adults ($<$ 29 years) is cerebral edema. This complication occurs in 0.7–1% of DKA episodes. A practical clinical consequence is that all persons older than 50 years of age or children younger than age 5 with DKA should be considered "high-risk" patients. Furthermore, during treatment of DKA, careful bedside assessment of the patient at regular intervals is mandatory, because deterioration in mental status is viewed as a medical emergency.

There are certain groups of people with diabetes, young women or urban and rural poor, who may be at higher risk for hyperglycemic emergencies. These groups require earlier and more intensive outpatient education and intervention to prevent morbidity and mortality. For example, young women were almost three times as likely to be admitted for DKA than men in surveys done 10 years ago, and in recent surveys, women outnumber men in terms of recurrent admissions (more than three per year). Risk factors that increase DKA in women include fear of gaining weight and eating disorders, fear of hypoglycemia, and the influence of menstrual cycles and emotional stress. A recent study by Rydall et al. (1997) reported the sad reality that up to 34% of young women (ages 12–18 years) omit insulin to maintain weight. These women generally have higher hemoglobin A_{1c} levels, more serious retinopathy, more emergency room visits, and recurrent DKA.

Minority urban populations, particularly African Americans, have a subset of individuals who appear to have type 2 diabetes, yet become critically ill with severe insulin deficiency and DKA, mimicking the typical presentation of type 1 diabetes. In their study of urban blacks, Umpierrez et al. (1997) showed that obesity (body mass index $>$ 28 kg/m^2) was present in 29% of those admitted with DKA, and in 56% of those with newly diagnosed diabetes and DKA. Most of the patients were older ($>$ 37 years), male, and had a family history of diabetes. In those with a known history of diabetes before admission, poor compliance with insulin therapy triggered DKA in about 50%. Omission of insulin was often due to inability to obtain medication or pay for the drug, poor appetite, or confusion about taking medication when ill, and use of drugs or alcohol. This study underlines three important clinical points: (a) DKA can occur in patients without chronic insulin dependence; (b) type 2 diabetes has a wide spectrum of clinical presentations; and (c) to avoid death and morbidity, there must be improved access to medical care and implementation of educational programs tailored to meet community needs.

In comparison with DKA, most surveys show fewer episodes of NKH, but NKH may be underreported because of difficulties recognizing this syndrome. In one survey of nearly 5000 adult urban blacks hospitalized for diabetes between 1993 and 1994, 156 patients met criteria for moderate or severe DKA and 23 had NKH. Another urban center diagnosed NKH in 17.5:100,000 person-years, whereas DKA occurred in 14:100,000 person-years. Because DKA and NKH likely represent a continuum of hyperglycemic diabetic emergencies, a subset of patients can present with a syndrome that is a mixture of the two. A review of admissions to a large city hospital found pure NKH in 32% of patients with uncontrolled diabetes and mixed hyperosmolarity and ketoacidosis in another 18%.

NKH is usually thought of as a disease of older patients with NIDDM, but it may occur in younger patients or those with IDDM. The reported mean age of patients with NKH is 57–69 years. Newly diagnosed diabetes is present in 33–60%. NKH can occur during hospitalization for other illnesses, and in one study 18% of cases were transferred from skilled nursing facilities. To increase recognition and reporting of this diabetic emergency, clinicians should think of this cause of "coma" when evaluating any elderly patient with mental status changes or obtundation. Characteristics that favor NKH are female gender, new-onset diabetes, and infection.

The mortality rate for NKH events is 10–60%, and reviews performed within the last 15 years, report a lower rate of 10–17%. Yet the syndrome may go unrecognized, so that mortality from NKH is likely underreported. Death may be attributed to a complication of the syndrome, thromboembolism or cardiovascular failure. The risk of death is higher when the patient has greater hyperosmolarity (> 340 mOsm/kg), and is more likely to occur within the first 72 h of treatment because of progressive shock or cardiovascular failure. It is important to recall that the severe hyperglycemia and the concomitant shift of water from the intracellular to the intravascular compartment prevent vascular collapse at this time of profound fluid depletion. Vascular collapse can subsequently occur if there is correction of the hyperglycemia without adequate expansion of the intravascular space with fluid. Later mortality is usually due to thromboembolic events. The risk of thromboembolism is increased in NKH because of dehydration, increased blood viscosity and coagulation abnormalities. Because of dehydration, rhabdomyolysis and acute tubular necrosis may also occur.

II. PATHOGENESIS OF DKA

One way to classify tissues in the body is by how they transport glucose. Accordingly, tissue may require insulin for glucose uptake and thus is insulin-sensitive, or it may not require insulin and is classed as insulin-insensitive. Figure 1 depicts the metabolism of glucose, amino acids, and fatty acids in the fed state, during fasting and during DKA in the major insulin-sensitive tissues: liver, muscle, and fat. This is compared with glucose metabolism in the nervous system (brain), which is an insulin-insensitive tissue in terms of glucose uptake. The brain's need for glucose, which is essential for mentation, remains relatively constant during feeding and in times of stress, fasting, and DKA. In contrast, insulin-sensitive tissues are deprived of glucose during times of insulin deficiency, such as fasting. Instead, they alter their intermediary metabolism from carbohydrate, which predominates in the fed state, to metabolizing fat. This alteration to fat mobilization and utilization as energy is a consequence of two hormonal shifts: one, the lack of effective levels of insulin allows lipolysis to occur; and two, the increased

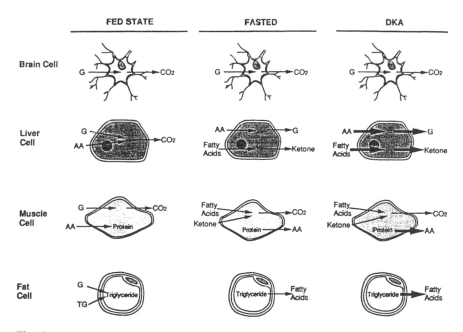

Fig. 1 Substrate metabolism during feeding, fasting, and ketoacidosis in insulin-insensitive tissue (brain) is compared with insulin-sensitive tissues (liver, muscle, and fat). G, glucose; AA, amino acids; TG, triglycerides. (From Kitabchi and Wall, 1995.)

levels of the counterregulatory hormones—glucagon, catecholamines, and corti-sol—contribute to hyperglycemia and ketonemia. The counterregulatory hor-mones do this by inhibiting insulin secretion; by activating lipolysis, glycogeno-lysis, and gluconeogenesis; and by inhibiting insulin-mediated glucose uptake by muscle (peripheral utilization).

Catecholamines promote lipolysis through the breakdown of triglycerides to free fatty acids and glycerol when the level of insulin is low (Fig. 2). The free fatty acids (FFA) along with the glycerol provide carbon fragments for gluconeo-genesis by the liver, thereby promoting hyperglycemia. Gluconeogenesis is also stimulated by the fall in insulin level and the increased glucagon level. With these hormonal changes, the rate-limiting enzyme of gluconeogenesis, phosphoenolpyr-uvate carboxykinase is stimulated, and hyperglycemia results from the accelerated production of glucose by the liver. A last critical element for sustaining hypergly-cemia is the inadequate utilization of glucose by peripheral tissue because of the increased levels of catecholamines and low insulin level.

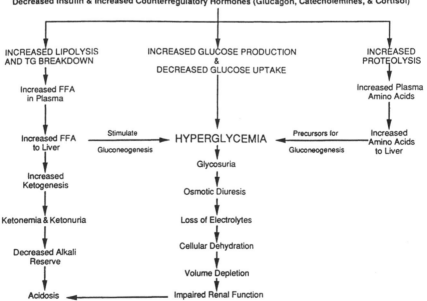

Fig. 2 Increased lipolysis and increased glucose production with decreased glucose uptake by insulin-sensitive tissues leads to an osmotic diuresis, loss of electrolytes, ke-tonemia, acidosis, and volume depletion in diabetic ketoacidosis. (From Kitabchi and Wall, 1995.)

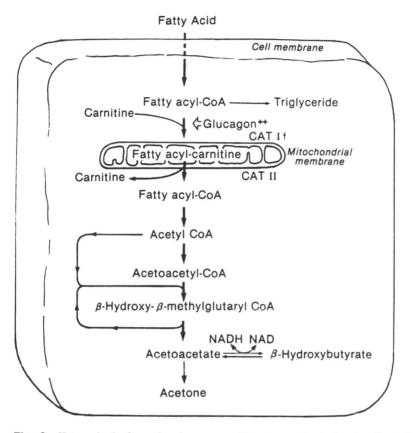

Fig. 3 Ketone body formation increases within liver cells during insulin deficiency. CAT I and CAT II are carnitine acyl transferases 1 and 2. (From Alberti 1995.)

The increased release of FFAs, in combination with an accelerated keto-genic capacity of the liver, lead to an increase in ketone body formation by β-oxidation (Fig. 3). Ketogenesis is enhanced by decreased availability of malonyl-coenzyme A (CoA), which occurs as a result of the increased glucagon levels. Malonyl-CoA inhibits carnitine palmitoyl acyl transferase (CAT1), the rate-limiting enzyme of ketogenesis. Thus, a reduction in malonyl-CoA, leads to stimulation of CAT1, effectively increasing ketogenesis. Insulin deficiency and higher levels of stress hormones then lead to a clinical picture in which catabolism with inherent depletion of cellular substrates and stores is the predominant feature.

The hormonal milieu of NKH is similar to that in DKA. There is a relative lack of insulin; insulin is present, but at levels inadequate to prevent hyperglycemia. The counterregulatory hormones are also increased in NKH, but their concentrations are not as high as that in DKA. The major difference between the syndromes is absence of significant ketogenesis in NKH, reflecting the lower concentrations of counterregulatory hormones and the higher intraportal insulin level, preventing FFA mobilization. NKH events are thus characterized by severe dehydration, higher levels of blood urea nitrogen (BUN) and glucose than in DKA, and absence of acidosis.

A. Fluid and Electrolyte Losses and Metabolic Acidosis

The major cause of dehydration in both DKA and NKH is osmotic diuresis, which is brought about by the excess excretion of glucose in the urine. As a result of this polyuria, sodium, chloride, and potassium, along with glucose and water, are lost in the urine. Fluid and electrolyte deficits per kilogram body weight in DKA are typically 100 mL water, 7–10 mEq Na^+, 3–5 mEq K^+, and 5–7 mEq Cl^- (Table 2); this is equivalent to a 10% loss of body weight from dehydration. As osmotic diuresis continues, progressive volume depletion leads to a decreased glomerular filtration rate, increasing hyperglycemia and ketonemia in DKA. The effect of osmotic diuresis is most pronounced in NKH and is the major cause of profound dehydration and increased osmolality. Thus, the most important first step in treating hyperglycemic emergencies is volume replacement.

Glucose in DKA is mostly extracellular, driving water from intracellular to the extracellular compartments. At first, the extracellular compartment is expanded and plasma sodium is diluted. To correct sodium for this dilution, the following formula is used: for every 100 mg/dL rise in plasma glucose, plasma sodium decreases by 1.6 mEq/L. Thus, for example, a plasma glucose of 700 mg/dL with a plasma sodium of 128 mEq/L implies a "true" sodium of 138 mEq/L. In addition, glucose in the intravascular compartment preserves intravascular volume and prevents cardiovascular collapse.

Table 2 Fluid and Electrolyte Deficits

	DKA	NKH
Water (mL/kg)	100	100–200
Na (mEq/kg)	7–10	5–13
K (mEq/kg)	3–5	5–15
Cl (mEq/kg)	3–5	3–7
PO_4 (mM/kg)	1–1.5	1–2

Source: Ennis and Kreisburg, 1996.

Potassium lost is usually 5 mEq/kg body weight (see Table 2), and can be as high as 10 mEq/kg. Hyperglycemia and the lack of insulin shift water and potassium from the intracellular to the extracellular compartment. Excess hydrogen ions, created by the accumulation of ketones, also act to displace potassium from its usual intracellular sites. Depletion of potassium is subsequently due to excessive losses in the urine. As the osmotic diuresis leads to an increased delivery of fluid and sodium to potassium secretory sites in the distal renal tubule, losses of sodium lead to secondary hyperaldosteronism, increasing potassium excretion. In addition, the negatively charged ketoanions in the tubular fluid enhance the loss of potassium.

Acidosis evolves owing to a buffer deficit caused by the enhanced production of ketoacids. The H^+ ions are at first buffered by extracellular (mostly HCO_3^-) and intracellular anions. Excess hydrogen ions are then eliminated by hyperventilation and by urinary excretion with loss of phosphate and ammonia. When the buffering capacity is outpaced by enhanced ketogenesis, metabolic acidosis occurs. Furthermore, the retention of ketoacids (β-hydroxybutyrate and acetoacetate) in the plasma results in an increase in the plasma anion gap.

The anion gap is calculated by subtracting the sum of chloride (Cl^-) and bicarbonate (HCO_3^-) anions from the sodium (Na^+) concentration: $Na - (Cl + HCO_3)$. The normal anion gap is 12 ± 2 mEq/L, and represents the normal quantity of unmeasurable anions. Because HCO_3^- is replaced by acetoacetate and β-hydroxybutyrate in DKA, and these ketone bodies are not measured as anions in electrolyte panels, the sum of HCO_3^- and Cl^- is reduced, increasing the anion gap.

B. Measurement of Urinary Ketones

Ketone bodies, acetoacetate, acetone, and β-hydroxybutyrate, are formed during periods of insulin deficiency by hepatic fatty acid oxidation. The ketone bodies then accumulate in the blood and some portion is also excreted in the urine with the cation sodium. The measurement of urinary or blood ketones is usually performed by the nitroprusside method, which detects acetoacetate and acetone, but not β-hydroxybutyrate. In severe acidosis or anoxia, the β-hydroxybutyrate/acetoacetate ratio is greatly elevated, so ketone measurement using test strips or tablets might yield a false-negative result. As DKA improves with therapy, there is a conversion of β-hydroxybutyrate to acetoacetate, leading to a seemingly "paradoxical" increase in measurable ketones during DKA treatment. Because a proportion of the ketone bodies is undetected by present techniques, changes in acid–base parameters are more reliably obtained from measurements of venous pH and plasma bicarbonate levels. Ketones should be measured only initially to confirm the diagnosis of DKA and at the end for control of DKA.

Table 3 Effects of DKA

Hyperglycemia	Dehydration	Ketogenesis
Primarily from gluconeogenesis in the liver, but also due to increased glycogen breakdown in the liver as well as a lack of glucose utilization by muscle and fat.	From polyuria (osmotic diuresis) with progressive loss of fluid and electrolytes. This can be exacerbated by obtundation or impaired access to fluids.	From increased lipolysis that increases free fatty acids, providing substrate, and counterregulatory hormones increasing ketogenic capacity of the liver.

The effects of alterations in the metabolism of fat, protein, and carbohydrate in DKA are summarized in Table 3.

C. Hypertonicity in Uncontrolled Diabetes

Effective osmolarity (effective Osm = 2 (Na + K) + glucose/18), rather than the total osmolarity (total Osm = 2 (Na + K) + glucose/18 + BUN/2.8) is important in the evolution of NKH and obtundation. The significant osmotically active substances in the body include those that freely pass the cell membranes, such as urea and alcohols, and those that are impermeable, including glucose (in the absence of insulin), Na, K, and mannitol. Substances that are permeable such as urea, are no longer thought to cause major changes in intracellular volume because of their lack of osmotic gradient across cell membranes. Elevated osmolarity can occur from renal failure (elevated urea) without a change in mental state. Mental status changes occur owing to a rise in tonicity, and thus only impermeable substances, Na, K, and glucose, should be considered in this calculation.

Hypertonicity occurs with uncontrolled diabetes because of the additive effects of the impermeable solute glucose and the hypotonic osmotic diuresis from glucosuria. Modest elevations in glucose alone cannot cause the significant hypertonicity of NKH, because the osmotic contribution of glucose is only 5 mOsm/L for every 90 mg/dL elevation in glucose levels. Sodium in comparison adds 2 mOsm/L for every 1 mEq/L increase. As blood levels of glucose increase during DKA or NKH, water is lost from the intracellular compartment and moves extracellularly. Thus hyperglycemia helps preserve intravascular volume and maintains perfusion of essential organs. Eventually the diuresis decreases all body water compartments. Thus an important clinical consequence follows that treatment of DKA or NKH with insulin before adequate fluid resuscitation, will result in vascular collapse. This is particularly true for patients with NKH.

Elevations in blood glucose, usually above 180 mg/dL, surpass the capacity for renal tubular reabsorption of glucose. Continued loss of sodium and water results in volume contraction, causing a decrease in glomerular filtration of glucose, leading to greater hyperglycemia and hypertonicity. Furthermore, glomerular filtration rate decreases with age, and aging increases the renal threshold for glucose. Thus, an important clinical observation is that elderly persons with diabetes may reach higher blood glucose levels before osmotic diuresis starts. This also means that the older diabetic may not have glucosuria when blood glucose levels are elevated, so that screening elderly patients for diabetes by checking their urine for glucose is not very sensitive, nor is the absence of glucosuria an indication of optimal diabetes control.

III. DIAGNOSIS AND INITIAL EVALUATION

Both DKA and NKH develop as progressive polyuria and polydipsia, with a prodromal period of usually 3–7 days of dehydration before hospital presentation. There may be a more rapid onset, literally overnight, if patients have been ingesting a modest amount of alcohol. Presenting features of DKA (Table 4) are polyuria, polydipsia, nausea and vomiting, mental status changes, hyperventilation, and abdominal pain. The ketonemia is likely responsible for the abdominal pain and nausea, but hypokalemia can also worsen gastroparesis and cause an ileus. Clinical findings include dehydration and hypotension, Kussmaul respiration (deep, sighing hyperventilation), tachycardia, warm skin, and confusion or coma. Hyperventilation is more obvious when the pH is less than 7.2, and is present as respiratory compensation for the metabolic acidosis. There may be symptoms and signs of sepsis and shock.

Table 4 Signs and Symptoms of DKA

Polyuria, polydipsia, and polyphagia
Weight loss
Abdominal pain, nausea, and vomiting
Drowsiness or profound lethargy, coma is rare
Rapid, deep respirations (Kussmaul)
Fruity breath, poor skin turgor, dry mucous membranes
Tachycardia and orthostatic hypotension
Blood glucose level is usually 400–500 mg/dL

DKA can be diagnosed at the bedside if the patient has a high blood glucose level (determined by fingerstick) and urine positive for ketones. Commonly associated findings that are not required for diagnosis are fruity breath, increased serum amylase, or increased anion gap (usually ≥ 15). The diagnosis is verified with arterial blood gas assessment to confirm the presence of metabolic acidosis. The definitive diagnosis of DKA consists of (a) hyperglycemia (> 250 mg/dL), (b) low serum bicarbonate (< 15 mEq/L), and (c) a low pH (< 7.3) with ketonemia (positive at 1:2 dilution) and moderate ketonuria. Virtually all patients who are admitted to hospital for DKA treatment have an increased anion gap; those who have been able to prevent dehydration by taking insulin and drinking fluids may present with a normal anion gap and hyperchloremic acidosis (see further discussion of hyperchloremic acidosis in Sec. VIII.E). Most patients will have a high white cell count, usually with a left shift, but less than 25,000/mm³ unless there is a coexistent bacterial infection. The presence of pneumonia may be difficult to confirm until the patient is better hydrated. Initial evaluation (Fig. 4) consists of blood chemistries, glucose by fingerstick, blood and urine ketones

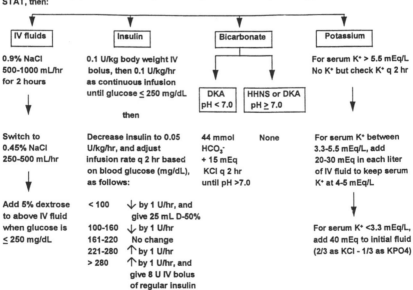

Lab follow-up: Measure glucose by finger stick q 2 hr and serum glucose, electrolytes, Mg⁺⁺, PO4⁻, and venous pH q 4 hr until resolution of ketoacidosis

Fig. 4 Algorithm of history, physical and treatment with intravenous fluid, insulin and electrolyte replacement in diabetic ketoacidosis. (From Umpierrez, et al., 1996.)

by nitroprusside reaction, complete blood cell counts with differential, arterial blood gas levels, and urinalysis. Patients with hyperglycemia often have low sodium and high potassium levels. However, the diagnosis of DKA is not dependent on finding a serum glucose value of 400 mg/dL or higher, which is a common misperception of many clinicians. A lower blood glucose level is likely to occur in pregnant women or in those who have been unable to eat, had vomiting, or took insulin in the prodromal phase. A careful physical examination is performed looking for any evidence of infection. This is followed by infusion of 1 L of 0.9% NaCl, while the bacterial cultures (when appropriate) and electrocardiogram (ECG) are obtained to evaluate possible precipitating factors. Transferring the patient before stabilization for noninvasive or invasive procedures should be avoided if possible. Treatment goals for DKA (Table 5) are, in order: (a) improve circulatory volume and tissue perfusion; (b) correct electrolyte abnormalities; (c) decrease serum glucose; and (d) clear the serum and urine of ketoacids at a steady rate.

It is usually not difficult to differentiate among the different causes of diabetic coma. Whereas acidosis causes a negative inotropic effect and peripheral vasodilation, such that patients in DKA have warm skin, those in NKH have normal skin temperature, higher blood glucose levels, and more profound dehydration, with no or trace ketones found in the blood. Alternatively hypoglycemic coma can be distinguished by the lower blood glucose level (usually less than 50 mg/dL) and the presence of cold and clammy extremities. If there is any doubt about the cause of coma, low or high glucose levels, 20 mL of 50% glucose can be given intravenously. Other causes of acidosis with an increased anion gap include lactic acidosis, uremia, and ingestion of salicylates or methanol. Plasma ketones may be mildly positive in severe lactic acidosis, but in these other causes of acidosis including lactic acidosis, the blood glucose is not as elevated as those values found in DKA.

Signs of NKH are those of profound dehydration. Patients have dry mucous membranes, absent sweating, and poor skin turgor, as well as postural hypotension. Cardiac and respiratory examinations are typically normal in the absence

Table 5 Treatment Stages of DKA and NKH

Goals of therapy are reached in three stages.

1. Volume restoration (hours 0–12)
2. Treatment of the underlying cause (hours 12–48)
   Restoration of tonicity to normal
   Correction of acid–base imbalance
3. Replenishment of water, electrolytes (Mg, Phos)

of pneumonia. Tachypnea, hypotension, or fever may indicate a gram-negative infection. Gastroparesis is often present, owing to the hypertonic state; thus nausea and vomiting may mistakenly suggest an underlying gastrointestinal pathology precipitating the event.

Neurological symptoms are common in NKH and can consist of focal findings that mimic cerebrovascular accident to frank coma. The cause of coma is unknown, but it is postulated that dehydration, changes in neurotransmitter levels, and microvascular ischemia are all operative. Lethargy and confusion are more common than frank coma, which usually does not occur unless the plasma osmolarity is 340 mOsm/L or higher. Most of the patients with coma have a relative or absolute increase in serum sodium levels, rather than hyperglycemia to explain the increased osmolarity.

If focal or diffuse mental status changes persist after hydration, CNS lesions or infection should be suspected. Seizures occur in 25% and can be focal. NKH-related seizures may be resistant to anticonvulsant therapy. Phenytoin should be used with caution, as it may exacerbate hyperglycemia by inhibiting insulin release. Cerebral edema is rare and is almost always due to rapid overcorrection of blood glucose concentration or when large amounts of insulin are given with large amounts of hypotonic fluids.

NKH is characterized by extreme fluid and electrolyte depletion (see Table 2) with total body water losses of 22–25%, which considerably exceeds that of fluid losses in DKA. The more profound water loss in NKH is likely due to a longer prodromal period and greater limited access to water. Osmotic diuresis leads to hypotonic fluid loss with electrolyte losses equivalent to roughly one-half of the water loss. Because hyperglycemia usually dilutes plasma Na, actual levels of Na are higher at presentation than the measurable cation (1.6 mEq/L increase in Na^+ for each 100 mg/dL increase in glucose: corrected Na = measured Na + 1.6 × plasma glucose (mg/dL) − 100/100). A clinical consequence of this is that a patient with severe hyperglycemia from NKH with a normal or elevated serum sodium level at diagnosis has had massive water loss.

A further loss of K may be present in NKH if there was a prior history of diuretic use, and total body potassium may be profoundly low. A mild metabolic acidosis may be present (pH > 7.3), but is no means typical owing to the accumulation of lactate from tissue hypoperfusion or uremic acids from renal hypoperfusion. A mixed ketoacidosis and NKH (pH < 7.3, strongly positive serum acetone, and effective osmolarity > 320 mOsm/L) may occur in as many as 33% of patients with uncontrolled diabetes.

Other serum markers may be abnormal during NKH, including liver transaminases, LDH, and CPK-MM; these changes are transient and are due to dehydration. Hypercholesterolemia and hypertriglyceridemia are usually present. There may be false elevations of the albumin, amylase, bilirubin calcium, total protein, SGOT, SGPT, and BUN. Leukocytosis with elevated granulocytes is common and may not imply infection, but rather, is a response to stress and dehydration with white blood counts usually 12–15,000. Hemoglobin and hematocrit are also elevated owing to dehydration.

IV. TREATMENT

A. Hydration

Numerous studies have demonstrated the safety and efficacy of giving hydration therapy in the treatment of DKA and NKH before initiation of insulin therapy. The use of fluid leads to a significant reduction in BUN, blood glucose, and potassium levels, but is less effective at reversing the metabolic acidosis from insulin deficiency, as opposed to the beneficial effect on lactic acidosis from dehydration and decreased tissue perfusion. Fluids are rapidly administered to restore normal circulatory volume, and to decrease the concentrations of the counterregulatory hormones, which improves insulin sensitivity. Rehydration lowers glucose by augmenting glucose excretion in the urine and diluting the extracellular compartment. In contrast, failure to give adequate fluid can exacerbate hypovolemia and shock if insulin is used to lower glucose, which is paradoxically maintaining the intravascular volume.

Initial fluid therapy should be isotonic saline because this fluid more rapidly corrects plasma volume than hypotonic fluid. For most patients with DKA, 10% dehydration is common, and 1 L of 0.9% saline is given in the first hour. This rate is continued for an additional hour if hypotension is not corrected or urine flow is less than 50–100 mL/h. If the patient is in shock, colloids should also be used, as these are retained in the intravascular space. Dehydration is judged by the physical examination (postural blood pressure changes, tachycardia, poor skin turgor, lack of sweating, and dry mucous membranes), the corrected sodium concentration, and the calculated effective plasma osmolarity. Corrected sodium concentrations higher than 140 mEq/L or calculated osmolalities of more than 340 mOsm/kg H_2O are associated with the largest fluid deficits, and they also correlate inversely with mental status; stupor or coma is seen with osmolalities higher than 340. In NKH, 0.9% saline is also used at 1 L/h until blood pressure and pulse, along with urine output, improve. Patients with coexisting cardiac or renal disease or those resuscitated with large fluid volumes require central vein pressure measurements to avoid under- or overhydration.

After hypotension is corrected by the use of isotonic saline and vital signs are stable, subsequent fluid therapy is given as hypotonic saline (0.45% NaCl) at 250–500 mL/h. Water losses exceed that of NaCl during DKA and NKH, and the administration of 0.45% saline leads to a gradual replacement of fluid, adjusting the rate of ongoing renal losses, plasma sodium levels, and clinical response.

The greatest danger to the patient with NKH is hypovolemia and progressive shock or thromboembolism; volume restoration is essential for patient survival. Initial fluid replacement is 1–2 L in first 2 h of treatment, then 7–9 L over the next 2–3 days, because the fluid deficit is usually 20–25% of body stores. Most use isotonic fluid replacement, as rapid correction of hypernatremia can lead to diffuse myelinolysis and death. Normal saline is used initially until the effective arterial blood volume is restored to maintain perfusion and glomerular filtration rate. Intravenous fluid is then changed to 0.45% normal saline; one-half of the free water deficit is replaced in the first 12 h of therapy, and the remainder is replaced in the next 24 h. Colloids are not recommended, as they can contribute to elevated plasma viscosity. Anuria or oliguria not responsive to fluid resuscitation may predispose the patient to congestive heart failure or adult respiratory distress syndrome (ARDS). Many of these patients have prior histories of renal insufficiency. Cardiovascular monitoring and dialysis may be necessary during this initial stage of treatment.

B. Insulin Replacement

The only form of insulin used traditionally during hyperglycemic diabetic emergencies is regular crystalline human insulin, although Humalog may also be appropriate if treatment is initiated using the subcutaneous route. For moderate to severe DKA (bicarbonate value less than 10), insulin is given intravenously as a continuous drip of 0.1–0.15 U/kg/h^{-1}, usually 10 U/h. This is the preferred regimen, although intermittent iv or im insulin can be used in emergent situations for which continuous intravenous insulin is not practical. When intravenous insulin cannot be given, sq injections 0.3–0.4 U/kg of regular or Humalog insulin can be given initially, followed by 5–10 U each hour. Studies differ on the use of a loading dose before a continuous iv infusion is used. It is our practice to give 10–20 U intravenously before starting the continuous infusion.

In comparative studies, low-dose insulin therapy (0.1 U/kg/h) given without a loading dose led to the same improvements in glycemia and ketonemia as high-dose insulin therapy (50 U/h) without the same risk of hypoglycemia and hypokalemia. It is expected that blood glucose should fall by 80–200 mg/dL/h during DKA treatment with low-dose iv insulin. If a decrease in glucose levels is not seen within 2–3 h, it should be assumed that the patient has an insulin-resistant state, likely because of infection. The insulin infusion rate should be doubled every hour until the blood glucose level starts to fall, and it is important to monitor blood glucose and electrolyte values.

During DKA, the urinary loss of ketoanion represents the loss of potential bicarbonate. When insulin is given and DKA is reversed, ketoanion metabolism is facilitated and hydrogen ions are consumed as bicarbonate is regenerated. Nonetheless, acidosis often does not fully correct, and there is frequently a posthyperchloremic, rather then anion gap, acidosis in this phase (see "hyperchloremic acidosis").

C. Potassium Therapy

During hydration and treatment of DKA with insulin, there is a rapid decline in potassium, particularly in the first 3 h. The most life-threatening electrolyte derangement in DKA is hypokalemia during the treatment. Most of the decline in serum potassium is due to the insulin-mediated reentry of potassium into the intracellular compartment. Nonetheless, potassium is not usually added to the initial first liter of 0.9% saline, because the addition of potassium to an already hyperkalemic patient may dangerously increase extracellular potassium and precipitate cardiac arrhythmias, especially if fluid is being rapidly administered. With subsequent fluid therapy, the serum potassium is checked every 1–2 h, and if it is less than 5.5 mEq/L and the patient is urinating, 20–30 mEq K$^+$ is given per liter. The goal is to maintain the K$^+$ between 4 and 5 mEq/L. Patients who present in DKA with low or normal K$^+$ levels have the greatest total body potassium deficit. Insulin therapy without aggressive potassium replacement can lead to profound hypokalemia, which can induce life-threatening arrhythmias, respiratory muscle weakness, and impaired cardiovascular function. These patients should receive potassium in the first liter of fluid, with the rate of intravenous K$^+$ administration never exceeding 40 mEq/h. When the patient is not nauseated and able to drink, potassium supplements can be given orally.

D. Bicarbonate Therapy

We do not recommend the use of bicarbonate except in life-threatening states of acidosis. Many retrospective studies show no significant difference in mental status or in the correction of hyperglycemia or in eventual outcome in the presence or absence of bicarbonate therapy. The use of alkali in treating DKA may be counterproductive. The use of bicarbonate therapy is based on the assumption that acidosis contributes to the morbidity of DKA. Intracellular acidosis could lead to abnormal organ and cellular function. Nonetheless, there are no clinical studies documenting the benefits of the use of bicarbonate. A recent review looked at seven patients with DKA with serum pH of 6.9–7.14. Three received bicarbonate and four did not. The group that received alkali had a 6-h delay in improvement of ketosis, compared with those who did not receive bicarbonate. Both acetoacetate and β-hydroxybutyrate increased in those given bicarbonate, showing that the presence of alkali increased ketone production. The use of bicarbonate during DKA is now eschewed, as it could lead to worsening hypokalemia, prolongation of ketoanion metabolism, and production of paradoxical central nervous system acidosis.

Bicarbonate therapy has not been withheld in studies of patients with severe acidosis: pH lower than 6.9. Until more studies are conducted, most authors suggest using bicarbonate in the treatment of DKA if the pH is lower than 7.0. If the pH is 6.9–7.0, 44 mEq of sodium bicarbonate is recommended, whereas for pH lower than 6.9, 88 mEq sodium bicarbonate is used. It is also recommended that 15 mEq KCl be given with each ampule (44 mEq) of bicarbonate to avoid hypokalemia.

E. Phosphorus Therapy

Phosphate is an intracellular ion that shifts to the extracellular compartment during DKA, so that serum levels are usually normal or increased. Phosphate, similar to glucose and potassium, reenters the intracellular compartment during insulin therapy, resulting in a fall in serum phosphate level. Arguments for the replacement of phosphorus during DKA are based on assumptions that hypophosphatemia can lead to respiratory depression, skeletal muscle weakness, hemolytic anemia, and cardiac dysfunction. Phosphate replacement would replete 2,3-diphosphoglycerate (2,3-DPG), which is decreased during DKA, thus shifting the O_2 dissociation curve to the right, enhancing tissue oxygen delivery. Nonetheless, because loss of phosphorus during DKA is minimal compared with body stores, and excessive phosphate replacement can produce hypocalcemia, tetany, and soft tissue calcification, many view phosphorus repletion as an unnecessary risk. Whereas selected clinical studies have shown that phosphate replacement during DKA is associated with an improved mental status or decreased mortality, the majority of randomized and controlled studies have been unable to demonstrate clinical benefits for the routine use of phosphate. The current recommendation is that any patient with a serum phosphate less than 1 mg/dL should receive phosphate, usually replaced as the anion (K-phos) in one-third the potassium deficit.

V. MANAGEMENT

Monitoring during treatment of DKA and NKH involves taking postural blood pressure, pulse, tracking urine flow, jugular vein distention, and auscultation of heart and lungs for signs of fluid overload. Nasogastric intubation may be needed for those with nausea and vomiting or obtundation. It is recommended that the clinical and laboratory data be properly recorded in a flowsheet and if possible logged into the medical chart for easy access (Fig. 5). Blood glucose determinations should be performed hourly, especially to detect those rare patients with insulin resistance, who do not respond to 0.1 U/kg/h. Once the acute situation has passed, fingerstick glucose values are continued at least every 4 h. Similar

HR	EKG	Wt	T	P	R	BP	UO	Ace	Glu	Ace	Glu	pH	CO2	Na	K	Cl	Osm	Ins	H2O	Na	K	PO4	HCO3	Glu

Abbreviations: HR, hour; EKG, electrocardiogram; Wt, weight; T, temperature; P, pulse; R, respirations; BP, blood pressure; UO, urinary output (mls.); Ace, acetone; Glu, glucose; pH, hydrogen ion concentration; CO2, carbon dioxide; Na, sodium; K, potassium; Cl, chloride; Osm, serum osmolarity; Ins, insulin (units); H2O, fluid resuscitation (L); PO4, phosphorus, HCO3, bicarbonate.

Fig. 5 Flowsheet for DKA. (From Davidson, 1986.)

guidelines are followed for electrolytes, particularly potassium. Electrolytes are checked every 2 h until the emergent situation is passed, then every 4–6 h until full recovery. Following the initial arterial blood gas measurement, venous blood can be used to follow the pH because it is easier to obtain, and less painful for the patient. Venous pH is about 0.03 lower than the arterial pH.

Intravenous fluid is hypotonic after the initial first liter of 0.9% normal saline. The average amount of fluid given during the first 6–8 h is about 5 L. Overzealous hydration can lead to edema, congestive heart disease, or ARDS. Antibiotics are often used, because most cases of NKH and DKA are due to infections, although it is our opinion that their use should not be considered routine. Low-grade fever is often seen in NKH, and leukocytosis is common in both DKA and NKH. Thus, it is appropriate to wait for clear evidence of infection before beginning antibiotic coverage. It is also prudent to withhold anticoagulation for the first 1–2 days to allow gastroparesis to remit (which when present increases the risk of gastrointestinal bleeding with heparin). Prophylactic heparin, given subcutaneously (5000 U every 12 h) should be used if prolonged bed rest is likely.

The range of time for patients to reverse DKA depends to a large extent on the initial degree of metabolic derangement. Recovery of DKA is defined as blood glucose value less than 200 mg/dL, bicarbonate more than 15 mEq/L, pH higher than 7.3, and ketonemia-negative at 1:2 dilution. For a patient with an initial glucose of 800 mg/dL and bicarbonate less than 10 mEq/L and pH under 7.1, it is estimated that it takes about 7.5 h for the blood glucose to reach 250 mg/dL, as a physiological dose of insulin lowers the blood glucose at a rate of 80 mg/dL/h. For bicarbonate and pH to reach these recovery levels, it is estimated that it takes twice the time, about 15 h. Because it does take longer to correct the acidosis, which is achieved with insulin treatment, it is necessary to supply glucose as a 5% dextrose solution (substituting D5NS or D5-1/2NS for the intravenous solution) after the glucose value reaches 250 mg/dL to prevent hypoglycemia.

Studies have shown that obtunded or comatose patients usually have a plasma osmolality of 340 mOsm/kg H_2O or higher. Thus, patients with an osmolality less than 340 mOsm/kg who are obtunded should be investigated by computed tomography (CT) scanning for CNS lesions, or for drug intoxication, or for other coexisting illnesses to account for the change in mental status, such as sepsis or hypercalcemia. A patient with obtundation caused by DKA needs the same amount of time to clear the sensorium as that needed for normalization of plasma bicarbonate. In obtunded patients, the blood glucose level should be maintained at 300 mg/dL with dextrose until the patient is alert.

Patients who do not respond to low-dose insulin therapy (0.1 U/kg/h) and blood glucoses remain elevated should be investigated for unrecognized sites of infection. These include skin and rectal abscesses, pleural or chest lesions, cervicitis, prostatitis, or decubitus ulcers. Other diseases that increase insulin resistance should be eliminated, including thyrotoxicosis, acromegaly, and Cushing's syndrome.

The half-life of insulin given intravenously is only 5–10 min, so that any interruption of insulin delivered by this method can lead to a lower level of insulin and recurrence of DKA. Often this occurs when the patient is changed from the intravenous insulin drip to the subcutaneous coverage with insulin, either because of delays in writing the orders during transfer from the intensive care setting to the general ward, or because of delays in obtaining the doses. When the patient is able to take food by mouth, all intravenous fluid is stopped. The patient is given a meal plan of an ADA diet of three meals and a bedtime snack. Regular or Humalog insulin, based on fingersticks or carbohydrate exchanges, is given before each meal, and NPH or Ultralente at bedtime. Alternatively, Ultralente or NPH is given before breakfast and supper with regular or Humalog before meals (Table 6). To prevent recurrence of hyperglycemia and ketoacidosis, it is imperative to plan in advance the switch over from intravenous to subcutaneous insulin. This is best done before a meal—breakfast or supper. The fingerstick is obtained about 20 min before the meal, intermediate or long-acting (NPH, Lente, or Ultralente) and short-acting insulins (regular or Humalog) are given subcutaneously, and 15–30 min later, the intravenous insulin is stopped to avoid insulin interruption. If the patient is given only intermediate-acting insulin, the intravenous insulin is stopped 2 h later.

VI. SPECIAL CASES

A. Pregnancy

The incidence of DKA in pregnant women with IDDM is 1.7%, whereas, in those with gestational diabetes, the occurrence is rare at 0.7%. In the last half of pregnancy, changes in carbohydrate and fat metabolism occur, increasing the risk of DKA. This change is due to the rise in placental hormones, estrogen and placenta-produced insulinase, which all combine to cause marked insulin resistance. DKA can mimic hyperemesis gravidarum and because blood sugars levels may not be grossly elevated, DKA is unrecognized in 30% of pregnant women with metabolic decompensation. The precipitants of DKA in pregnancy are, in order of frequency, emesis owing to gastroenteropathy or infection (42%), noncompliance (25%), and physician mismanagement (17%).

The presentation and diagnostic features of diabetic ketoacidosis are similar in women who are pregnant or nonpregnant. The signs and symptoms are abdominal pain, nausea and vomiting, polyuria and polydipsia, acetone breath, Kussmaul respirations, and finally, hypotension and changes in mental status. The glucose

Table 6 Subcutaneous Insulin Regimens after DKA

Calculate 0.6 U × wt (kg) for 24-h dose of insulin. Use 0.5 U if patient is young or thin and 0.7 U if patient is obese. Use 1 U/kg if patient is receiving steroids.
  Give 4/9 dose as NPH before breakfast, and 1/6 of dose as NPH before bedtime.
  Give 2/9 of dose as regular before breakfast and 1/6 of dose as regular before supper.
Example: 26-year-old male weighing 70 kg would require a total insulin dose of 42 U. He would receive 19 NPH and 9 regular before breakfast, 7 regular before supper and 7 NPH at bedtime.
Before meals, the dose of regular can be adjusted as follows.

Glucose ≤ 70 mg/dL	Subtract 3% of total requirement from usual dose
Glucose 71–140 mg/dL	No change in dose
Glucose > 140 mg/dL	Add 6% of total requirement to usual dose

Example: if this man has a glucose level of 68 before breakfast, he would receive 8 U of regular. If his glucose before breakfast is 220, he would receive 12 U regular. If his glucose before supper is 68, he would receive 6 U regular. Finally, if his glucose before supper is 200, he receives 10 U regular.

Advantages of program	Disadvantages of program
No insulin taken at lunchtime, physicians are familiar with the use of NPH and regular insulins.	Predisposes to late morning and early afternoon hypoglycemia, patient may need to take snacks at 10–11 AM and again at 3–4 PM.

More intensive insulin programs may be started under the guidance of a diabetes care team or endocrinologist.
Ultralente insulin can be started (50% of total dose) before breakfast and supper with Humalog (50% of dose or about 0.15 U/kg) before every meal. Alternatively, regular insulin (80% of total dose) can be used before meals with NPH (20% of total dose) at bedtime.

Advantages of program	Disadvantages of program
More closely mimics normal insulin secretion, flexibility for mealtimes, allows tight control	Must take insulin before every meal, and if this is regular, it is taken 20–30 min before meals. Tight control increases risk for hypoglycemia.

value is usually more than 300 mg/dL, bicarbonate is less than 15, and pH is less than 7.3, although there are a significant number of pregnant women who present in diabetic ketoacidosis with plasma glucose values less than 200. In a recent paper, 36% of pregnant women in DKA had glucose levels of less than 200, and in 90% the presenting signs were nausea, vomiting, and decreased caloric intake.

During DKA, there is a decrease in uterine blood flow in the pregnant woman. Thus, fetal hypoxemia may result and be compounded by maternal phosphorus deficiency that occurs in DKA. Loss of potassium by the fetus can cause fetal cardiac arrest. In one study of 11 women with DKA during pregnancy, there was one fetal death and 2 women underwent emergent cesarian sections because of fetal distress. Thirty years ago, a survey reported a fetal loss rate of 30% during maternal DKA, and the rate rose to 64% if the pregnant woman was comatose during the metabolic derangement. A more recent survey done in 1993 found that 35% of women presenting with DKA during pregnancy had fetal death on admission. Fetal loss was more likely if the serum glucose was lower and gesta- tional age less than 7 months. Another 1993 survey estimated that 22% of pregnant women with DKA sustained loss of the fetus, and that this loss was more likely if it occurred during the first trimester. These statistics mean DKA in pregnancy should be treated aggressively with the concerted effort of a designated team of Ob/Gyn and medical (diabetologists) physicians and nurses.

Treatment of DKA in pregnancy is no different from that in nonpregnant patients, but it is very important to recognize the occurrence of normoglycemic DKA. Fluid is given to replace the deficit, which is usually 4–10 L. During the first hour, 1–2 L of NS are given, then the replacement rate is decreased to 300–500 mL/h. Insulin is started as a low dose intravenous drip at 5–10 U/h. This rate is doubled if the blood glucose does not show a 30% fall within the first 2–3 h. Glucose is added to the intravenous solution when the blood glucose value is 200–250 mg/dL. Finally, potassium is started 2–4 h after fluid resuscita- tion at 10–40 mEq/h to ensure there is adequate urine production, thereby, avoid- ing hyperkalemia.

B. Pediatric DKA

Admissions of patients for DKA in the pediatric age group often result from a new diagnosis of diabetes. Other reasons include acute stress, poor sick-day management, and teenage rebellion, during which failure to take insulin may indicate, especially in young women, an eating disorder and fear of weight gain. Symptoms and diagnostic criteria are similar to adults, and treatment has the same goals: restoration of volume; stopping ketogenesis by giving insulin; correction of electrolyte losses; and avoidance of complications, particularly hypoglycemia, hypokalemia, and cerebral edema. The details of diagnosis and treatment of keto- acidosis in children are discussed in a separate chapter in this volume.

VII. ISSUES TO BE DISCUSSED BEFORE DISCHARGE

Morbidity and mortality from DKA and NKH continue to be troublesome issues, and avoidance of hyperglycemic emergencies is key to reducing costs of diabetes care and loss of employment. Episodes of DKA and NKH may be decreased by

Table 7 Early Symptoms and Signs of Diabetes

Polyuria and nocturia
Recurrent urinary or genital tract infections
Recurrent skin infections or poor wound healing
Candidiasis or thrush
Pruritus
Weight loss
Plantar ulcers

enacting screening programs to identify those with undiagnosed diabetes or glucose intolerance who are at risk for decompensation (Table 7). Discharge planning
for patients admitted for DKA or NKH should focus on preventing future episodes. Recognizing the symptoms and signs of uncontrolled diabetes (Table 8)
will allow caregivers and patients to take corrective action, thereby avoiding
hyperglycemic emergencies and metabolic derangements. Patients must be educated on ''sick day'' management, particularly how to adjust medications, increase fluid intake, and when to alert their caregivers if hyperglycemia persists
despite attempts to keep it under control. Nurses and other caregivers of the
elderly, especially those employed in nursing homes, need to be educated about
the signs and symptoms of hyperglycemia, dehydration, and infection. New onset
of nocturia or bed-wetting, or urogenital rash (candidiasis), or poorly healing skin
ulcers, is an often overlooked, but important, clinical correlations for hyperglycemia. In addition, elderly patients who are lethargic or unresponsive should be
evaluated for hyperglycemia and NKH.

Patients who have been hospitalized for DKA or NKH need to receive
before discharge a complete educational program from their diabetes team regard-
ing diet, exercise, insulin dosage, glucose monitoring, emergency care, sick day
rules, treatment of hypoglycemia, and follow-up outpatient care. Individualized
educational sessions and group sessions outlining and emphasizing ''survival

Table 8 Risk Factors for Diabetes

Strong family history for type 2 diabetes
History of gestational diabetes or babies weighing over 4 kg
Body mass index > 30
Autoimmune diseases
Sedentary lifestyle
Hypertension, hyperlipidemia, and gout

skills'' are essential if the incidence of DKA and NKH is to be reduced and repeated episodes avoided. Also, these issues should be discussed again during outpatient visits to ensure educational goals are retained and implemented.

VIII. COMPLICATIONS OF THERAPY

A. Hypoperfusion with Thromboembolic Disorders

Severe dehydration results in decreased perfusion of organs and promotes coagulation, which can lead to myocardial, bowel, or brain infarctions. This is the reason for the rapid administration of crystalloid or colloid solutions to replace extracellular volume following the diagnosis of NKH or DKA. The risk of hypotension and ischemia increases with treatment delay; thus, to reduce stroke and heart attack, patients and caregivers (family, visiting nurses, primary care doctors, and nurses) should be educated how to recognize the prodromal symptoms of diabetes, hyperglycemia, and dehydration. By earlier recognition of premorbid states, DKA and NKH can be prevented and morbidity and mortality caused by ischemia often is avoided.

B. Cerebral Edema

Patients with DKA typically are hyperosmolar, presenting with plasma osmolalities usually higher than 295 mOsm/kg H_2O. During the treatment of DKA, the resolution of hyperglycemia leads to a progressive decrease in plasma osmolality that favors a shift of water from the extracellular to the intracellular space. The use of insulin further promotes entry of osmotically active particles (i.e., glucose and K^+) into the cell. Brain cells maintain cellular volume by producing new intracellular peptides, called idiogenic osmoles, which prevent cellular shrinkage. Idiogenic osmoles cannot be rapidly disposed of, so if the extracellular space is rapidly expanded, leading to a fall in extracellular osmolality, there is an accentuated shift of water into brain cells, with subsequent swelling of the cells.

Retrospective studies have shown patients at risk for cerebral edema are those who receive fluid resuscitation at a rate greater than 4 L/m^2 per day. Additionally, those patients who usually present with low sodium values and during treatment have a decrease in serum sodium concentration or fail to show a rise in serum sodium level as blood glucose falls are at increased risk. Symptomatic or fatal cerebral edema is rare but can occur in pediatric patients with DKA, particularly those younger than 5 years of age or those with a new diagnosis of diabetes. It is rarer in adults, although it is surprisingly common to see CT evidence of subclinical cerebral edema during the first 24 h of DKA treatment.

Importantly, subclinical edema spontaneously resolves and is unassociated with any clinical findings.

Signs of cerebral edema include loss of alertness or a sudden and severe headache. Incontinence, vomiting, disorientation, and agitation, or changes in vital signs, such as a decrease in body temperature, hypotension or hypertension, periods of apnea, or cardiac arrhythmias can occur. As the swelling increases, opthalmoplegia, asymmetrical pupils, or a sluggish or fixed pupil, posturing, and seizures ensue. Mannitol is given as 1 g/kg body weight over 15 min and repeated at 2 g/kg body weight as needed. Intubation with hyperventilation is also performed, although most studies conclude that the use of dexamethasone or hyperventilation have not been helpful. The diagnosis is clinical and does not depend on CT scanning, for which findings may lag behind the clinical state. A lumbar puncture should not be performed, but rather neurological and neurosurgical consultations are required, as this is a medical emergency that is too often fatal or leads to extensive loss of sensory and motor functions.

Cerebral edema may occur as soon as within 2–24 h of treatment of DKA in about 1:100 children. The clinical picture is one of a young patient who initially improved while receiving fluids or insulin for DKA who suddenly develops a headache and becomes lethargic or obtunded. Neurological deterioration progresses over several hours, with pupils become asymmetrical heralding eventual herniation of the brain stem. Mortality is about 70%, and in those who recover, only 14% have no permanent deficits. Unfortunately, many studies show that biochemical findings, age of the patient, duration of ketoacidosis, and management protocols do not successfully predict which patients will have or will survive cerebral edema. Most centers now use slow rates of rehydration with isotonic saline in hopes of reducing the occurrence of cerebral edema.

C. Adult Respiratory Distress Syndrome

Also called noncardiogenic pulmonary edema, ARDS is a rare, but again, potentially fatal complication of DKA. ARDS occurs during the treatment phase of DKA, and although it is tempting to speculate that ARDS occurs because of rapid and excessive fluid replacement, its cause is unknown. It may occur because of an underlying infection or coexistent cardiogenic shock.

Most patients with DKA have normal arterial partial pressures of oxygen and normal alveolar to arterial O_2 (A–a) gradients. Hyperpnea (Kussmaul respiration) is due to severe metabolic acidosis, rather than pulmonary dysfunction.

Colloid osmotic pressure, the pressure within vessels owing to particulate matter, is initially increased by DKA. During rehydration with normal saline, the left atrial pressure increases and the colloid osmotic pressure often decreases to levels lower than those seen in normal healthy subjects. Both of these changes favor edema formation in the lung, even in the presence of normal heart function.

There is also a progressive decrease in PaO_2 and an increase in the $A-aO_2$ gradient. In most patients, these changes are not clinically significant, and chest radiographs remain normal. Only a small set of patients appear to progress to ARDS; namely, those patients who present in DKA with a widened $A-aO_2$ gradient or those with rales on clinical examination. It is prudent to decrease the rate of fluid replacement in these high-risk patients, monitor the PaO_2 by pulse oximetry, and use colloid (such as albumin) and not crystalloids to treat hypotension that is not responsive to moderate crystalloid replacement. In addition, central venous monitoring should be used to assist with fluid replacement.

D. Pancreatitis

Diabetic ketocidosis is not known to directly induce pancreatitis. There have been autopsy-proved findings of pancreatitis in patients who have died during episodes of DKA, but the sequence of events are unclear. Recently, Nair and Pitchumoni (1997) describe three cases in whom transient but severe hyperlipidemia during DKA caused acute pancreatitis. These patients had an underlying defect in lipoprotein metabolism, described best as type 2B hyperlipidemia. It is thus hypothesized that hypertriglyceridemia causing pancreatitis occurs mostly in patients with deficiencies of lipoprotein receptors and apoproteins. In addition, DKA may cause pancreatitis by enhancing the concentration of free fatty acids, causing a toxic reaction within pancreatic acini, or forming fat emboli within the pancreas.

Diagnosis of pancreatitis from the history, physical, and laboratory findings may be difficult during DKA. Most patients with DKA present with nausea, vomiting, and abdominal pain; all these symptoms can be suggestive of pancreatitis. Serum amylase may be elevated in DKA, but is usually transient and unrelated to pancreatic damage, reflecting instead salivary gland activity. There are also elevations in serum lipase, which may not specifically represent pancreatic inflammation. Furthermore, there are reports of pancreatitis and DKA in which the serum amylase is not elevated owing to the presence of an inhibitor in the serum that suppresses amylase activity. Thus, the diagnosis of pancreatitis during an episode of ketoacidosis is based first on suspicion by history and second, clinical examination (abdominal findings), and then is confirmed by radiographic means. A CT scan of the abdomen, looking for edema of the pancreas, is confirmatory.

E. Hyperchloremic Acidosis

In DKA, a large amount of ketone bodies are excreted in the urine, and thus there is an insufficient quantity of ketoanion available to be converted back to bicarbonate and correct the metabolic acidosis. In most cases, near the end of DKA treatment, there is a normal anion gap metabolic acidosis with relative hyperchloremia and a buffer deficit of 300–400 mEq after resolution of ke-

Table 9 The Delta Anion Gap/Delta HCO$_3$ Ratio in Defining Diabetic States

Delta gap/delta HCO$_3$	< 0.4	0.4–0.8	> 0.8
On admission	11%	43%	46%
4 h later	46%	36%	17%
8 h later	72%	19%	9%

Delta gap = calculated anion gap − 16; delta HCO$_3$ = 25 − measured HCO$_3$ (arterial blood).
Source: Adrogue et al., 1982.

tonemia. This buffer deficit is due to the urinary loss of ketoanions unaccompanied by hydrogen ions. This acidosis has no adverse clinical effects and is gradually corrected over the subsequent 24–48 h by enhanced renal acid excretion.

Hyperchloremic acidosis is also a direct effect of infusion of standard NaCl intravenous fluids containing a concentration of chloride that exceeds the plasma chloride level, volume expansion with bicarbonate-free fluids, and intracellular shifts of NaCHO$_3$ during correction of DKA. Sodium losses exceed chloride losses during DKA; thus, the use of NaCl-containing fluids results in a relative hyperchloremia, occurring during the first 2–4 h of treatment when ketonuria is maximal. During this period, plasma chloride concentrations increase disproportionately to the concomitant changes in plasma sodium and bicarbonate.

Clinicians can use the delta anion gap/delta HCO$_3$ ratio, which represents the fraction of the plasma bicarbonate deficit that is accounted for by the retention of anions, to define the type of acid–base disorder seen in DKA. A ratio of 0.8 or higher represents increased anion gap acidosis and DKA, a ratio of 0.4–0.8 is a mixed acidosis, whereas a ratio less than 0.4 indicates hyperchloremic acidosis. For example, a patient admitted for ketoacidosis will have a pH of 7.06, a bicarbonate of 5, and an anion gap of 37. The delta anion gap is 21 and the delta HCO$_3$ is 20, so the ratio is greater than 1. Eight hours later, the pH will be 7.2, with a bicarbonate of 9, and an anion gap of 17. Here the delta anion gap is 1 and the delta HCO$_3$ is 16 for a ratio of 0.06. Table 9, taken from Adrogue et al. (1982), shows how fluid and insulin therapy over 8 h convert those with ketoacidosis and dehydration to hyperchloremic acidosis.

F. Hypokalemia

During DKA, total body K is depleted 3–5 mM/kg body weight. Therapy of DKA shifts K$^+$ from the extracellular to the intracellular compartment by correction of the acidosis, repletion with sodium and insulin effects on glycogen synthesis, and K$^+$ transport into cells. The continued renal loss of K$^+$ and the shift into cells can lead to profound hypokalemia and death if not treated prospectively. There is also an increased risk for hypokalemia during treatment of DKA or NKH if the patients used diuretics before presentation, or if patients were following a restricted caloric intake. Thus potassium has to be given prospectively, and to avoid cardiac arrhythmias, it is best to give the supplementation orally, rather than intravenously, if the patient is not nauseated or obtunded.

G. Hypoglycemia

Treatment regimens using high-dose subcutaneous insulin lead to significantly more early and later hypoglycemia than the modern protocols using 0.1 U/kg/h. *Hypoglycemia* is defined as a blood glucose value lower than 60 mg/dL. Umpierrez et al. (1997) reviewed the treatment of inpatients with hyperglycemic emergencies admitted to an urban hospital. If patients were treated without using a protocol (see Appendix for DKA treatment protocol) for insulin adjustments during DKA or NKH, hypoglycemia occurred almost five times more often. Most episodes of hypoglycemia occurred during the second 12 h of treatment, with 75% described as mild (40–60 mg/dL) and 25% had severe hypoglycemia (< 40 mg/dL). This review states that the most frequent cause of hypoglycemia during treatment was the failure to reduce the insulin infusion rate by 50% once blood glucose levels are lower than 250 mg/dL. Patients with NKH had less hypoglycemia than those with DKA. Permanent neurological damage can occur from prolonged (> 4 h) severe hypoglycemia.

APPENDIX: PROTOCOL FOR MANAGEMENT OF DIABETIC KETOACIDOSIS

1. Careful history and physical with attention to mental status, cardiovascular and renal status, sources of infection and state of hydration.
2. Initial biochemical evaluation: blood ketones, glucose (fingerstick), urine ketones, plasma glucose, blood gases and pH, serum electrolytes, BUN, amylase, CBC, urinalysis, CXR, ECG, bacterial cultures if appropriate.
3. After blood draws, give 1 L 0.9% NS then 0.45% NS 200–1000 ml/h, unless there is a concern about cardiac or renal dysfunction. Do not exceed 5 L/8 h. If initial K^+ < 3.5 mEq/L, K^+ supplements should be given at the rate of 40 mEq/L. Give 20–30 mEq K^+ after first liter of NS if K^+ > 3.5, but < 5.5 mEq/L, and urinary output is adequate. Potassium should be given orally if the patient is not nauseated and is not vomiting. Give no K^+ if K^+ > 5.5 mEq/L, but repeat K^+ every 1–2 h.

4. No bicarbonate is given for pH > 7, if pH < 7 but > 6.9, give 1 ampule (44 mEq), for pH < 6.9 give 88 mEq $NaHCO_3$. Each ampule of $NaHCO_3$ runs in 30 min with 15 mEq KCl. Repeat above every 2 h until pH > 7.0.

5. When DKA is confirmed, give 0.4 U regular insulin per kilogram body weight (half as IV push and half as SQ). If DKA is severe or patient is comatose, give 7–10 U (0.1 U/kg) insulin per hour as continuous infusion. When the plasma glucose value reaches 250 mg/dL, change to 100–300 ml/h D5-1/2 NS if sodium level is higher than 140. Use D5-NS at 100–300 ml/h if sodium value is less than 140. Decrease iv insulin infusion to 0.05 $U/kg/h^{-1}$ and adjust the infusion every 2 h based on blood glucose concentration

< 100 mg/dL	Decrease by 1 U/h and give 25 ml 50% dextrose
100–160 mg/dL	Decrease by 1 U/h
161–220 mg/dL	No change
221–280 mg/dL	Increase by 1 U/h
> 280 mg/dL	Give 8 U iv bolus and increase by 1 U/h

6. When DKA is controlled (glucose under 200 mg/dL, $HCO_3 > 15$ mEq/L and pH > 7.3 and serum ketone negative at 1:2 dilution), patient is changed to subcutaneous insulin. (Adapted from Kitabchi AE, Wall BM, 1995.)

BIBLIOGRAPHY

Adrogue HJ, Wilson H, Boyd AE, Suki WN, Eknoyan G. Plasma acid–base patterns in diabetic ketoacidosis. N Engl J Med 307:1603–1610, 1982.

Alberti KGMM. Diabetic acidosis, hyperosmolar coma and lactic acidosis. In: Becker KL, ed. Principles and Practice of Endocrinology and Metabolism. 2nd ed. Philadelphia: J.B. Lippincott 1995:1316–1329.

Davidson JK. Diabetic ketoacidosis and hyperglycemic hyperosmolar state. In: Davidson JK, ed. Clinical Diabetes Mellitus: A Problem Oriented Approach. New York: Thieme, Inc., 1986:310–311.

Ennis ED, Kreisberg RA. Diabetic ketoacidosis and the hyperglycemic hyperosmolar syndrome. In: Leroith D, Taylor SI, Olefskyn JM, eds. Diabetes Mellitus: A Fundamental and Clinical Text. Philadelphia: Lippincott-Raven, 1996:276–287.

Genuth SM. Diabetic ketoacidosis and hyperglycemic hyperosmolar coma. Curr Ther Endocrinol Metab 5:400–406, 1994.

Kitabchi AE, Wall BM. Diabetic ketoacidosis. Med Clin North Am 79:9–37, 1995.

Lebovitz HL. Diabetic ketoacidosis. Lancet 345:767–772, 1995.

Lorber D. Nonketotic hypertonicity in diabetes mellitus. Med Clin North Am 79:39–52, 1995.

Rosenbloom AL, Hanas R. Diabetic ketoacidosis (DKA): treatment guidelines. Clin Pediatr 35:261–266, 1996.

Rydall AC, Rodin GM, Olmsted MP, Devenyi RG, Daneman D. Disordered eating behavior and microvascular complications in young women with insulin-dependent diabetes mellitus. N Engl J Med 336:1849–1854, 1997.

Umpierrez GE, Khajavi M, Kitabchi AE. Review: diabetic ketoacidosis and hyperglycemic hyperosmolar nonketotic syndrome. Am J Med Sci 311:225–233, 1996.

Umpierrez GE, Kelly JP, Navarrete JE, Casals MMC, Kitabchi AE. Hyperglycemic crises in urban blacks. Arch Intern Med 157:669–675, 1997.

Whiteman VE, Homko CJ, Reece EA. Management of hypoglycemia and diabetic ketoacidosis in pregnancy. Obstet Gynecol Clin North Am 23:87–107, 1996.

41

Diabetes and Polycystic Ovary Syndrome

Carolyn H. Kreinsen and Andrea Dunaif
Brigham and Women's Hospital, Boston, Massachusetts

I. INTRODUCTION

Polycystic ovary syndrome (PCOS) is the most common endocrine disorder impacting women of reproductive age. The current diagnostic criteria for the endocrinopathy are hyperandrogenism and chronic anovulation in premenopausal women without underlying androgen-secreting neoplasms, nonclassic adrenal hyperplasia, pituitary or thyroid disease. It is a disorder of exclusion and one of unknown etiology. However, strong evidence of familial clustering suggests a genetic component to the development of PCOS. A recent population-based study showed a prevalence in premenopausal white and African American women of about 5%. For over seven decades, investigators have recognized and scrutinized various aspects of the syndrome. More recently, it has become apparent that the syndrome has major metabolic consequences secondary to insulin resistance and that insulin resistance plays an important role in the pathogenesis of the reproductive abnormalities. The syndrome is a major risk factor for type 2 diabetes mellitus (DM) in premenopausal women, with prevalence rates sevenfold greater than the $\sim$1% prevalence in reproductively normal premenopausal women. Overall prevalence rates of glucose intolerance and type 2 DM of 40% have been reported in several U.S. studies of PCOS women.

Many of the clinical signs and symptoms apparent in PCOS stem from the associated chronic anovulation and hyperandrogenism. Reproductive morbidity manifests as dysfunctional uterine bleeding, oligomenorrhea, amenorrhea, and infertility. Endometrial hyperplasia and adenocarcinoma may be subsequent long-term sequelae of chronic anovulation. Onset of PCOS frequently occurs at or

687

around menarche with inability to establish regular menstrual cycles. The spectrum of more overt problems, including hirsutism, acne, diffuse or male-pattern alopecia, seborrhea, and abdominal obesity, sequelae of hyperandrogenism, may present at puberty or later, during the second and third decades of life. Increased androgen production, biological availability, and target tissue utilization in PCOS represent an interplay of three "compartments": the ovaries, the adrenals, and the periphery. Phenotypic presentation also reflects the influence of environmental factors, such as obesity and genetic differences in number of hair follicles and target tissue androgen receptors. Generalized obesity and abdominal obesity are more prevalent in PCOS women than in appropriately matched reproductively normal control women. Acanthosis nigricans is frequently present on the back of the neck and in the axillae. Acromegaloid features may be present on occasion.

Given the anovulatory state, progesterone levels are acyclic and chronically low in PCOS. Appropriate uterine withdrawal bleeding does occur in PCOS women after administration of a course of exogenous progesterone. In the normal ovulatory ovary, follicles synthesize androgens, primarily testosterone, in the theca cells under the modulation of luteinizing hormone (LH). Androgens diffuse into adjacent ovarian granulosa cells and undergo aromatization to estradiol (E_2) under the regulatory influence of follicle stimulating hormone (FSH). In PCOS women, there is an increase in LH secretion without concurrent increased FSH release. An acyclic, static, low-normal level of FSH persists. With greater LH-induced androgen production and limited capacity for conversion to estradiol, a hyperandrogenic state evolves. The adrenals contribute somewhat to overall hyperandrogenemia; however, the ovaries are usually the major source. Acyclic production of estrogen ensues, including peripheral aromatization of circulating androstenedione to estrone (E_1). In obese individuals, there is a substantially higher degree of extraovarian estrogen production in the adipose tissue. A chronic hyperestrogenic situation results with an increased ratio of E_1/E_2 levels.

Anovulation ultimately results from failure of follicular maturation and subsequent atresia in the context of relative FSH deficiency. Ovaries become enlarged and atretic with capsular thickening. The follicles contained are largely cystic and atretic with hyperplastic theca and stroma. A condition termed hyperthecosis, islands of luteinized theca cells in the stroma, may be present. Importantly, polycystic ovaries, while typical of PCOS, are not specific to the syndrome. Any condition producing hyperandrogenism and chronic anovulation may cause polycystic ovaries. Conversely, they have been found in asymptomatic women with ovulatory cycles.

II. INSULIN RESISTANCE

Various health disorders have been associated with PCOS, some affecting young women, most with long-term ramifications for the life span. Insulin resistance and glucose intolerance have emerged as common findings in PCOS. Indeed, it now appears that insulin resistance is a critical element underlying the complex endocrine and metabolic abnormalities that comprise the syndrome. All PCOS women, particularly those within the obese subset, are at increased risk for developing type 2 DM, with presentation as early as adolescence, as opposed to the more usual sixth to seventh decades typifying the general population.

Insulin resistance, independent of obesity, is a unique feature of PCOS but not of hyperandrogenic states in general. Obesity is a common cause of insulin resistance and hyperinsulinemia; it also occurs more frequently in PCOS women than in age- and sex-matched control women in the general population. Obesity has a major synergistic negative effect with PCOS on insulin resistance, such that obese PCOS women are at greater risk for glucose intolerance and dyslipidemia. There also appears to be a direct relation between the chronically anovulatory state and insulin resistance. Therapies that improve insulin sensitivity may restore ovulation in PCOS women. Although hyperandrogenemia may contribute somewhat to the insulin resistance, there is an intrinsic defect in insulin action in PCOS. Several rare disorders have been identified in which extreme insulin resistant diabetes mellitus in females has been found in conjunction with hyperandrogenism. These include the type A syndrome in adolescent women and the type B syndrome in pre- and postmenopausal women, associated with anti-insulin receptor antibodies. Other studies noted insulin receptor gene mutations as the cause of leprechaunism, Rabson-Mendenhall syndrome, and some cases of type A syndrome. All of these disorders have insulin-resistant diabetes mellitus, acanthosis nigricans, and hyperandrogenism in common.

While the classic target tissues for insulin action on glucose metabolism are liver, muscle, and adipose, receptors are present in most tissues, including the human ovary. Although insulin can stimulate ovarian production of testosterone and androstenedione, it does not appear to regulate ovarian androgen secretion in normal women. Conversely, hyperinsulinemia does appear to alter steroidogenesis in PCOS, independent of changes in gonadotropin secretion. A postbinding defect in insulin receptor signaling appears to underlie insulin resistance in PCOS women. This defect is most likely genetic, for it persists in cultured cells. It remains to be seen whether a single genetic defect with variable penetrance may explain the association of PCOS and insulin resistance, or whether there are additional genetic or environmental factors.

Obesity not only is more prevalent in PCOS women, with ramifications for increased insulin resistance and hyperinsulinemia, but also exerts a direct negative effect on insulin sensitivity, glucose tolerance, and lipid levels. Studies in premenopausal PCOS women have failed to show a positive association between insulin resistance and blood pressure. However, an increased tendency for the development of hypertension later in life has been noted. Dyslipidemias, including decreased high-density lipoprotein (HDL) cholesterol, as well as increased low-density lipoprotein (LDL) cholesterol and triglycerides have been associated with PCOS. However, obesity, not the syndrome itself, may be the more instrumental factor underlying the first two. Again, insulin levels correlate directly with lipid abnormalities.

Women with PCOS may be at increased risk for cardiovascular disease. The epidemiological literature reports somewhat conflicting results relative to this. Controlling for weight has been one major problem limiting studies to date. Recent data indicate that these women have increased circulating levels of plasminogen activator inhibitor (PAI-1) with subsequent diminished fibrinolytic activity. Insulin stimulates the production of PAI-1; elevated levels of PAI-1 are associated with insulin resistance and represent elevated risk for intravascular thrombosis. PAI-1 levels in women with PCOS have decreased with improved insulin sensitivity stemming from weight loss or insulin-sensitizing medications. Several cross-sectional studies have raised concern that women with PCOS may be at increased risk for coronary and carotid artery disease. The atherogenic properties of insulin, especially chronically elevated levels of insulin, may play a pivotal role.

III. CLINICAL PRESENTATION

Women with PCOS often seek initial medical advice for menstrual irregularities or dermatological problems stemming from chronic anovulation and hyperandrogenism, respectively. Course and chronology of the presenting problem as well as a detailed health, gynecological, medication, and family history are critical to accurate diagnosis of the disorder. PCOS is not sudden in onset. Subtle signs and symptoms are often evident at the time of menarche or within the following years. Oligomenorrhea and hirsutism represent the most frequent early concerns of affected women. Infertility, amenorrhea, dysfunctional uterine bleeding, acne, alopecia, and seborrhea are also common. Abdominal obesity is noted in many women with PCOS, but certainly not all. Family histories of infertility, menstrual problems, hyperandrogenic manifestations, early diabetes mellitus, dyslipidemia, and hypertension are often present.

Signs of true virilization are not usually consistent with a diagnosis of PCOS. Marked deepening of the voice, increasing unexplained or disproportionate muscle mass, and clitorimegaly (clitoris larger than 1 cm in width) are more often harbingers of a severely hyperandrogenic state, indicative perhaps of an ovarian or adrenal androgen-secreting tumor.

Physical examination must include blood pressure measurement, height and weight determination, and circumference recording of waist and hips. Obesity, if present in women with PCOS, is frequently abdominal and not gynecoid, with a waist/hip ratio of > 0.8. Dermatological examination should focus on the presence of acne or seborrhea. Alopecia may be present even with mild hyperandrogenism. Often the hairline is preserved and there is a diffuse decrease in density in the frontal and parietal areas. Acanthosis nigricans, a brownish hyperpigmentation of skin folds of the neck, axillae, and intertriginous areas, is often present in obese PCOS women. Histologically characterized by papillomatosis and hyperkeratosis, this phenomenon is often seen in association with insulin resistance, hyperinsulinemia, and diabetes mellitus.

Hirsutism is the term for excessive growth of androgen-dependent terminal hair. These terminal hairs are medullated with dense cores and tend to be darker, thicker, and coarser than vellus hair. The majority of hirsutism in women is attributable to PCOS. Ultimately, the degree of hirsutism present in the hyperandrogenic state depends on the peripheral activity of 5α-reductase and subsequent conversion of androgen to dihydrotestosterone and the number of hair follicles. PCOS women occasionally are not hirsute, despite hyperandrogenism.

On physical examination, hirsutism can be noted on the face and neck, along the midline distribution of the chest, back, upper and lower abdomen, and in the axillary, thigh, and pubic regions. In the absence of obvious hair, it is necessary to look for signs of shaving, plucking, or other depilatory activity, as well as resultant ingrown hairs and folliculitis caused by hair removal attempts. Vellus hypertrichosis should be ruled out.

Overall muscle bulk must be evaluated in the context of personal lifestyle. Gynecological examination should entail inspection of the external genitalia for abnormalities and question of clitoromegaly as well as bimanual palpation seeking ovarian enlargement or mass, unilateral or bilateral.

IV. DIAGNOSES

To reiterate, PCOS in women is a common disorder with diagnostic criteria of hyperandrogenism and chronic anovulation; it is also a diagnosis of exclusion. Whenever menstrual irregularities are a presenting complaint, it is first necessary to rule out pregnancy. Given a normal human chorionic gonadotropin (hCG), it is imperative to rule out androgen-secreting neoplasm of the ovaries or adrenals, prolactin-secreting pituitary adenoma, and nonclassic congenital adrenal hyperplasia. Hyper- and hypothyroidism also merit consideration and exclusion.

Polycystic ovaries are not pathognomonic for PCOS. Therefore, while most women with PCOS have polycystic ovaries on ultrasound, the finding is neither specific to or necessary for the diagnosis of PCOS. Single LH and FSH values have little practical use in this process. An elevated LH/FSH ratio, while quite common in PCOS, is often undetectable owing to pulsate secretion of LH.

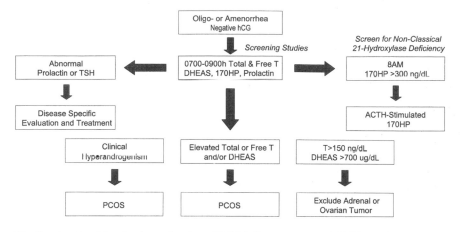

Fig. 1 An algorithm for the evaluation of PCOS. T, testosterone; 170 HP, 17-hydroxypro-
gesterone; DHEAS, dehydroepiandrosterone sulfate; TSH, thyroid stimulating hormone.

A reasonable diagnostic approach to women with evidence of chronic anovulation and hyperandrogenism is delineated in the algorithm depicted in Fig. 1.
Initial screening involves serological testing at 0700–0900 h of prolactin, free and
total testosterone, thyroid-stimulating hormone (TSH), dehydroepiandrosterone
sulfate (DHEAS), and 17-hydroxyprogesterone (17-OHP) levels. The
0700–0900-h timing is to allow for accurate measurement of 17-OHP, screening
for the most common cause of congenital adrenal hyperplasia–nonclassic adrenal
21-hydroxylase deficiency. If the level is less than 300 ng/dL, the diagnosis
is unlikely. If more than 300 ng/dL, an adrenocorticotropic hormone (ACTH)
stimulation test and referral to an endocrinologist are warranted. Abnormal prolactin or TSH requires disease-specific evaluation.

If testosterone or DHEAS are elevated without evidence of nonclassic 21-
hydroxylase deficiency, the differential narrows to PCOS versus an androgen-
secreting tumor. Both levels are lower in PCOS, with testosterone ranging between 80 and 150 ng/dL and DHEAS between 360 and 700 μg/dL. Higher testosterone or DHEAS levels warrant a search for ovarian or adrenal neoplasms.

V. TREATMENT

Polycystic ovary syndrome incorporates complex neuroendocrine, metabolic,
physical, and cosmetic ramifications. Approach to treatment must be both compre-

hensive and integrative. Most affected women who seek medical advice during their early adult years do so for evaluation of menstrual irregularities, infertility issues, or dermatological problems. The associated underlying insulin resistance, while usually present, has not yet become clinically manifest in terms of overt adverse sequelae. However, the plan of treatment must reflect appreciation for the spectrum and chronic course of the disorder as well as patient priorities and concerns. Intervention may ameliorate one problem while exacerbating another. Inattention to early abnormalities may result in long-term health problems.

Once a diagnosis of PCOS has been established, the provider should obtain fasting lipid and lipoprotein levels. Fasting blood sugar levels fail to detect type 2 DM using the new American Diabetes Association criteria in approximately one-half of women with PCOS who have diabetes by 2-h post-75-g glucose challenge values using WHO criteria. Furthermore, only a few women with PCOS who have impaired glucose tolerance by WHO criteria have impaired fasting glucose by American Diabetes Association criteria. Since microvascular complications of diabetes correlate well with the new American Diabetes Association Diagnostic Criteria based on fasting glucose levels, glucose tolerance testing is not currently recommended in the general population. However, we recommend that it be considered in PCOS women, since close to 50% of women may be glucose intolerant and knowledge of this may assist the physician in motivating the patient to lose weight. All women with PCOS, pre- and postmenopausal, must be considered at risk for dyslipidemias, coronary artery disease, hypertension, and type 2 DM. Insulin resistance and hyperinsulinemia in PCOS are multifactorial. Obesity, although not causative, certainly imparts a negatively synergistic effect. If the initial glucose tolerance test is normal, it should be rechecked at least every 5 years, as well as after a substantial weight gain or pregnancy. If abnormal, appropriate intervention must ensue. The WHO criteria for glucose intolerance is the following: less than 140 mg/dL is normal; 140–199 mg/dL is impaired; 200 mg/dL or higher is type 2 DM. The American Diabetes Association Diagnostic Criteria for diabetes is a fasting blood glucose higher than 126 mg/dL. Lipids must be monitored for low HDL levels as well as elevated triglyceride and LDL levels. Fasting lipids and a fasting glucose should be checked annually, if initially within normal limits.

Weight loss and increased aerobic activity represent a cornerstone of therapy for women with PCOS, especially those who fall within the obese subset. This intervention, while critical, will remain one of the most challenging to institute. Weight loss decreases androgen levels and can restore ovulation. Fertility in obese women has been restored with as little as a 7% reduction in body weight. Reduced androgen levels tend to decrease problematic hirsutism, acne, and alopecia. Insulin resistance is lessened with weight loss, highlighting the negative effect of obesity on glucose tolerance in PCOS. Reduced circulating insulin levels appear to be the underlying factor for weight loss-associated reproductive benefits.

Treatment for lipid abnormalities should address the particular element of concern with the appropriate drugs available, if dietary and exercise measures prove inadequate. The dyslipidemias associated with PCOS require monitoring and intervention similar to those indicated for lipid derangements of other etiologies. Conversely, select pharmaceutical agents that lower insulin levels by improving insulin sensitivity, rather than by triggering increased insulin production, may represent the most efficacious modality for treating type 2 DM in women with PCOS. Metformin, a biguanide, reduces hepatic gluconeogenesis and glycogenolysis. It interrupts a key physiological mechanism of type 2 DM—increased hepatic glucose output—with no effect on the pancreas, while improving peripheral glucose utilization. Results of studies examining metformin in women with PCOS have varied from noting significant reductions in insulin and androgen levels to no change at all with use of the agent. One study noted a decrease in hyperandrogenism due to weight loss, potentially metformin-mediated. Troglitazone, a thiazoidenedione, improves insulin sensitivity primarily in peripheral muscle and fat cells, with only minor hepatic activity and no pancreatic effect. The improved insulin sensitivity in women with PCOS who are taking troglitazone has occurred without weight loss. Androgen, estrogen, and LH levels also decreased. Further studies are underway.

Menstrual irregularities ranging from dysfunctional uterine bleeding to oligomenorrhea and amenorrhea represent some of the more distressing issues for PCOS women of reproductive years. From a clinical perspective, unopposed exposure of the uterine endometrium to estrogen without cyclic progesterone and periodic shedding of the lining predisposes to endometrial hyperplasia and increased risk of uterine cancer. Oral contraceptives are a widely employed treatment modality that provide cyclic endometrial shedding and control of excess androgen production by decreasing circulating LH. Exogenous estrogens also induce synthesis of sex hormone-binding globulin, often low in women with PCOS. These globulins bind circulating testosterone, thereby diminishing its biological activity. These oral contraceptive-mediated changes in androgen metabolism reduce hirsutism, acne, and alopecia over time. Progestins exert a direct peripheral target organ effect as well, by competing for androgen receptors and inhibiting 5-α-reductase activity.

Although there are many benefits to oral contraceptive (OCP) use in women with PCOS, they may exert harmful effects as well. Agents containing the androgenic progestin levonorgestral are highly inadvisable in the context of a preexisting hyperandrogenic state. A potentially more limiting issue is that OCPs can produce insulin resistance in "normal" women, with one study demonstrating notable resistance with a combination pill containing triphasic progestin. This effect is a serious consideration for all women with PCOS, especially for obese women with a greater baseline propensity for insulin resistance. Recent studies, however, suggest that the long-term metabolic effects of combination oral contraceptives are beneficial in women with PCOS.

An alternative means of ensuring endometrial protection is the use of medroxyprogesterone acetate, taken intermittently at low dosage, 13–14 days each month, to induce subsequent cyclic endometrial shedding. Although the drug does decrease insulin sensitivity, at the low dosage of 5 mg/day orally on the aforementioned schedule, adverse effects are minimal.

There are a variety of other pharmaceuticals that decrease hyperandrogenism, do not worsen, and may actually improve insulin sensitivity in women with PCOS. The adverse effects of hyperandrogenism were recounted earlier. Antiandrogenic agents block the peripheral effects of excess androgen production by competing with testosterone and dihydrotestosterone for androgen receptors. These are often given in combination with OCP therapy. Some of these drugs also manifest teratogenic potential, to varying degrees, rendering concomitant OCP usage essential. There is no U.S. Food and Drug Administration (FDA) approved agent for the treatment of hyperandrogenism in women.

The most frequently employed and preferred antiandrogenic agent in the United States is spironolactone, with initial dosage of 75 mg/day orally, and maintenance dosage usually ranging from 100 to 200 mg/day. This drug, which is also an aldosterone receptor antagonist, in higher doses decreases glandular production of testosterone and competitively inhibits androgen receptor binding. Side effects do exist and must be considered in its use. Another pharmaceutical, flutamide, has similar effect, but is costly and has been associated with hepatic failure in a small number of recipients. Finasteride, a 5α-reductase inhibitor, blocks the conversion of testosterone to dihydrotestosterone, but is not recommended owing to a range of side effects, including marked teratogenicity. Ketoconazole interferes with androgen biosynthesis and thereby lowers circulating androgen levels. It is not recommended because of numerous side effects, including hepatotoxicity. Glucocorticoids suppress adrenal androgen production, but can induce or exacerbate insulin resistance and should be avoided.

Analogues of GnRH have been used on occasion to reduce hyperandrogenism by suppressing FSH and LH secretion from the pituitary. These may be helpful for a select subgroup of women unable to take oral contraceptives. However, this treatment is costly and must be given with hormone replacement doses of estrogen and progestin to prevent the development of osteoporosis.

In addition to treating the underlying disorder, women may opt for cosmetic approaches, particularly for hirsutism, ranging from bleaching, plucking, shaving, and waxing to more permanent interventions of electrolysis or laser therapy. It is worthwhile to have some acquaintance with the benefits and drawbacks of each.

VI. REFERRAL

The move to refer a patient with PCOS to a subspecialist, in this instance to an endocrinologist or a reproductive endocrinologist, is a variable and provider-specific decision, resting on several criteria. These include the provider knowledge of and comfort with the condition itself; the severity of a patient's clinical presentation and her individual concerns and priorities; the level of diagnostic ease versus uncertainty; and the plethora of questions on optimal treatment approach.

PCOS is a common disorder and affected women most frequently present first to their primary care provider. Therefore, possession of a working knowledge of the disorder, ability to recognize or question its possible presence based on patient complaints, history, and physical, and the subsequent capability to initiate a diagnostic evaluation based on the algorithm previously presented are essential.

It is appropriate to refer at any point of the process in which direction is unclear and patient care conceivably compromised. Although it is necessary to appreciate the range and action of treatment options available, some are more straightforward than others. This may be an appropriate time to seek consultative opinion to ensure optimal care or to refer the patient to an endocrinologist for initiation of therapy and comanagement.

Infertility issues warrant appropriate referral. Women with PCOS have lower success and higher complications rates with ovulation induction. Weight loss, in an obese woman with PCOS, is an important first step, and concerted effort should be directed toward that goal early on. This action alone can restore ovulation and fertility. It can also enhance the efficacy of other fertility-fostering interventions.

BIBLIOGRAPHY

Azziz R, Redmond G, Wheeland RG. Excessive hair growth: diagnosis and therapy. Patient Care April 15:157–168, 1998.

Barth JH. Investigation in the assessment and management of patients with hirsutism. Reprod Endocrinol 9:193–201, 1997.

Carr BR, Wilson JD. Disorders of the ovary and female reproductive tract. In: Isselbacher KJ, et al., eds. Harrison's Principles of Internal Medicine. 13th ed. New York: McGraw Hill, 1994:2017–2036

Dunaif A. Hyperandrogenic anovulation (PCOS): a unique disorder of insulin action associated with an increased risk of non–insulin-dependent diabetes mellitus. Am J Med 98(suppl 1A):33–39, 1995

Dunaif A. Insulin resistance and the polycystic ovary syndrome: mechanism and implications for pathogenesis. Endocr Rev 18:774–800, 1997.

Dunaif A, Green G, Phelps RG, Lebwohl M, Futterweit W, Lewy L. Acanthosis nigricans, insulin action, and hyperandrogenism: clinical, histological, and biochemical findings. J Clin Endocrinol Metab 73:590–595, 1991.

Franks S. Polycystic ovary syndrome. N Engl J Med 333:853–861, 1995.

Hershlag H, Peterson CH. Endocrine disorders. In: Berek JS, ed. Novak's Gynecology 12th ed. Baltimore: Williams & Wilkins, 1996:837–845.

Kessel B, Liu J. Clinical and laboratory evaluation of hirsutism. Clin Obstet Gynecol 34: 805–816, 1991.

Legro R, Dunaif A. The role of insulin resistance in polycystic ovary syndrome. Endocrinologist 6:307–321, 1996.

Lobo RA. Hirsutism in polycystic ovary syndrome: current concepts. Clin Obstet Gynecol 34:817–826, 1991.

Pierpoint T, Mckeigue PM, Isaacs AJ, Wild SH, Jacob HS. Mortality of women with polycystic ovary syndrome at long-term follow-up. J Clin Epidemiol 51:581–586, 1998.

Price TM, Bates GW. Ovarian endocrine disorders. In: Leppert PC, Howard FM, eds. Primary Care for Women. Philadelphia: Lippincott–Raven, 1997:248–253.

Quintana B, Dunaif A. Insulin resistance and the polycystic ovary syndrome. AACC Endocrinol 13:359–366, 1995.

Schwartz S, Raskin P, Fonseca V, Graneline KF. Effect of troglitazone in insulin-treated patients with type II diabetes mellitus. N Engl J Med 338:861–866, 1998.

Speroff L, Glass RH, Kase NG. Clinical Gynecologic Endocrinology and Infertility. 5th ed. Baltimore: Williams & Wilkins, 1994:457–482.

42
Polyendocrine Syndromes

K. Patrick Ober
*Wake Forest University School of Medicine, Winston-Salem,
North Carolina*

I. INTRODUCTION

Diabetes mellitus does not always occur as an isolated endocrine disorder. Not infrequently, diabetes is associated with other endocrine disorders, and these associated endocrinopathies may have a substantial influence on the nature, severity, course, and management of the diabetes.

By definition, diabetes itself is an endocrine disorder. Thus, strictly speaking, a patient who has diabetes mellitus concomitantly with any other endocrine disease could be said to have a polyendocrine disorder. Some endocrine disorders have been linked with diabetes as fairly well-defined "pluriglandular deficiency syndromes," with the connection based on shared autoimmune etiology and the finding of an increased risk for specific endocrine disorders in susceptible patients. These are well-defined syndromes, however; clearly, not all possible combinations of diabetes mellitus and other endocrine diseases should be considered to be classic polyendocrine syndromes. Nonetheless, there are several quite common endocrine disorders that are frequently encountered in patients with diabetes mellitus (a circumstance that is due more to the frequency with which these conditions occur in the general population, rather than any specific genetic predisposition), in addition to the "classic" pluriglandular associations of diabetes mellitus. All of these endocrine associations, whether classic or not, can have a major effect on the management of the patient with diabetes, and the most important of these will be reviewed in this chapter.

There are several mechanisms by which diabetes might be associated with other endocrine disorders, and the organization of this chapter will be based on this classification:

1. Diabetes may result from another endocrine disorder.
2. Diabetes may coexist with other endocrine diseases because of a shared etiological mechanism.
3. Diabetes itself may cause another endocrinopathy.
4. Diabetes and another endocrine disorder may occur together as coincidence.

Each of this categories will be discussed separately.

II. DIABETES AS A CONSEQUENCE OF ANOTHER ENDOCRINE DISORDER

This category includes *secondary forms of diabetes* that develop as the result of specific endocrine diseases, and includes disorders such as Cushing's syndrome, acromegaly, and glucagonoma. These associated endocrine disorders frequently cause insulin resistance, which then promotes the development of diabetes mellitus. The primary challenge in such situations is to recognize and appropriately treat the underlying endocrine disorder. Recognition and effective treatment of these diseases typically results in substantial improvement, and sometimes resolution, of the diabetic state. Causes of secondary diabetes are discussed on Chapter 14 and will not be covered further in this chapter.

III. DIABETES ASSOCIATED WITH OTHER ENDOCRINE DISEASES ON THE BASIS OF A SHARED ETIOLOGICAL MECHANISM

The polyendocrine syndromes in this category usually involve type 1 diabetes mellitus. The same autoimmune processes that are responsible for the β-cell destruction which leads to the development of type 1 diabetes may similarly destroy other endocrine cells. Common targets include adrenal, gonadal, thyroid, or parathyroid tissues. In some situations, medical management of each of the separate endocrinopathies is not much more complicated than the separate therapy for each individual disorder (as with diabetes and hypoparathyroidism). In many other cases, however, the metabolic consequences of the additional endocrine disorder can profoundly alter the stability and control of the diabetes. For example, the development of severe hyperthyroidism caused by Graves' disease in a previously well-controlled patient with type 1 diabetes may lead to pronounced metabolic decompensation and ketoacidosis, and the advent of Addison's disease in the patient with preexisting type 1 diabetes may cause dramatically lowered insulin requirements and frequent hypoglycemia.

Not all patients with diabetes have β-cell loss on the basis of autoimmune processes; some have lost β-cell function because of systemic infiltrative diseases, and the infiltrative disorder may also lead to damage to other endocrine tissues. An illustration of such shared etiology would be hemochromatosis, in which a common infiltrative process impairs the function of multiple endocrine tissues, including (but certainly not limited to) beta cells.

In many patients, of course, diabetes mellitus is not caused by islet cell loss, but instead, insulin resistance is the major factor that has resulted in the development of diabetes. In such patients, the same insulin resistance that provoked the initiation of the diabetic state may also promote the development of endocrinopathies, such as polycystic ovary disease through the effects of the associated hyperinsulinemia. This is discussed in detail in Chap. 41.

A. Addison's Disease (Primary Adrenal Insufficiency)

Primary adrenal insufficiency is most commonly the result of autoimmune adrenalitis. As such, it may occur as an isolated entity, or it may occur in association with other autoimmune endocrine disorders, including type 1 diabetes mellitus. Addison's disease is seen in two major autoimmune polyglandular syndromes (Table 1). Type I autoimmune polyglandular syndrome includes Addison's disease, hypoparathyroidism, and chronic mucocutaneous candidiasis, and type 1 diabetes mellitus is infrequently seen in this syndrome. Type II autoimmune polyglandular syndrome is manifest as Addison's disease, autoimmune thyroid disease (Graves' disease or Hashimoto's disease), or type 1 diabetes mellitus. Type II is also known as Schmidt's syndrome; the age of onset ranges from

Table 1 Diseases Associated with Pluriglandular Deficiency Syndrome

Type I	
Hypoparathyroidism	~ 90%
Mucocutaneous candidiasis	~ 75%
Adrenal insufficiency	~ 60%
Gonadal failure	~ 50%
Autoimmune thyroid disease	~ 10%
Type 1 diabetes mellitus	~ 1%
Type II	
Adrenal insufficiency	100%
Autoimmune thyroid disease	~ 70%
Type 1 diabetes mellitus	~ 50%
Gonadal failure	Variable

Table 2 Clinical Manifestations of Primary Adrenal Insufficiency

Glucocorticoid deficiency
    Nausea, vomiting, anorexia, weight loss
    Asthenia, weakness
    Hyperpigmentation
    Hypoglycemia, decreased insulin requirement
Mineralocorticoid deficiency
    Sodium wasting
        Hyponatremia (90%)
        Hypovolemia
        Hypotension
        Azotemia (prerenal)
    Hyperkalemia (65%)
    Metabolic acidosis

childhood to late adulthood, and is more common in females by a ratio of 1.8:1. The disorder appears to be associated with HLA-B8 (DW3) haplotypes.

The presentation of Addison's disease is often nonspecific (Table 2). The progression of the disorder is slow and insidious in many cases, with major features including weight loss, fatigue, generalized weakness, and malaise. Hyperpigmentation of the skin reflects the increase in melanocyte-stimulating activity which is associated with increased levels of corticotropin (adrenocorticotropic hormone; ACTH). The increased pigment can be generalized, but is more likely to occur on extensor surfaces, such as elbows, knuckles, and knees, in palmar creases, on the lips or buccal mucosa, or on scars of recent origin. Vitiligo, when present, is a strong indicator for an autoimmune process as the underlying etiological process.

Hypotension is very common in Addison's disease, and usually presents clinically as postural hypotension. This is the result of volume depletion (on the basis of aldosterone deficiency) and decreased vascular resistance (owing to cortisol deficiency).

> *Key clinical point:* Postural hypotension is a common feature in the patient with longstanding diabetes mellitus, and is usually caused by autonomic neuropathy. The possibility of Addison's disease should always be considered as an alternative explanation if the patient has other clinical features that are consistent with adrenal insufficiency (see Table 2).

Gastrointestinal symptoms are also prominent in patients with Addison's disease, with major manifestations being anorexia, nausea, and vomiting in almost all advanced cases, weight loss in a vast majority, and chronic nonspecific abdominal pain in a sizable minority.

Key clinical point: These manifestations are similar to those of diabetic gastroparesis, and the possibility of Addison's disease should be kept in mind when these symptoms occur in the diabetic patient.

Electrolyte disturbances are common features of adrenal insufficiency. Hyponatremia (seen in over 90% of cases of Addison's disease) may occur with either primary or secondary adrenal insufficiency, although the mechanisms are probably different in the two settings, with sodium wasting and volume contraction occurring in the former, as opposed to the dilutional hyponatremia of the latter. Hyperkalemia (seen in 50–60% of cases of Addison's disease) is the result of aldosterone deficiency and thus is rarely found in patients with secondary adrenal insufficiency.

Key clinical point: Many patients with diabetes of long duration will have aldosterone deficiency owing to impaired production of renin (a condition that is discussed in detail later), and this hypoaldosterone state results in the electrolyte changes of hyperkalemia or hyponatremia; these same changes are also compatible with Addison's disease. The ultimate cause of these electrolyte findings—impaired aldosterone production—is present in both the hyporeninemic hypoaldosteronism of diabetes and in Addison's disease. However, the clinical implications are considerably different in the two disorders: the production of cortisol is normal in the diabetic patient who has low aldosterone production, but cortisol secretion is significantly impaired (with potentially life-threatening consequences) in the patient with adrenal insufficiency. Cortisol production should be assessed in any patient in whom adrenal insufficiency is suspected.

Adrenal insufficiency is associated with increased sensitivity to insulin, and should be considered as a diagnosis in the patient who experiences frequent problems with hypoglycemia or has a significant decrease in insulin requirement without other apparent explanation.

Evaluation of the patient with features of adrenal insufficiency is relatively straightforward. Normally, cortisol levels vary considerably throughout the day owing to central nervous system (CNS)-driven diurnal patterns, the superimposed effects of stress, and numerous other factors, and because of this variability the measurement of a single cortisol value is unlikely to give useful information unless extremely low or extremely high serum cortisol levels are found. However, the diagnosis can be established readily by documenting low serum cortisol levels, with a failure of the adrenals to respond appropriately to stimulation by ACTH or an ACTH analogue.

The most useful test for adrenal insufficiency mimics the normal control system for stimulating adrenal function. Under physiological circumstances, stress will promote pituitary production of ACTH, which then stimulates adrenal

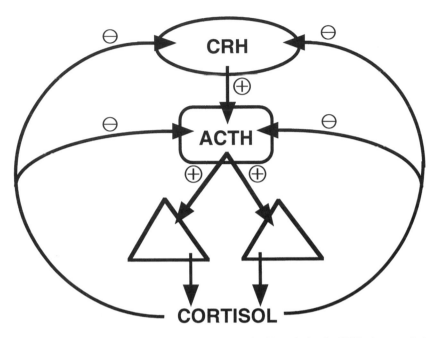

Fig. 1 The hypothalamic–pituitary–adrenal axis. Hypothalamic CRH triggers pituitary production of ACTH, which then stimulates adrenal production of cortisol. Cortisol suppresses CRH and ACTH by a negative-feedback mechanism.

production of cortisol (Fig. 1). If a patient is injected with an ACTH analogue (cosyntropin; Cortrosyn), an increase in the serum cortisol level to the level of 18–20 μg/dL is sufficient to adequately document the presence of responsive adrenal tissue and effectively rule out the diagnosis of Addison's disease (Fig. 2). The cosyntropin can be injected either intramuscularly or intravenously at a standard dose of 0.25 mg (250 μg), with cortisol measurements at baseline and 30 and 60 min after the injection.

If there is an impaired response to the stimulation test, the following issues should be considered:

1.   Differentiate between primary and secondary adrenal insufficiency (either of which may give blunted responses to the cosyntropin test). Clinical findings of hyperpigmentation in association with features of aldosterone deficiency point to primary adrenal failure, and are not

ADRENAL INSUFFICIENCY

EVALUATION

■ *Cosyntropin (Cortrosyn) stimulation test*
  ● **0.25 mg IM or IV**
■ *Normal response:*
  ● *peak cortisol @ 30-60 min*
  ● *peak cortisol > 18-20 µg/dl*

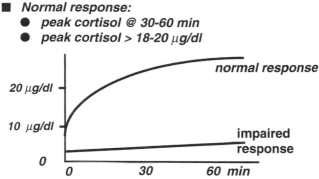

Fig. 2 Intramuscular or intravenous injection of an ACTH analog (cosyntropin) will lead to an increase in serum cortisol to the level of 18 µg/dL or higher by 30–60 min in the normal individual. A blunted response is indicative of adrenal insufficiency.

expected in patients with secondary adrenal failure. Thus, the distinction between primary and secondary adrenal failure can usually be made on a clinical basis. Additional testing may be needed for clarification in some cases.

2. Determine a specific etiological factor (which could include autoimmune disease, a variety of infections, hemorrhage, and metastatic cancer) if primary adrenal insufficiency is confirmed. If the patient has type 1 diabetes, an autoimmune cause of the adrenal insufficiency is likely, and positive titers of adrenal antibodies would be supportive of an immunological process, as would the finding of small atrophied adrenal glands or computed tomography (CT). Other causes, such as hemorrhage, chronic granulomatous disease, or neoplasm, are possible, and CT would probably show bilateral adrenal enlargement or areas of high density or calcification in such cases.

3. Further evaluate other aspects of hypothalamic and pituitary function (including thyroid function, and in some cases, gonadal function, growth hormone status, and possibly ADH status) if secondary adrenal insufficiency is found.

4. Define an appropriate therapeutic program for the patient.

5. Educate the patient about dosage adjustment for various intercurrent illnesses and related problems.

Treatment consists of replacement of the steroid deficiencies. Although glucocorticoid insufficiency can be treated by prescribing cortisol (hydrocortisone) itself, this is relatively expensive; prednisone is equally effective and much less costly. The typical dosage of prednisone that is used for replacement purposes is 5–7.5 mg daily, with higher doses (up to tenfold the maintenance dose of prednisone or its equivalent) required during significant stressful illnesses or with surgery. Regardless of the specific glucocorticoid used, mineralocorticoid replacement is also typically needed in the patient with primary adrenal failure, usually as fludrocortisone 0.1 mg daily (with some variation based on response in blood pressure, volume retention, and electrolytes).

B. Hyperthyroidism

The thyroid is a frequent target in autoimmune endocrine disease. The result may be a state of either increased or decreased thyroid hormone production, with effects on metabolic processes that may be quite dramatic at times.

Graves' disease, an autoimmune disorder seen most often in young women, is the most common cause of hyperthyroidism. It is generally associated with diffuse and symmetrical enlargement of the thyroid gland. Ophthalmopathy and, less frequently, dermopathy (in the form of pretibial myxedema), are accompaniments of the thyroid disorder. As an autoimmune disorder with clear links to HLA markers, Graves' disease should not be an unexpected problem in the patient with type 1 diabetes mellitus. Other causes of thyrotoxicosis include subacute thyroiditis, postpartum thyroiditis (which also has an immunological basis), toxic thyroid adenomas, toxic multinodular goiters, and iatrogenic thyrotoxicosis from excessive doses of exogenous thyroxine therapy. Regardless of etiology, the metabolic consequences will be the same.

Thyrotoxicosis causes increases in glucose absorption, utilization, and production. Gluconeogenesis by the liver is accelerated. Peripheral tissues have increased rates of glucose uptake. Thyroid hormone stimulates both glucose production and glucose disposal, independently of insulin levels. These interrelations of thyroid hormone and glucose metabolism are made more complex because thyroid hormone can cause not only insulin resistance, but also it promotes accelerated insulin degradation. The resultant increase in insulin clearance is in turn, associated with a compensatory increase in insulin secretion.

When a nondiabetic individual develops hyperthyroidism, the oral glucose tolerance test is frequently abnormal, although the fasting blood sugar value usually remains in the normal range. There may be an early or exaggerated glucose peak in the hyperthyroid patient, reflecting alterations in glucose absorption caused by the thyrotoxic state. Glucose intolerance has been reported in over 50% of thyrotoxic patients, although overt diabetes related to the hyperthyroid condition itself is unusual.

In the patient with known diabetes, the development of thyrotoxicosis will virtually always lead to decompensation of diabetic control, and sometimes will result in frequent episodes of ketoacidosis in type 1 diabetes. In general, insulin requirements are increased. The patient with latent diabetes may be unmasked with development of thyrotoxicosis. The thyrotoxic patient who requires insulin for adequate glucose control should always be assumed to have underlying diabetes, and it is very unlikely that such a patient will have a reversible disorder of glucose regulation that will clear with control of the hypermetabolic condition.

The more common clinical features of hyperthyroidism are listed in Table 3. The measurement of thyroid-stimulating hormone (TSH; thyrotropin) has emerged as the best single test for evaluating thyroid function. This measurement takes advantage of the negative feedback loop between the thyroid and the pituitary (Fig. 3). A suppressed TSH usually indicates that the thyroid gland is producing excessive thyroxine (T_4) or triiodothyronine (T_3); that is, the patient has hyperthyroidism. Less frequently, a low level of TSH can be evidence of impaired pituitary function, leading to inadequate stimulation of T_4 production (secondary hypothyroidism). These two conditions associated with low TSH concentrations are usually separated easily on the basis of the patient's clinical features (hyperthyroid vs. hypothyroid). Measurement of free thyroxine index (or free T_4) will also distinguish between hyperthyroidism and hypopituitarism as the cause of a low TSH. Even in the patient with clearcut hyperthyroidism and a suppressed TSH, measurement of the free thyroxine index or free T_4 may be of use in assessing the severity of the hyperthyroid condition. Patients with a suppressed TSH and a normal free thyroxine index are considered to have "subclinical hyperthyroidism," although nonetheless, they may be at increased risk for problems, such as osteoporosis and atrial fibrillation. In cases of apparent subclinical hyper-

Table 3 Symptoms of Hyperthyroidism

Nervousness and anxiety
Tremor
Increased sweating
Heat intolerance
Palpitations and tachycardia
Fatigue, weakness, impaired stamina
Weight loss in the setting of increased appetite
Hyperdefecation
Irritability

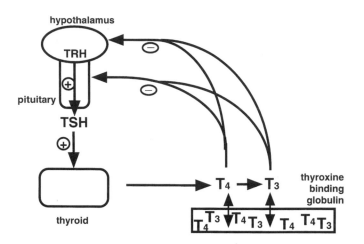

Fig. 3 Hypothalamic TRH triggers pituitary production of TSH, which then stimulates thyroid gland production of T_4 and T_3. T_4 and T_3 are predominantly bound to thyroxine-binding globulin, and only the unbound ("free") thyroid hormones have physiological activity. The free hormones suppress TRH and TSH by a negative-feedback mechanism.

thyroidism, it is advisable to monitor a serum T_3 level to determine whether the patient has "T_3-toxicosis."

Once the presence of a thyrotoxic state has been determined by laboratory criteria, it is essential to define the specific cause of the thyrotoxicosis before there can be any consideration of initiating therapy. Graves' disease, an autoimmune process in which the hyperthyroid state is associated with ophthalmological and (less commonly) dermatological changes, will be the most likely cause of hyperthyroidism in a patient with type 1 diabetes. Therapeutic options include definitive therapy with ablation by radioactive iodine (or, used much less in recent years, surgical removal of the gland), or medical control of the thyrotoxic state by thionamide drugs (propylthiouracil or methimazole), with the hope of attaining a remission of the underlying immunological process. While waiting for achievement of a euthyroid state, hyperadrenergic symptoms such as tachycardia and tremor can be controlled with the use of β-adrenergic blocking drugs (with the need to be aware that the effects of such agents on the patient with diabetes not only can reduce the recognition of low blood sugar, but also may impair the patient's counterregulatory response to the hypoglycemia).

In the young woman who develops thyrotoxicosis, another related immunologically based disorder—"silent" lymphocytic thyroiditis—may also cause hyperthyroidism. Unlike Graves' disease, this disorder is typically a self-resolving process that does not require definitive ablative therapy. It commonly occurs in postpartum women, and may evolve spontaneously to a state of hypothyroidism, which is usually self-limited and followed by return to euthyroid status; some patients will have permanent hypothyroidism as a result; hence, regular monitoring of such patients is essential once the diagnosis is established. This disorder, which is linked to HLA-DR3, can be differentiated from Grave's disease by radioactive iodine uptake, which will be elevated in the typical patient with Graves' disease, but will be suppressed in the patient with thyroiditis.

Patients with diabetes may also develop hyperthyroidism from etiologies that are unrelated to the diabetes, but instead represent the simultaneous occurrence of two unrelated but common processes. In the older patient with thyrotoxicosis, a toxic multinodular goiter will more commonly be the cause of a hyperthyroid state. The clinical setting and the physical examination of the thyroid gland will usually suggest the correct etiology. Radioactive iodine therapy is the preferred management of such patients, with use of thionamide agents being an alternative if there is need to control the thyrotoxic state more rapidly than can be accomplished with radioactive iodine.

Other possible causes of thyrotoxicosis include granulomatous (deQuervain's or "subacute") thyroiditis, which commonly presents during the course of a viral upper respiratory tract infection and is treated symptomatically with anti-inflammatory drugs; factitious thyrotoxicosis related to ingestion of exogenous thyroid hormone, managed by appropriate adjustment of dosage; hyperthyroidism from a solitary autonomous nodule; and numerous less common causes.

C. Hypothyroidism

Hypothyroidism is commonly the result of autoimmune thyroid dysfunction (Hashimoto's disease) and, as such, can be seen in conjunction with type 1 diabetes. Because the prevalence of hypothyroidism increases substantially after the age of 50, particularly in women, its greatest statistical association will be with type 2 diabetes, even though there is no specific etiological relation of the two disorders in such patients. As a result, hypothyroidism will be discussed in more detail later as a typical example of concurrence of two common, but etiologically unrelated, endocrine disorders.

D. Hypogonadism

Diabetes mellitus can develop as a result of iron overload in the beta cells in patients with hereditary hemochromatosis, and occurs in 50% of patients with the disorder who are not discovered by screening. Insulin and C peptide production are reduced, but alpha-cell function appears to be relatively spared, and glucagon levels are not significantly reduced. Skin hyperpigmentation occurs in 70% of affected individuals, resulting from cutaneous iron deposition and melanin; in combination with the development of diabetes mellitus, this pigmentation has led to the use of the term "bronze diabetes" to characterize patients with this disorder. Other associated abnormalities include liver disease, arthralgias, and cardiomyopathy.

Hemochromatosis in the male is also commonly associated with hypogonadism, resulting from iron deposition in both hypothalamic and testicular tissues that leads to inadequate testosterone production. About 45% of men with hemochromatosis will have impotence. Endocrine studies usually demonstrate low serum levels of testosterone, FSH, and LH, consistent with a hypothalamic or pituitary basis for the disorder. Hypogonadism on the basis of primary testicular failure (documented by the finding of low serum testosterone levels associated with elevated FSH and LH) is much less common.

> *Key Clinical Point:* Impotence is a common complication of diabetes, affecting about half of all men with diabetes. Typically, the sexual dysfunction of diabetes is related to neuropathy and vascular disease of diabetes, and the gonadal axis is intact, with normal testosterone levels. In general, measurement of serum testosterone in such patients is of extremely low yield and is not warranted as a routine test. However, in the diabetic patient whose impotence is associated with other clinical features that are consistent with hemochromatosis, it is essential to measure serum testosterone as well as pursue appropriate studies, as needed, to define the elevation of iron stores that defines hemochromatosis.

Premenopausal women are less likely to develop clinical problems from tissue iron overload owing to the menstrual loss of iron (in addition to iron loss with pregnancy and lactation); therefore, hypogonadism is not a common accompaniment of hemochromatosis in women. Although amenorrhea can occur, it is unusual for loss of libido or natural menopause to occur before the age of 45 years.

The diagnosis of hemochromatosis is made by demonstration of increased body iron stores. Serum transferrin saturation (serum iron concentration/total iron binding capacity) over 60% in men or 50% in women is 95% accurate in defining the presence of abnormal iron metabolism. Treatment consists of iron removal by phlebotomy.

Repeated phlebotomy may reverse the hypogonadism. This primarily occurs in men younger than 40 years. Otherwise, hypogonadism can be treated with testosterone replacement. Testosterone per se cannot be effective administered orally; the testosterone congeners that are administered by mouth are associated with a risk of hepatic dysfunction, and should be avoided in hypogonadal patients in general (and certainly in the patient with hemochromatosis who is likely to have significant liver disease already because of the underlying disorder). Testosterone can be effectively restored by intramuscular injection of long-acting agents, such as testosterone enanthate or testosterone cypionate, either of which can be administered at a dose of 200 mg every 2 weeks. This will result in serum levels in the normal physiological range for men after a steady state is achieved following the initial rise after the injection. Alternatively, testosterone can be administered by transdermal systems (patches), with a typical dose being one 5 mg patch to be replaced daily.

IV. DIABETES AS AN ETIOLOGY FOR OTHER ENDOCRINOPATHIES

There is a less apparent link between diabetes mellitus and other endocrinopathies. In some of these situations, the second endocrine disorder is not a direct result of the diabetes, but instead, it usually occurs as an indirect result of diabetes. For example, there is an increased risk for pituitary infarction and resultant hypopituitarism in patients with diabetes mellitus; this is very likely a manifestation of *diabetes-related vascular disease.* Similarly, patients with long-standing diabetes commonly have impaired aldosterone production owing to reduced production of renin in the juxtaglomerular apparatus of the kidney on the basis of renal microvascular disease ("hyporeninemic hypoaldosteronism").

A. Hypopituitarism

Hypopituitarism can be caused by pituitary tumors, hypothalamic tumors, trauma, infiltrative diseases involving the hypothalamus such as sarcoidosis, central nervous system radiation therapy, metastatic malignancy, or pituitary infarction or hemorrhage. There is not a single predictable or consistent presentation of hypopituitarism. Depending on the specific causative process and its extent, the loss of endocrine function may be total or partial, and the development of symptomatology may be sudden or insidious.

Sheehan's syndrome classically results from the insult of postpartum blood loss and hypotension, leading to necrosis of a pituitary that has become highly vascularized during pregnancy. Failure to lactate, failure to resume menses, and development of symptoms of hypothyroidism or hypoadrenalism are typical clinical manifestations. The diagnosis may not be made for several years following the original hypotensive event, especially if the pituitary insufficiency is incomplete and some residual pituitary function is preserved.

Pituitary apoplexy is a syndrome associated with acute pituitary hemorrhage, and is typically associated with an undiagnosed pituitary tumor. It usually presents with sudden severe headache, visual loss, cranial nerve palsies, and decreased mentation. Associated secondary adrenal insufficiency may be life-threatening if the diagnosis is not recognized and treated appropriately. Evidence of pituitary hemorrhage is usual readily seen on computed tomography (CT) or magnetic resonance imaging (MRI) scans. Management should include the administration of stress level glucocorticoid therapy; in addition, neurosurgical decompression may be a consideration in the patients with the greatest degree of mental status change and largest amount of hemorrhage, although the specific indications for such intervention remain debatable.

Diabetes mellitus is a well-recognized risk factor for pituitary infarction. This is presumably on the basis of the vascular disease that is associated systemically with diabetes.

Symptomatology of hypopituitarism may vary, depending on the degree and severity of pituitary impairment. Hypogonadism may be manifested as impaired libido or impotence in the male.

> *Key clinical point:* These complaints of sexual dysfunction might mistakenly be attributed to the neuropathy and vascular disease of diabetes, which are most likely to occur in the patient with long-standing diabetes (who is also the individual who is at greatest risk for pituitary infarction), and formal assessment of the pituitary–gonadal axis should be undertaken if the patient also has other features of hypopituitarism.

Patients with diabetes-related sexual dysfunction should have normal testosterone levels; the finding of a low serum testosterone measurement should trigger the ordering of an LH level, and the finding of an LH value that is not elevated is indicative of pituitary disease. Hypogonadism in a woman of reproductive age is usually associated with amenorrhea and a low serum estradiol level in the setting of a nonelevated (i.e., low or inappropriately "normal") FSH. The postmenopausal woman with hypopituitarism will similarly have a level of FSH that is low or inappropriately within the normal range, in contrast to the elevation of FSH that is the expected marker for the loss of ovarian function that defines the normal menopause.

The patient with hypopituitarism may also have features of the associated hypothyroidism, and these will be no different from those that occur in primary hypothyroidism: fatigue, weight gain, lethargy, dry skin, swelling, impaired memory and concentration, constipation, cold intolerance, bradycardia, delayed relaxation of deep tendon reflexes, and periorbital edema. Laboratory studies may show mild hyponatremia and mild microcytic anemia. Laboratory confirmation of hypothyroidism is based on the finding of a low free thyroxine index. The half-life of thyroxine is about 1 week; thus, in the patient who has had an acute insult to the pituitary (e.g., pituitary apoplexy), the free thyroxine index may still be within the normal range if measured shortly after the acute event, and repeat measurement a couple of weeks later will give a more accurate assessment of the functional capacity of the pituitary–thyroid axis. Compared with primary hypothyroidism, in which the TSH measurement is elevated, the patient with hypopituitarism and secondary hypothyroidism will have a TSH that is either low or "normal" (the latter finding being inappropriate to the low circulating level of free thyroxine, and thus indicative of pituitary dysfunction).

The clinical features of secondary hypoadrenalism of hypopituitarism are similar to, but not identical with, the manifestations of primary hypoadrenalism. In both primary and secondary hypoadrenalism, patients will have the relatively nonspecific problems of weakness, malaise, fatigue, anorexia, nausea, weight loss, and lethargy. The patient with secondary hypoadrenalism will lack the hyperpigmentation seen in the patient with primary adrenal failure, which is related to the elevation of ACTH. The patient with secondary adrenal insufficiency will not have the hyponatremia, hypovolemia, hypotension, or hypokalemia that result from the failure to produce aldosterone in the patient with primary adrenal insufficiency; aldosterone production is primarily dependent on the renin–angiotensin system and, therefore, remains functional in the absence of ACTH. The patient with secondary hypoadrenalism may have hyponatremia, however, from other mechanisms that are related to increased vasopressin (ADH) secretion.

> *Key clinical point:* In the patient with secondary hypoadrenalism (hypopituitarism), just as in the patient with primary hypoadrenalism, increased insulin sensitivity and increased susceptibility to hypoglycemia (with decreasing insulin requirement) in the patient with diabetes mellitus is a major manifestation of hypadrenalism.

The diagnosis of secondary adrenal insufficiency can be made in several fashions. The gold standard test is the stimulation of insulin-induced hypoglycemia ("insulin tolerance test") with monitoring of the subsequent cortisol response; this test, which effectively assesses the integrity of the entire hypothalamic–pituitary–adrenal axis, is involved, time-consuming, and potentially dangerous, and will not be discussed further here. Similarly, measurement of the pituitary and adrenal response to suppression of cortisol synthesis with metyrapone is not free of risk, and is certainly not essential for the accurate diagnosis of secondary adrenal insufficiency. In fact, the cosyntropin stimulation test, described previously, is virtually as good a test for secondary adrenal insufficiency as it is for primary adrenal insufficiency. The rationalization for the test is similar in both conditions: in primary adrenal insufficiency, there is not enough functioning adrenal tissue to respond to the ACTH analogue. In secondary adrenal insufficiency of any significant duration, there has been adrenal atrophy owing to the chronic lack of ACTH, and thus the response to cosyntropin is blunted. There are a couple of caveats relevant to using the cosyntropin test for diagnosis of secondary adrenal insufficiency, however:

1. If the pituitary insult has been recent (such as the woman who had postpartum pituitary hemorrhage 1 week ago), not enough time has passed to cause atrophy of the adrenal glands, and thus a normal response to stimulation would be expected (although the baseline cortisol may be lower than expected, which as an isolated measurement may be an undependable parameter of adrenal function). In such a setting, use of an insulin tolerance test or metyrapone test should be considered as more accurate ways to assess the entire axis.

2. In some patients, the ACTH deficiency will be incomplete, and there will not be total atrophy of the adrenal glands. In such a case, the adrenal response to exogenous cosyntropin may be misleadingly normal (in part because the test uses a very large and nonphysiological dose of 250 μg, far more than the normal amount of normal ACTH secretion). It appears that use of a much smaller amount of cosyntropin (1 μg rather than 250 μg) will give a subnormal response in such cases, and this low-dose cosyntropin test may be a much more sensitive method of identifying the patient who has secondary adrenal insufficiency.

B. Hypoaldosteronism

The possibility of aldosterone deficiency should be considered in any patient who has persistent hyperkalemia in the absence of an obvious cause such as renal failure or the use of potassium-sparing diuretics. Although there are many potential causes of deficient aldosterone production, including primary adrenal insufficiency (as discussed earlier), patients with diabetes mellitus are particularly predisposed to hyporeninemic hypoaldosteronism, in which impairment of aldosterone production is the result of inadequate renal production of renin.

Hyperkalemia is the major clinical feature of hyporeninemic hypoaldosteronism. Although sodium wasting is also theoretically expected, in reality it is not a usual clinical accompaniment of the disorder because of compensatory action of other sodium-retaining substances, such as angiotensin II and norepinephrine. Similarly, the hyponatremia that might be anticipated is rarely seen; in the absence of hypovolemia, there is no stimulation of vasopressin to promote free water retention. The disorder is usually seen in patients with diabetes who have mild renal insufficiency, accompanied by modest elevations in serum creatinine that are substantially lower than the levels that exemplify the advanced renal failure in which hyperkalemia is the norm. Low plasma renin activity in these patients is due to impairment of the conversion of precursor prorenin to renin, as well as to the suppression of renin secretion by the volume expansion that is associated with diabetic renal disease.

> *Key clinical point:* If hyponatremia and volume contraction are present in a hyperkalemic diabetic patient with mild renal dysfunction, the possibility of primary adrenal failure should be considered, as described previously.

The diagnosis of hyporeninemic hypoaldosteronism can reasonably be made on the basis of clinical criteria alone. The finding of persistent potassium elevation in the 5.0–6.5 mEq/L range with a mild metabolic acidosis, with mild to moderate renal insufficiency (serum creatinine value in the 1.5–3.0 mg/dL range), in a 50- to 70-year-old patient with long-standing diabetes who is not taking potassium supplements or using (ACE) inhibitors or angiotensin II receptor blockers, represents a very typical presentation. Further laboratory testing is not essential with such a presentation. If there is any doubt about the diagnosis, it can be confirmed by demonstrating that the patient is incapable of generating increased production of renin and aldosterone by stimulation testing. In normals, renin and aldosterone levels increase after upright posture for 3 h or administration of a loop diuretic, whereas the patient with hyporeninemic hypoaldosteronism cannot respond appropriately to this challenge to the effective circulating volume. The patient with Addison's disease will demonstrate a high plasma renin activity with a low serum aldosterone; this combination of test results places the pathophysiological process in the adrenal glands, rather than in the kidneys, and points to the need to formally assess cortisol production.

In theory, treatment of hyporeninemic hypoaldosteronism can be accomplished by mineralocorticoid replacement in the form of fludrocortisone 0.5–2.0 mg daily. In reality, however, this is not suitable therapy for most diabetic patients with the disorder. By the time patients develop hyporeninemic hypoaldosteronism, they have frequently had diabetes and associated renal disease long enough that they are likely to have hypertension, edema, or other volume-overload problems, and as a result the use of a sodium-retaining (and thus volume-retaining) agent, such as fludrocortisone, is counterproductive. Instead, preferred options for managing the hyperkalemia include dietary potassium restriction, avoidance of drugs that cause potassium retention, avoidance of severe hyperglycemia, treatment of acidosis with bicarbonate, use of a cation-exchange resin (Kayexalate), and use of a loop diuretic for the volume excess state.

V. COINCIDENTAL ASSOCIATION OF DIABETES MELLITUS WITH OTHER ENDOCRINE DISEASES

The old adage of "common things are common" applies here. As discussed elsewhere in this volume, type 2 diabetes mellitus affects millions of individuals in this country and throughout the world. Primary hypothyroidism is also a very common disease. Both type 2 diabetes and hypothyroidism are seen in increasing frequency as populations age and, as a result, the coexistence of type 2 diabetes and hypothyroidism is common.

A. Hypothyroidism

As might be expected, hypothyroidism may cause some slowing of the metabolic processes that involve glucose and insulin regulation. Absorption of glucose from the gastrointestinal tract is slowed; glucose utilization in peripheral tissues is lowered; availability of gluconeogenic substrate is decreased. Similarly, insulin half-life is prolonged, insulin levels tend to be lower, and insulin secretion may be reduced.

In the nondiabetic subject, these hypothyroid-related changes in glucose and insulin metabolism are not clinically important. There may be some flattening of the oral glucose tolerance test curve because of the decreased rate of glucose absorption, in spite of the decrease in peripheral glucose utilization. Hypoglycemia is not an expected complication of hypothyroidism, and any finding of hypoglycemia in a hypothyroid individual should lead to concern about possible secondary hypothyroidism, in which hypoglycemia would be more directly related to the concomitant hypoadrenal state (as discussed earlier) than to thyroid function. Within the normal range of blood sugar values, insulin sensitivity appears to be normal with hypothyroidism, and the rate of fall in glucose levels after an insulin challenge is close to normal. There may some decrease in glucose utilization after administration of a large bolus of glucose to the hypothyroid subject, even in the setting of coincident insulin administration; this impairment, however, may well represent the impaired metabolic activity of hypothyroid tissues, rather than true insulin resistance.

In the patient with diabetes mellitus, the development of hypothyroidism may cause a decreased insulin requirement owing to decreased insulin degradation and decreased appetite. As hypothyroidism is corrected in an insulin-dependent patient, an increase in insulin requirement should be anticipated as the hypometabolic state resolves.

The more common clinical features of hypothyroidism are listed in Table 4. An elevation of TSH is the most accurate method for identifying the presence

Table 4 Symptoms of Hypothyroidism

Weakness, fatigue, lethargy
Dry and coarse skin
Coarse hair
Slow speech and mentation, poor concentration
Cold intolerance
Edema (facial, periorbital, and lower extremity)
Constipation
Weight gain
Hoarseness
Depression

of primary hypothyroidism, representing the negative-feedback relation between the thyroid gland's production of the thyroid hormone and the response of the hypothalamic–pituitary unit in the regulatory process (see Fig. 3). By far the most common causes of hypothyroidism are related to primary thyroid failure. However, a smaller number of patients will have hypothyroidism on the basis of hypothalamic or pituitary disease, in which case the TSH level will not be elevated (see the previous discussion of hypopituitarism).

Hypothyroidism is treated with replacement of *l*-thyroxine. On average, the expected full replacement dose will usually be in the range of 0.1–0.15 mg daily, although specific individuals may require more or less. In older patients, or in patients who are at a high risk for atherosclerotic cardiovascular disease, it is advisable to start at a relatively small dose and titrate the levels up gradually. In such a situation, an initial dose of 0.05 mg daily (or even as low as 0.025 mg daily) would be reasonable. If possible, the goal in the patient with primary hypothyroidism is to bring the TSH into the normal range; an elevated TSH indicates inadequate dosing, and a suppressed TSH reflects excessive therapy (and increased long-term risks for osteoporosis). Because of the long half-life of thyroxine (approximately 7 days), TSH should not be monitored more frequently than every 6–8 weeks. More frequent monitoring or dosage adjustment leads to a risk of making inappropriate dosage adjustments before a steady state is reached.

BIBLIOGRAPHY

Kelly TM, Edwards CQ, Meikle AW, Kushner JP. Hypogonadism in hemochromatosis: reversal with iron depletion. Ann Intern Med 101:629–632, 1984.

Loeb JN. Metabolic changes in hypothyroidism. In Braverman LE, Utiger RD, eds. The Thyroid, a Fundamental and Clinical Text. 6th ed. Philadelphia: JB Lippincott, 1991:1064–1071.

Loeb JN. Metabolic changes in thyrotoxicosis. In Braverman LE, Utiger RD, eds. The Thyroid, a Fundamental and Clinical Text. 6th Ed. Philadelphia: JB Lippincott, 1991:845–853.

Matsumoto AM. Hormonal therapy of male hypogonadism. Endocrinol Metab Clin North Am 23:857–875, 1994.

Vance ML. Hypopituitarism. N Engl J Med 330:1651–1662, 1994.

Werbel SS, Ober KP. Acute adrenal insufficiency. Endocrinol Metab Clin North Am 22: 303–328, 1993.

Index